Uniquest Series
PHYSIOLOGY

Uniquest Series
PHYSIOLOGY

A Compilation of All India University Questions 2011–2021

Second Edition

V Suganthi MD (Physiology)
Professor and Head
(Department of Physiology)
Vinayaka Mission's Kirupananda Variyar Medical College and Hospitals
Salem, Tamil Nadu, India

Executive Editor
National Journal of Basic Medical Sciences

Foreword
Milind V Bhutkar

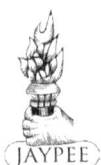

JAYPEE BROTHERS MEDICAL PUBLISHERS
The Health Sciences Publisher
New Delhi | London

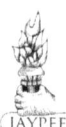
Jaypee Brothers Medical Publishers (P) Ltd

Headquarters
Jaypee Brothers Medical Publishers (P) Ltd
EMCA House, 23/23-B
Ansari Road, Daryaganj
New Delhi 110 002, India
Landline: +91-11-23272143, +91-11-23272703
+91-11-23282021, +91-11-23245672
Email: jaypee@jaypeebrothers.com

Corporate Office
Jaypee Brothers Medical Publishers (P) Ltd
4838/24, Ansari Road, Daryaganj
New Delhi 110 002, India
Phone: +91-11-43574357
Fax: +91-11-43574314
Email: jaypee@jaypeebrothers.com

Overseas Office
J.P. Medical Ltd
83 Victoria Street, London
SW1H 0HW (UK)
Phone: +44 20 3170 8910
Fax: +44 (0)20 3008 6180
Email: info@jpmedpub.com

Website: www.jaypeebrothers.com
Website: www.jaypeedigital.com

© 2023, Jaypee Brothers Medical Publishers

The views and opinions expressed in this book are solely those of the original contributor(s)/author(s) and do not necessarily represent those of editor(s) and publisher of the book.

All rights reserved. No part of this publication may be reproduced, stored or transmitted in any form or by any means, electronic, mechanical, photocopying, recording or otherwise, without the prior permission in writing of the publishers.

All brand names and product names used in this book are trade names, service marks, trademarks or registered trademarks of their respective owners. The publisher is not associated with any product or vendor mentioned in this book.

Medical knowledge and practice change constantly. This book is designed to provide accurate, authoritative information about the subject matter in question. However, readers are advised to check the most current information available on procedures included and check information from the manufacturer of each product to be administered, to verify the recommended dose, formula, method and duration of administration, adverse effects and contraindications. It is the responsibility of the practitioner to take all appropriate safety precautions. Neither the publisher nor the author(s)/editor(s) assume any liability for any injury and/or damage to persons or property arising from or related to use of material in this book.

This book is sold on the understanding that the publisher is not engaged in providing professional medical services. If such advice or services are required, the services of a competent medical professional should be sought.

Every effort has been made where necessary to contact holders of copyright to obtain permission to reproduce copyright material. If any have been inadvertently overlooked, the publisher will be pleased to make the necessary arrangements at the first opportunity.

Inquiries for bulk sales may be solicited at: jaypee@jaypeebrothers.com

Uniquest Series: Physiology

First Edition: 2019

Second Edition: **2023**

ISBN: 978-93-5465-812-9

Dedication

I dedicate this book for the loving memory of my parents Mr D Vajiravelu and Mrs V Chandra, who had inspired me to take up this career and had been a moral support all through my life and also to my husband and children who had been a great support in my career.

FOREWORD

It gives me immense pleasure to note that Dr V Suganthi, MD (Physiology) Professor and Head (Department of Physiology) at Vinayaka Mission's Kirupananda Variyar Medical College Salem, Tamil Nadu, India, and Executive Editor at National Journal of Basic Medical Sciences, has written a book titled *Uniquest Series: Physiology*.

Today's first MBBS students face a peculiar problem. Officially first MBBS duration is one year but practically students get only about nine months to prepare for the examinations. Combine this with an ever-expanding syllabus and falling standards of English language in students fraternity, they really have a tough job at their hands.

Considering this scenario, a book like this one will prove to be invaluable for the students. Dr V Suganthi has more than ten years of teaching experience and she has distilled her experience and expertise in penning this book.

I am sure *Uniquest Series: Physiology* will be of great help for first MBBS students in facing their examination confidently.

Milind V Bhutkar MD MNAMS
Former Dean
Vinayaka Mission's Kirupananda Variyar
Medical College & Hospitals
Salem, Tamil Nadu, India
Vice-Principal, Professor and Head
Department of Physiology
Swamy Vivekanandha Medical
College Hospital and Research Institue,
Tiruchengode, Namakkal District
Tamil Nadu, India

PREFACE TO THE SECOND EDITION

Physiology, a study of normal functions of the body is a basic science in medicine. A thorough knowledge in physiology is needed for understanding the other subjects in medicine. Physiology is a constantly evolving field in medicine.

The new revised curriculum of Medical Council of India (MCI) has introduced more clinically-oriented, skill-based, analytical and application-oriented learning objectives and assessment methods. This new edition of the book provides appropriate answers for the questions which are based on the new curriculum and will definitely help the students to present the appropriate answers for the questions in the exam and also acquire knowledge in physiology. This edition has the solved question papers of the past 11 years (20011-2021).

This question-answer book in physiology is unique in its form as it has solved question papers with patterns of essays, short notes and short answers. It has been prepared with utmost care and concern of undergraduate students.

The contents presented in this book are from my lecture notes and from latest editions of standard physiology textbooks.

I hope this book is useful for the student community for improving their knowledge and to present their answers in a perfect form in their exams.

I would like to welcome suggestions on improving the utility of this book in future.

V Suganthi

PREFACE TO THE FIRST EDITION

Physiology, a study of normal functions of the body, is a basic science in medicine. A sound knowledge of physiology is needed to understand deranged body functions in disease conditions and to learn the physiological basis of treating diseases.

This book has been written for the benefit of undergraduate students to acquire knowledge and guide them to give appropriate answers to questions in their examinations and to help them clear the exams. Answers are given in three forms: Essays, Short notes and Short answers.

The contents presented in this book are taken from my lecture notes and updates from standard physiology textbooks.

This question-answer book in physiology is first of its kind and has been prepared with utmost care and concern for the students.

I would like to welcome suggestions on improving the utility of this book in future.

V Suganthi

ACKNOWLEDGMENTS

I extend my gratitude to my teachers of physiology for guiding me in my academic career.

I wish to thank the administrators (Past and present) of our institution, Vinayaka Mission's Kirupananda Variyar Medical College and Hospitals, Salem, Tamil Nadu, India, a Unit of Vinayaka Missions Research Foundation (Deemed to be University), Salem, for their constant encouragement and guidance.

I thank my family members for supporting me in this venture.

I thank my colleagues who had been a great support in all the departmental activities.

I thank all my students who have inspired me to write this book.

I am thankful to the whole team of M/s Jaypee Brothers Medical Publishers (P) Ltd, New Delhi, India, who helped and guided me, Shri Jitendar P Vij (Group Chairman), Mr Ankit Vij (Managing Director), Mr MS Mani (Group President), Dr Madhu Choudhary (Director-Educational Publishing), Ms Pooja Bhandari (Production Head), Ms Sunita Katla (Executive Assistant to Group Chairman and Publishing Manager), Ms Samina Khan (Executive Assistant to Director-Educational Publishing), Mr Rajesh Sharma (Production Coordinator), Ms Seema Dogra (Cover Visualizer), Mr Vakil Khan (Proofreader), Mr Ajeet Rathor (Typesetter), Mr Sharvan Kumar (Graphic Designer) and their team members, for all their support to work in this project and make it a success.

CONTENTS

1. Answers to 2011 Question Paper — 1
2. Answers to 2012 Question Paper — 68
3. Answers to 2013 Question Paper — 131
4. Answers to 2014 Question Paper — 212
5. Answers to 2015 Question Paper — 272
6. Answers to 2016 Question Paper — 329
7. Answers to 2017 Question Paper — 362
8. Answers to 2018 Question Paper — 405
9. Answers to 2019 Question Paper — 448
10. Answers to 2020 Question Paper — 485
11. Answers to 2021 Question Paper — 529

Physiology Topic-wise University Questions (from 2011–2021 Papers) — 593

ND
Answers to 2011 Question Paper

ANSWER ALL QUESTIONS

I. Essay Questions (15 Marks each)

1. Write in detail the electron microscopic structure of skeletal muscle and the molecular mechanism of muscular contraction.
2. Discuss the composition, mechanism and regulation of gastric secretion.
3. Define cardiac output. Discuss the factors regulating the cardiac output. Add a note on Fick's principle.
4. Trace the visual pathway and the effects of lesion at various points in the pathway.
5. Define GFR. Explain briefly about mechanism of factors regulating GFR.
6. Define Hemostasis. Describe briefly about the mechanism of clotting. Add a note on hemophilia.
7. Name the functional division of cerebellum. Describe the structure, connections and functions of cerebellum. Mention any two signs of cerebellar lesion.
8. Describe the structure and function of the conducting system of the Heart. List the properties of cardiac muscle.

II. Short Notes (5 Marks each)

1. Neuromuscular junction.
2. Regulation of salivary secretion.
3. Functions of pancreatic juice.
4. Erythropoiesis.
5. Micturition reflex.
6. Spermatogenesis.
7. Glucagon.
8. Fetoplacental unit.
9. Secondary active transport.
10. Fibrinolytic system.
11. Normal ECG in lead II.
12. Regulation of coronary blood flow.
13. Compliance of lung.
14. Carbon dioxide transport.
15. Dysbarism.
16. Functions of thalamus.
17. Rapid eye movement (REM) sleep.
18. Decerebrate rigidity.
19. Taste pathway.
20. Theories of hearing.
21. Resting membrane potential.
22. Negative feedback mechanism with example.
23. Pathophysiology of diabetes mellitus.
24. Small intestinal movements.
25. Neuroendocrine reflex.
26. Functions of placenta.
27. Describe the phases of gastric juice secretion
28. Hormonal regulation of menstrual cycle.
29. Dwarf.
30. Composition and functions of saliva.
31. Non-respiratory functions of lung.
32. What is FRC? How will you measure FRC and its clinical importance?
33. Artificial respiration.
34. Referred pain and its theories.
35. Special features of coronary circulation.
36. Color vision.
37. Taste pathway.
38. Explain dark adaptation.
39. What is myasthenia gravis? Explain the biological basis of its treatment.
40. Brown-Séquard syndrome.

III. Short answers (2 Marks each)

1. Milieu interior.
2. Functions of large intestine.
3. Steatorrhea.

4. Dietary fiber.
5. Multi-unit smooth muscle.
6. Sarcomere.
7. Cytokines.
8. Autoimmune disease.
9. Na^+-K^+ pump.
10. EMG.
11. State Frank-Starling's Law of the heart.
12. List short-term regulation of blood pressure.
13. Intrapleural pressure.
14. State dead space and its normal value.
15. Define histotoxic hypoxia with an example.
16. What is Bell-Magendie Law?
17. Four functions of reticular activating system.
18. Functions of prefrontal lobe.
19. What is endocochlear potential?
20. Delta waves in EEG.
21. Four functions of plasma protein.
22. Helper cells.
23. Kernicterus.
24. Secondary active transport.
25. Rigor mortis.
26. Name the second messengers.
27. Name the hormones involved for the growth.
28. What is Turner's syndrome—three features?
29. APUD cells of its secretion.
30. Law of intestine.
31. Double Bohr effect.
32. Aldosterone escape.
33. What are different types of water absorption?
34. What is Houssay animal?
35. Name the hormones involved in calcium homeostasis, and the main organs that will act.
36. Draw the diagram of alveolocapillary membrane and write the thickness of it.
37. What is SCUBA?
38. Who discovered J receptors? What is its physiological significance?
39. What are otolith organs?
40. What is alpha block?
41. Define Frank-Starling Law.
42. What is Monro-Kellie Doctrine Law?
43. What is stereognosis? Where is its center?
44. What are the functions of frontal lobe?
45. Precentral cortex.
46. What are mechanoreceptors? Give example.
47. What is summation? Mention its types.
48. What are cholinergic and adrenergic receptors?
49. Draw the structure of rods and cones.
50. What is the difference between spasticity and rigidity?
51. Define histotoxic hypoxia.

I. ESSAY QUESTIONS

1. Write in detail the electron microscopic structure of skeletal muscle and the molecular mechanism of muscular contraction.

Structure of Skeletal Muscle

❏ Skeletal muscle is made up of muscle fibers, which are the basic unit of muscles and surrounding connective tissues (*refer* **Fig. 1**).
❏ Each muscle fiber is surrounded by connective tissue—endomysium.
❏ Many muscle fibers are bundled up to form fasciculi and each fasciculus is surrounded by—perimysium.

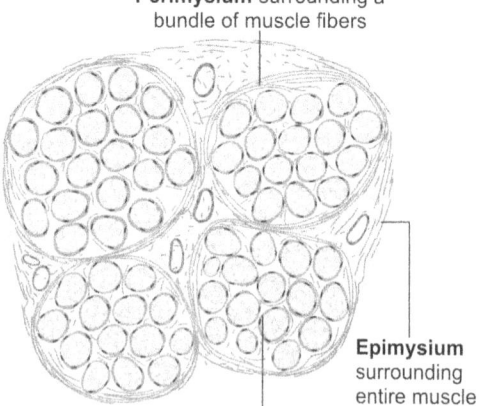

Fig. 1: Skeletal muscle with the surrounding connective tissues.

- The fasciculi are bundled to form the muscle and it is surrounded by—epimysium.
- All these connective tissues join to form the tendon.
- Each muscle fiber has many myofibrils and the muscle fiber is surrounded by Sarcolemma—the cell membrane (**Figs. 2A and B**).
- The myofibrils have thick and thin filaments.
- The Filaments are made of proteins—actin, myosin, troponin and tropomyosin.
- Actin and myosin are the contractile proteins and troponin and tropomyosin are regulatory proteins.
- The arrangement of thick and thin filaments appears as light and dark striations (bands) under light microscope due to the refractive indices of the various parts.
- The *dark band* is A band and is 1.5 µm in length and is made of *thick filaments and overlapping thin filaments*. The center of A band has a lighter H zone with a M line in the middle of it. H zone is the area where thin filaments do not overlap thick filaments and therefore appears as lighter area. The thick filament is made of myosin molecules.
- The *light band* is made of *thin filaments* with a dark line—Z line in the middle of it. The thin filament is made of the proteins—actin, tropomyosin and troponin with 3 subunits—I, C and T.

Sarcomere

- The segment of myofibril between two Z lines is the **sarcomere**.
- It includes ½ of I band and A band and ½ I band.
- It is 2.5 µm in length.
- This forms the structural and functional unit of the muscle fiber.
- On contraction of the muscle, the length of sarcomere decreases and on relaxation it is increased.

Thick Filament

- Under electron microscope, a transverse section of the A band, it is seen that each thick filament is surrounded by 6 thin filaments in a hexagonal pattern.
- The type of myosin in skeletal muscle is myosin II. Myosin has two globular heads and a tail.
- It is made of 2 heavy chains and 4 light chains. The light chains and the amino terminals of heavy chains form the head. The rest of the heavy chains are wound on each other to form the tail (**Fig. 3A**).
- Each head of the myosin molecule has two binding sites, one for actin and the other is the ATPase site which hydrolyses ATP.
- The myosins are arranged symmetrically in the thick filament and in the center part, on either sides of M line there is a small zone where there is absence of myosin heads and it appears lighter. It is the pseudo-H zone.

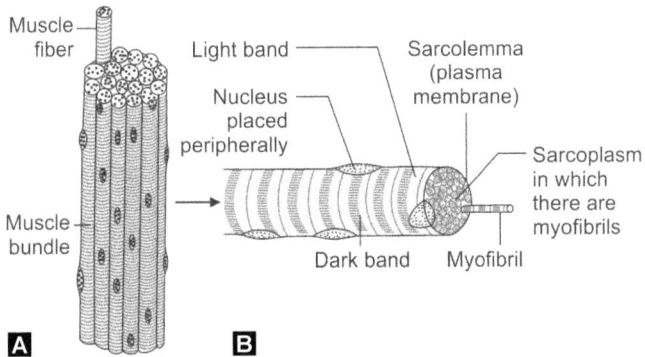

Figs. 2A and B: Structure of muscles: Muscle bundle (A) and muscle fiber (B). Arrangement of thick and thin filaments in the muscle fiber (B).

- M line is the site of reversal of polarity of myosin molecules in each of the thick filaments.

Thin Filament

- It is made of actin, troponin and tropomyosin **(Fig. 3B)**.
- There are 300–400 actin molecules are present in each thin filament. The actin molecule is made of two chains of globular units of G actin. The chain is said to be F-actin. The actin forms a double helix.
- There are 40–60 tropomyosin molecules in each thin filament. It is in the form of strands and lies in the groove between the actin helix. It covers the myosin binding site on actin.
- Troponin molecules are globular units which are present on tropomyosin at intervals. There are 3 subunits—troponin T, I and C.
- **Troponin T:** Attaches other components of troponin to tropomyosin
- **Troponin I:** Inhibits myosin head binding with actin
- **Troponin C:** Binds to calcium ion following which muscle contraction is initiated.

Other Proteins in Skeletal Muscle

There anchoring proteins: Actinin, titin and desmin

Sarcotubular System

- Under electron microscope, the myofilaments in sarcoplasm are surrounded by vesicles and tubules which make up the sarcotubular system **(Fig. 4)**.
- This system is made up of T-tubules and the sarcoplasmic reticulum (SR).
- T-tubules are invaginations of sarcolemma.

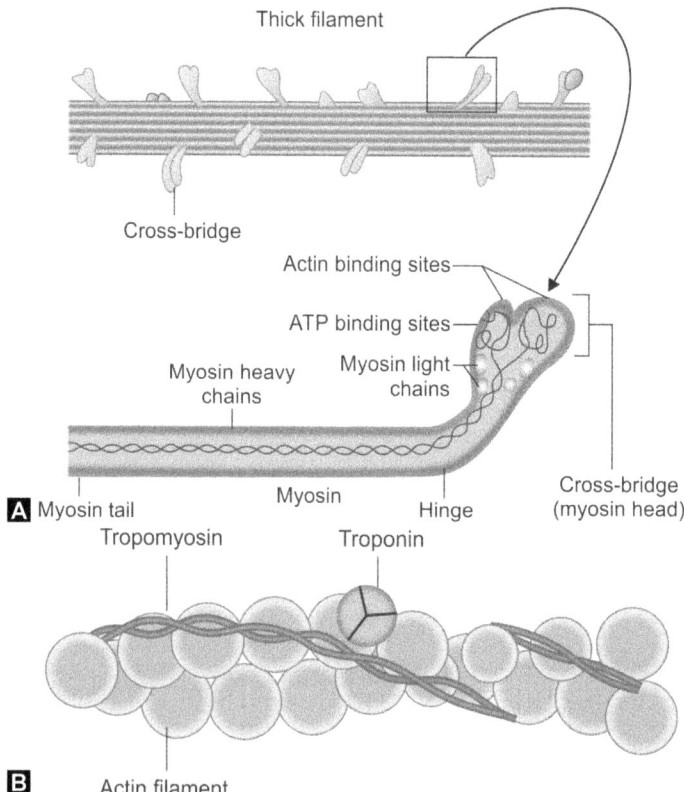

Figs. 3A and B: Structure of myosin in thick filament (A) and structure of actin, tropomyosin and troponin molecules in thin filament (B).

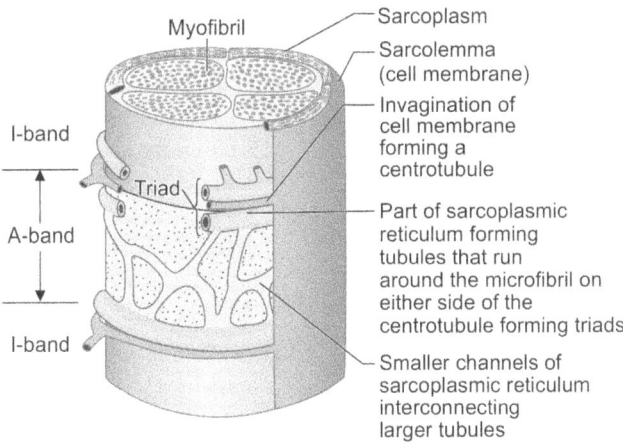

Fig. 4: Arrangement of sarcotubular system in the myofibril.

- Sarcoplasmic reticulum covers the myofibrils and they enlarge as cisterns and are in contact with the T-tubules at the junction of A-I bands.
- The T-tubule with the cistern of SR on either side forms the **triad**.
- T-tubule helps in spread of impulse into the muscle membrane and causes release of Ca^{2+} from SR.

Molecular mechanism of muscle contraction:
- Muscle, on excitation by action potential results in contraction.
- So the electrical phenomenon has leads to a mechanical response.
- The linking of the electrical event to a mechanical response is given as excitation-contraction coupling.

Excitation—Contraction Coupling

When the motor nerve to the skeletal muscle is excited, the neurotransmitter acetylcholine (ACh) is released at the neuromuscular junction.
↓
The ACh binds to **Nicotinic ACh receptors** in the muscle membrane below the nerve—*the motor end plate*.
↓
On binding of ACh with receptor (which by itself is a channel) results in opening of the non-specific cation channels followed by influx of sodium ions and there is a local depolarization of motor end plate—*end plate potential (EPP)*.
↓
The EPP excites the neighboring muscle membrane and action potential is generated in the muscle membrane.
↓
The AP spreads to the T-tubule and activates dihydropyridine receptors (DHP) which in turn triggers the calcium release channels called the Ryanodine receptors in SR and calcium ions are released.
↓
Calcium diffuses into the cytoplasm and gets attached to the troponin C. Binding of calcium with troponin C triggers many events resulting in muscle contraction.

Muscle Contraction

- Sliding theory or Ratchet theory had been put forward to explain muscle contraction by AF Huxley and HE Huxley in 1954.
- This theory postulates that the actin filament slide over the myosin filament following the formation of actin-myosin complexes and cross-bridge cycling.
- At rest, the myosin binding site on actin is covered by tropomyosin and inhibits binding of actin and myosin.
- On binding of calcium with troponin C, tropomyosin molecule changes its configuration and moves out, exposing myosin binding sites on actin.

- For each tropomyosin molecule moving out, 7 actin molecules are exposed.

Cross-bridge Cycling (refer Fig. 5)
- Each myosin head has two binding sites.
- One for binding with actin and other one is an ATPase which hydrolysis ATP.
- On attaching with one ATP, the ATPase hydrolyses the ATP molecule and the energy is stored in the head and thereby it is energized.
- ADP and Pi are also attached to the head.
- The energized head is 90° perpendicular to thin filament.
- **Power stroke:** When the troponin C binds with Ca^{2+}, the actin binding sites for myosin are exposed and the perpendicular energized head binds to actin.
- Immediately after binding, the head flexes from 90° to 45° and ADP and Pi are released. This is said to be the power stroke or cross-bridge cycling.
- The bent head is detached from actin molecule when another ATP molecule binds to the myosin head.
- This ATP is again hydrolyzed and the head is re-energized and ready to undergo the next cycle.
- As a result of repeated cross-bridge cycling, the actin filament from either side is moved towards the center of A band and there is muscle contraction.

Muscle Relaxation
- After the excitation process, Ca^{2+} in the cytosol is pumped back into the SR by calcium ATPase pump on SR membrane.
- On removal of Ca^{2+}, troponin C realigns tropomyosin back to the position of covering of myosin binding sites in actin and the muscle relaxes.

Changes Happening in the Sarcomere following Muscle Contraction
- H zone disappears
- Sarcomere shortens

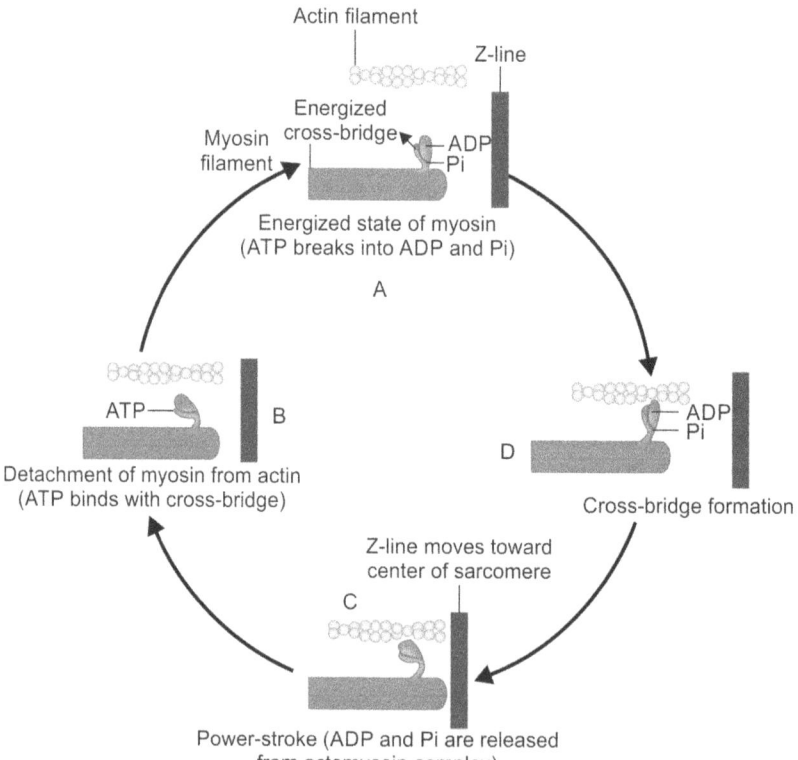

Fig. 5: Cross-bridge cycling in skeletal muscle contraction.

- A-band width remains same
- I-band width decreases
- Z-lines are brought closer

2. Discuss the composition, mechanism and regulation of gastric secretion.

Composition of Gastric Juice

- 2-2.5 L/day
- pH 1-2
- Water—99.45%
- Solids—0.55%
- Electrolytes—Na^+, K^+, Mg^{2+}, Cl^-, HCO_3^-, HPO_4^-, SO_4^-
- Enzymes—pepsin, lipase, gelatinase
- Mucus—insoluble and soluble
- Intrinsic factor

Mechanism of HCL Secretion

- In stomach, hydrochloric acid is secreted by the parietal cells which are present in the main gastric glands in body of the stomach.
- Pure secretion from the parietal cell has a pH of 0.82 and is isotonic (150 mEq of H^+ and 150 mEq of Cl^+).
- Parietal cell is polarized with an apical side facing the lumen and a basolateral side facing the interstitium.
- There are many tubulovesicular structures in the parietal cell which are studded with H^+-K^+ ATPase which pump H^+ into the lumen in exchange for K^+.
- These cells are highly metabolizing and they put out lot of CO_2. The cell is also rich in the enzyme carbonic anhydrase.

HCl secretion from the parietal cells happens in 2 steps:

1. Secretion of H^+ into the lumen
2. Secretion of Cl^- into the lumen

The steps involved in HCl secretion are:

1. CO_2 in the cell is hydrated in the presence of carbonic anhydrase, $CO_2 + H_2O \rightarrow H_2CO_3$
2. $H CO_3 \rightarrow H^+ + HCO_3^-$
3. The H^+ is pumped into the lumen by the H^+-K^+ ATPase pump on the apical side. For one H^+ pumped out of cell one K^+ is taken into the cell which later diffuses back into the lumen
4. HCO_3^- is extruded in the basolateral side through an anion exchanger in exchange for one Cl^- (refer **Fig. 6**).
5. The Cl^- which enters the cell will diffuse across the apical membrane into the lumen.
6. So for every H^+ secreted, one Cl^- is also secreted into the lumen and one HCO_3^- is absorbed into the blood.

So when gastric secretion is increased after a meal, the HCO_3^- getting added to the blood is increased, thereby raising the pH of blood—***Post-prandial alkaline tide.***

Regulation of Gastric Secretion

Neural, humoral and reflex regulation of secretion.

Factors that stimulate:
1. Vagus N
2. Gastrin
3. Histamine (refer **Fig. 7**)

Factors that inhibit:
1. Low pH in the stomach
2. Somatostatin
3. Prostaglandin E_2

Regulation is discussed in terms of:

1. Cephalic phase
2. Gastric phase
3. Intestinal phase

Cephalic phase:
- Nearly 500 mL/h (45% of total secretion)
- Initiated by thought, sight, smell, taste of food through Vagus N
- Emotions also affect secretion (refer **Fig. 8**).

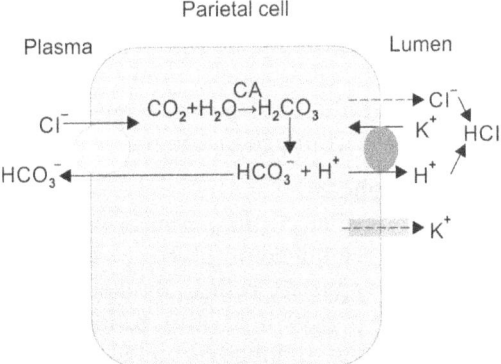

Fig. 6: Mechanism of HCl secretion.
(CA: carbonic anhydrase)

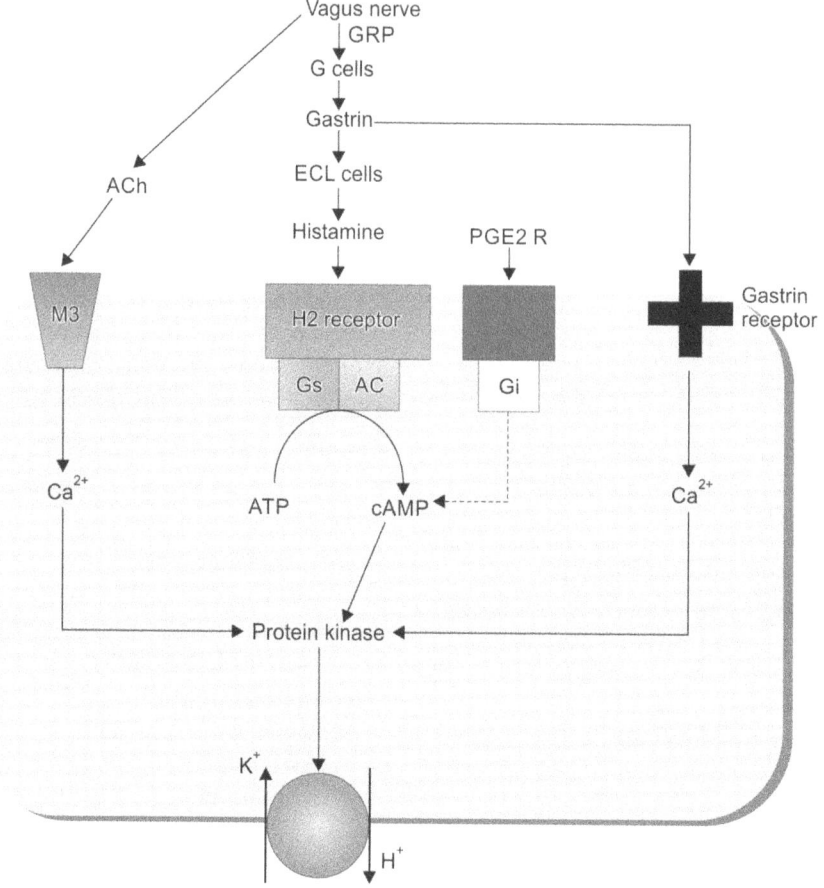

Fig. 7: Parietal cell with the regulating factors for HCl secretion.
(PGE2 R: prostaglandin E2 receptor; M3: muscarinic receptor)

Gastric phase:
- In this phase, it amounts to about 50% of the secretion. Food in stomach induces secretion by:
  - Distension of body of stomach (by reflexes—vagal reflex)
  - Distension of antrum (by gastrin secretion)
  - By products of partial digestion of protein (through gastrin secretion)

Intestinal phase:
- It begins when chyme enters the intestine.
- Intestinal influence is inhibitory. By:
  - **Enterogastric reflex:** By distension, presence of acid and products of digestion—inhibits secretion.
  - Hormonal mechanism—CCK, Secretin, GIP, neurotensin, etc.,—enterogastrone.

3. Define cardiac output. Discuss the factors regulating the cardiac output. Add a note on Fick's principle.

- Cardiac output (CO) is defined as the amount of blood ejected by each ventricle per minute.
- CO = Stroke volume (SV) X hear rate (HR) (*refer* **Fig. 9**)
- NV = 70 mL/beat X 70/min = 4900 mL/min

Determinants of Cardiac Output
- CO = Stroke volume (SV) X heart rate (HR)
- So factors affecting either of them will alter CO.

Factors Affecting SV
- Preload
- After load
- Contractility

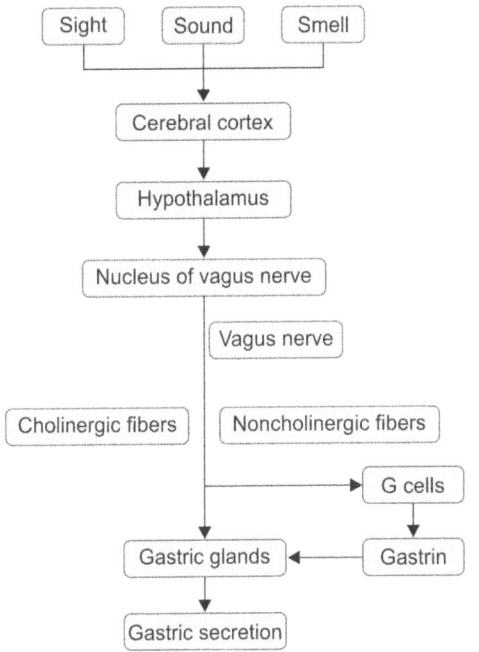

Fig. 8: Cephalic phase of regulation of HCl secretion. This phase of gastric secretion is regulated through vagu nerve.

Factors Affecting HR

HR is affected by nerves supplying heart (Sympathetic and parasympathetic nerves) and cardiac centers.

Preload

- The initial muscle length is the **preload** (the extent to which the muscle is stretched before contraction).
- Preload is decided by the **end diastolic volume (EDV).**
- EDV is decided by the **venous return (VR).**
- Preload affecting stroke volume is based on the Frank-starling's Law:
- It states that within physiological limits, the force of contraction is directly proportional to the initial length of the muscle.

Causes for Application of Frank-Starling's Law

- Increase in EDV →↑ stretch of muscle fiber → interaction of thick and thin filament increases →↑ force of contraction.
- Stretch of muscle fibers → opens stretch sensitive Ca^{2+} channels on sarcolemma →↑ Ca^{2+} influx →↑ force of contraction
- ↑Ca^{2+} influx →↑ Ca^{2+} release from SR (CICR) →↑ force of contraction.
- ↑ stretch of muscle fiber →↑ affinity of troponin for Ca^{2+}

EDV is dependent on:

- **Venous return,** Which is dependent on:
  - *Skeletal muscle pump:* Contraction of limb muscles press on the veins and

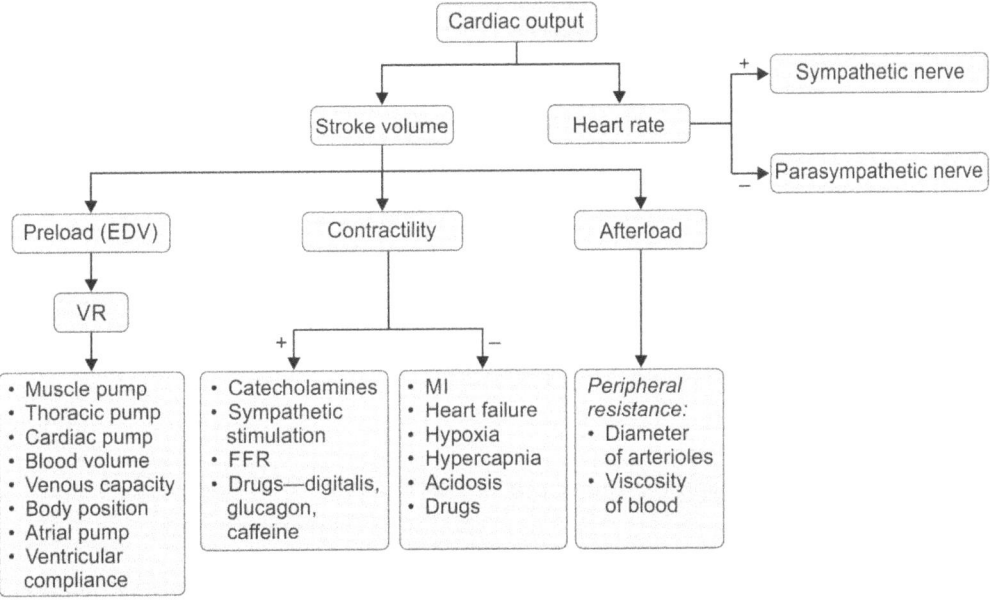

Fig. 9: Regulation of cardiac output.

increases forward movement of blood in the veins
- *Thoracic pump:* Increase in respiration depresses the diaphragm and decreases intrathoracic pressure and thereby it acts, such as a suction force to increase VR
- *Abdominal pump:* During respiration compression of abdominal muscles press on the veins and favors venous emptying
- *Cardiac pump:* Vis A Tergo (Force from behind), Vis A Fronte (Force from front)
- *Total blood volume:* As the blood volume increases VR increases and vice versa
- *Capacity of venous system:* Sympathetic stimulation to the veins causes venoconstriction and thereby increases venous emptying
- *Body position:* On standing, there is venous pooling due to gravity and it may decrease the VR.

❏ **Atrial pump activity:** Contributes 20% ventricular filling and stimulated by sympathetic stimulation.
❏ **Ventricular compliance:** Affected by damage to myocardium as in MI, pericardial effusion, cardiac tamponade.

This type of regulation of stroke volume in relation to change in initial length of muscle fiber is said to be **heterometric regulation**.

Contractility

Contractility is increased in force of contraction and thereby increase in stroke volume without increase in initial muscle length:
❏ Ventricles are able to do more work per stroke at a given EDV.
❏ Factors which affect contractility—inotropic agents.
❏ There are positive and negative inotropic agents.

Contractility is increased by:
❏ Autonomic activity (Sympathetics are positively inotropic)
❏ **Muscle mass:** Increase in myocardial mass increases contractility as after regular exercise
❏ Concentration of hormones and chemicals
❏ **Heart rate:** Force frequency relationship

Factors increasing contractility, positive inotropic agents:
❏ Sympathetic stimulation
❏ Circulating catecholamines
❏ Force frequency relationship
❏ Digitalis
❏ Glucagon
❏ Insulin
❏ Thyroxine
❏ Chemicals, such as xanthine, theophylline

Factors decreasing contractility, negative inotropic agents:
❏ Loss of myocardium as in myocardial infarction
❏ Hypoxia
❏ Hypercapnia
❏ Acidosis
❏ Acetylcholine

Regulation of stroke volume by affecting contractility of myocardium is **homometric regulation**. Here the force of contraction is affected without much change in muscle length.

Afterload
❏ It is the force against which the heart muscle shortens
❏ Cardiac output is inversely proportional to After load
❏ **Cardiac output α 1/after load (Anrep effect)**
❏ It is decided by peripheral resistance
❏ **Peripheral resistance is decided by:**
  - Vessel diameter
  - Viscosity of blood
❏ **This is also included in homometric regulation.**

Regulation of Heart Rate
❏ Heart rate is also a factor affecting CO.
❏ HR is in turn regulated by autonomic nerves.
❏ Sympathetics $\rightarrow \uparrow$ heart rate
❏ Parasympathetics $\rightarrow \downarrow$ HR
❏ Normally $\uparrow$ HR $\rightarrow \uparrow$ CO
❏ But in severe tachycardia $\rightarrow \downarrow$ duration of diastole $\rightarrow \downarrow$ ventricular filling $\rightarrow \downarrow$ CO

Measurement of Cardiac Output

Fick's Principle

- Fick's principle is defined as the amount of substance taken up by an organ or the whole body per unit of time and is equal to the arteriovenous difference of the substance times the blood flow.
- Substance taken by an organ = A-V difference X blood flow
- Blood flow = Substance taken by the organ/A-V difference
- Here the substance taken up is oxygen consumed by the whole organ
- Output of left ventricle = O_2 consumption (mL/min)/$A_{(O2)} - V_{(O2)}$
- O_2 Consumed is derived with spirometry
- Arterial blood sample is taken from peripheral artery
- Venous sample is collected from pulmonary artery
  = 250 mL/min/200 mL/L - 150 mL/L
  = 250 mL/min/50 mL/L
  = 5 L/min
- **Advantage:** Accurate and no chemical is injected
- **Disadvantage:** Needs hospitalization, catheterization, etc.

---

4. Trace the visual pathway and the effects of lesion at various points in the pathway.

Visual Pathway

- The visual pathway starts in the retina.
- Retina has ten layers. Rods and cones are in the innermost close to choroid.
- The light passes through all the layers and fall on rods and cones.
- The layer close to vitreous chamber is made of ganglion cells. The axons of these cells form the optic nerve.
- The optic nerve leaves the eye through the optic disc, the blind spot.
- The fibers from temporal part of retina receive impulses from nasal field of vision and travels in the lateral half of the nerve and the fibers from nasal part of retina receive impulses from temporal field of vision and travels in medial half of the nerve.
- The optic nerves cross in the optic chiasma. The medial fibers alone cross over and join the uncrossed fibers of the opposite optic nerve.
- On each side medial crossed fibers and lateral uncrossed fibers join to form the optic tract.
- The optic tract reaches the lateral geniculate body of the thalamus and relays there.
- The next order of fibers which originate in the LGB is termed the geniculocalcarine fibers and they reach the primary visual area in the occipital cortex (area 17).
- From here impulses reach the visual association areas (areas 18 and 19).

Lesions

Injury in the visual pathway leads to visual field defects. The type of lesion depends on the site of lesion.

1. Complete loss of vision—**Anopia**
2. Loss of vision in one half of the visual field—**Hemianopia**
   a. **Lesion in optic nerve:** There is complete loss of vision (Anopia) on the same side visual field.
   b. **Lesion in optic chiasma (crossed fibers)**—Bitemporal hemianopia
   c. **Lesion in optic chiasma (uncrossed fibers):** Damage happens due to Carotid artery aneurysm—leads to binasal hemianopia.
   d. **Lesion in optic tract:** Lesion in one side will cause homonymous hemianopia of the opposite side, such as lesion in left optic tract will cause right homonymous hemianopia.
   e. **Lesion in geniculocalcarine tract:** Homonymous hemianopia
   f. **Optic radiation (medial fibers):** Homonymous lower quadrantanopia.
   g. **Optic radiation (Lateral fibers):** Homonymous upper quadrantanopia.
   h. **Lesion in visual cortex:** Homonymous hemianopia with macular sparing. Macula is spared because it has a larger area of representation in the visual cortex (*refer* **Figs. 10A to D**).

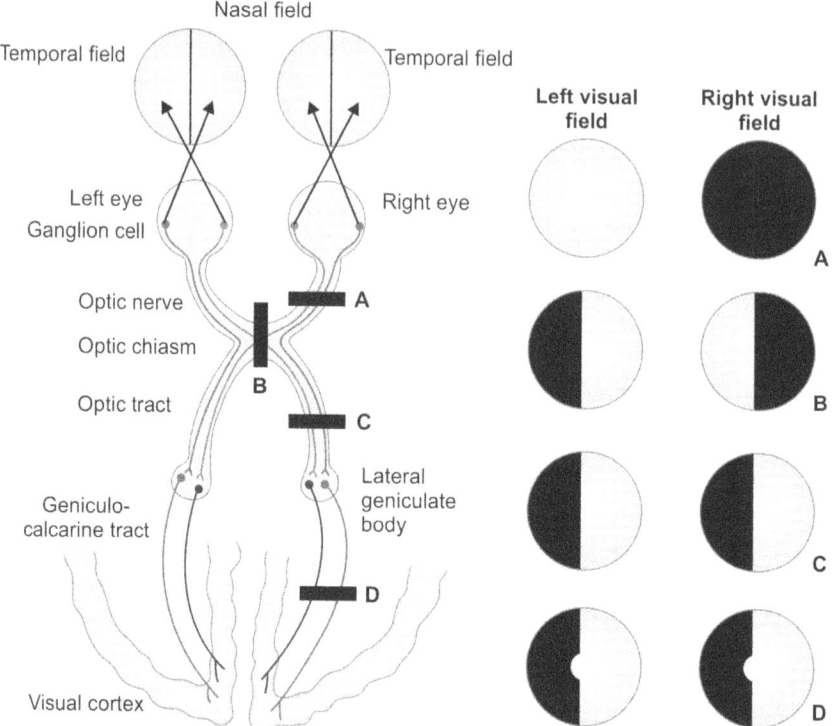

Figs. 10A to D: Visual pathway and lesions: (A) Lesion in right optic nerve causes right anopia; (B) Lesion of nasal fibers of optic chiasm causes bitemporal heteronymous hemianopia; (C) Lesion of right optic tract, causes left homonymous hemianopia; (D) Lesion in geniculocalcarine tract causes left homonymous hemianopia with macular sparing.

---

5. Define GFR. Explain briefly about mechanism of factors regulating GFR.

- GFR refers to the volume of the glomerular filtrate formed each minute by all the nephrons in both the kidneys. The normal value is 125 mL/min or 7.5L/h or 180L/day.
- Mechanism of filtration across the glomerular capillary is similar to the mechanism of filtration across any of the systemic capillaries.
- So filtration is dependent on the Starling's forces across the capillary membrane and characteristics of the membrane and renal blood flow and arterial blood pressure.
- Filtration across the membrane is decided by the balance of the starling's forces. (*refer* Fig. 11)
- **GFR is expressed as:**
  - **GFR** = $K_f [(P_{GC} - P_T) - (\pi_{GC} - \pi_T)]$
  - **GFR** = Glomerular filtration rate

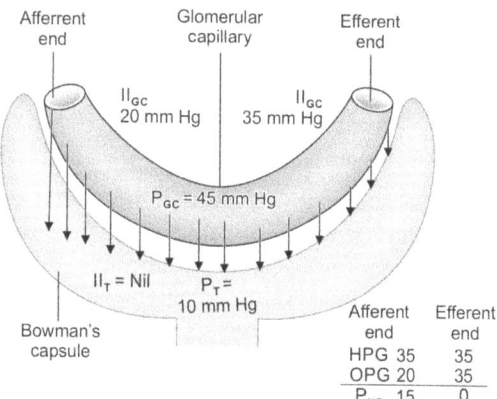

Fig. 11: Mechanism of filtration along the glomerular capillary. In contrast to systemic capillaries filtration happens along the entire capillary.

(P_{GC}: capillary hydrostatic pressure; P_T: bowman's space hydrostatic pressure; π_{GC}: glomerular capillary oncotic pressure; π_T: osmotic pressure in Bowman's space)

- K_f = Filtration coefficient of the membrane and it is 12.5m²/min/mm Hg. It is the product of glomerular

capillary wall conductivity and effective filtration surface area.
- P_{GC} = Glomerular capillary hydrostatic pressure
- P_T = Hydrostatic pressure in Bowman's space
- π_{GC} = Glomerular capillary oncotic pressure
- π_T = Oncotic pressure in Bowman's space

Factors Regulating GFR

- **Surface area of filtration membrane** is altered by the contraction or relaxation of the mesangial cells. Contraction of mesangial cells decreases the surface area of filtration and relaxation increases it. Contraction is induced by Angiotensin II, endothelin, ADH, etc., and relaxation is stimulated by ANP, dopamine, cAMP and PGE_2.
- **Permeability of glomerular membrane** for neutral substances of less than 4 nm molecular diameter is favored and neutral substances above 8 nm are not filtered. Between 4 to 8 nm the filtration is inversely proportional to diameter of substances. There are negatively charged sialoproteins lining the glomerular membrane which prevents negatively charged particles, such as albumin from getting filtered even though it is 6 nm in diameter. Permeability is increased in hypoxia and presence of toxic substances.
- **Hydrostatic pressure in glomerulus:** It is higher than in other capillaries in the body as the efferent arterioles (the outlet of glomerulus) is more constricted and offers more resistance than the afferent arterioles (the inlet for glomerulus) which are short and straight branches. So, factors which increase efferent arteriolar constriction will increase the hydrostatic pressure in the glomerulus. Changes in the systemic blood pressure will affect renal perfusion and thereby the filtration. The hydrostatic pressure in the glomerulus at the afferent and efferent end is 45 mm Hg.
- **Hydrostatic pressure in Bowman's space:** This is the pressure exerted by the filtered fluid in the bowman's space and it opposes filtration. Normally, it is 10 mm Hg. It increases in conditions of obstruction of urinary tract as in ureteric calculi blocking the flow of fluid in the tubule.
- **Oncotic pressure in the glomerulus:** GFR is inversely proportional to oncotic pressure. It is exerted by the plasma proteins. The capillary oncotic pressure at afferent end is 25 mm Hg and at efferent end, it is 35 mm Hg. This is because as the fluid leaves the capillary from afferent to efferent ends of capillaries the concentration of plasma proteins increases and thereby oncotic pressure increases. So in conditions of hyperproteinemia or hemoconcentration oncotic pressure rises and GFR decreases. In hypoproteinemia, GFR is increased.
- **Oncotic pressure in Bowman's space:** It is very negligible because no protein is filtered into the bowman's space.
- **Effective filtration pressure:** It is the net outward pressure which favors filtration and is calculated as the difference between the outward and inward forces
  - $GFR = K_f [(P_{GC} - P_T) - (\pi_{GC} - \pi_T)]$
  - $GFR = 12.5 (45 - 10) - (25 - 0)$
  - $= 12.5 \times 10 = 125$ mL/min
- **Other factors affecting GFR:**
  - Sympathetic stimulation of renal vessels leads to marked vasoconstriction and thereby decreases GFR.
  - Hormones, such as norepinephrine, endothelin and angiotensin II cause intense vasoconstriction and thereby decrease RBF and GFR. Ang II at low concentrations cause only constriction of efferent arteriole and thereby increases GFR. ANP, dopamine, nitric oxide, prostaglandins cause vasodilatation and increase RBF and GFR.

---

6. Define Hemostasis. Describe briefly about the mechanism of clotting. Add a note on hemophilia.

- Blood while flowing in the vessels is fluid in nature, but when the vessel wall is injured

or the blood is removed from the body and collected in a test tube it becomes a jelly, such as mass—the Clot.
- Clotting or coagulation of blood involves a series of cascade of events in which many clotting factors (Proteins in the plasma) are activated in a serial manner. There are many such clotting factors.

They are:
- **Factor I:** Fibrinogen
- **Factor II:** Prothrombin
- **Factor III:** Thromboplastin
- **Factor IV:** Calcium
- **Factor V:** Labile factor or proaccelerin
- **Factor VI:** Non-existent
- **Factor VII:** Stable factor or proconvertin
- **Factor VIII:** Antihemophilic factor
- **Factor IX:** Christmas factor or plasma thromboplastic component (PTC) or antihemophilic factor B
- **Factor X:** Stuart-Prower factor
- **Factor XI:** Plasma thromboplastin antecedent (PTA) or antihemophilic factor C.
- **Factor XII:** Hageman factor or glass factor or contact factor
- **Factor XIII:** Laki-Lorand factor or fibrin stabilizing factor
- **HMW-K:** High molecular weight kininogen or Fitzgerald factor
- Pre-Ka (Prekallikrein or Fletcher factor)
- **Kallikrein:** Ka
- **PL:** Platelet phospholipid

The coagulation process involves three major steps:
- Formation of prothrombin activator
- Conversion of prothrombin to thrombin
- Conversion of fibrinogen to fibrin

Formation of Prothrombin Activator is by 2 Mechanisms

1. Extrinsic pathway
2. Intrinsic pathway

Intrinsic Pathway

This pathway is activated when there is injury to vessel wall and exposure of collagen or blood itself.

Steps involved are:
- Injury to vessel wall exposes collagen activates factor XII to XIIa
- Factor XIIa activates factor XI to XIa
- Factor XIa activates factor IX to IXa
- Factor IXa in the presence of VIII, Ca^{2+} and platelet phospholipids (PPL) activates Factor X to Xa.
- The activated factor Xa, platelet phospholipids, factor Va and Ca^{2+} forms the **prothrombin activator**. (*refer* **Fig. 12**)

Extrinsic Pathway

The extrinsic pathway is triggered when the injury involves damage to the blood vessels and the surrounding tissues. The damaged tissue releases tissue thromboplastin, a protein-phospholipid mixture which activates factor VII. This triggers the extrinsic pathway.
- Inactive factor VII is activated to active factor VIIa
- VIIa in the presence of Ca^{++}, platelet phospholipid (PL) and tissue thromboplastin, activates factors IX and X.
- Active factor Xa, Va, Ca^{++} and PL, forms the prothrombin activator.
- Prothrombin activator converts prothrombin to thrombin.
- Thrombin catalyzes the conversion of fibrinogen to fibrin

Conversion of Prothrombin to Thrombin

Prothrombin activator in the presence of Ca^{2+} converts prothrombin to thrombin. This happens at the surface of platelets. Thrombin is a proteolytic enzyme.

Conversion of Fibrinogen to Fibrin
- Thrombin, a proteolytic enzyme removes two pairs of polypeptide chains from each fibrinogen molecule and converts it to fibrin monomer.
- The fibrin monomers now polymerize to form long fibrin threads. The fibrin is initially a loose mesh of interlacing strands. This meshwork traps the blood cells
- It is later converted to a dense tight aggregate by formation of covalent cross-linkages. This is catalyzed by factor XIII

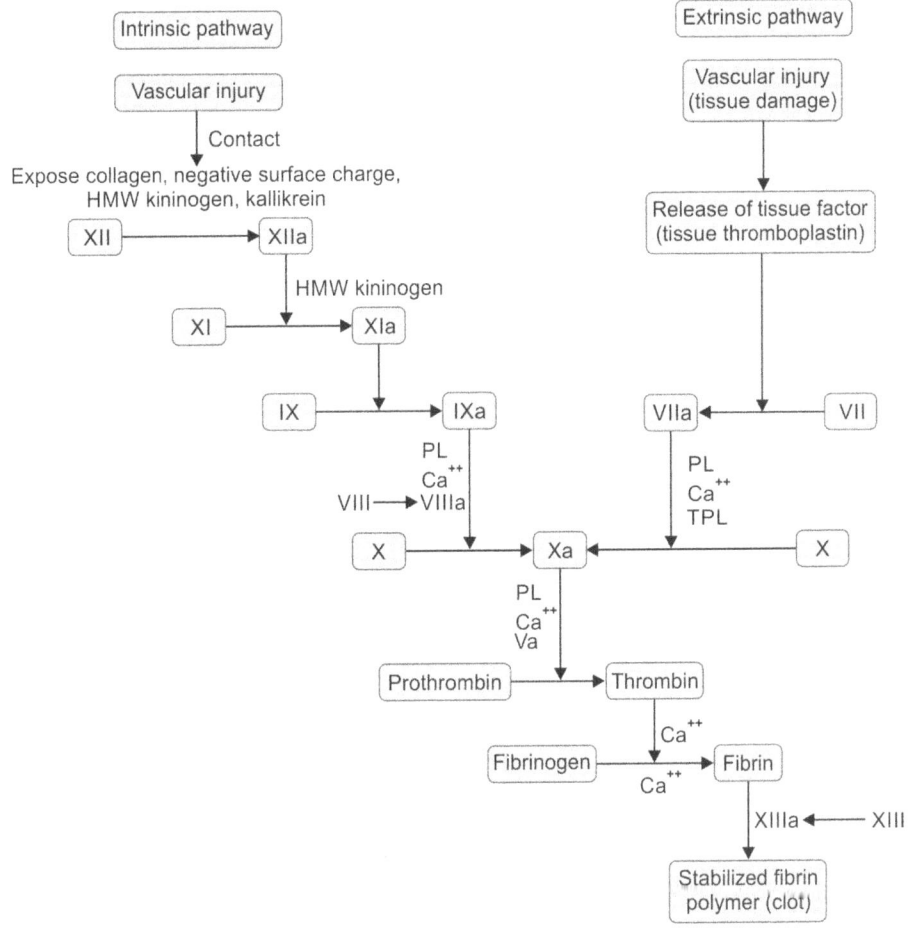

Fig. 12: Mechanism of Clotting.
(TPL: tissue phospholipid; PL: platelet phospholipid)

and Ca^{2+}. The stabilized fibrin mesh with the trapped blood cells forms the clot.

---

7. Name the functional division of cerebellum. Describe the structure, connections and functions of cerebellum. Mention any two signs of cerebellar lesion.

- Also called as small brain
- It is located posterior and inferior to the cerebral hemispheres.
- Cerebellum is connected to the brainstem by superior, middle and inferior cerebellar peduncles.
- Cortex is extremely folded and has a surface area 75% as that of cerebral cortex.
- It has a central body called vermis and 2 lateral hemispheres.
- Vermis is so called as it resembles a worm. It is bent on itself. It has a superior and inferior surface.
- The vermis consists of the following divisions from above downwards—lingula, central lobule, culmen, declive, folium, tuber, pyramis, uvula and nodule.
- In the hemisphere each part is related to the vermis.

Anatomical Divisions

Each hemisphere is divided by two transverse furrows into lobes—anterior, posterior and flocculonodular lobes.

Phylogenetical Divisions

- **Archicerebellum:** Flocculonodular lobe
- **Paleocerebellum:** Consists of vermis and paravermal portions
- **Neocerebellum:** Consists of cerebellar hemispheres

Functional Divisions

- The main functions of cerebellum are to maintain posture and balance and coordinate voluntary movements.
- Based on the functions it is divided into three parts:
  1. *Vestibulocerebellum:* Made up of the Flocculonodular lobe.
  2. *Spinocerebellum:* Consists of vermis and the intermediate part of the cerebellar hemispheres (Paravermal portion).
  3. *Neocerebellum:* Consists of the lateral parts of the hemispheres (*refer* **Fig. 13**).

Connections and functions of cerebellum:

- Connections include the afferents and efferents to cerebellum which enter cerebellum and leave, through the cerebellar peduncles.
- There are 3 cerebellar peduncles—superior, inferior and middle cerebellar peduncles.

Afferent Connections

The afferents to cerebellum come through the climbing fibers and mossy fibers.

Climbing Fibers

- They contain the olivocerebellar tract which arises from the inferior olivary nucleus in medulla.
- The olivary nucleus in turn receives proprioceptive inputs from all over the body.
- The climbing fibers end on the dendrites of Purkinje cells and they make one-to-one connection with the Purkinje cells and excite them.
- Collaterals from climbing fibers also excite the golgi cells and the deep nuclei of cerebellum.
- Climbing fibers enter the cerebellum through the inferior cerebellar peduncle.

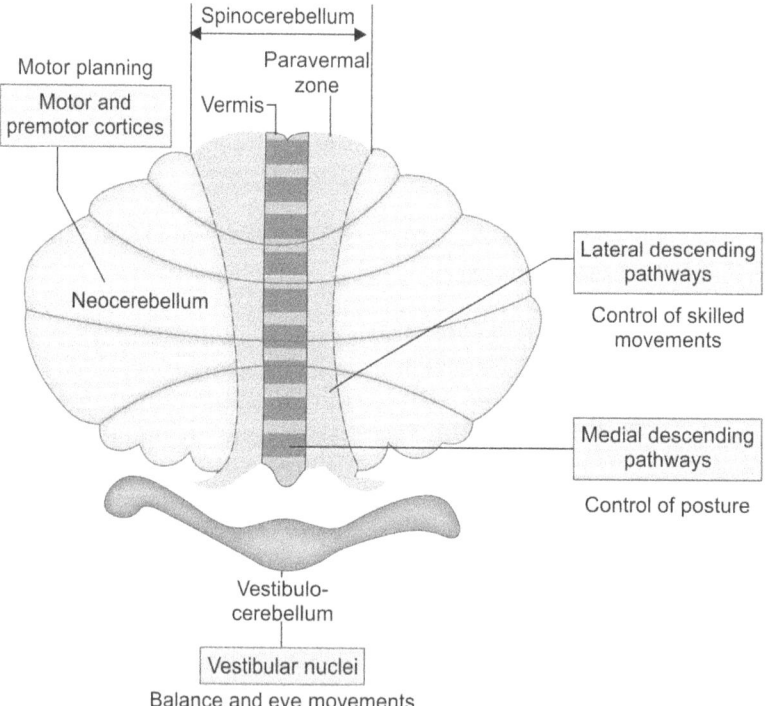

Fig. 13: Functional divisions of cerebellum with their connections and functions.

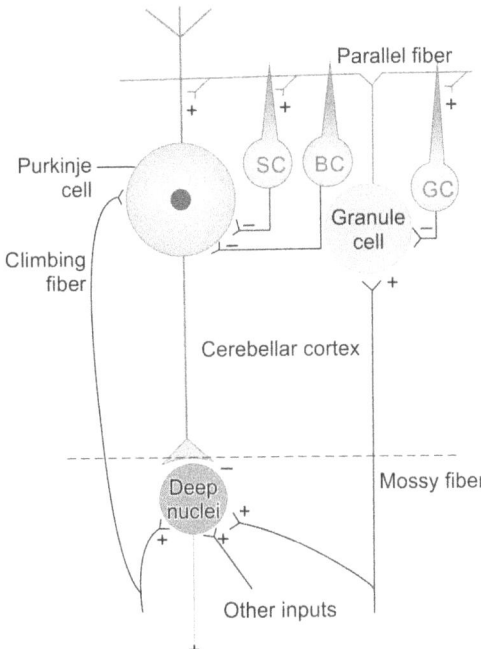

Fig. 14: Afferents to cerebellum through climbing and Mossy fibers.
(SC: stellate cells; BC: basket cells; GC: golgi cells; (-) inhibition; (+) stimulation)

This peduncle brings in most of the other afferent fibers to cerebellum (*refer* **Fig. 14**).

Mossy Fibers

☐ Mossy fibers include all the other afferents entering the cerebellum other than olivocerebellar tract.
☐ It includes—dorsal and ventral spinocerebellar tracts, vestibulocerebellar tract, reticulocerebellar tract, cuneocerebellar tract, tectocerebellar tract, rubrocerebellar tract and pontocerebellar tract.
  • *Dorsal spinocerebellar tract:* It carries unconscious proprioceptive inputs and exteroceptive inputs from same side limbs and trunk of same side and they enter cerebellum through ipsilateral Inferior cerebellar peduncle. It ends on the spinocerebellum.
  • *Ventral spinocerebellar tract:* It carries cutaneous and proprioceptive inputs from opposite side of the lower limbs and enters cerebellum through ipsilateral superior cerebellar peduncle and they are distributed to the hind limb area of spinocerebellum.
  • *Vestibulocerebellar tract:* It carries impulses from the same side vestibular nucleus about information regarding the position of head in relation to body posture. It enters the cerebellum through ipsilateral inferior cerebellar peduncle. It ends in the flocculonodular lobe (Vestibulocerebellum).
  • *Reticulocerebellar tract:* It arises from the lateral reticular nucleus and enters through inferior cerebellar peduncle and is distributed to all areas of cerebellar cortex.
  • *Cuneocerebellar tract:* It arises from external arcuate nucleus and carries proprioceptive information from head, neck, upper limb and upper part of the body. It enters through ipsilateral inferior cerebellar peduncle and distributed to spinocerebellum.
  • *Tectocerebellar tract:* It carries visual and auditory information from superior and inferior colliculi. It enters through superior cerebellar peduncle.
  • *Rubrocerebellar tract:* It arises from the red nucleus. It contains information from cerebral cortex. It has both crossed and uncrossed fibers. It enters through superior cerebellar peduncle and ends on dentate nucleus (One of the deep nuclei of cerebellum).
  • *Pontocerebellar tract:* These are fibers arising from motor area of cerebral cortex and end on pontine nuclei. From here they arise to form the pontocerebellar fibers. They cross to opposite side and enter through the opposite middle cerebellar peduncle and are distributed to all areas of cerebellar cortex.

Efferent Connections

☐ All the efferents from cerebellar cortex are through the Purkinje fiber output which ends on the deep cerebellar nuclei. Purkinje cell output is inhibitory in nature.

- The deep nuclei are—dentate, emboliform, fastigial and globose. Emboliform and globose are together called as nucleus interpositus.
- The deep nuclei also receive collaterals from climbing and mossy fibers and both are excitatory in nature.
- The net effect of output from deep nuclei is excitatory to brain stem and thalamus.
- All parts of cerebellum, except the vestibulocerebellum exit the cerebellum through deep nuclei.
  - *Cerebellovestibular pathway-vestibulospinal tract:* It leaves the vesti-bulo-cerebellum and projects to the vestibular nuclei directly. It controls the activity of vestibulospinal tract
  - *Cerebelloreticular pathway-reticulospinal tract:* The vermal portion of spinocerebellum projects to pontine reticular formation through fastigial nucleus. From here the reticulospinal tract arises and through this tract cerebellum controls the anterior horn cells.
- *Paravermal portion of spinocerebellum* project to nucleus interpositus and this in turn projects to the red nucleus. Thereby cerebellum controls the rubrospinal tract.
- *Dentato-thalamo-cortical pathway:* Impulses from cerebrocerebellum end on dentate nucleus and from here it goes through thalamus and reaches motor cortex. From motor cortex corticospinal tract arises and ends on alpha motor neurons. Through this pathway cerebellum fine tunes the activity of corticospinal tract (*Refer* **Fig. 15**).

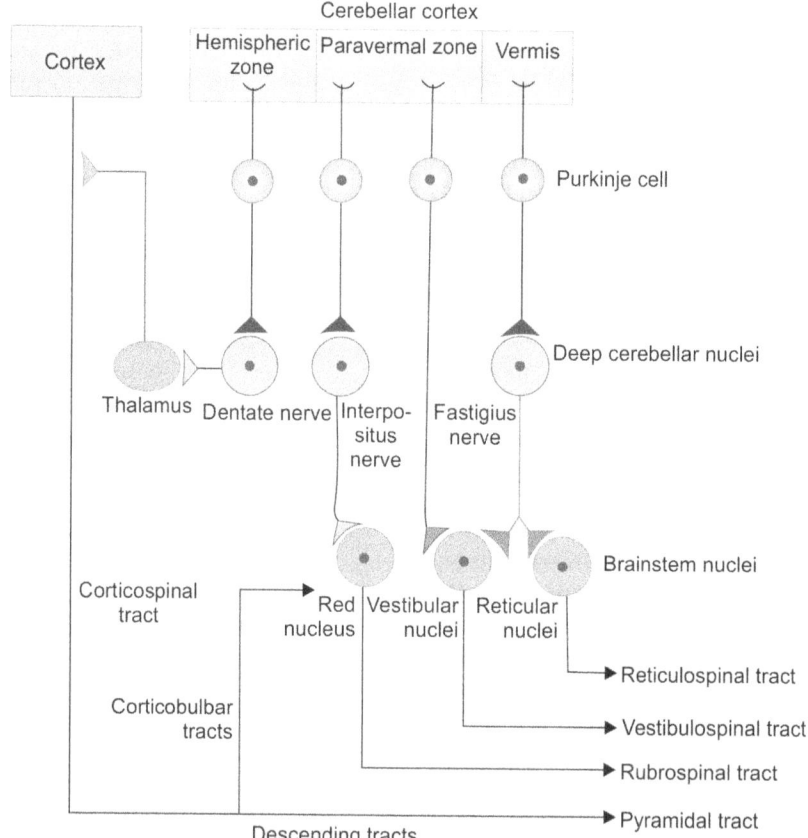

Fig. 15: Efferent connections from cerebellum through deep nuclei to brainstem. They are vestibulospinal tract, reticulospinal tract, rubrospinal tract. Through thalamic connections controls corticospinal tract.

Functions of Cerebellum

- **Control of posture and equilibrium:**
  - Vestibulocerebellum or the flocculonodular lobe controls posture and equilibrium.
  - It receives inputs from vestibular apparatus directly and also through vestibular nuclei about position of head and body.
  - It sends efferents to vestibular nuclei from which the vestibulospinal tract arises to regulate posture.
  - Vestibulocerebellum is also concerned with regulating vestibulo-ocular reflex.
- **Control of muscle tone and stretch reflex:**
  - Spinocerebellum influences the muscle tone through its output via fastigial nucleus which in turn controls the vestibulospinal and reticulospinal tract (arising from pontine reticular formation).
  - The major influence of cerebellum on tone is facilitatory.
  - Vestibulospinal tract is facilitatory to α motor neurons and reticulospinal tract is facilitatory to γ motor neurons.
  - Since control of cerebellum is on both α and γ motor neurons it has an important role in α-γ linkage.
- **Control of voluntary movements:**
  - Paravermal portion of spinocerebellum controls skilled voluntary movements.
  - It does not initiate movements but it coordinates voluntary movements.
  - Coordination of movements is by regulating the time, rate, range, force and direction of movements.
  - All three functional divisions of the cerebellum work together as "comparator of servo mechanism".

Comparator-servo mechanism
  - Impulses for voluntary movements are planned and programmed in the premotor cortex and it is sequenced in primary motor area and the command to skeletal muscles is sent through the corticospinal tract.
  - A copy of the plan or intended movement is also sent to the spinocerebellum.
  - Cerebellum also gets feedback from the proprioceptors about the actual movement performed by the muscles and joints.
  - It also receives other sensory inputs from eye, ear and vestibular apparatus.
  - Now the cerebellum compares the intended movement and the executed movement along with other sensory inputs mentioned above.
  - It thereby modifies appropriately the ongoing movement.
  - If any corrections have to be done in programming of movements the error signals are sent to the motor cortex.
- **Control of body movements of one side:**
  - Motor cortex of one side is connected to opposite cerebellum through a closed feedback loop; cerebral-cerebellar-ccerebral circuit, the cortico-ponto-dentato-thalamo-cortical pathway.
  - So each cerebellar hemisphere controls the opposite cerebral cortex.
  - But the corticospinal tract descending down from the motor cortex decussates in medulla and controls the opposite side of the body.
  - Since there is double decussation, it is that cerebellum controls same side of the body.
- **Planning and programming of movements:** Cerebrocerebellum has extensive connections with motor cortex and therefore is involved in planning and programming of movements.
- **Learning of skills:**
  - Cerebellum always tends to make changes in ongoing movements and therefore it improves by learning.
  - Another evidence is that there are increased activities in the climbing fibers when a new skill is learnt.
  - So cerebellum has a great role in learning skills.

- **Eyeball movement:** Pyramid of cerebellum is concerned with eyeball movement.

Signs of Cerebellar Lesions
- No paralysis
- No sensory deficits
- Deep reflexes not affected much except for **pendular knee jerk.**
- Hypotonia
- All movements are characterized by Ataxia.
- **Ataxia:** Defect in coordination due to errors in the rate, range, force and direction of movement.

It manifests as:
- Drunken gait
- Scanning speech
- Dysmetria
- Intention tremor
- Rebound phenomenon—Pendular knee jerk
- Dysdiadochokinesia
- Decomposition of movements
- Nystagmus

---

8. Describe the structure and function of the conducting system of the heart. List the properties of cardiac muscle.

Properties of Cardiac Muscle
- Automaticity
- Rhythmicity (Chronotropism)
- Conductivity (Dromotropism)
- Excitability (Bathmotropism)
- Contractility (Inotropism)

Conducting System of the Heart
- Ability to conduct an impulse (action potential)
- Conduction of impulse is by sequential depolarization of adjacent membrane.
- In the heart, there is a specialized conducting system.
- It starts in the SA node and reaches the ventricles.
- It consists of the SA node, internodal tracts, AV node, bundle of His, right and left branches of bundle of His, Purkinje fibers and the ventricular muscles.

SA Node
- It is located in the wall of the right atrium close to the opening of SVC.
- It is made up of modified muscle fibers with more rounded cells with indistinct borders and less striations. They are called as P cells.
- Such cells are present in the AV node also.
- In the heart, the SA node, AV node, His bundle and ventricles can generate their own impulses.
- But SA node is called the pacemaker as it generates impulses at a faster rate than the other tissues. So, it is called the pace maker.
- The pacemaker cells do not have a stable resting membrane potential.
- They tend to depolarize and repolarize in a continuous fashion in spite of nerve supply.
- The potential developed here is called as the **pacemaker potential**.

Pacemaker Potential
- The RMP in SA node is around –55 to –60 mV.
- But it is not a stable potential. There is a slow depolarization till –40 mV. Once –40 mV is reached, there is a rapid depolarization (Phase 0) to +5 mV and there is a rapid repolarization to –55 mV (Phase 3).
- Then it reaches the RMP (Phase 4)
- Once again, there is a slow depolarization, the process continues.
- This slow rising phase before the rapid depolarization is called as the prepotential or pacemaker potential.

Ionic Events Responsible for Pacemaker Potential
- The prepotential is divided into 3 sections based on the ionic events—the first part of slow depolarization is due to decay of K^+ current (Closure of K^+ channels), followed by Na^+ influx through 'h' or 'f' channels and the last part is due to Ca^{2+} influx through transient type Ca^{2+} (T type) channels (*refer* **Fig. 16**).

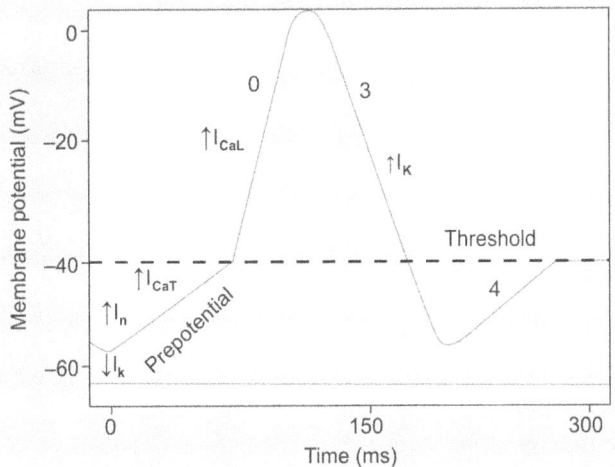

Fig. 16: Pacemaker potential. Slope of pacemaker potential (Phase 4), the prepotential is due to 3 events; first part of depolarization is due to closure of K⁺ channels, 2nd part is due to Na⁺ influx through sodium channel and last part of depolarization is due to Ca²⁺ influx through T-type Ca²⁺ channels. Rapid depolarization (Phase 0) is due to opening of L-type Ca²⁺ channels and repolarization (Phase 3) due to opening of K⁺ channels.

- The rapid depolarization which starts at –40 mV is due to Ca²⁺ influx through long lasting Ca²⁺ channels (L type).
- Rapid repolarization is due to K⁺ efflux through K⁺ channels resulting in repolarization to –55 to –60 mV.

Conducting Pathway

- These impulses originated in the SA node are conducted down through the specialized conducting system as mentioned above.
- The impulses from SA node are transmitted to the AV node through 3 internodal bundles which are specialized tissues for conduction of impulses from SA node to AV node in a faster way.
- The atrial tissues also conduct impulses but they are slower.

The three internodal bundles are:
1. Anterior internodal tract of Bachman
2. Middle internodal tract of Wenckebach
3. Posterior internodal tract of Thorel
4. Through these bundles the impulses reach the AV node.

Interatrial Tract of Bachman

- This bundle starts in the SA node and ends in the left atrium.

- The left atrium is also depolarized simultaneously.

AV Node

- It is located beneath the endocardium on the right side of lower part of atrial septum near the tricuspid valve.
- The conduction velocity through the AVN is very slow because the fibers are smaller with less number of gap junctions.
- There is a delay of 0.1 s
- The delay provides time for atrial contraction and final ventricular filling.
- It also prevents transmission of all impulses from atria to ventricles in supraventricular tachycardia.
- It is supplied by sympathetic and parasympathetic (PS) nerves which alter the conduction rate.

Atrioventricular Bundle of His

- This bundle starts in the AV bundle and descends down the fibrous skeleton and divides into right and left branches and they supply the right and left ventricles.
- The bundles divide into many small branches, the Purkinje fibers (*refer* **Fig. 17**).

Purkinje Fibers

They are present in the endocardium and reaches all parts of ventricles.

Ventricles

- The spread of depolarization in the ventricular muscles are from the AVN to the His bundle → Purkinje fibers → ventricles.
- The conduction velocity of the AP through ventricular muscles are 0.3–0.4 msec.
- This results in depolarization of both ventricles at the same time and leads to contraction of both ventricles at the same time.
- In ventricle, the spread of depolarization is from endocardium to epicardium.

In humans, depolarization of ventricle starts in the left side of interventricular septum
↓
Then moves to right side across the mid part of interventricular septum
↓
Then the wave spreads downwards to the apex
↓
Then it turns back along the ventricular muscle towards the AV groove from endocardium to epicardium
↓
The last part to be depolarized are the posterobasal part of left ventricle, pulmonary conus and uppermost portion of septum
↓

- Repolarization starts in the epicardium and spreads towards endocardium.
- Ability to contract follows the excitation of atrial and ventricular myocardium.
- The function of conducting system is to excite the myocardium following which intracellular calcium is increased and thereby contraction of the muscle follows.

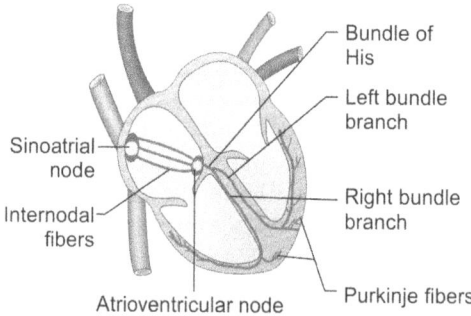

Fig. 17: Conducting system of the heart.

II. SHORT NOTES

1. Neuromuscular junction.

It is the junction between the motor neuron and the muscle fiber it supplies.

Structure of NMJ

- The neuromuscular junction (NMJ) is formed by the axon terminal of the motor neuron.
- On approaching the muscle fiber, the axon loses its myelin sheath and divides into many branches and the nerve terminals bulge to form the terminal buttons which approaches the muscle fiber at its center.
- NMJ has a presynaptic membrane, synaptic cleft and postsynaptic membrane. (*refer* **Fig. 18**)

Presynaptic Terminal

- It is the membrane of the terminal button of the axon.
- It has many ACh vesicles and mitochondria within the membrane.
- The membrane is studded with many voltage-gated Ca^{2+} channels.

Synaptic Cleft

- It is a space of 50–100 nm width between the presynaptic and postsynaptic membranes.

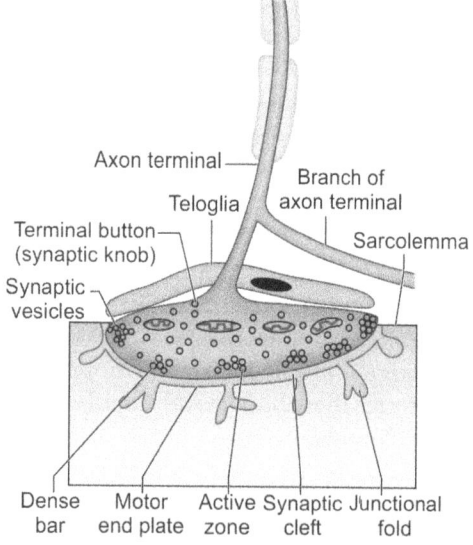

Fig. 18: Neuromuscular junction.

- It has ECF in it and acetylcholinesterase enzyme is present in it.

Postsynaptic Membrane
- It is the muscle membrane in contact with the nerve terminal and it is thrown into many folds—junctional folds and is thickened and deepened—synaptic trough.
- The muscle membrane here is called as the **motor end plate.**
- It contains the nicotinic acetylcholine receptors.

Impulse Transmission in NMJ

Stimulation of nerve fiber
↓
AP generated in nerve fiber
↓
Conduction of AP in nerve fiber
↓
Impulse reaches nerve terminal
↓
Voltage-gated Ca^{2+} channels in nerve terminal open
↓
Ca^{2+} influx into presynaptic membrane
↓
Exocytosis of ACh vesicles and ACh is released into synaptic cleft
↓
ACh moves across the cleft and binds to nicotinic ACh receptors in muscle membrane
↓
The receptor is a non-specific cation channel which opens on binding with ACh
↓
Influx of Na^+ ions into postsynaptic membrane
↓
Local depolarization of muscle membrane—**end plate potential**
↓
Generation of action potential in the neighboring muscle membrane by the EPP

Drugs Acting on NMJ

Blockers of NMJ
- **Curare:** It binds with the ACh receptors and prevents binding of ACh to their receptors. This blocks the neuromuscular transmission.
- **Bungarotoxin:** This is acquired from snake venom. It also prevents impulse transmission by binding the ACh receptors.
- **Succinylcholine:** They act just like ACh and make the muscle membrane depolarized. But the choline esterase does not have any effect on these substances and therefore the muscle is continuously depolarized and cannot be stimulated again.
- **Botulinum toxin:** They are derived from the bacteria *Clostridium tetani* and it prevents release of ACh vesicles from terminal buttons.

Stimulators of NMJ
- **Drugs having ACh like action:** Drugs, such as carbachol, nicotine, etc., act on ACh receptors like ACh but cannot be removed or slowly removed by ACh esterase. This makes the muscle to have repeated depolarizations resulting in muscle spasm.
- **Drugs that inhibit choline esterase: Drugs**, such as neostigmine, physostigmine, diisopropyl fluorophosphate (DFP) stimulate the NMJ by inactivating cholinesterase. This results in continuous activation of ACh on receptors and repeated muscle spasm. It takes weeks together for removal of ACh and therefor it has a fatal poisoning effect.

Diseases Affecting NMJ

Myasthenia Gravis
- It is an autoimmune disease.
- Antibodies are formed against the nicotinic ACh receptors in NMJ.
- There is weakness, fatigue and the muscles become weak with use and therefore symptoms worsen towards the evening.
- Antibodies not only combine with ACh receptors, they also flatten the postsynaptic membrane and cause endocytosis of ACh into presynaptic membrane.
- Because of these effects, the muscle response to stimulation gradually decreases.

- Symptoms improve after rest and are better on getting up in the morning.
- The extraocular and facial muscles are the first to be affected and ptosis and diplopia are present.

Treatment:
- **Acetylcholinesterase (ACh E) inhibitors:** ACh E inhibitors increase the amount of ACh in the NMJ and they can displace the antibodies and improve functions.
- **Thymectomy:** Decreases the immune response by inhibiting T cell activation.
- Immunosuppressants
- Plasmapheresis

Eaton-Lambert Syndrome
- It is also an autoimmune disease.
- Antibodies are formed against voltage gated Ca^{2+} channels in the presynaptic membrane.
- Here the symptoms of muscle weakness improve with repeated stimulation, as Ca^{2+} levels increase with each stimulus.

2. Regulation of salivary secretion.

- There are major and minor salivary glands.
- They can be classified as mucous and serous salivary glands based on the type of secretory cells in the salivary acini.
- There are 3 pairs of major salivary glands situated in the oral cavity—parotid, sublingual and submandibular salivary glands.
- Parotid glands are purely serous in nature and they secrete watery saliva.
- Sublingual gland is a mucous gland secretes thick viscous saliva.
- Submandibular glands are mixed glands; they have both serous and mucous types of secretory cells lining the acini.
- Minor salivary glands are present in the mucosa of oral cavity, buccal mucosa, etc.

Regulation of Salivary Secretion

Salivary secretion is under neural regulation. It is controlled by the autonomic nerves.

Parasympathetic stimulation increases salivary secretion which is watery and low in organic content. Along with acetylcholine released at the nerve terminal, VIP is also released by some postganglionic parasympathetic nerves which causes vasodilation and increases blood flow to the gland and thereby increases salivary secretion. Increased secretion through parasympathetic stimulation is by way of reflexes. The reflexes are conditioned and unconditioned reflexes.

Conditioned Reflexes

Salivary secretion is increased by thought, sight or smell of food and is by impulses coming from higher centers.

Unconditioned Reflex

Secretion is stimulated by placing substances in the mouth thereby stimulating the touch receptors in the oral cavity.

Sympathetic stimulation causes vasoconstriction of blood vessels supplying the glands and causes secretion of small amount of thick viscous saliva rich in organic contents.

3. Functions of pancreatic juice.

Pancreatic juice contains enzymes for digestion of lipids, proteins and carbohydrates.

Digestive Function of Pancreatic Juice

Digestion of Lipids
- Pancreatic lipase is the major fat digesting enzyme. It digests triglycerides into monoglycerides and fatty acids.
- **Colipase:** It exposes the active sites of pancreatic lipase and facilitates its lipolytic action.
- **Phospholipase A2:** It acts on phospholipids and converts it to fatty acids and lysophospholipids.
- Cholesterol ester hydrolase acts on cholesterol esters and splits it into cholesterol and fatty acids.

Digestion of Proteins

Proteolytic enzymes are secreted in the inactive forms—trypsinogen, chymotrypsinogen, proelastase and procarboxypeptidase A and B.
- Trypsinogen on secretion into duodenum is activated to trypsin by the enzyme enterokinase in the intestine.

- Trypsinogen trypsin, happens in presence of intestinal enzyme, enterokinase
- Chymotrypsinogen chymotrypsin, in presence of trypsin
- Proelastase and procarboxylase elastase and carboxylase, in presence of trypsin
- Trypsin and chymotrypsin act on proteins and polypeptides and cleaves the peptide bonds in basic and aromatic amino acids.
- Elastase acts on elastin and some other proteins.
- Carboxypeptidases also act on proteins and polypeptides
- Nucleases split ribose and deoxyribose nucleotides
- Collagenase digests collagen

Digestion of Carbohydrates

Pancreatic a amylase: It is secreted in active form and just like salivary amylase it hydrolysis glycogen, starch and other complex carbohydrates to form disaccharides.

Regulation of Intestinal pH

- Pancreatic juice is rich in HCO_3^-, and therefore alkaline in nature.
- HCO_3^- is secreted by the ductal cells of pancreas.
- The alkalinity created by HCO_3^- neutralizes the HCl derived from gastric juice as it enters the intestine.

4. Erythropoiesis.

- Erythropoiesis is production of RBCs. Life span of RBCs are 120 days.
- Hence continuous destruction and production of RBCs take place at a constant rate.

Site of Erythropoiesis

- **Mesoblastic stage:** In the embryonal stage—yolk sac.
- **Hepatic stage:** Later in the fetal stage up to 5 months—liver, spleen, thymus and lymph nodes.
- **Myeloid stage:** 3 months before birth—red bone marrow of all bones.
- **Adult life:** Red bone marrow of flat bones and epiphysis of long bones.

Changes during Maturation

- Reduction in size of the cell.
- Cytoplasm increases in amount and nucleus decreases in size.
- Cytoplasm changes from basophilic nature to polychromatophilic and then to acidophilic nature due to hemoglobinization of cytoplasm
- Disappearance of RNA
- Loss of nucleoli and then nucleus

Pronormoblast

- Large cell, diameter—20-25 µm.
- Cytoplasm is less.
- High concentration of polyribosomes.
- Large nucleus with multiple nucleoli
- Hemoglobin not formed

Early Normoblast

- Diameter of cell, 15-18 µm
- Cell exhibits mitosis
- Cytoplasm is still less, basophilic
- Nucleus large, occupies 3/4th of cell.
- Heterochromatin clumps present.

Intermediate Normoblast

- The cell is smaller in size, 12-15 µm.
- Cytoplasm changes from blue to pink as hemoglobin starts to appear.
- Nucleus small, occupies half the cell. No nucleoli.
- Hemoglobin formation makes the cell acidophilic also—Polychromatophilic cytoplasm.
- Mitosis is sluggish.

Late Normoblast

- Cell is smaller in size.
- Cytoplasm is deeply eosinophilic—Orthochromatic erythroblast.
- Nucleus is small and pyknotic.
- Cart-wheel arrangement of chromatin.
- Hb synthesis increases

Reticulocyte

- Cell size is 7.8 µm
- Nucleus is extruded
- Hemoglobin present
- Chromatin reticulum seen (*refer* **Fig. 19**)

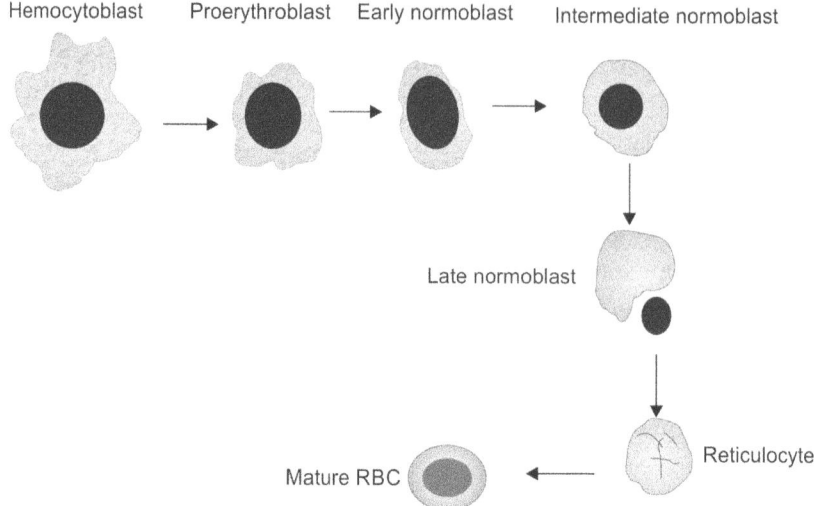

Fig. 19: Stages of erythropoiesis.

Mature RBC
- Cell size is 7.5 μm
- RBC is biconcave in shape
- Chromatin reticulum disappears

The whole process of maturation from Pronormoblast to reticulocyte takes 7 days. It takes 2 days for Reticulocyte to mature as an RBC.

Regulation of Erythropoiesis

There are general and special factors regulating erythropoiesis.

General Factor—Hypoxia
- Major function of RBC is to carry oxygen to the tissues.
- So, when there is decrease in tissue oxygen levels, it induces production of RBCs.
- Hypoxia stimulates the interstitial cells of the kidneys to synthesize the hormone **erythropoietin**.
- It acts on bone marrow to stimulate the erythropoietin sensitive stem cells to become proerythroblasts and thereby stimulates formation of RBCs.
- It also increases the release of reticulocytes from the bone marrow.

Factors Increasing Erythropoietin Production
- Hypoxia
- Catecholamines
- Thyroxine
- Testosterone

Special Maturation Factors

Dietary Factors
- Proteins help in globin formation
- Iron helps in heme formation
- Copper, cobalt and nickel also helps in heme formation
- Calcium helps in absorption of iron from GIT
- Vitamin C also helps in iron absorption
- Vitamin B12 and folic acid helps in synthesis of nucleic acids and final maturation of RBC
- Intrinsic factor synthesized in the stomach by the parietal cells help in absorption of vitamin B12.

5. Micturition reflex.

Nerve Supply of Urinary Bladder

- Urinary bladder is a triangular-shaped sac like structure. The bladder extends down as the urethra.
- The bladder wall is made of detrusor, a smooth muscle and there are two sphincters—internal and external urethral sphincters.
- Internal sphincter is at the neck of the bladder and is made of smooth muscle.

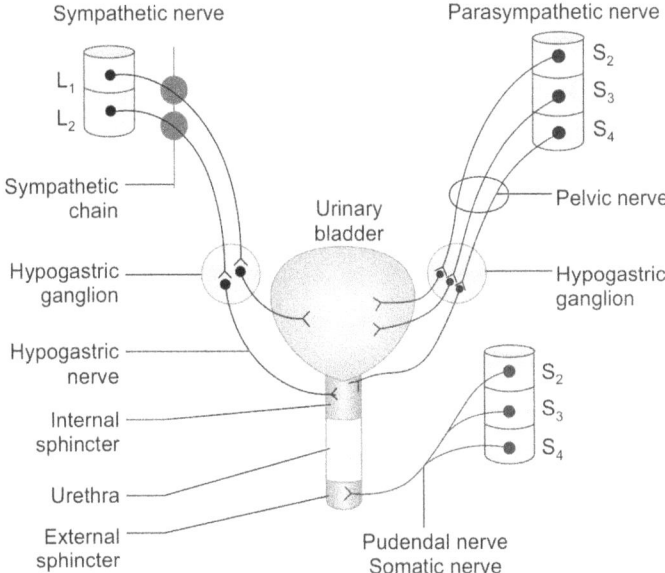

Fig. 20: Nerve supply of urinary bladder.

- It is supplied by sympathetic and parasympathetic nerves (*refer* **Fig. 20**).
- External sphincter is made of skeletal muscle and is supplied by somatic motor nerve (pudendal nerve).
- The bladder wall is also supplied by sympathetic and parasympathetic nerves.
- Parasympathetic nerves (pelvic nerve) have both afferents and efferents to bladder wall and Internal sphincter. They arise from S2–S4 segments of spinal cord. When they are stimulated, they cause contraction of bladder wall and relaxation of internal sphincter and therefore emptying of bladder.
- The sympathetic nerves (hypogastric nerve) also have afferents and efferents and they arise from L1–L3 segments of spinal cord. They also supply the bladder wall and internal sphincter. When stimulated, they cause relaxation of bladder wall and contraction of internal sphincter and therefore filling of bladder.
- Somatic nerve (pudendal nerve) to external sphincter arises from S2–S4 segments of spinal cord and have control from higher centers. It is under voluntary control.
- Once urine enters the renal pelvis, it flows through the ureters and enters the bladder, where urine is stored.

Micturition Reflex (*refer* Fig. 21)

- Micturition is the process of emptying the urinary bladder.
- **Two processes are involved:**
  1. The bladder fills progressively until the tension in its wall rises above a threshold level, and then
  2. A nervous reflex called the micturition reflex occurs that empties the bladder.
  The micturition reflex is an automatic spinal cord reflex; however, it can be inhibited or facilitated by centers in the brainstem and cerebral cortex.

The Reflex Pathway

- **Initiation:** Reflex initiated by stimulation of stretch receptors in bladder wall.
- **Stimulus:** Filling of bladder up to 300–400 mL
- **Afferents:** Through pelvic nerves (PS) to reach S2–S4 segments in spinal cord.
- **Efferents:** PS motor fibers from S2–S4 end in the detrusor muscle (excitatory) and internal sphincter (inhibitory).

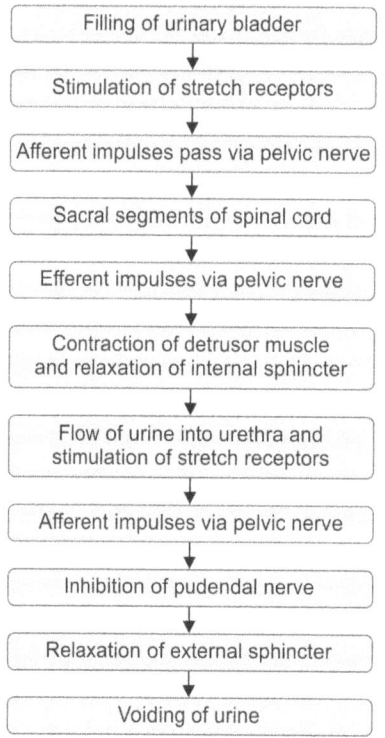

Fig. 21: Micturition reflex.

- **Response:** Causes contraction of bladder wall and relaxation of internal sphincter. Once it becomes powerful another reflex through pudendal nerve relaxes the ES → voiding.

---

6. Spermatogenesis.

- The process of formation of mature sperm is called spermatogenesis.
- It takes place in the seminiferous tubule. It happens in the wall of the tubule from basal lamina towards the lumen.
- The immature cells are present in the basal aspect of the tubule and the maturing cells move toward the adluminal compartment.
- Spermatogenesis involves both mitotic and meiotic divisions and Spermiogenesis.

Mitotic Division

- The primitive germ cell, spermatogonia, in the basal lamina of the seminiferous tubule undergoes mitotic divisions to form Primary spermatocytes.
- Each spermatogonium divides 5 times to produce 32 spermatogonia.
- 32 spermatogonia (44+X+Y) reach the adluminal side of the tubule and undergo mitosis to become 64 Primary spermatocytes (44+X+Y).
- Primary spermatocytes are large cells with diploid number of chromosomes (2n).

Meiotic Divisions

- The primary spermatocytes with diploid number of chromosomes undergo the first meiotic division to form the secondary spermatocyte which is haploid in nature.
- The second meiotic division results in formation of spermatids (22+X or Y).
- A total of 512 spermatids are derived from single spermatogonia.

Spermiogenesis

- The spermatids do not undergo further divisions but structural changes takes place as the spermatids mature into sperm— Spermiogenesis.
- This process happens in the deep folds of Sertoli cells.

The changes taking place are:
- The amount of cytoplasm is reduced in spermatids
- The nucleus elongates to become the head of sperm
- The acrosomal cap is formed
- The tail and middle piece are formed.

Spermiation

- After the maturation the sperms stay attached to the Sertoli cells.
- The release of sperms into the tubule is called Spermiation.

Factors Regulating Spermatogenesis

Hormones regulating spermatogenesis are— androgens, gonadotropins and estrogen

- **Androgens:** A high concentration of testosterone in the tubular fluid is essential for spermatogenesis. LH stimulates Leydig cells to secrete testosterone. Sertoli cells secrete androgen binding protein (ABP) to which testosterone binds and its levels are kept elevated.

Spermiogenesis is androgen dependent.

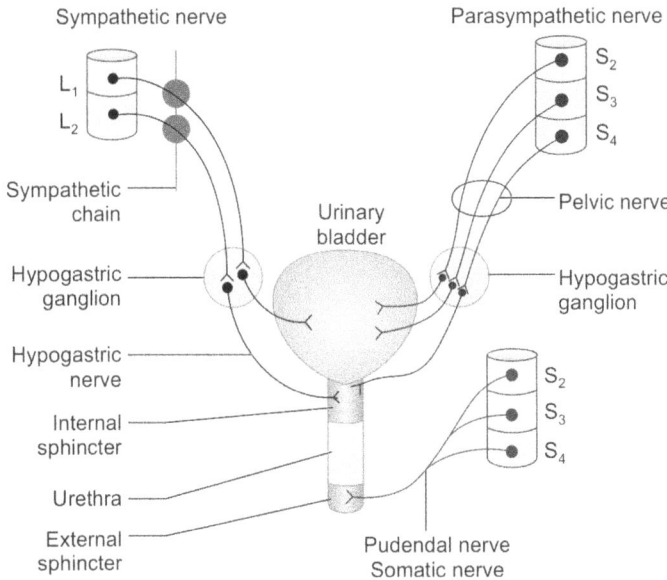

Fig. 20: Nerve supply of urinary bladder.

- It is supplied by sympathetic and parasympathetic nerves (*refer* **Fig. 20**).
- External sphincter is made of skeletal muscle and is supplied by somatic motor nerve (pudendal nerve).
- The bladder wall is also supplied by sympathetic and parasympathetic nerves.
- Parasympathetic nerves (pelvic nerve) have both afferents and efferents to bladder wall and Internal sphincter. They arise from S2–S4 segments of spinal cord. When they are stimulated, they cause contraction of bladder wall and relaxation of internal sphincter and therefore emptying of bladder.
- The sympathetic nerves (hypogastric nerve) also have afferents and efferents and they arise from L1–L3 segments of spinal cord. They also supply the bladder wall and internal sphincter. When stimulated, they cause relaxation of bladder wall and contraction of internal sphincter and therefore filling of bladder.
- Somatic nerve (pudendal nerve) to external sphincter arises from S2–S4 segments of spinal cord and have control from higher centers. It is under voluntary control.
- Once urine enters the renal pelvis, it flows through the ureters and enters the bladder, where urine is stored.

Micturition Reflex (*refer* Fig. 21)

- Micturition is the process of emptying the urinary bladder.
- Two processes are involved:
  1. The bladder fills progressively until the tension in its wall rises above a threshold level, and then
  2. A nervous reflex called the micturition reflex occurs that empties the bladder.
     The micturition reflex is an automatic spinal cord reflex; however, it can be inhibited or facilitated by centers in the brainstem and cerebral cortex.

The Reflex Pathway

- **Initiation:** Reflex initiated by stimulation of stretch receptors in bladder wall.
- **Stimulus:** Filling of bladder up to 300–400 mL.
- **Afferents:** Through pelvic nerves (PS) to reach S2–S4 segments in spinal cord.
- **Efferents:** PS motor fibers from S2–S4 end in the detrusor muscle (excitatory) and internal sphincter (inhibitory).

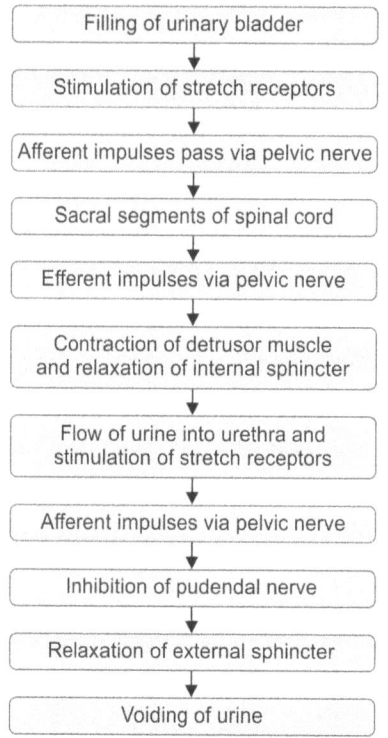

Fig. 21: Micturition reflex.

- **Response:** Causes contraction of bladder wall and relaxation of internal sphincter. Once it becomes powerful another reflex through pudendal nerve relaxes the ES → voiding.

---

6. Spermatogenesis.

- The process of formation of mature sperm is called spermatogenesis.
- It takes place in the seminiferous tubule. It happens in the wall of the tubule from basal lamina towards the lumen.
- The immature cells are present in the basal aspect of the tubule and the maturing cells move toward the adluminal compartment.
- Spermatogenesis involves both mitotic and meiotic divisions and Spermiogenesis.

Mitotic Division

- The primitive germ cell, spermatogonia, in the basal lamina of the seminiferous tubule undergoes mitotic divisions to form Primary spermatocytes.
- Each spermatogonium divides 5 times to produce 32 spermatogonia.
- 32 spermatogonia (44+X+Y) reach the adluminal side of the tubule and undergo mitosis to become 64 Primary spermatocytes (44+X+Y).
- Primary spermatocytes are large cells with diploid number of chromosomes (2n).

Meiotic Divisions

- The primary spermatocytes with diploid number of chromosomes undergo the first meiotic division to form the secondary spermatocyte which is haploid in nature.
- The second meiotic division results in formation of spermatids (22+X or Y).
- A total of 512 spermatids are derived from single spermatogonia.

Spermiogenesis

- The spermatids do not undergo further divisions but structural changes takes place as the spermatids mature into sperm— Spermiogenesis.
- This process happens in the deep folds of Sertoli cells.

The changes taking place are:
- The amount of cytoplasm is reduced in spermatids
- The nucleus elongates to become the head of sperm
- The acrosomal cap is formed
- The tail and middle piece are formed.

Spermiation

- After the maturation the sperms stay attached to the Sertoli cells.
- The release of sperms into the tubule is called Spermiation.

Factors Regulating Spermatogenesis

Hormones regulating spermatogenesis are— androgens, gonadotropins and estrogen

- **Androgens:** A high concentration of testosterone in the tubular fluid is essential for spermatogenesis. LH stimulates Leydig cells to secrete testosterone. Sertoli cells secrete androgen binding protein (ABP) to which testosterone binds and its levels are kept elevated.

Spermiogenesis is androgen dependent.

- **LH:** It stimulates Leydig cells to secrete testosterone and thereby is needed for spermatogenesis.
- **FSH:** Stimulates Sertoli cells and Sertoli cells help in conversion of spermatids to sperms, secretion of ABP and secretion of inhibin. It also increases LH receptors in Leydig cells. It maintains gametogenic function of testis.
- **Estrogen:** Content is high in the fluid in rete testis and estrogen acts to increase fluid reabsorption and spermatozoa is concentrated. This is essential for fertility of an individual.
- **Body temperature:** Spermatogenesis takes place in a temperature less than the inner body temperature. The testes are kept at a temperature of 32°C. If the testes are exposed to higher temperatures the tubular walls degenerate and sterility results.

7. Glucagon.

- It is a polypeptide hormone secreted by the a cells of islets of Langerhans of endocrine pancreas.
- It circulates in plasma unbound and its half-life is 6 minutes.
- Normal fasting level is 100–150 pg/mL
- Mechanism of action—since it is a protein hormone it has a membrane receptor and on binding, it activates the second messenger cascade and its actions are mediated through cAMP. It has metabolic effects on various substrates.

Effects on Carbohydrate Metabolism

- It increases blood glucose levels by various mechanisms, such as glycogenolysis and gluconeogenesis.
- In liver, it activates the enzyme phosphorylase and breaks down glycogen.
- Glycogenolysis is favored by activating phospholipase C and increasing cytoplasmic Ca^{2+} in the hepatocytes.
- It has no glycogenolytic action on muscles.
- It increases gluconeogenesis with the help of pyruvate, lactate, glycerol and amino acids.

Effect on Lipid Metabolism

- It is lipolytic and ketogenic in nature.
- It stimulates action of lipase in adipose tissue and release of fatty acids and glycerol.
- In the liver the fatty acids are oxidized resulting in energy production and ketone body formation.

Effect on Protein Metabolism

- It increases amino acid uptake by liver and increases gluconeogenesis.
- It has calorigenic effects.
- It is positively inotropic as it increases myocardial cAMP.
- Stimulates secretion of insulin, growth hormone and pancreatic somatostatin

Insulin: Glucagon Ratio

- Insulin is glycogenic, anti-gluconeogenic, anti-lipolytic and anti-ketogenic.
- It is a hormone of storage/abundance and stores the absorbed nutrients.
- Glucagon has the opposite actions of insulin and is the hormone of energy release. So the levels of both the hormones must be kept in consideration.
- It is given as molar ratio of insulin and glucagon (I: G).
- I: G ratio in balanced diet is 2.3.
- On fasting, the ratio drops to 0.5.
- This helps in mobilization of substrates and supply of glucose to vital organs.
- In conditions after carbohydrate load or after a meal the I:G ratio reaches 10.

Regulation of Glucagon Secretion

Factors Which Stimulate Glucagon Secretion

- Amino acids (amino acids which are gluconeogenic, such as arginine, alanine, serine, cysteine, etc.)
- Hormones, such as CCK, gastrin and cortisol
- Exercise
- Infections
- Stress
- β adrenergic stimulators
- Theophylline
- Acetylcholine

Factors Which Inhibit Glucagon Secretion
- Glucose
- Somatostatin
- Secretin
- FFA
- Ketones
- Insulin
- α adrenergic stimulators
- GABA

8. Fetoplacental unit.

- Placenta produces steroidal hormones; estrogen and progesterone with the interaction of the fetal adrenals.
- Placenta forms pregnenolone and progesterone from cholesterol
- Some of this pregnenolone enters the fetal circulation and along with the pregnenolone from fetal liver, forms the substrate for formation of Dehydroepiandrosterone (DHEA) and 16-OH DHEAS in fetal adrenals.
- DHEAS and 16-OHDHEAS are transported back to the placenta where DHEAS forms estradiol and 16-OHDHEAS forms estriol. (*refer* **Fig. 22**)
- Estriol is the major estrogen and since its formation requires fetal adrenals, urinary excretion of estriol by mother is a good indicator of well-being of fetus.

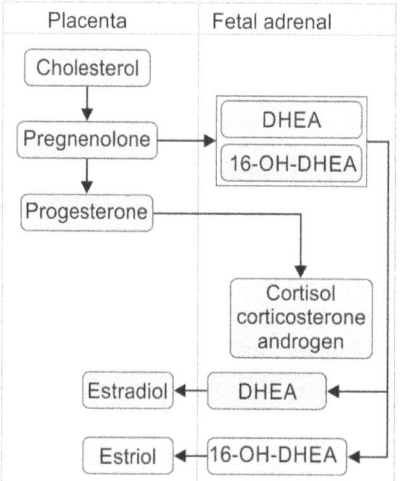

Fig. 22: Fetoplacental unit. Placenta and fetal adrenals, together synthesize progesterone and estrogen.

9. Secondary active transport.

- Active transport across cell membrane involves use of energy and is an uphill transport.
- The substances move against the concentration and electrical gradient.
- Primary active transport derives the energy directly from hydrolysis of ATP. Therefore, the carrier molecules are ATPases, such as Na^+-K^+ ATPase.
- Secondary active transporter uses energy from ATP hydrolysis indirectly. The Na^+-K^+ ATPase which is present in all cells, carries 3 molecules of Na^+ from ICF to ECF and 2 K^+ from ECF to ICF. By the action of this pump there is a concentration gradient established for Na^+ to move into the cell. This inward Na^+ gradient is coupled to transport other ions, such as glucose; the Na-glucose transporter (SGLT) in epithelial cells in intestines and kidneys.
- Secondary active transporters can be symports or antiports
- Low sodium concentration in the cell favors Na^+ influx and the symport will move glucose into the cell only when both Na^+ and glucose binds to it. So the Na^+ gradient is used to transport glucose across the membrane.
- In cardiac myocytes, the Na^+ gradient is used to transport Ca^{2+} to the ECF. So Na^+-Ca^{2+} exchanger is an antiport moving Na^+ into the cell and Ca^{2+} out of the cells.
- There are also Na^+-Amino acid symport, Na^+-I^- symport, Na^+, K^+, $2Cl^-$ symport, etc.

10. Fibrinolytic system

- Tendency to form clot in an injured vessel is at the same time balanced by anticlotting or fibrinolytic pathways in the vessel to keep the lumen of blood vessel patent.
- Fibrinolytic system involves an important protease enzyme plasmin which is present in an inactive form as plasminogen in plasma.
- On activation, plasmin lyses the fibrin and fibrinogen to produce fibrin degradation products (FDP) which in turn inhibits thrombin.

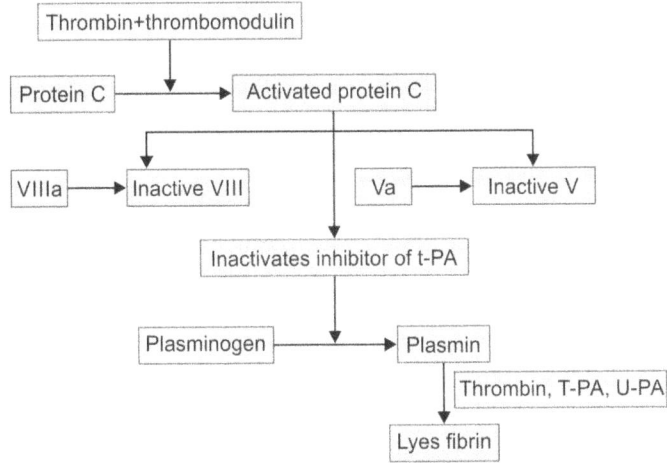

Fig. 23: Fibrinolytic system and its regulation.

- Plasminogen is activated by thrombin, and there are plasminogen activators—the tissue type plasminogen activator (t-PA) and urokinase-type plasminogen activator (u-PA).
- Plasminogen receptors are also located on the endothelial cells and binding to the receptor, plasminogen is activated and prevents clot formation in intact vessels.
- There are also tissue plasminogen inhibitors in plasma which are regulated by protein C and its co-factor protein S (*refer* Fig. 23).

11. Normal ECG in lead II.

Normal ECG in Lead II

- Lead II is a bipolar limb lead between right arm (negative electrode) and left arm (positive electrode).
- The ECG tracing in lead II shows both negative and positive deflections equally and therefore used as a standard recording.
- There are intervals and segments in the ECG

ECG Waves

- There are positive and negative waves are deflections in the ECG tracing.
- There are 4 waveforms—P wave, QRS complex, T wave and U wave (*refer* Fig. 24).
  a. *P wave:* This is the first positive wave in ECG and is due to atrial depolarization. Duration is 0.1 second

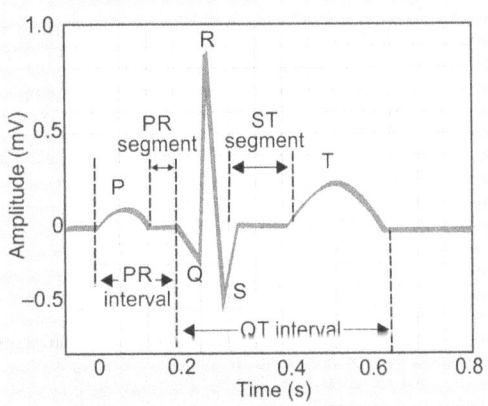

Fig. 24: Normal ECG in Lead II with waves, segments and intervals.

  b. *QRS complex:* Consists of a negative Q wave, positive R wave and negative s wave. This complex is due to ventricular depolarization. Normal duration is 0.08 seconds.
  c. *T wave* is a positive deflection following QRS complex and is due to ventricular repolarization. Normal duration is 0.27 seconds
  d. *U wave* is also positive deflection and is normally not seen. It is seen in slow depolarization of the papillary muscle. Duration is 0.08 seconds.

ECG Segments

- These are isoelectric lines seen in between the ECG waves.

- There are two segments—PR segment and ST segment
  a. *PR Segment:* It starts at the end of P wave to beginning of QRS complex.
  b. *ST segment:* It begins in the end of QRS complex and is up to the beginning of T wave.

ECG Intervals

- Intervals in ECG include waves and segments.
- The intervals are—PR interval, QT interval, ST interval, PP interval and RR interval.
- **J point:** This is an indicator of end of ventricular depolarization and start of ventricular repolarization. It is at the end of QRS and is at the isoelectric line.
  - *PR interval:* It is between beginning of P wave to beginning of Q wave.
    - The normal duration is 0.12-0.2 sec (average 0.18 sec).
    - This denotes atrial depolarization and conduction to AV node.
    - Prolonged PR interval signifies AV conduction block
  - *QT interval:* It starts at Q wave and ends with T wave.
    - Normal duration is 0.4 seconds.
    - It denotes the systolic phase of the ventricle
    - It is prolonged in ventricular conduction defects, hypocalcemia and myocardial ischemia.
  - *ST interval:* It is from the end of S wave to the end of T wave.
    - Normal duration is 0.32 seconds.
    - It denotes ventricular repolarization.
  - *PP interval:* It is the interval between two successive P waves.
    - It is used to calculate atrial rate
  - *RR interval:* It is the interval between two successive R waves.
    - It is used to calculate the heart rate.

12. Regulation of coronary blood flow.

Regulation of coronary blood flow is by autoregulation, neural regulation and by metabolic regulation.

Autoregulation

- Well developed in heart but autoregulation falls when the BP falls below 70 mm Hg and coronary blood flow is decreased.
- Autoregulation is between 70-110 mm Hg

Neural Regulation

By sympathetic and parasympathetic nerves.

Sympathetic stimulation: Norepinephrine secreted from sympathetic nerve terminal acts on α and β adrenergic receptors. There is a direct effect and an indirect effect following stimulation of sympathetic nerves to heart.

- **Direct effect:** It is the effect of norepinephrine (NE) on α receptors—resulting in vasoconstriction and thereby decreases coronary blood flow.
- **Indirect effect:** Effect of NE on σ receptors leads to -↑HR and contractility → production of vasodilator metabolites → vasodilatation → Increased blood flow in coronary vessels.

Effect of parasympathetic stimultion: Decreased heart rate → No metabolites formed → Decreased blood flow in coronary vessel

Metabolic Regulation

- This is the most important mechanism by which coronary blood flow is regulated.
- Metabolic regulators are -↓PO_2, ↑PCO_2, ↑H^+, prostaglandins, ↑lactate, adenosine and adenine nucleotides.
- Adenosine is a major factor regulating blood flow. Adenosine is released from myocardium during hypoxia and it causes vasodilation.
- ↓PO_2—directly produces vasodilatation

Regulation by Endothelium

Endothelium derived relaxing factors like nitric oxide, prostaglandins, prostacyclin and endothelium derived hyperpolarizing factors (EDHF) also cause vasodilatation and increase coronary blood flow.

13. Compliance of lung.

- Stretchability or the recoiling tendency due to the elastic property of the lung is said to be the compliance.

- Compliance of the respiratory system is defined as the change in the lung volume per unit change in the airway pressure.
- It is given as C = ΔV/ΔP
  - C = Compliance
  - ΔV = Change in volume
  - ΔP = Change in pressure
  - It is expressed in L/cm H_2O

Compliance in Respiratory System is Given Under Two Headings

- Compliance of lungs only
- Compliance of lungs and thoracic wall

Compliance of Lungs and Thoracic Cavity

Both the lungs and thoracic cavity are elastic and viscous in nature and therefore each of them has their own recoiling tendencies.

Normal value of thoracic cavity and lungs together is 0.13 L/cm H_2O.

It means, when there is an increase in airway pressure by 1 cm H_2O the volume of the lungs increases by 0.13 liters.

Compliance of Lung Alone

- Normal value is around 0.22 L/cm H_2O
- So compliance of lung is twice that of lung and thoracic cavity together.

Measurement of Compliance of Lungs and Chest Wall

- The interaction of recoiling of lung and chest wall is demonstrated in living subjects by using the spirometer.
- After clipping the nose, the subject is asked to breathe in from a spirometer from end expiratory position in increments of volumes.
- There is a valve beyond the mouth piece, through which he breathes and also a pressure recording device is attached to the mouth piece.
- The person inhales a given volume of air and the valve is shut and the person is asked to relax the respiratory muscles and the change in airway pressure is noted.
- This procedure is repeated after inhaling and exhaling various volumes of air and also recording of airway pressures.
- The airway pressures are plotted against the lung volumes to get the relaxation pressure curve of the respiratory system. (refer **Fig. 25**)
- From the curve, it is noted that at zero pressure the lung volume is equal to FRC

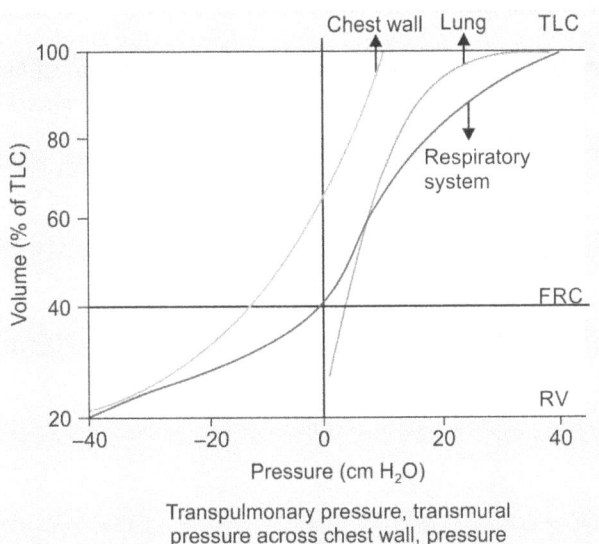

Fig. 25: Relaxation pressure-volume curve of lung and chest wall. It gives the relation between intrapulmonary pressure and volume. Curve in gray color is the curve of total respiratory system. At FRC, the transmural pressure is zero and above it the pressure is positive and below it, negative.

and this volume is said to be the relaxation volume.
- It is the volume at which the recoiling of lungs is exactly balanced by the recoiling of the thoracic wall.
- The measurement of compliance can be made using the curve especially where it is the steepest.
- Above the relaxation volume as the volume increases the pressure also increases and it reaches about +30 mm Hg.
- Below the relaxation volume as the volume decreases the pressure also decreases and reaches –30 mm Hg.

Factors Affecting Compliance of Lungs and Chest Wall

- Compliance when decreased shifts the pressure-volume curve to the right and downwards, as in—pulmonary edema, congestion and pulmonary fibrosis
- Compliance when increased the curve is shifted to the left and above as in: Emphysema and old age.

Measurement of Compliance of Lungs Alone

- The compliance of lungs alone can be measured by measuring the intrapleural pressures (IPP) at various lung volumes.
- IPP gives an idea about the distensibility of the lungs.
- As the lung expands the IPP becomes more negative as the recoiling forces are more.
- IPP can be recorded by measuring intra-esophageal pressures.
- The person is asked to breathe in from a spirometer from the end expiratory position up to end inspiratory position and holds the breath.
- The IPP is measured in this manner for various lung volumes inhaled and exhaled and a graph is plotted.
- The observation is that the curves of change in pressure to change in volume is different for inspiration and expiration and is curved.
- The curve depicts that at similar IPP, the lung volume is less in inspiratory phase than in expiratory phase. The curve is said to be the **"hysteresis curve"** (*refer* **Fig. 26**).
- The difference in pressure volume-relationship in inspiration and expiration is due to—viscous resistance and Airway resistance.
- Compliance is greater when measured during deflation than when measured during inflation.
- Lung compliance is calculated by taking a point on the graph at the end of inspiration when there is no air flow and so there is no viscous and elastic resistance.

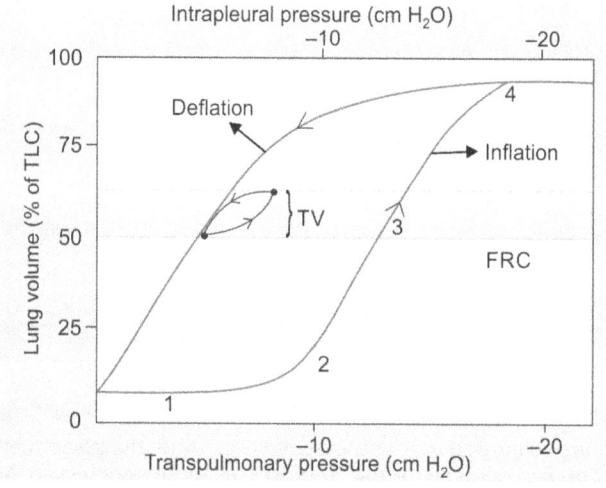

Fig. 26: Pressure-volume relations in the lungs. Pressure changes in inflation and deflation are different.

- Lung compliance is calculated as $\Delta V/\Delta P$ = 0.22 L/cm H_2O.
- This amount of lung compliance is affected by the elastic tissues in the lungs and also the surface tension of the fluid lining the alveoli.
- The contribution of each factor is studied by removing the lungs of an experimental animal and distending them with air and water alternately while measuring the intrapulmonary pressure.
- While distension with air, the pressure-volume curve measures both tissues elasticity and surface tension, whereas while using saline surface tension becomes zero and the curve measures only tissue elasticity.
- In the curve with saline, there is not much difference in inspiratory and expiratory curves. The elasticity due to surface tension is much smaller at small lung volumes than at large lung volumes. This may be due to the effect of surfactant.

Factors Affecting Lung Compliance Alone

- **Lung volume:** A person with one lung, will have the change in volume to change in pressure.
- Compliance is more during deflation of lung than while inflating the lungs.
- Due to effect of gravity in standing position compliance is less in the apex of the lung.

Specific Compliance

- As mentioned above, in a person with one lung (even though compliance of that lung is normal) the compliance is decreased as the lung volume is decreased. To overcome this, compliance can be calculated as a function of FRC.
- Specific compliance = compliance/FRC.

---

14. Carbon dioxide transport.

CO_2 is Transported in 4 Forms

1. As dissolved form in plasma
2. As carbamino-compound—combination with plasma proteins.
3. As bicarbonate
4. As carbamino-hemoglobin—combination with hemoglobin.

As Dissolved Form

- CO_2 in dissolved form in plasma is proportional to the partial pressure of CO_2.
- It has 20 times more solubility than O_2 in blood.
- Some amount of CO_2 combines with plasma proteins to form **carbamino-protein** complex.

As Bicarbonate

- The major form by which CO_2 is transported is as bicarbonate. Nearly 70% is transported as HCO_3^-.
- As the CO_2 enters the blood, it saturates the plasma and quickly diffuses into the RBCs.
- In the RBC, the enzyme carbonic anhydrase catalyzes the reaction of CO_2 combining with water to form H_2CO_3 (refer **Fig. 27**).
- $H_2CO_3 \rightarrow H^+ + HCO_3^-$
- As the HCO_3^- levels increase within the RBC, it starts leaving the RBC in exchange for Cl^-.
- This exchange happens through the band 3 protein which is an anion exchanger. It is present on the membrane of RBC.
- This is called as the "**chloride shift**" or "**hamburger shift**".
- So in the venous blood the RBCs have more osmotically active particles which causes water retention in the RBC and increases its size.
- Therefore, hematocrit of venous blood is 3% more than the arterial blood.
- The H^+ is buffered by hemoglobin within the RBC.

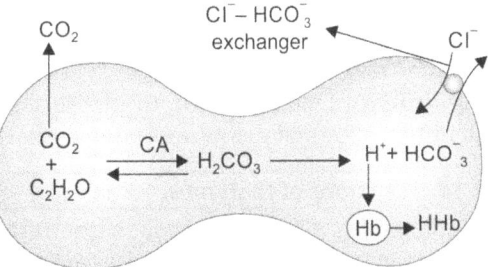

Fig. 27: Chloride shift.

- As Hb binds with H⁺ the Oxy-Hb curve shifts to the right and O_2 is released to the tissues.
- As the venous blood reaches the lungs the reverse process of all the above happens and CO_2 is released and blown out.
- High O_2 levels in the lungs helps in unloading of CO_2.

As Carbamino-Compound

- CO_2 in RBC binds to hemoglobin to form Carbamino-hemoglobin.
- About 23% of CO_2 is transported in this form.

---

15. Dysbarism.

- Also called as "Decompression sickness, The bends, Caissons disease, Divers palsy".
- This happens when a person breathing compressed air ascends up rapidly.
- At high pressures, N_2 dissolves in body fluids and stays dissolved.
- When the person ascends up to sea level gradually N_2 is converted to air gradually and is blown out.
- But when he ascends up rapidly the dissolved N_2 does not have enough time to be converted to air and to be blown out and therefor it stays in the tissues as N_2 bubbles.
- N_2 dissolved in tissues forms bubbles while escaping from tissues due to rapid ascent.
- Gas bubbles block the blood vessels and stay in tissues to create symptoms.

Symptoms are:
- Pain in joints and muscles of legs or arms.
- Sensation of numbness
- The chokes–shortness of breath, pulmonary edema, etc.
- Paralysis of muscles
- Coronary ischemia
- Neurological symptoms

Treatment: Recompression in pressurized chamber followed by slow decompression.

---

16. Functions of thalamus.

- Thalamus functions as a major relay station for most sensory impulses reaching the cortex.
- Thalamus acts as a crude center for sense perception, such as crude touch, pain, crude form of temperature sensation.
- It also contributes to motor function by relaying impulses from cerebellum and basal ganglia to motor cortex.
- Relays impulse between different areas of cortex.
- Contributes to regulation of autonomic activities and maintenance of consciousness.
- Due to the intimate connections of thalamus with frontal cortex and hypothalamus it is involved in various emotions.
- It is an integrating center for sleep, intralaminar nuclei for NREM sleep and lateral geniculate body for REM sleep.
- Concerned with recent memory and emotions due to its involvement in Papez circuit.
- Concerned with language.
- Important role in genesis of synchronization of EEG waves and alertness of the individual. Induces alertness due to its connections with RAS.

---

17. REM sleep.

- Sleep is said to be a state of altered consciousness or partial unconsciousness from which a person can be aroused.
- Sleep deprivation results in impaired attention, learning and performance.
- Sleep has two components—non-rapid eye movement (NREM) and rapid eye movement (REM) sleep

REM Sleep

- In a period of sleep of 7–8 hours, REM and NREM sleep phases alternate.
- REM sleep occurs 3–5 times during the sleep period alternating with NREM sleep.
- Initial episode of REM sleep will be lasting for 10–20 minutes. Then with each episode, it prolongs and the final episode is for 50 minutes.
- In adults REM sleep totals for about 90–120 minutes. With increasing age, period of REM sleep decreases.

- About 50% of an infants' sleep is REM sleep. 35% for 2-year-old infant and 25% for adults.
- REM sleep is thought to be important for maturation of brain in infants. This has been identified by the high percentage of REM sleep in infants.

Physiological Changes in REM Sleep

- Most of the dreaming occurs in REM sleep. These dreams can be remembered.
- Eyes move rapidly back and forth under the eyelid.
- Neuronal activities are higher—brain blood flow and O_2 use is high.
- EEG recordings are similar to that of an active and awake person.
- Excepting the motor neurons governing respiration and eye, impulses in most of them are inhibited.
- Inhibition of motor neurons results in loss of muscle tone and even some time paralysis.
- Parasympathetic activity increases and sympathetic activity decreases → decrease in HR and BP.
- Periodically sympathetic activity is also increased.
- Bruxism, erection of penis and twitching of facial muscles are seen in REM sleep.

Control of REM Sleep

- NREM and REM sleep are mediated by different parts of the brain.
- REM sleep—neurons in pons and mid brain.

---

18. Decerebrate rigidity

- Decerebration is a procedure where the medulla is separated from the brainstem by making a mid-collicular transection (Between superior and inferior colliculi). It is done experimentally in animals to study the role of medulla in posture regulation.
- Muscle tone is exaggerated in the decerebrate animal.
- Righting reflexes are lost.
- There are no features of shock immediately after the transection.
- Immediately after transection, there is marked rigidity in the muscles especially in the extensor group of muscles and the back muscles.
- So limbs and spine are hyperextended.
- The rigidity is due to hyperactive stretch reflex in the extensor groups of muscles.

It happens by two mechanisms:
1. Increased excitability of alpha motor neurons supplying the muscles
2. Increased activity in gamma motor neurons supplying the muscle spindles of extensors.
   - For understanding the cause of increase in activity of the above two groups of neurons we need to understand the higher centers controlling the stretch reflex.
   - There are two major areas in the brain stem controlling the excitability of anterior horn cells in the spinal cord:
     a. A large facilitatory area in the pontine reticular formation which gives rise to the pontine reticulospinal tract. (*refer* Fig. 28)
     b. A small inhibitory area in the medullary reticular formation, giving rise to the medullary reticulospinal tract.

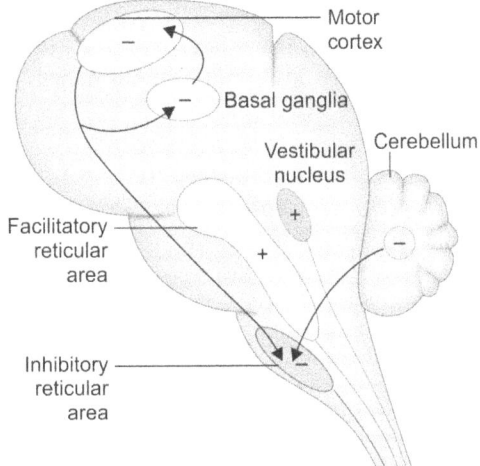

Fig. 28: Higher control of muscle tone; inhibitory areas—cerebral cortex, basal ganglia, cerebellum and inhibitory medullary reticular area. Facilitatory area—pontine facilitatory reticular formation.

- The facilitatory area discharges spontaneously whereas the inhibitory medullary area is under the control of higher centers—cerebral cortex, basal ganglia and cerebellum.
- The basal ganglia acts through cerebral cortex and from the cortex the cortical fibers control the medullary inhibitory area.
- So the net effect of stimulation of 3 inhibitory areas and one facilitatory area is overall inhibition of stretch reflex in normal condition.
- In mid-collicular section two of the inhibitions are removed and the facilitation continues resulting in rigidity and hypertonia.

19. Taste pathway.

The taste receptors are present in the taste buds which are located on the tongue in the papillae:
- There are 10,000 taste buds.
- Taste buds are located in—fungiform, foliate and vallate papillae.
- Cells in taste buds—type 1 and 2—supporting cells.
- Type 3 cells—receptor epithelial cells has microvilli projecting into taste pore.
- They are receptors are replaced constantly in 10 days.
- Each bud is innervated by 50 nerves at bases of receptor cells.
- Each nerve innervates 5 taste buds.
- The sensory fibers from the taste buds travel through 3 nerves—*Chorda tympani* branch of facial nerve (from anterior 2/3rd of the tongue), glossopharyngeal nerve (from posterior 1/3rd of the tongue) and vagus N from epiglottis, pharynx and palate.
- They all reach the medulla and terminate on the same side nucleus tractus solitarius of the same side (*refer* **Fig. 29**).
- From here the second order neurons travel along with medial lemniscus to reach ventral posteromedial nucleus of ipsilateral thalamus.

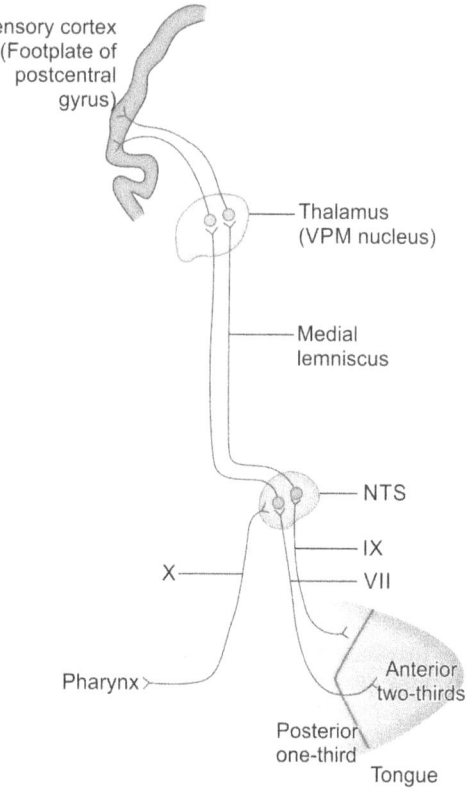

Fig. 29: Taste pathway. Sensation of taste is carried through VIIth cranial nerve from anterior 2/3rd of tongue, by glossopharyngeal nerve (IX) from anterior 1/3rd of tongue, from pharynx, epiglottis by vagus nerve (X) to nucleus tractus solitarius (NTS).

- Some fibers from medulla go to the vomiting center, hypothalamus, limbic system and salivary nucleus.
- The 3rd order neurons arise from the thalamus and they reach the foot of postcentral gyrus on the same side (area 43).
- From there impulses are also transmitted to the insula and lateral orbitofrontal cortex.

20. Theories of hearing.

Rutherford Telephone Theory
- According to this theory, the ear acts like a telephone and transmits the same number of impulses as that of the frequency of sound.

- For example, if the sound is of 6000 Hz frequency, the auditory nerve transmits 6000 impulses.
- But it is not acceptable, as the nerves cannot transmit at this high frequency.
- But lower frequency sounds, less than 2000 Hz/sec can produce a volley of similar number of impulses.

Place Theory
- According to this theory, sound waves of different frequencies stimulate the basilar membrane of organ of corti in different areas.
- Sound waves of higher frequency stimulate the structures near the base of the cochlea and low frequency waves stimulate the structures near the apex.

Resonance Volley Theory
- This theory combines both the above theories and it proposes that the volley theory is acceptable for low frequency sounds below 2000 Hz and higher frequency sounds are encoded by the place at which the organ of corti and basilar membrane are stimulated.
- This is the most accepted theory.

21. Resting membrane potential.
- There is a potential difference across the membrane of all cells and the inside of the cell is more negative than the outside of the cell. This is said to be the membrane potential. The membrane potential at rest in a cell is said to be the resting membrane potential (RMP).
- The RMP in excitable cells like the nerve and muscle cells are important as the change in the potential makes the cell to become more excited or inhibited.
- RMP is due to unequal distribution of ions on either side of the membrane and various forces acting on the membrane.

They are:
- Unequal distribution of ions across the cell membrane
- Differences in the permeability of the membrane to various ions.
- Na$^+$ K$^+$ pump or Na$^+$ K$^+$ ATPase

The RMP of various cells:
- RMP of the nerve is –70 mV
- RMP of skeletal membrane is –90 mV
- RMP of cardiac muscle is –90 mV
- RMP of smooth muscles is variable

Selective permeability of the membrane to ions:
The membrane allows certain molecules to move freely across and restrict movements of certain. It is highly permeable to K$^+$ and chloride at rest and only moderately permeable to Na$^+$. It is totally impermeable to intracellular proteins and phosphates which are anions. The high permeability for K$^+$ allows it to move out of the cells and the anions are impermeable and they line up along the interior of the membrane to create the negative membrane potential.

There are gated channels for other ions in the membrane which allows movements of ions in various situations.

Concentration of ions in ICF and ECF:
- **Cations:** Na$^+$ are high in the ECF (140 mEq/L) and K$^+$ are high in the ICF (150 mEq/L) (*refer* **Fig. 30**).
- **Anions:** Cl$^-$ and HCO$_3^-$ are high in ECF and in ICF proteins and PO$_4^-$ are high.

Na$^+$-K$^+$ pump
This pump, by creating a gradient for Na$^+$ helps to maintain the RMP. It also contributes

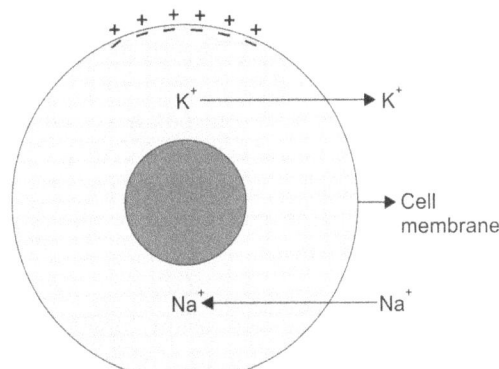

Fig. 30: Genesis of RMP. At rest, an electrical potential difference exists across the membrane of a cell with the inside being negative than the outside of a cell. This is because the cell membrane is more permeable to K$^+$ at rest than to Na+. So K$^+$ efflux is more than Na$^+$ influx. This is responsible for the RMP.

minimally for genesis of RMP as the pump extrudes 3 Na⁺ ions out of the cell and 2 K⁺ ions into the cell. So a loss of a single positive ion creates a net negativity inside the membrane.

Factors responsible for genesis of RMP:
- **Permeability of membrane to K⁺:** Membrane is highly permeable to K⁺ at rest and K⁺ gradient is outward and the outward movement creates negativity inside the cell.
- **Permeability of membrane to Na⁺:** At rest, there is always an inward gradient for Na⁺ and the membrane is less permeable to Na⁺ than K⁺ and therefore the Na⁺ influx will not balance K⁺ efflux and so inside the cell the potential is negative.
- **Permeability of membrane to anions:** The membrane is totally impermeable to anions and therefore they remain inside the cell to create negativity along the inner aspect of the membrane.
- **Na⁺-K⁺ Pump:** They offer minimum role in genesis of RMP but they help to maintain RMP.

22. Negative feedback mechanism with example.

- Most of the control systems in the body are negative feedback regulations.
- In negative feedback regulation, if a particular activity is increased or decreased, the control system initiates a chain of actions by which the activity returns back to normal.
- So the control system has a sensor to sense the change, a control center that receives signals from the sensor and sends command to the effector which will bring about the change.

Examples:
Body temperature regulation, regulation of pH, regulation of blood glucose levels, regulation of thyroid hormone secretion.

Blood Pressure Regulation

Increase in mean arterial pressure
↓
Sensed by baroreceptors
↓
Impulses are carried by IXth and Xth cranial nerves
↓
Inhibits vasomotor center and stimulates cardiac vagal center
↓
Decreases heart rate and stroke volume
↓
Decreases cardiac output
↓
Decreases mean arterial pressure

23. Pathophysiology of diabetes mellitus.

Deficiency of insulin is diabetes mellitus.

Causes

Diabetes mellitus occurs due to destruction of β cells of islets in the pancreas or due to decreased sensitivity of receptors for insulin. Based on the causes and features diabetes is classified into two types—type 1 and type 2 diabetes mellitus—**primary diabetes mellitus**.

Secondary diabetes mellitus: Diabetes is secondary to some other diseases, such as Cushing's syndrome, acromegaly, pancreatitis, etc.

Type 1 Diabetes Mellitus
- This is due to autoimmune destruction of β cells and insulin is not secreted.
- Plasma insulin levels are low and undetectable
- This condition is treated with only insulin and therefore also called as Insulin dependent diabetes mellitus (IDDM).
- Antibodies are present against b cell surface antigens.
- It is usually seen in children and adults of <45 years of age.
- They are prone for ketoacidosis and are thin.
- Chance of developing the disease in identical twins is 50%

Type 2 Diabetes Mellitus
- This is due to decreased sensitivity of insulin receptors for insulin.
- Insulin levels are normal or even elevated

- Therefore, it is also called as non-insulin dependent diabetes mellitus (NIDDM).
- The individuals with NIDDM are obese and the disease occurs usually after >45 years of age.
- This is the most common type of DM
- The chance of developing the disease in identical disease is 100%.

Symptoms of DM

- DM is characterized by polyphagia, polydipsia, polyuria, weight loss, hyperglycemia and glycosuria. In severe condition, it leads to ketoacidosis and coma.
  - *Polyphagia:* Increased food intake. This is due to inability of usage of glucose by the neurons in satiety center of hypothalamus due to absence of insulin. So, the low glucose in these cells leads to stimulation of the feeding center and thereby increased food intake.
  - *Polyuria:* Passage of large amounts of urine. As the plasma glucose levels increase, the amount of glucose filtered is also increased. The SGLT transporter in renal tubular cells of PCT gets saturated and is not able to reabsorb glucose from the filtrate and glucose starts appearing in the urine. The glucose when retained in tubule holds back water and other electrolytes in the tubule and results in osmotic diuresis. Other ions, such as Na^+, K^+ and phosphates are also lost in urine
  - *Polydipsia:* When water is lost excessively, thirst mechanism is stimulated because of cellular dehydration and water intake is increased.
  - *Weight loss* is due to loss of calories in the urine and mobilization of other stores, such as fats and proteins resulting in weight loss.
  - *Hyperglycemia* is due to decreased peripheral utilization of glucose by skeletal muscles, adipose tissues and liver. There is also increased glucose output from liver.
  - *Glycosuria* is excessive loss of glucose in urine. This happens when the renal threshold (>180 mg/dL) is reached. Glycosuria leads to all the symptoms mentioned above.

Physiological Basis of Treatment of DM

- *Sulfonylurea derivatives,* such as tolbutamide, acetohexamide, glipizide, glyburide are hypoglycemic agents and they decrease blood glucose levels by increasing production of insulin. So they are effective in people with some amount of working β cells. It cannot be used in type 1 DM. They act by inhibiting ATP-inhibited K^+ channels and decrease K^+ efflux thereby depolarizing the membrane and favors Ca^{2+} influx and release of insulin.
- The other groups of drugs are *biguanides,* such as phenformin, metformin which act in the absence of insulin. They decrease the hepatic output of glucose and thereby decreases blood glucose levels. Metformin can be used in combination with sulfonylureas in treatment for type 2 DM.
- *Thiazolidinediones,* such as troglitazone are hypoglycemic agents which increase the insulin-mediated peripheral utilization of glucose. They act by binding to peroxisome proliferator-activated receptor (PPARγ).
- *Exercise:* It is a very effective strategy to decrease blood glucose levels in type 1 and type 2 DM. Exercise increases glucose entry into skeletal muscle by inserting an insulin independent GLUT 4 glucose transporter in muscle cell membranes. This increases glucose uptake by muscle cells for a prolonged duration after exercise also and therefore regular exercise can increase insulin sensitivity.

---

24. Small intestinal movements.

Movements of the Small Intestines

Five types of movements in the normal state:
1. **Peristalsis:** Propulsive movement
2. **Mixing movements:** Segmentation contraction and tonic contraction
3. **Migrating motor complexes (MMC)**

4. Movements of villi
5. Contractions of muscularis mucosa

Abnormal movements: Peristaltic rushes.

MMC

- Migrating motility complexes are motility present in the interdigestive period.
- These are bursts of electrical and mechanical activities in GIT.
- It starts in the esophagus and spreads through the stomach and ileum to the ileocecal valve
- Occurs once in 90 minutes and lasts for 10-20 minutes.
- It clears the GIT for the next meal.
- Occurs in 3 phases—phases I, II and III:
  - *Phase I:* No spike potential, no contractions
  - *Phase II:* Irregular spike potentials and contractions
  - *Phase III:* Regular spike potentials and contractions

Mixing Movements

Segmentation Contractions

- These are ring like contractions present in short segments of the intestine of 1-2 cm.
- They are present in regular intervals.
- Their frequency matches the slow wave frequency.
- Slow waves are waves generated in the pace maker cells located in the wall of duodenum and it spreads through the muscular wall of the intestines.
- Strength of the contraction depends on the spike waves superimposed on the slow waves.
- These ring like contractions appear in one segment and the nearby segment relaxes, this is followed by another set of contractions in the segments between the previous contractions.
- These contractions appear sausage shaped and they cut into the bolus and move it to and fro and increase their exposure to the absorptive surface of the mucosa.
- Therefore, these contractions help in mixing the bolus with digestive juices and in digestion and absorption of food.

Tonic Contractions

- These are prolonged contractions of one segment of intestine and the segment appears to be isolated from the rest of the ileum.
- Segmentation and tonic contractions delay the passage of chyme and thereby allow contact of chyme with enterocytes and favor absorption.

Peristalsis

- This is a type of propulsive movement which helps to move the chyme forward. It is a reflex initiated by the stretch of the intestinal wall following the entry of food.
- Stretch of the intestinal wall initiates a ring of constriction behind the bolus and a relaxation in front of the bolus.
- The ring of contraction behind pushes the bolus to the relaxed segment in front of the bolus.
- Next ring of contraction now appears in the previous relaxed segment and the bolus is pushed further.
- These waves always propel the contents from the oral to caudal direction and never in the opposite direction—*law of the gut*.
- These waves appear even in the absence of nerve supply but they can be modified by the autonomic nerves, parasympathetic nerves increase the activity and sympathetic nerves decrease the activity.
- The propelling speed varies from 2-25 cm/s.
- Sometimes, the peristaltic waves can be very fast and they empty the contents faster—peristaltic rushes, seen in acute diarrhea.
- Antiperistalsis happens in vomiting.

25. Neuroendocrinal reflex.

- In this type of reflex, the afferent limb of the reflex is neural and the efferent limb is humoral or endocrine.
- Examples of this reflex are milk ejection or milk let down reflex and the parturition reflex.

Milk Ejection Reflex

Oxytocin is a hormone secreted from the hypothalamus and released from posterior

pituitary gland. It acts on the myoepithelial cells lining the ducts of breast and expels milk through a reflex.
- The receptors for this reflex are touch receptors around the nipple. When the infant suckles at the breast the touch receptors are stimulated.
- Impulses are relayed through somatic afferent pathways to the supraoptic (SO) and paraventricular (PV) nuclei of hypothalamus.
- These nuclei secrete the hormone oxytocin which is transported through blood and acts on the myoepithelial cells lining the ducts of the breast resulting in expulsion of milk (*refer* **Fig. 31**).

Parturition Reflex
- Towards the term of pregnancy, estrogen levels in the blood rise and increases the sensitivity of oxytocin receptors in the uterine myometrium, to oxytocin.
- As a result of action of oxytocin, the uterus contracts and fetal head is pushed down stretching the cervix. There are stretch receptors in the cervix.
- As the cervix is stretched the stretch receptors are stimulated and impulses are transmitted through sensory afferent fibers to SO and PV nuclei of hypothalamus.
- These nuclei secrete oxytocin.
- Oxytocin binds to the receptors in the uterine myometrium and induces further contractions. This further pushes the fetal head down, further stretching the cervix and more oxytocin is released.
- This continues as a positive feedback mechanism till the fetus is born.

26. Functions of placenta.
- Synthesis of hormones (endocrine function of placenta)
- Transport of substances across the placenta between the mother and fetus
- Protection of fetus

Hormones Synthesized by Placenta
- Human chorionic gonadotropin (hCG)
- Human chorionic somatomammotropin (hCS)
- Placental progesterone
- Placental estrogen
- Relaxin

Human Chorionic Gonadotropin (hCG)
- It is synthesized by syncytiotrophoblasts of placenta
- It is a glycoprotein with α and β subunits
- It starts appearing in the blood of the mother by 6 days after fertilization and reaches a peak by 10-12 weeks.
- Clinically, presence of hCG in urine of a female is "the indicator" of pregnancy.
- It stimulates the corpus luteum to secrete progesterone till the placenta is fully formed.
- hCG helps in sexual differentiation of male fetus.
- It induces hyperemesis in the first trimester.

Human Chorionic Somatomammotropin (hCS)
- It is also secreted from the syncytiotrophoblast of placenta.
- Its secretion starts by 5th week of pregnancy and reaches a peak towards term.
- It is similar to growth hormone and has growth promoting actions, so called as "Maternal growth hormone of pregnancy"
- It stimulates lipolysis, N, K^+ and Ca^{2+} retention and decreases glucose utilization by the mother so that the substrates are diverted to the fetus.

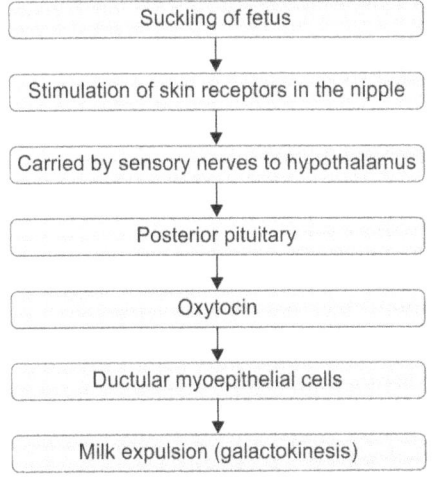

Fig. 31: Milk ejection reflex.

- Amount of hCS secreted is equal to size of placenta and therefore level of hCS indicates placental viability.

Placental Progesterone

- In the early weeks of pregnancy, progesterone is produced by corpus luteum and later the function is taken over by placenta.
- It is produced by coordination between the mother and the fetus—the fetoplacental unit.
- It makes the endometrium secretory and thereby nourishes the fertilized ovum.
- It keeps the myometrium of the pregnant uterus quiescent which is essential for the survival of the fetus.
- It acts on the alveolar system of the maternal breast and facilitates development of maternal breast.
- It has an immunosuppressive role in protecting the fetus.

Placental Estrogen

- The major estrogen in pregnancy is estriol.
- It stimulates development of the ductular system of the maternal breast
- The levels of estrogen rises during pregnancy but on nearing term estrogen progesterone ratio rises and estrogen makes the myometrium excitable.
- On decrease of levels of estrogen after delivery of fetus, prolactin stimulates milk secretion from the breast.

Relaxin

- Its level in the early pregnancy is high to relax the uterine wall to favor implantation of fetus.
- In later weeks, it causes relaxation of pubic symphysis and pelvic ligaments to facilitate delivery of fetus.

Other hormones secreted are:
CRH, β endorphin, α-MSH, GnRH, inhibin, prolactin, etc.

Transport Functions of Placenta

- **Transport of nutrients:** Placenta transports nutrients from the mother to the fetus. The nutrients transported are glucose, fats, amino acids and Ca^{2+}, inorganic phosphates, K^+, Na^+.
- **Transports of waste products** from the fetus to the mother—substances transported are urea, uric acid and creatinine.
- **Transport of gases:** Dissolved O_2 is transported from maternal side of placenta to the fetus along the pressure gradient. Fetus receives its O_2 from maternal venous sinuses and therefore is living in a hypoxic environment. But the fetal Hb with 2a and 2 g chains have higher affinity for O_2. CO_2 is also eliminated from fetal circulation into maternal blood by diffusion across the placenta.
- **Transport of antibodies:** Maternal antibodies are transferred to the fetus and are responsible for innate immunity.

Protection of Fetus

- It acts as a barrier for prevention of transport of toxic substances from the mother to fetus.
- Progesterone produced by placenta helps to maintain pregnancy.

27. Describe the phases of gastric juice secretion.

Regulation of Gastric Secretion

Neural, humoral and reflex regulation of secretion

Factors that Stimulate

- Vagus N
- Gastrin
- Histamine

Factors that Inhibit

- Low pH in the stomach
- Somatostatin
- Prostaglandin E2 (*refer* **Fig. 32**)

Regulation is Discussed in Terms of:

- Cephalic phase
- Gastric phase
- Intestinal phase

Cephalic Phase

- Nearly 500 mL/h (45% of total secretion)

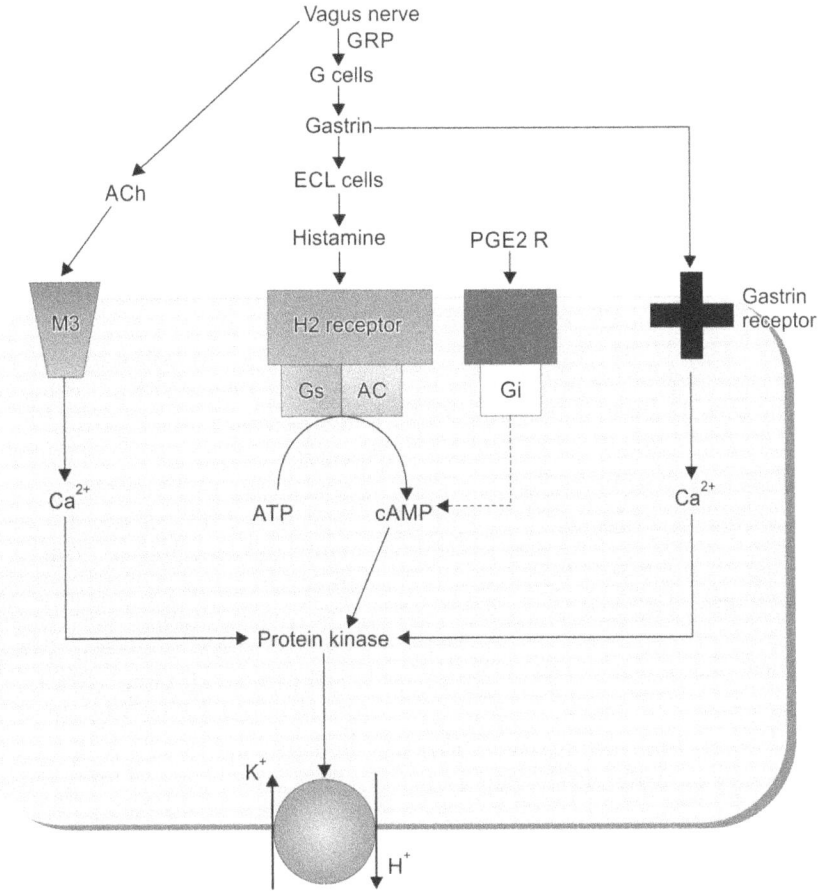

Fig. 32: Parietal cell with the regulating factors for HCl secretion
(PGE2 R: prostaglandin E2 receptor; M3: muscrinic receptor)

- Initiated by thought, sight, smell, taste of food through vagus nerve
- Emotions also affect secretion

Gastric Phase
- About 50% of total secretion. Food in stomach induces secretion by:
  - Distension of body of stomach (through reflexes—vagal reflex)
  - Distension of antrum (through gastrin secretion)
  - By products of partial digestion of protein (through gastrin secretion)

Intestinal Phase
- It begins when chyme enters the intestine.
- Intestinal influence is inhibitory. By:
  - **Enterogastric reflex:** By distension, presence of acid and products of digestion—inhibits secretion.
- **Hormonal mechanism:** CCK, secretin, GIP, neurotensin, etc.,—enterogastrone.

28. Hormonal regulation of menstrual cycle.

- Menstrual cycle is the female sexual cycle and it happens once in 28-30 days. It is associated with uterine bleeding—menstruation.
- It is a preparatory cycle for fertilization and implantation of the fertilized ovum
- Therefore, cyclic changes happen in the uterus, ovaries, cervix and vagina.
- All these changes are under the control of various hormones.
- The hormones regulating menstrual cycle are hypothalamic hormones (GnRH), anterior pituitary hormones (FSH and LH)

and ovarian hormones (estrogen and progesterone).
- GnRH from hypothalamus is the key controller of gonadotropin released from anterior pituitary.
- GnRH is secreted in pulsatile fashion and the pulsatility of GnRH is very important in regulating secretions of LH and FSH.
- GnRH pulsatility is in turn kept in check by levels of estrogen and progesterone. Just before LH surge, pulsatility of GnRH is increased by high levels of estrogen.
- We will be now discussing the hormonal regulation for ovarian changes and endometrial changes separately.

Regulation of Ovarian Changes

Ovarian changes happen in 3 phases:
1. Follicular phase
2. Ovulatory phase
3. Luteal phase

Follicular Phase
- This phase starts from day 1 of menstruation to the day of ovulation (usually 14th day).
- Day 1 onwards the FSH and LH levels start increasing. Due to the actions of FSH, 10-20 follicles start to grow in size.
- The granulosa cells of the follicles acquire FSH receptors and start secreting estrogen. Only one follicle continues to grow and become the dominant follicle and this is the follicle which secretes estrogen maximally. Other follicles become atretic.
- The estrogen levels start increasing. Estrogen along with FSH induces LH receptors on granulosa cells and theca cells.
- LH acts on theca cells to increase androgen synthesis and this androgen is diverted to granulosa cells for synthesis of estrogen.
- Now the rising estrogen levels have a **positive feedback** effect on LH secretion from the anterior pituitary resulting in LH peak or LH surge. LH stimulates granulosa cells to synthesize progesterone.
- Nine hours after the LH surge, ovulation happens on the 14th day.
- As LH increases, progesterone levels increase and the proteolytic enzyme activity (plasmin) is enhanced resulting in distension of follicle and the rupture of follicle is stimulated by prostaglandins and leukotrienes. This results in ovulation.

Luteal Phase
- This phase starts after the ovulation and lasts for 14 days. This time period is a constant one.
- Following ovulation the follicle is filled with blood and is called as corpus hemorrhagicum.
- Soon after the release of ovum, granulosa and theca cells of the follicle proliferate and become lipid laden and are now yellow in color and are called as luteal cells. Now the follicle is called as—corpus luteum.
- Corpus luteum, under the influence of LH, starts secreting progesterone, estrogen and inhibin. High levels of these hormones negatively inhibit the secretion of FSH and LH.
- The maintenance of corpus luteum function is by the action of LH.
- If ovum is not fertilized, corpus luteum reaches a peak secretion of steroidal hormones by 7 days following ovulation and then begins to undergo degeneration and luteolysis and becomes a scar tissue—corpus albicans.
- Now the hormone production of corpus luteum drops and progesterone, estrogen and inhibin levels decrease.
- The inhibition over FSH and LH is lifted and there is a rise in FSH levels which induces the next cycle with the development of new set of follicles.

Regulation of Changes in the Uterine Endometrium

The uterine changes are given in 3 phases:
1. Proliferative phase
2. Secretory phase
3. Menstrual phase

Proliferative Phase
- This phase correlates with the follicular phase of ovarian cycle.

- Estrogen secreted from the follicle stimulates growth of uterine endometrium and therefore it thickens.
- Glands in the endometrium and the blood vessels in endometrium also grows.
- This phase is from day 5 till the day of ovulation.

Secretory Phase
- This phase is from the day of ovulation to 25th day of the cycle.
- It correlates with the luteal phase in the ovarian cycle.
- Progesterone levels are high and they make the endometrium secretory by acting on the glands. Maximum action is 5–7 days after ovulation.
- The secretion from the endometrial glands is rich in glycogen and can nourish the fertilized ovum.
- The secretory endometrium is favorable for implantation of fertilized ovum.
- If fertilization does not happen, corpus luteum starts to regress and the progesterone and estrogen levels decrease.
- Withdrawal of hormonal support of the endometrium and release of prostaglandins result in vasoconstriction of the spiral arteries → uterine ischemia happens and endometrial necrosis and shedding of endometrium happens resulting in bleeding.

Menstrual Phase
It starts with the menstrual bleeding with the shedding of outer 2/3rd of endometrium, unfertilized ovum and continues for 5 days.

29. Dwarf.

Dwarfism is due to deficiency of growth hormone or GRH, deficiency of IGF-1, receptor insensitivity, thyroid hormone deficiency.

Causes for Dwarfism
- Isolated growth hormone deficiency may be due to GRH deficiency or due to abnormalities of GH secreting cells.
- Sometimes, the GH levels may be normal or even elevated, but the GH receptors are insensitive to GH due to loss-of function mutation of the genes for GH receptors—this is Laron dwarfism.
- African Pygmies are a type of dwarfism and are due to reduction of plasma level of growth-hormone binding protein and there is also absence of rise in IGF-1 at the time of puberty.
- Cretinism is hypothyroidism in children and it results in stunted growth and mental retardation.
- Dwarfism is also seen in conditions of precocious puberty.
- Gonadal dysgenesis is also a cause of dwarfism
- Various bone and metabolic disorders also result in dwarfism.
- **Psychosocial dwarfism:** This type of dwarfism is seen in children who are subjected to chronic abuse and neglect. It is also called as Kaspar Hauser syndrome.
- **Achondroplasia:** It is the most common type of dwarfism. Here the trunk is normal and short limbs. It is an autosomal dominant condition caused by mutation in the gene that code for Fibroblast growth factor receptor 3.

Symptoms
- In a hypothyroid dwarf, there is short stature, pot belly, enlarged tongue and delayed sexual maturity. There is definite mental retardation, idiotic facies.
- **In pituitary dwarfism:** There is short stature, proportionated growth retardation, normal mental development, sexual maturation may/may not be delayed and immature facies is seen.

30. Composition and functions of saliva.

Composition of Saliva
- **Rate of secretion:** 1000–1800 mL/day.
- **pH:** 6 to 7.4
- **Water:** 99.95%
- **Solids:** 0.5%
- **Solids:** Organic and inorganic
- **Organic:** Enzymes, such as ptyalin, lysozyme, lingual lipase, carbonic

anhydrase, RNAse, DNAse, others, such as kallikrein, blood group antigens, IgA, etc. Urea, uric acid, cholesterol and mucin
- **Inorganic:** Na^+, K^+, Ca^{++}, PO_4, Mg^{++}, Cl^-, HCO_3^-, sulfate, bromide, etc.
- **Saliva is hypotonic:** Tonicity depends on the rate of salivary secretion

Functions of Saliva

- Ptyalin (α-amylase) in saliva splits starches. Action of amylase is maximum at a pH of 6.8. Digestion continues in stomach for some time till the pH becomes less than 4.
- **Protective function:** Saliva cleans the mouth after a meal and prevents growth of harmful bacteria.
- Saliva contains lysozyme, IgA and lactoferrin for protection. Lysozymes are bactericidal and lactoferrin is bacteriostatic in action.
- Saliva facilitates speech.
- It helps in taste of food.
- Mucus in saliva helps in lubrication of food, mastication and swallowing
- It buffers the gastric juice in stomach.
- Proline rich proteins in the saliva protect the enamel of tooth.
- Saliva dilutes hot and irritant foods and protects buccal mucosa. It also dilutes regurgitated bile and HCl
- In animals it helps in temperature regulation.
- Helps in excretion of heavy metals, alcohol, morphine, thiocyanate, etc.

31. Non-respiratory functions of lung.

Non-respiratory Functions

- **Acts as a reservoir for blood:** The pulmonary vessels are highly compliant and therefore can store blood without much increase in pressure. In cases of imbalance in left ventricular output and systemic venous return, the stored blood in the pulmonary circulation helps to regulate cardiac output
- **Filters** small emboli, particles in blood, detached cancer cells, fat cells, air emboli in blood.
- **Processes inhaled air:** The atmospheric air which enters the airways is hydrated as it passes through the airways.
- **Olfactory function**
- **Metabolic function:**
  - Synthesizes and secretes surfactant
  - Pulmonary capillary endothelial cells secrete angiotensin converting enzyme (ACE) and thereby converts angiotensin I to angiotensin II.
  - Synthesizes, stores and secretes substances, such as prostaglandins, histamine and kallikrein
  - Partially removes prostaglandin, bradykinin, adenine nucleotides, serotonin, norepinephrine and acetylcholine.
- **Helps in defense:** With the help of pulmonary alveolar macrophages, IgA, mucus secretion, beating of cilia, cough reflex.
- **Helps in speech**
- **Helps in absorption** of drugs, such as anesthetic gases, aerosols and bronchodilators.
- **Fibrinolytic mechanism** present in the lungs lyses the clot.

32. What is FRC? How will you measure FRC and its clinical importance?

- It is the volume of air remaining in the lung at the end of tidal expiration.
- It is equal to residual volume + expiratory reserve volume
- Normal value is 2.5 L

Measurement of FRC

It can be measured by two methods:
1. Nitrogen washout method
2. Helium dilution method

Nitrogen Washout Method

- It is based on the fact that alveoli contain 80% N_2 (got from breathing atmospheric air which has 80% N_2).
- The subject is asked to breathe 100% O_2 for 5 minutes.
- Then he is asked to expire into the Douglas bag (Which is washed with 100% O_2)

- The volume of air expired and the concentration of N_2 in the expired air is measured and with these values FRC is calculated.

For example:
The volume of air expired into the bag = 40 L
- N_2 concentration is 5%
- So 100 mL of air contains 5 mL of N_2 and therefore 40,000 mL of air will contain
  = 5 × 40,000/100
  = 2000 mL of N_2
- The 2000 mL of N_2 has been washed out from the alveoli and there is 80% N_2 in the air, i.e., 80 mL of N_2 in 100 mL of air.
- So 2000 mL would have been present in = 2000 × 100/80 = 2500 mL
- 2500 mL is the FRC.

Helium Dilution Technique
- Here the subject is made to breathe from the spirometer containing a mixture of air and helium.
- He is asked to exhale, till the tidal expiration and then he breathes in and out of the spirometer continuously till the amount of helium in spirometer and lungs are equilibrated.

Then FRC is calculated by using the formula:
- Initial volume (V_1) X initial concentration of helium (He_i) = final volume (V_1 +FRC) X final concentration of helium (He_f)
- Therefore FRC = V_1 (He_i - He_f)/He_f
- If V_1 = 2000 mL
- He_i = 12%
- He_f = 5%
- Then FRC = 2000 (12-5)/5 = 2000 X 7/5 = 2800 mL
- FRC = 2800 mL

Significance of FRC
- FRC acts as a buffer and allows continuous exchange of gases in inspiration as well as expiration.
- Without FRC, the pO_2 in alveoli will increase to 150 mm Hg and in expiration it may reach even zero.
- Presence of FRC maintains pO_2 at 100 mm Hg.
- FRC dilutes the toxic gases, as the FRC (2300 mL) is always present in lungs
- Helps in breath holding
- Work of breathing is minimized by the FRC as the presence of this volume of air in lungs prevent the collapse of the alveoli
- FRC prevents collapse and thereby decreases pulmonary vascular resistance.

33. Artificial respiration.

When there is respiratory deficiency or respiratory arrest artificial respiration is given.

Conditions: Drowning, gas poisoning, electric shock, anesthesia, accidents, etc.

Methods: Instrumental and manual methods.

Instrumental Methods

Used when there is a need for prolonged support.

Three types:
1. Positive pressure method
2. Negative pressure method
3. Boyles apparatus

Positive Pressure Method
- Used in operation theaters
- Here air or O_2 mixture is used to inflate the lungs at positive pressures either continuously or intermittently.
- It impairs venous return.

Negative Pressure Method
Achieved by alternate compression and relaxing the chest wall.

They are:
- Drinker's method (iron lung chamber)
- **Bragg-Paul method:** Use of hollow elastic rubber bag.
- Others

Drinker's Method (Iron Lung Method)
- The instrument contains an airtight iron chamber with a bellow on one side of the instrument.
- When the bellow moves in and out it creates a rise and fall of pressure inside the chamber.
- The person is placed inside the chamber with the head and neck outside the chamber.
- When the pressure rises inside the chamber expiration happens for the

patient and when the pressure falls in the chamber there is inspiration.

Bragg-Paul Method
- Here an elastic rubber bag is tied around the chest of the patient.
- The bag is connected to a pump which can inflate and deflate the bag.
- When the bag is inflated it compresses the chest and air is expired.
- When the pressure is released, the chest enlarges passively and air is drawn in.

Boyles Apparatus

This apparatus is used in the hospitals for artificial ventilation. It is an automatic instrument in which rate and depth of ventilation and composition of inspired can be altered.

Manual Methods

Holger-Nielsen Method
- The subject is made to lie prone and the head is turned to one side (**Fig. 33A**).
- The shoulder is abducted and flexed at the elbow and the hands are placed under the cheek.
- The operator is in kneeling position at the head of the patient and he places his hands spread on the back of the subject and bends forward to press on his back (**Fig. 33B**).
- The pressure on the back of the subject and compresses on the chest and expels the air out (**Fig. 33C**).
- Then he holds the arm above the elbow of the subject and pulls the arm forward (**Fig. 33D**).
- This enlarges the chest and results in inspiration. It is repeated 12/min. This is an exhaustive method for the examiner.

Eve's Rocking Method
- Here the subject is made to lie prone on board which is rocketed on a pivot so that it can move up and down like a see-saw.
- When the board is tilted head down the abdominal organs push on the diaphragm resulting decrease in thoracic volume and expiration happens.
- When the board is tilted in the opposite direction the inspiration happens.

Mouth-to-Mouth Respiration
- It can be direct or indirect method. In direct method, the operator places his mouth directly on the subject's mouth and in indirect method it is done with a small tube.
- The subject is made to lie supine; the airway is kept clean from vomitus, foreign body, etc.
- The subject's head is extended, the operator sits on the side of the subject

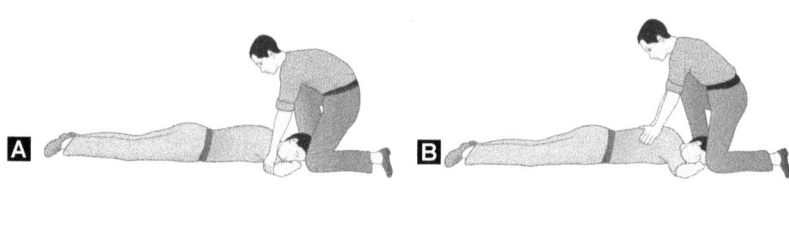

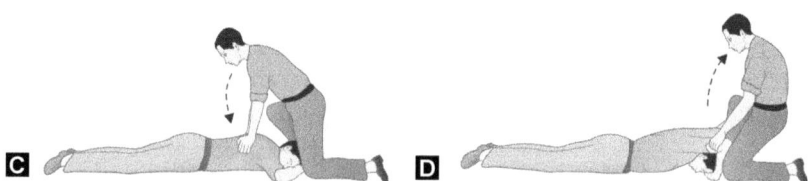

Figs. 33A to D: Holger-Nielsen method of artificial respiration.

holds the lower jaw with his left hand and opens the mouth and with his right hand clips the nostrils.
- The operator then inhales deeply and places his mouth on the subject's mouth or the tube placed in the subject's mouth and blows into the subject's mouth smoothly, volume twice that of the tidal volume.
- This inflates the lungs of the subject and then the examiner removes his mouth from the subject's mouth and the lungs recoil resulting in expiration.
- It is repeated 12 times a minute.
- **Advantages:** Can be applied immediately, can achieve large tidal volumes, CO_2 stimulates respiration, simple technique.
- **Disadvantages:** Infection may spread, Volunteer may get exhausted.

34. Referred pain and its theories.

Irritation of a vicus or viscera usually produces pain which is not usually felt in the location of the viscus but in a somatic structure that is in a distance from the viscus. This is *refer* **red pain**.

For example:
- Cardiac pain is usually referred to the inner aspect of the left arm or to the neck.
- When there is an irritation of central region of diaphragm there is pain in the tip of the shoulder.
- Pain in the testicle due to distension of ureter as in ureteric calculus.

Theories of Referred Pain

The pain in viscera is usually referred to a somatic structure that has developed from the same embryonic segment or dermatome as the structure in which the pain originates—**dermatomal rule**.

Theories of referred pain are—convergence theory and facilitation theory.

Convergence Theory
- Peripheral nerve fibers from the somatic and visceral structures converge on the same second order neuron present in lamina V of dorsal gray horn.
- The second order neuron is common for impulses from somatic and visceral structures.
- So the tract carrying pain sensation from somatic structures also carry pain fibers from visceral structures (*refer* **Fig. 34**).
- Cortex sometimes cannot differentiate from somatic and visceral inputs and so pain from visceral structure is referred to the somatic structure.

Facilitation Theory
- The visceral afferent fibers on entering spinal cord give collaterals to afferents coming from the somatic structures.
- So impulses coming from the visceral afferents facilitate and strengthen the impulses coming from the somatic structure (*refer* **Fig. 35**).

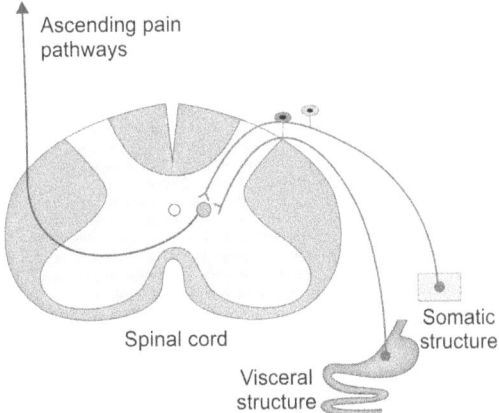

Fig. 34: Convergence theory of referred pain. Note the afferents from somatic and visceral structures converge on the same second order neuron.

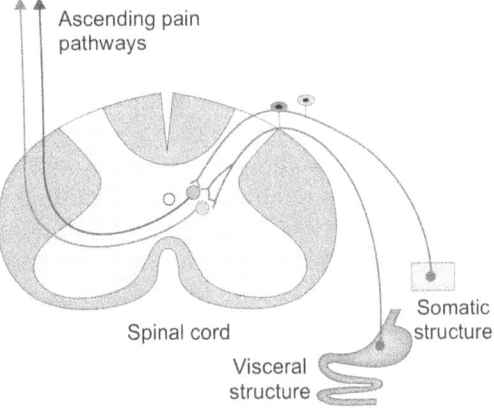

Fig. 35: Facilitation theory of referred pain. Note the visceral afferents give a collateral to second order neurons of somatic structure.

- So a minor activity in the somatic afferents is facilitated by the visceral afferents and therefore pain is referred to the somatic structure.

35. Special features of coronary circulation.

- There are 2 coronary arteries—right and left. Right artery supplies the right atrium and right ventricle and left coronary artery supplies left atrium and ventricles.
- There is no anastomoses between the two arteries and therefore they are end arteries. Therefore, blockage of vessels results in ischemia or infarction supplied by those arteries.
- There are phasic changes in blood flow through coronaries. In systole as the myocardium contracts, the blood vessels are compressed and there is no blood flow through the coronaries. In diastole as the myocardium relaxes the vessels dilate and blood flow increases through the vessels.
- The endocardial vessels show the maximum phasic variation in blood flow. Therefore, these areas suffer from hypoxia and are prone for ischemia in compromised states.
- Metabolic regulation is well-developed in coronary vessels. The blood flow increase is based on the need of the myocardium.
- Coronary circulation is adjustable based on the activities of the myocardium as in exercise the coronary blood flow can increased by 4–5 times to meet the body's demand. So it has adequate blood flow reserve.
- The myocardium extracts nearly 80% of O_2 from arterial blood and therefore the AV difference of O_2 is high. So it increases O_2 supply the blood flow should increase.
- The rate of blood flow through the coronary vessels is the second highest next to the renal blood flow. It is 250 mL/min.
- The rate of O_2 consumption is the highest of all the organs in the body. It is about 9.7 mL/100 g of tissue/min.

36. Color Vision.

- **Color has 3 attributes:** Hue, intensity and saturation.
- Each color has a complementary color and when it is mixed with it, produces white color.
- Cones are the receptors for color vision.
- There are 3 primary colors—red (723-647 nm), green (575-493 nm), blue (492-450 nm).
- Young-Helmholtz have postulated that there are 3 types of cones each responding to a particular wavelength of light.
- They are maximally sensitive to each of the primary colors due to presence of 3 types of photopigments and therefore 3 types of cones—S (Blue), L (Red) and M (Green) cones.
- The L, M and S cones show maximal response to wavelengths of 560 nm, 530 nm and 420 nm respectively (refer **Fig. 36**).
- Different color sensations are perceived by determining the relative frequencies of impulses from each cone system.
- The color perceived is also dependent on the level of illumination and also the background color.
- Different shades of colors perceived also depend on the intensity of the color.
- Based on young-Helmholtz theory, for perceiving a color at least two cone types are needed.
- The visual cortex compares the relative frequency of action potentials in the

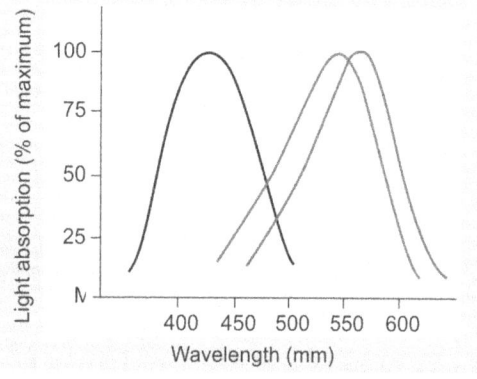

Fig. 36: Three cones and their sensitive wavelength.

activated cone pathways and finds the wavelength and thereby identifies the color.
- Change in intensity is appreciated by change in wavelength
- Color vision is a function of fovea as it has densely packed cones and this are can get details of the object rather than discrimination of colors.
- Gene for rhodopsin is on chromosome 3 and gene for S cone pigment is on chromosome 7 and for green and red pigment it is on X chromosome.

Neural Mechanisms

- Color impulses are mediated by P type of ganglion cells by subtracting input from one cone type to other.
- From lateral geniculate body (LGB) impulses travel to cortex in 3 pathways:
  1. **A red-green pathway:** Signals differences between L and M cones.
  2. **A blue-yellow pathway:** Signals differences between S and sum of L and M cones.
  3. **Luminance pathway:** Signals sum of L and M cones.
- They project to 4C layer and blobs in layer 2 and 3 of area 17 (V1) → then projects to V8.
- **Color blindness** may be only for some colors—due to absence of one or more types of cones.
- The suffix 'anopia' is used for color blindness.
- The suffix 'anomaly' is used to denote color weakness.
- The prefixes 'Prot, deuter, trit' are used to for 'red, green and blue' colors.
- If only 2 cones are present and one cone is absent (**dichromats**)—**protanopia** (red blindness), **deuteranopia** (green color blindness) or **tritanopia** (blue color blindness).
- **Trichromats:** Have all 3 cones, but one is weak
- **Monochromats** are individuals with only one cone system. They do not appreciate any colors. They see only black, white and shades of gray.

37. Taste pathway.

The taste receptors are present in the taste buds which are located on the tongue in the papillae.
- There are 10,000 taste buds.
- Taste buds are located in—fungiform, foliate and vallate papillae.
- Cells in taste buds—type 1 and 2—supporting cells.
- Type 3 cells—receptor epithelial cells has microvilli projecting into taste pore.
- They are receptors are replaced constantly in 10 days.
- Each bud is innervated by 50 nerves at bases of receptor cells.
- Each nerve innervates 5 taste buds.
- The sensory fibers from the taste buds travel through 3 nerves—choda tympani branch of facial nerve (from anterior 2/3rd of the tongue), glossopharyngeal nerve (from posterior 1/3rd of the tongue) and Vagus N from epiglottis, pharynx and palate.
- They all reach the medulla and terminate on the same side nucleus tractus solitaries of the same side. (*refer* **Fig. 37**)
- From here the second order neurons travel along with medial lemniscus to reach ventral posteromedial nucleus of ipsilateral thalamus.
- Some fibers from medulla go to the vomiting center, hypothalamus, limbic system and salivary nucleus.
- The 3rd order neurons arise from the thalamus and they reach the foot of postcentral gyrus on the same side (area 43).
- From there impulses are also transmitted to the insula and lateral orbitofrontal cortex.

38. Explain dark adaptation.

- The dark adaptation happens in two phases.
- The first phase is due to cone adaptation and it happens in the first 5-10 minutes.

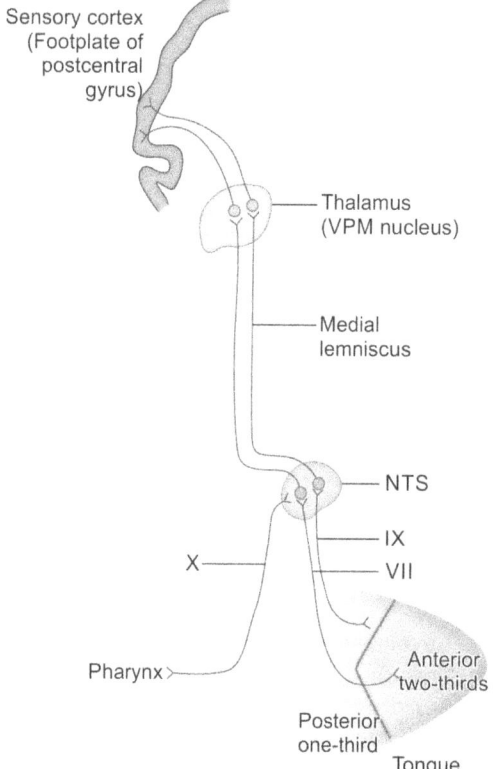

Fig. 37: Taste pathway. Sensation of taste is carried through VIIth cranial nerve from anterior 2/3rd of tongue, by glossopharyngeal nerve (IX) from anterior 1/3rd of tongue, from pharynx, epiglottis by vagus nerve (X) to nucleus tractus solitarius (NTS).

- This increases the retinal sensitivity to light 100 times.
- In the second phase of adaptation, the rod sensitivity to light increases and the retinal sensitivity increases by 1000–10,000 times.
- Once rod adaptation has happened even a single photon of light is visible to the eye.

Chemical Adaptation

- When a person stays in bright light, the rod pigment rhodopsin is bleached and is converted to all-trans-retinal and opsin.
- Therefore rods are insensitive to light and do not respond to light.
- The rod sensitivity can increase only when the rhodopsin is re-synthesized and this takes several minutes to happen.
- That is why, the dark adaptation by rods takes 20 minutes. (*refer* **Fig. 38**)

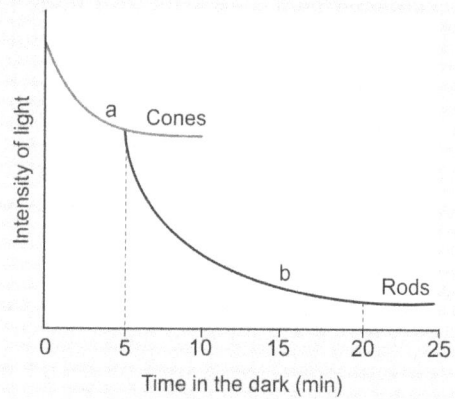

Fig. 38: Dark adaptation curve. There are two curves, curve (a) shows cone adaptation and curve (b) shows rod adaptation.

- The rods are present in the retina 15–20 degrees away from the fovea. That is the reason there is dilatation of the pupil to expose the retina rich in rods to light.
- The time taken for dark adaptation depends on the degree of brightness of light to which the eye is exposed and for how long it is being exposed.
- Brighter the light and longer the duration later it takes for dark adaptation.

39. What is myasthenia gravis? Explain the biological basis of its treatment.

- It is an autoimmune disease.
- Antibodies are formed against the nicotinic ACh receptors in neuromuscular junction.
- There is weakness, fatigue and the muscles become weak with repeated use and therefore symptoms worsen towards the evening.
- The antibodies not only combine with ACh for the receptors but they also flatten the postsynaptic membrane and cause endocytosis of ACh into presynaptic membrane.
- Because of these effects, the muscle response to repeated stimulation gradually decreases.
- Symptoms improve after rest and are better on getting up in the morning.
- The extraocular and facial muscles are the first to be affected and ptosis and diplopia are present.

Treatment

- **Acetylcholine esterase (ACh E) inhibitors—** ACh E inhibitors increase the amount of ACh in the NMJ and they can displace the antibodies and improve functions.
- **Thymectomy:** Decreases the immune response by inhibiting T cell activation.
- **Immunosuppressants**
- **Plasmapheresis**

40. Brown-Séquard syndrome.

Hemi-section of spinal cord is called Brown-Séquard syndrome. It involves lesion of one lateral half of spinal cord.

Following injury to the spinal cord there are these following stages:
I. Stage of spinal shock
II. Stage of reflex activity
III. Stage of reflex failure

Immediately after the lesion, there is complete loss of function below the level of lesion. This happens because of sudden removal of impulses from higher centers.

The symptoms of Brown-Séquard are seen in the second stage. Symptoms are explained as the features above the level of lesion, at the level and below the level of lesion, on the same side and opposite side of lesion.

	Sensory		Motor	
	Same side	Opposite side	Same side	Opposite side
Above the level of lesion	Small area of hyperasthesia	Normal	Normal	Normal
At the level of lesion	Complete loss of sensation (anesthesia)	Not affected	Lower motor neuron type of paralysis	Not affected
Below the level of lesion	**Damage to dorsal column fibers:** Loss of fine touch, tactile localization, two point discrimination, vibration sense, stereognosis and position sense	**Damage to lateral and anterior spinothalamic tract:** Loss of pain, temperature and crude touch sensations. All other sensations are intact	Upper motor neuron type of paralysis as the inhibition from higher centers is removed. Temporary loss of vasomotor tone	Not usually affected

III. SHORT ANSWERS

1. Milieu interior.

- Milieu interior was the term coined by Claude Bernard.
- It denotes the internal environment of the body.
- Cells can perform their functions properly only when the internal sea/environment of the body is kept a constant.
- Internal sea is the extracellular fluid (ECF).
- Homeostasis was the term coined by WB Cannon and it denotes the maintenance of a constant internal environment.

Following factors should be regulated for homeostasis:
- Regulation of plasma pH
- Regulation of body temperature
- Regulation of water and electrolyte balance
- Supply of nutrients, O_2, enzymes and hormones
- Removal of metabolites and waste products

It is regulated by negative and positive feedback mechanisms.

Example of negative feedback: Regulation of blood pressure is an example of negative feedback regulation:

Increase in blood pressure
↓
Sensed by baroreceptors
↓
Stimulation of cardiac vagal center and inhibition of vasomotor center
↓
Decrease in heart rate and stroke volume
↓
Decrease in cardiac output
↓
Decrease in blood pressure

Example of positive feedback: Parturition reflex is an example of positive feedback regulation:

At the end of term pregnancy
↓
Increase in sensitivity of oxytocin receptors
↓
Oxytocin binds to its receptor and induces contraction of uterine muscles
↓
Contraction of uterus and descent of fetal head
↓
Stretch of cervix
↓
Stimulation of stretch receptors in cervix
↓
Impulse travels through afferent sensory nerves
↓
Impulses reach hypothalamus
↓
Secretion of oxytocin from hypothalamus
More contraction of uterus

Further descent of head and the cycle continues till the fetus is born.

2. Functions of large intestine.

- It acts as a **reservoir** for undigested food material and they are stored here till they are expelled as feces.
- **Absorption:** The most important components absorbed in the colon are water and electrolytes. The large absorptive capacity of colon can be used to instill certain drugs, such as anesthetics, analgesics, etc., through the colon.
- **Formation of feces:** The undigested residue of the food substances is made into formed fecal matter in the colon.
- **Colonic bacteria:** Colon has large numbers of beneficial bacteria which helps to form many useful substances, such as vitamin K, B complex vitamins and folic acid.
- **Short-chain fatty acids** are also synthesized in the large intestine by action of intestinal bacteria on complex carbohydrates, resistant starch and other dietary fibers.
- Goblet cells in the mucosa of large intestine produce large volume of **mucus** which helps in smooth passage of feces.
- Alkaline nature (pH 8) of large intestinal secretion **neutralizes acids** formed by bacteria on feces.
- Undigested cellulose, hemicellulose and some fats are digested by the colonic bacteria.
- **Heavy metals like lead, mercury, etc., are excreted through feces.**

3. Steatorrhea.

- Excretion of fats in stools is called steatorrhea. Stools in steatorrhea, are fatty, bulky and clay-colored because of impaired digestion and absorption of fats.
- It usually happens following pancreatectomy or damage to exocrine pancreas.
- Indigestion of fats is due to deficiency of lipase, lack of alkaline secretion from the pancreas or lowering of intestinal pH.
- Hypersecretion of gastric acids also causes steatorrhea.
- Other important cause is improper absorption of bile salts and therefore loss of bile salts in stools. Loss of bile salts beyond the capacity for production by liver leads to defective absorption of fats and results in steatorrhea.

4. Dietary fiber.

- Dietary fibers include cellulose, hemicellulose, lignin, etc.
- These substances when ingested are not digested due to lack of microorganisms for digesting them.
- So they pass out without getting digested.

Functions of dietary fibers are:
- The undigested fibers when they are present in the colon they tend to hold water and increase the bulk of feces and therefore can be **used for treating constipation**.
- It **decreases the rate of absorption** of nutrients form intestines and thereby prevents sudden increase in blood glucose levels after food intake. Due to slow absorption of carbohydrates, insulin demand is also decreased. So it can be used as a **supplementary treatment in diabetes mellitus**.
- It **decreases blood cholesterol levels** by excreting bile salts. Bile salts get trapped in the fiber and is excreted. The rate of formation of bile salts are increased and cholesterol is used for it. So it is used for controlling hypercholesteremia, obesity, etc.
- It **prevents colon cancer** by diluting the carcinogens and minimizing their contact with the colon.

5. Multi-unit smooth muscle.

- There are two types of smooth muscles—single unit and multi-unit muscles
- **Multi-unit smooth muscle:** These types of muscles are present in ciliary body of eye, iris, precapillary sphincters, piloerector muscles, large airways of lungs, etc.
- There are no gap junctions between these muscle fibers, whereas gap junctions are present in single-unit muscles.
- Single-unit muscle with the gap junctions act as a syncitium, but the multi-unit muscles do not act as syncitium.
- Multi-unit muscles like the skeletal muscles are dependent on neural control but are not under voluntary control as it is supplied by autonomic nerves.

6. Sarcomere.

- It is the structural and functional unit of a myofibril. In the myofibril, thick and thin filaments are arranged in repeating pattern; **the sarcomere**.
- It is the portion of muscle fiber between two Z lines (*refer* **Fig. 39**).
- The average length is 2 µm.

7. Cytokines.

- These are hormone-like substances that regulate immune response.
- They are secreted by lymphocytes, macrophages, endothelial cells, neurons, glial cells and other cells.
- Cytokines are named after their actions, such as B cell-differentiating factors,

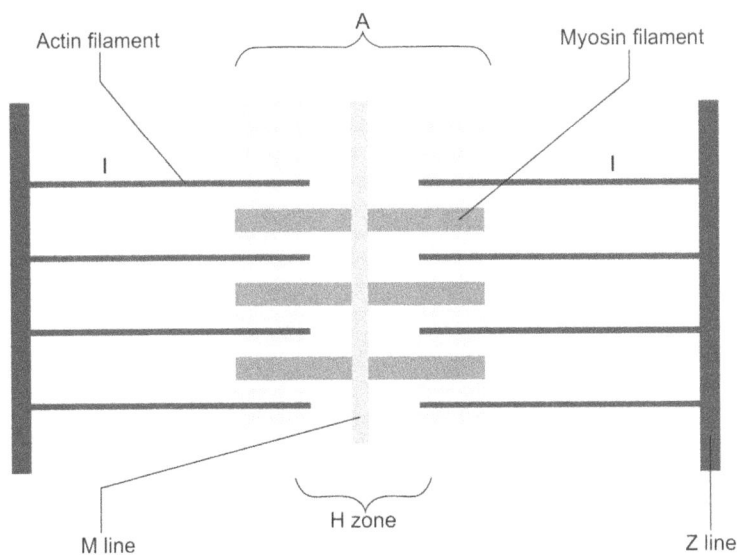

Fig. 39: Sarcomere.

B cell-stimulating factor. Once the amino acid sequence of cytokine is identified it is named as **interleukins**.
- B cell differentiating factor is now named as interleukin-4.
- There are interleukins-1, 2, 4, 5, 6, 8, 11, 12, tumor necrosis factor α, lymphotoxin (tumor necrosis factor β), transforming growth factor β, granulocyte-macrophage CSF, interferons α, β and γ.
- The cytokines have both systemic and paracrine actions. IL-1, 6 and TNF-α cause fever and IL-1 increases slow wave sleep and reduces appetite.
- Chemokines, which attract WBCs towards site of inflammation, are also belonging to the cytokine family.

Some of the actions of cytokines are:
- **IL-1 and 2:** Activation of T cells and macrophages, promotes inflammation
- **IL-4:** Activation of lymphocytes, monocytes and IgE
- **IL-5:** Differentiation of eosinophils
- **IL-6:** Differentiation of B cells, stimulates production of acute phase proteins
- **IL-8:** Chemotaxis

8. Autoimmune disease.

- During the processing of development of immunity, lymphocytes are presented with self- and non-self-antigens and the cells and antibodies responding to self-antigens are eliminated—tolerance.
- Sometimes antibodies against self-antigens are not eliminated and it results in *autoimmune diseases*.
- It can be B cell or T cell mediated, it can be organ-specific or systemic in nature.

Examples are:
- **Type 1 diabetes mellitus:** Antibodies against B cells in Islet of pancreas.
- **Myasthenia gravis:** Antibodies for nicotinic acetylcholine receptors in NMJ.
- **Multiple sclerosis:** Antibodies against myelin basic protein and several other components of myelin.
- **Graves' disease:** Antibodies for TSH receptors and the receptors are activated resulting in hyperthyroidism.
- **Molecular mimicry:** Antibodies against certain bacteria will cross-react with body constituents, as in rheumatic fever where antibodies against *Streptococcus* attacks the cardiac myosin and induces damage to heart.

9. Na^+-K^+ pump.

- It is present in all cells of the body.
- It is an electrogenic pump as it pumps $3Na^+$ out of the cell and $2K^+$ into the cell. It catalyzes hydrolysis of ATP and uses the energy to move the ions across cell membrane.
- Its activity is inhibited by chemicals, such as Ouabain and digitalis used for heart failure.
- It has α and β subunits.
- Na^+ and K^+ are transported through α subunit.
- α subunit is larger and has intracellular Na^+ and ATP binding sites and a phosphorylation site.
- When Na^+ binds to a subunit, ATP also binds and is converted to ADP and the Pi is added to phosphorylation site.
- This changes the configuration of the pump and extrudes Na^+ into ECF. K^+ then binds extracellularly, dephosphorylating a subunit and comes back to original configuration and releases K^+ intracellularly.
- β-subunit is a glycoprotein and has no transport action but its presence is needed for pump activity (*refer* **Fig. 40**).
- Extracellularly there are binding sites for K^+ and ouabain.
- Pump activity is regulated by 2nd messengers and hormones.
- Thyroid hormone, aldosterone and insulin increase the pump activity, whereas dopamine decreases the pump activity.

10. EMG.

- The process of studying the electrical activity of the muscles on a cathode ray oscilloscope is called as **electromyography**.
- It gives an idea about the activation of motor units.

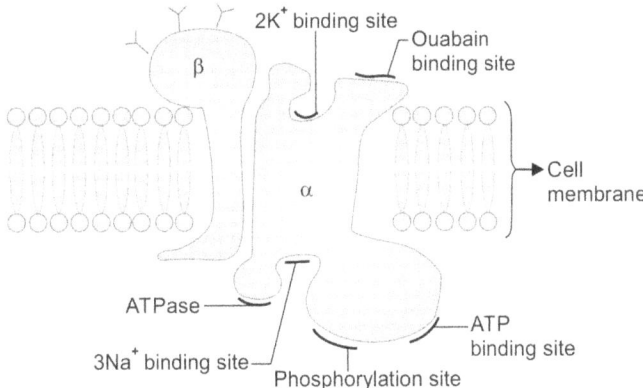

Fig. 40: Sodium-potassium pump. The pump has 2 subunits—α and β subunits. α-subunit has the binding sites for Na+ (intracellularly) and extracellular binding sites for K+ and ouabain. Intracellularly there are Phosphorylation and ATP binding sites.

- It can be recorded in humans by placing small metal disks on the skin over the muscle to be examined as the recording electrode or by using a hypodermic needle electrode.
- The record obtained with these electrodes is electromyogram.

Activities Normally Seen in a Muscle

At Rest

There is no spontaneous activity at rest:
- **Insertion activity:** On insertion of the needle, there will be small depolarization due to mechanical stimulus and is short lived. It may be prolonged in denervated muscle and absent when it is not kept in a muscle.
- **On voluntary action:** During activation of one motor unit, the electrical potential recorded is the motor unit potential (MUP). It lasts for 5 msec and amplitude is 0.5 mV.
- **Minimal stimulation:** Only few motor units close to needle give off electrical discharge.
- **On increasing stimulation:** Firing rate of small units increase till larger units start firing.
- **During maximal stimulation:** Many motor units are contracting and MUPs are superimposed on each other and it is not possible to identify individual components.

Abnormal Activities in a Muscle

- **Fasciculation potentials** are abnormal involuntary contractions in muscle fibers of single motor unit and they resemble MUPs
- **Fibrillation potentials** are of short duration and low amplitude.
- **Uses of electromyogram:** Used to diagnose neuromuscular diseases, myopathies and peripheral nerve lesion.

11. State Frank Starling's law of the heart.

It states that within the physiological limits, the force of contraction is directly proportional to the initial length of the muscle.

12. List short-term regulation of blood pressure.

- Short-term regulatory mechanisms come into action within few seconds of changes in mean arterial pressure (MAP).
- It lasts for few seconds to few minutes.
- For example, regulation of BP when a person stands up from supine position, the decrease in BP due to venous pooling is immediately corrected by baroreceptor mechanism.
- This mechanism can correct the BP when MAP is between 60–110 mm Hg.
- **They are:**
  - **Baroreceptor reflex**
  - **Chemoreceptor reflex**
  - **CNS ischemic response**

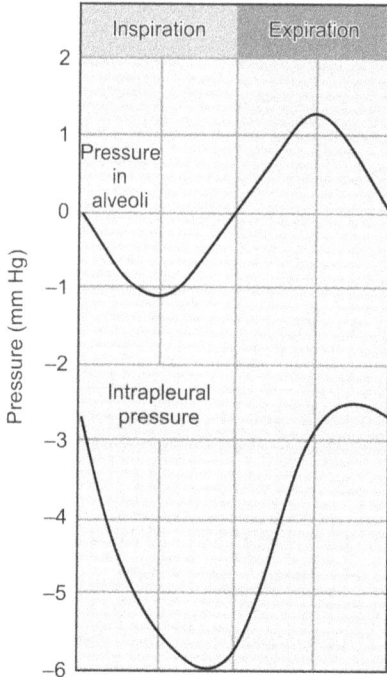

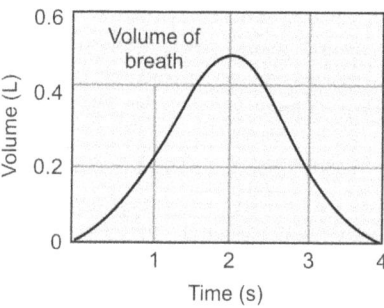

Fig. 41: Intrapleural pressure, intra-alveolar pressure and lung volume in inspiration and expiration.

13. Intrapleural pressure.

- It is the pressure in the space between the two pleurae—visceral and parietal pleura.
- It is negative or subatmospheric.
- At rest, when the respiratory muscles are relaxed and airways are kept open it is around −2.5 mm Hg.
- The negative pressure is due to two opposing forces acting on each other.

They are:
- The recoiling tendency of the lung towards inwards due to the presence of elastic tissue in the lungs and surface tension of the fluid which cause collapse of lungs.
- The recoiling tendency of the muscle of the thoracic cage towards outward results in expansion of thorax.
- These two forces act opposite to each other pulling apart the two layers of the pleurae and thereby creating a negative pressure in the space.
- During inspiration, as the chest wall expands, the negative pressure becomes more (−6 mm Hg) negative and thereby pulls on the lungs to create a negative intrathoracic pressure.
- During expiration, the inspiratory muscle activity is cut off and the chest wall begins to recoil back to expiratory position and the lungs recoil inwards and the intrapleural pressure is back to −2.5 mm Hg (*refer* **Fig. 41**).

14. State dead space and its normal value.

Dead space volume is the part of the pulmonary ventilation that does not take part in gaseous exchange.

They are of three types:
1. **Anatomical dead space:** It is the volume of air present in the conducting zone of airways where no gaseous exchange takes place. It is from the nose to terminal bronchioles. Normal volume is 150 mL.
2. **Alveolar dead space:** It is the volume of air in the alveoli which do not take part in gas exchange as in lung disorders. But in normal condition this volume is zero.
3. **Physiological dead space or total dead space** = Anatomical dead space + Alveolar dead space.
   = 150 + 0 = 150 mL

15. Define histotoxic hypoxia with an example.

- Hypoxia is O_2 deficiency at the tissue level.
- Histotoxic hypoxia is a condition in which the amount of O_2 delivered to the tissue is adequate but the tissue is unable to utilize O_2 due to toxic poisoning as in **cyanide poisoning**.
- Here tissue oxidative process is affected by inhibition of cytochrome oxidases and other oxidative enzymes.

- It is treated with methylene blue or nitrites which form methemoglobine and this reacts with cyanide to form cyanmethemoglobin which is a less toxic compound.

16. What is Bell-Magendie Law?

Bell-Magendie Law states that in the spinal cord the dorsal nerve roots are sensory and ventral nerve roots are motor.

17. Four functions of reticular activating system.

- RAS plays a role in sleep-wakefulness. It also induces alertness.
- It plays a role in development of EEG waves, learning and memory.
- Controls muscle tone—mainly through the descending reticular formation.
- Since many visceral areas are located here it regulates visceral functions.

18. Functions of prefrontal lobe.

- In animals, it is considered to be the seat of intelligence but in humans, it is the seat of mind.
- It controls the mood and feelings of the subject
- It is involved in higher functions, such as emotions, learning and memory
- It controls various intellectual activities, such as planning of future, concentration on actions, solving mathematical problems, etc.
- It helps in appreciation and discrimination of odors
- It initiates movements in relation to emotions.
- It plans the sequence of movements for an action along with motor cortex for actions.

19. What is endocochlear potential?

- The fluids in the cochlear compartments are responsible for the endocochlear potentials.
- Endolymph in the scala media contains high K^+ concentration than the perilymph in the scala vestibuli and scala tympani.
- There is a potential of + 80 mV due to this difference in ionic concentration.
- This potential is the endocochlear potential.

20. Delta waves in EEG.

- Frequency of these waves is 1–5 Hz.
- Amplitude is 20–200 µV
- Delta waves occur in sleep in adults but present in infants during wakefulness.
- When present in an awake adult it indicates brain damage.

21. Four functions of plasma protein.

- Albumin regulates plasma colloidal oncotic pressure.
- Albumin helps in transport of bilirubin, hormones, ions, fatty acids, metals, etc.
- Globulins act as transport proteins as in transferrin transports iron, ceruloplasmin copper, lipoproteins lipids, etc.
- Fibrinogen helps in coagulation of blood and provides viscosity of blood.

22. Helper cells.

There are 4 types of T lymphocytes—helper T cells, cytotoxic T cells, suppressor T cells and memory T cells.

Helper T Cells

- These are the major types of T cells.
- As the name implies they help the immune system; both cell-mediated and humoral immunity.
- They secrete many interleukins and thereby help the immunity.
- They are also called as CD 4 cells.

Helper T cells are activated in the following mechanisms:

- Antigen which has entered the body is phagocytosed, digested and processed inside the macrophages and the peptide fragment of the antigen in the phagosome combines with the vesicle containing MHC II.
- After fusion of the vesicles, the antigen binds with MHC II and both are incorporated in the cell membrane of antigen presenting cell (macrophage).
- The APC with the antigen and MHC II circulate in blood or in lymphatic tissues

and the T cells with the receptor for the antigen recognize the antigenic fragment.
- The T cell gets activated and undergoes differentiation and proliferation to form Helper T cells.
- Helper T cells secrete interleukin-2 which by autocrine and paracrine influence activate other helper T cells and also activate B cells and cytotoxic T cells.
- As the helper T cells activate cytotoxic T cells and B cells it has an important role in cellular immunity and humoral immunity.

23. Kernicterus.

- It is seen in hemolytic disease of the newborn.
- In this condition, there is Rh incompatibility between the Rh-negative mother and Rh positive fetus.
- The RBCs with Rh antigen from fetal blood enters mother's circulation at the time of delivery of first fetus.
- Mother's immune system produces Anti-D antibodies against D antigen and if the mother conceives for the second time with a Rh fetus, antibodies cross the placenta and affects the Rh-positive fetus.
- It results in massive hemolysis and the bilirubin levels increase and results in jaundice.
- In fetus, the blood brain barrier (BBB) is immature and the bilirubin crosses the BBB and affects basal ganglia since it has affinity for bilirubin.
- There are symptoms of motor dysfunctions.

24. Secondary active transport.

- Active transport across cell membrane involves use of energy and is an uphill transport.
- The substances move against the concentration and electrical gradient.
- Primary active transport derives the energy directly from hydrolysis of ATP. Therefore, the carrier molecules are ATPases, such as Na^+- K^+ ATPase.
- Secondary active transporter uses energy from ATP hydrolysis indirectly. The Na^+–K^+ ATPase which is present in all cells, carries 3 molecules of Na^+ from ICF to ECF and 2 K^+ from ECF to ICF. By the action of this pump there is a concentration gradient established for Na^+ to move into the cell. This inward Na^+ gradient is coupled to transport other ions, such as glucose; the Na-glucose transporter (SGLT) in epithelial cells in intestines and kidneys.
- Secondary active transporters can be symports or antiports
- Low sodium concentration in the cell favors Na^+ influx and the symport will move glucose into the cell only when both Na^+ and glucose binds to it. So, the Na^+ gradient is used to transport glucose across the membrane.
- In cardiac myocytes, the Na^+ gradient is used to transport Ca^{2+} to the ECF. So, Na^+-Ca^{2+} exchanger is an antiport moving Na^+ into the cell and Ca^{2+} out of the cells.
- There are also Na^+-Amino acid symport, Na^+-I^- symport, Na^+, K^+, $2Cl^-$ symport, etc.

25. Rigor mortis.

- Rigor mortis is stiffening of muscles after the death of an individual.
- Stiffness is due to sustained attachment of myosin heads to the actin filament due to loss of ATP.
- After myosin cross-bridge attachment to actin filament, removal of the cross-bridge needs attachment of an ATP molecule.
- After death, there is no more ATP synthesized therefore the myosin heads stay attached to actin filament resulting in stiffness of muscle.
- Rigidity disappears after some hours due to release of enzymes from lysosomes which will digest the muscle proteins.
- The appearance and disappearance of rigor mortis is used to identify the time of death.

26. Name the second messengers.

- cAMP
- cGMP
- Ca^{++}
- Inositol triphosphate (IP3)
- Diacylglycerol (DAG)

27. Name the hormones involved for the growth.

- Thyroid hormone, growth hormones, androgen and estrogen are essential for growth.
- Insulin is also essential for growth.

28. What is Turner's syndrome—three features?

- Turner's syndrome is a defect due to nondisjunction of chromosomes.
- It is a condition in which a pair of chromosomes fails to separate so both go to one daughter cell during meiosis.
- In individuals with XO chromosomal pattern, the gonads are rudimentary or absent so that the female external genitalia develops.
- There is short stature, no sexual maturity at puberty and congenital abnormalities are present.
- It is also called as gonadal dysgenesis or ovarian agenesis.

29. APUD cells of its secretion.

- APUD (amine precursor uptake and decarboxylation) cells are present in the GIT and they secrete amines and polypeptides.
- These cells are present in other organs, such as the lungs.
- They are also neuroendocrine cells and carcinoid tumor originates from these cells.

30. Law of intestine.

Peristaltic waves are stimulated by distension of intestines. The wave created by distension spreads on either directions but the wave towards the oral side dies out. Therefore the peristaltic waves proceed only form oral to aboral direction and moves chyme only in the aboral direction.

31. Double Bohr effect.

- The fetal blood coming back to placenta carries more CO_2 and the CO_2 is released into the maternal blood.
- The maternal blood pH drops because of the mixing of CO_2 and the maternal blood is more acidic than fetal blood.
- So in this situation, the hemoglobin—oxygen dissociation curve shifts to left in fetal blood and in maternal blood to right side—**double Bohr's effect**.
- This helps fetus to receive sufficient oxygen.

32. Aldosterone escape.

- Aldosterone acts on the renal tubules in the DCT and collecting duct.
- It increases Na^+ and water reabsorption in the renal tubules.
- Therefore aldosterone increases water reabsorption and increases ECF volume.
- However in hyperaldosteronism the increased retention of salt and water does not result in edema.
- The absence of edema in hyperaldosteronism is due to release of atrial natriuretic peptide (ANP) from right atrium following volume expansion.
- ANP acts on the kidneys and induces natriuresis, no edema occurs
- This is said to be **aldosterone escape phenomenon**.

33. What are different types of water absorption?

There are two types of water resorption in the kidneys—obligatory and facultative reabsorption.
1. **Obligatory reabsorption:** About 85% of the filtered water is reabsorbed by osmosis along with the solute reabsorption and this happens irrespective of body water balance. About 67% of this is reabsorbed from PCT and 15–18% from loop of Henle.
2. **Facultative reabsorption:** About 15% of water reabsorption may/may not happen and is based on the body water balance. It happens in the collecting duct by action of ADH.

34. What is Houssay animal?

- It is an animal that has been pancreatectomized and hypophysectomized.

- It is named after the discoverer of the principle that animals are more sensitive to insulin after removal of the pituitary, and that after this operation the intensity of diabetes in de-pancreatized animals is diminished.
- This is because of decreased effect of growth hormone on blood glucose levels.

35. Name the hormones involved in calcium homeostasis, and the main organs that will act.

The hormones involved in calcium homeostasis are:
- **Parathormone:** It acts on the bones and stimulates bone resorption and thereby increases blood calcium levels. It also acts on the kidneys and increases calcium reabsorption. PTH stimulates synthesis of 1,25-dihydroxycholecalciferol and thereby indirectly stimulates calcium absorption from the GIT.
- **1,25-dihydroxycholecalciferol:** Acts on the GIT and stimulates absorption of calcium from the GIT. It also acts on the kidneys to increase calcium reabsorption.
- PTH and 1,25-dihydroxycholecalciferol increase blood calcium levels.
- **Calcitonin:** It is the only hormone which decreases blood calcium levels. It acts on the bones and kidneys. On the bones, it decreases bone resorption and in kidneys it increases calcium excretion in urine.

36. Draw the diagram of alveolocapillary membrane and write the thickness of it.

- The alveolocapillary membrane is also called as the respiratory membrane.
- It separates the blood in the capillaries and the air in the alveoli
- The gases which have to move from alveoli to capillary or in the opposite direction they have to diffuse across this membrane.
- It is made up of alveolar epithelial lining, basement membrane and the capillary endothelial lining (*refer* **Fig. 42**).
- The thickness of the membrane is 0.2 to 0.5 mm.

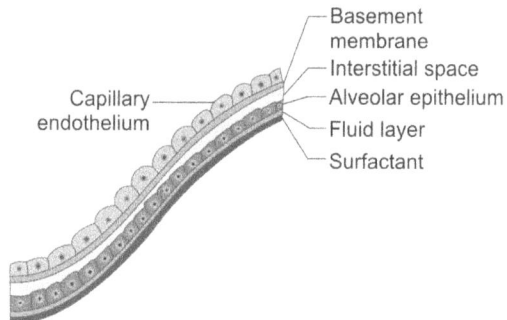

Fig. 42: Respiratory membrane.

37. What is SCUBA?

SCUBA is Self-contained Underwater Breathing Apparatus

The type used for commercial purpose is open-circuit demand system.

It contains the following parts:
- One or more tanks of compressed air or breathing mixtures
- A first stage reducing valve to reduce the high pressure in tank to low pressure
- An inhalation demand valve to create a small negative pressure for inhalation of air
- An exhalation valve to breathe out air into the sea
- A mask and a tube with dead space.

Operation of SCUBA
- During inhalation, the first step is operation of the first stage reducing valve to reduce the pressure of air from the tank and delivers air at a pressure minimally above the surrounding water pressure.
- Inspiration creates a negative pressure on the diaphragm of the demand valve and opens it to allow air to enter the mask and then to lungs.
- By this method only the amount needed enters the mask.
- Then the expiration follows and the air is breathed out into the sea.

38. Who discovered J receptors? What is its physiological significance?

- 'J' receptors are juxtapulmonary capillary receptors located adjacent to alveoli

and can be stimulated by substances in pulmonary capillary blood.
- They are the endings of unmyelinated C fibers in the alveoli
- It was discovered by an Indian Physiologist Dr AS Paintal.
- They are stimulated by hyperinflation of lungs and also by intravenous or intracardiac injection of chemicals, such as capsaicin.
- The immediate responses are apnea followed by rapid breathing, bradycardia and hypotension—These responses are called as **pulmonary chemoreflex**.
- Similar responses are seen in pulmonary edema, congestion and embolism due to chemicals released in these states.

39. What are otolith organs?

- There are two sac like structures in the vestibular apparatus, the utricle and saccule.
- These are called as the otolithic organs.
- Their receptor cells, hair cells are located in the receptor organs maculae.
- The hairs of these cells are embedded in a gelatinous mass containing crystals of calcium carbonate—the **otoliths or otoconia** (*refer* **Fig. 43**)
- So these organs are called as otolithic organs.

40. What is alpha block?

Alpha Waves
- Occurs at a frequency of 8-13 per second. Amplitude is 50-100 μV
- Present in all normal individuals when they are awake and resting with closed eyes.
- Disappears entirely during sleep.
- It is found in the parieto-occipital region.
- Alpha rhythm affected by blood glucose levels, body temperature and glucocorticoids.

Alpha Block
- Alpha rhythm disappears on opening the eyes. (*refer* **Fig. 44**)
- Also called as desynchronization.

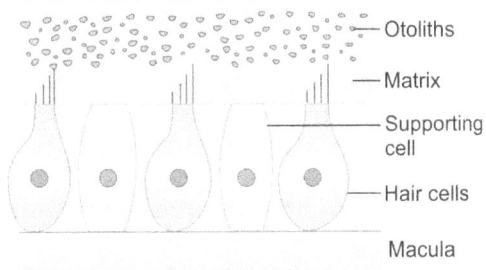

Fig. 43: Otolithic organ.

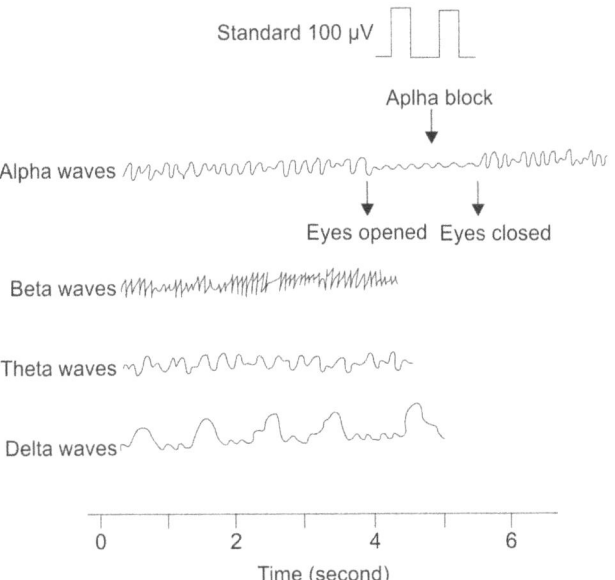

Fig. 44: EEG waves with alpha block in alpha waves.

41. Define Frank-Starling law.

Refer answers to question number 11, same section.

42. What is Monro–Kellie Doctrine law?

- **Monro-Kellie doctrine:** According to this phenomenon at any given time, the contents within the cranial cavity is a constant.
- It includes the brain, blood and CSF. So if any one component increases, it is at the expense of the other two.
- For example if there is an increase in cerebral venous pressure there is a similar increase in ICP and these two decrease the blood flowing through the arteries.

43. What is stereognosis? Where is its center?

- The ability to identify familiar objects by handling them and without seeing them is called **stereognosis**.
- The center is in the cerebral cortex, parietal lobe posterior to postcentral gyrus.

44. What are the functions of frontal lobe?

Frontal lobe is divided into two main areas—precentral cortex and prefrontal lobe.

Precentral Cortex

This consists of the areas—primary motor area (area 4), premotor area (area 6), supplementary motor area and frontal eye field (area 8).

Functions

- Primary motor area is responsible for initiation of voluntary movements in opposite half of the body and for speech. It also contributes 30% fibers for the corticospinal tract.
- Premotor area also contributes 30% fibers for CST. It programs the skilled motor activity and thereby directs area 4 for its execution.
- Supplementary area coordinates movements on both sides of the body.
- Frontal eye field controls voluntary conjugate movements of the eye.

Prefrontal Lobe

- This is the part of frontal lobe from which no motor responses are elicited.
- It contains the Brodmann areas—9, 10, 11, 12, 13, 14, 23, 24, 32 and 46.

Functions

- In animals, it is considered to be the seat of intelligence, but in humans, it is the seat of mind.
- It controls the mood and feelings of the subject
- It is involved in higher functions, such as emotions, learning and memory.
- It controls various intellectual activities, such as planning of future, concentration on actions, solving mathematical problems, etc.
- It helps in appreciation and discrimination of odors
- It initiates movements in relation to emotions.
- It plans the sequence of movements for an action along with motor cortex for actions.

45. What are mechanoreceptors? Give example.

- These are receptors which provide information about touch, pressure and vibration stimuli from the skin.
- They are nerve endings of unmyelinated axon surrounded by lamellated connective tissue.
- **For example:** Pacinian corpuscle (receptor for vibration), Meissner corpuscle (receptor for touch).

46. What is summation? Mention its types.

- Summation means adding up of impulses.
- In the synapse, following release of neurotransmitters there could be depolarization or hyperpolarization of the membrane.

- These are called as postsynaptic potentials and they belong to the category of graded potentials.
- These individual potentials from many synapses can summate and excite the membrane and take it to firing level.
- There are two types of summations—spatial and temporal summation.
- Temporal summation—the same input stimulates the postsynaptic neuron repeatedly and thereby excites it.
- Spatial summation—here many inputs stimulate simultaneously to excite it.

47. What are cholinergic and adrenergic receptors?

Cholinergic Receptors

- The receptors for acetylcholine are called as cholinergic receptors.
- They are present on the postsynaptic neurons or the muscle membrane or on the secretory glands.
- They are of two types—nicotinic and muscarinic receptors.

Adrenergic Receptors

- The receptors for adrenaline and noradrenaline are called as adrenergic receptors.
- They are of two main types—α and β receptors.
- There are subtypes for each one.
- They are $\alpha 1$, $\alpha 2$, $\beta 1$, $\beta 2$, and $\beta 3$ receptors.

48. Draw the structure of rods and cones.
Refer Fig. 45.

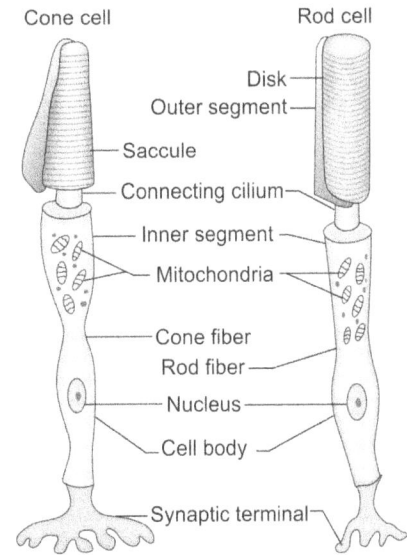

Fig. 45: Structure of rods and cones.

49. What is the difference between spasticity and rigidity?

Spasticity	Rigidity
Seen in pyramidal tract lesion	Seen in extrapyramidal lesion
Increased tone in only antagonistic muscles	Increased tone in both agonists and antagonists
Resistance to stretch is seen in initial phase and disappears later	Resistance is seen throughout the passive movement
Clasp-knife type	Cog wheel type and lead pipe rigidity

50. Define histotoxic hypoxia.
Refer answer to question 15, same section.

Answers to 2012 Question Paper

ANSWER ALL QUESTIONS

I. Essay Questions **(15 Marks each)**
1. Explain the sliding filament hypothesis and outline the main events in the cross-bridge cycle.
2. Draw an oxygen dissociation curve and describe how oxygen is transported in the blood. Depict the Bohr effect.
3. What are the components of gastric secretion? Explain the regulation of gastric secretion.
4. Classify pain. What are the receptors for pain? Describe the dual pathways for pain. What is analgesic system in the brain?
5. What are the normal blood sugar levels? Which hormones regulate the blood sugar level and how? Add a note on diabetes mellitus.
6. Discuss stages of erythropoiesis and the factors affecting it. Add a note on sickle cell anemia.
7. Define cardiac output. Discuss the factors affecting cardiac output and any one method of determination. What is the significance of ejection fraction in ventricular functioning?
8. List the ascending tracts in the spinal cord and discuss the tracts of posterior column with diagram.

II. Short Notes **(5 Marks each)**
1. Anticoagulants.
2. G protein.
3. Calcitriol.
4. Thyroid function tests.
5. Describe the reflex arcs involved in micturition.
6. Explain the renal contribution to pH control.
7. Tubuloglomerular feedback mechanism.
8. Functions of plasma proteins.
9. Hemophilia.
10. Counter current blood flow in the villi.
11. Frank-Starling Law of the heart.
12. Cardiac pacemaker potential.
13. Draw a labeled diagram of a normal ECG in lead II. Write a brief note on PR interval.
14. Non-progressive shock.
15. Traveling waves in the ear.
16. Ventilation-perfusion ratio.
17. Caisson disease.
18. Brown-Séquard syndrome.
19. Functions of ascending reticular activating system.
20. Role of Purkinje cells of cerebellum.
21. Functions of platelets.
22. Composition and functions of gastric juice.
23. Molecular basis of skeletal muscle contraction.
24. Sertoli cells.
25. Rh blood group.
26. Movements of small intestine.
27. Functions of placenta.
28. Functions of mitochondria.
29. Puberty.
30. Functions of glucocorticoids.
31. Chemical regulation of respiration.
32. Functions of middle ear.
33. Hypovolemic shock.
34. Ventilation-perfusion ratio.
35. Parkinson's disease with treatment.
36. Classification of nerve fibers.
37. Heart sounds.
38. Errors of refraction with correction.
39. Transport of oxygen in blood.
40. Waves of EEG.

III. Short Answers (2 Marks each)

1. Functions of Na^+-K^+ pump.
2. Saltatory conduction.
3. Conn's syndrome.
4. Laron dwarf.
5. Aquaporins.
6. Anion gap.
7. Macula densa.
8. Opsonization.
9. Immunological memory
10. Cholelithiasis
11. Enterogastric reflex.
12. Peristaltic rush.
13. Progeria.
14. Pills.
15. Permissive action.
16. Astigmatism.
17. Ocular dominance columns.
18. Dicrotic notch.
19. Cardiac reserve.
20. Reynolds number.
21. J point.
22. Extrasystole.
23. Bell-Magendie law.
24. Cogwheel rigidity.
25. Betz cells.
26. Homunculus.
27. Anomic aphasia.
28. Timed vital capacity.
29. Pneumotaxic center.
30. Asphyxia
31. Inulin clearance.
32. Oxytocin.
33. Fever.
34. Second messengers.
35. Functions of bile salts.
36. ESR.
37. Hypocalcemic tetany.
38. Placental hormones
39. Myasthenia gravis.
40. Immunoglobulins.
41. Summation.
42. Hering–Breuer inflation reflex.
43. Taste receptor.
44. PR interval in ECG.
45. Chronaxie.
46. CSF formation.
47. Phasic changes in coronary circulation.
48. FEV1.
49. Dopamine.

I. ESSAY QUESTIONS

1. Explain the sliding filament hypothesis and outline the main events in the cross-bridge cycle.

- Skeletal muscle is made up of muscle fibers, which are the basic unit of muscles and surrounding connective tissues.
- Each muscle fiber has many myofibrils and the muscle fiber is surrounded by Sarcolemma—the cell membrane.
- The myofibrils have thick and thin filaments.
- The filaments are made of proteins—actin, myosin, troponin and tropomyosin.
- Actin and myosin are the contractile proteins and troponin and tropomyosin are regulatory proteins.
- The arrangement of thick and thin filaments appears as light and dark striations (bands) under light microscope due to the refractive indices of the various parts.
- The dark band is A band and is 1.5 µm in length and is made of thick filaments and overlapping thin filaments. The center of A band has a lighter H zone with a M line in the middle of it. H zone is the area where thin filaments do not overlap thick filaments and therefore appears as lighter area. The thick filament is made of myosin molecules.
- The light band is made of thin filaments with a dark line—Z line in the middle of it. The thin filament is made of the proteins—actin, tropomyosin and troponin with 3 subunits—I, C and T.

Sarcomere

- The segment of myofibril between two Z lines is the **sarcomere**.
- It includes ½ of I band and A band and ½ I band.
- It is 2.5 µm in length.
- This forms the structural and functional unit of the muscle fiber (*refer* **Fig. 1**).

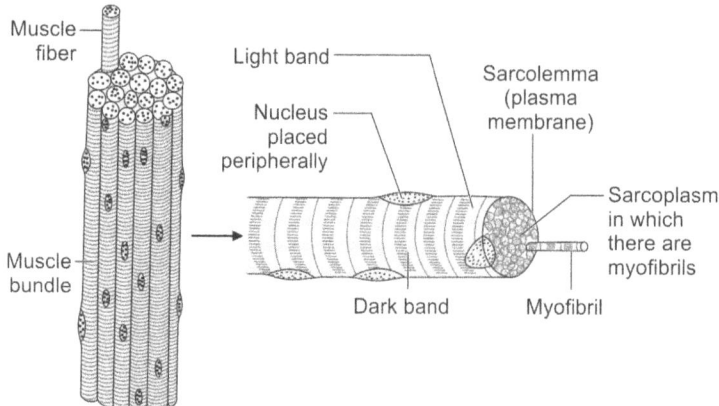

Fig. 1: Structure of muscles: Muscle bundle (A) and muscle fiber (B). Arrangement of thick and thin filaments in the muscle fiber (B).

- On contraction of the muscle, the length of sarcomere decreases and on relaxation it is increased.

Thick Filament

- Under electron microscope, a transverse section of the A band, it is seen that each thick filament is surrounded by 6 thin filaments in a hexagonal pattern.
- The type of myosin in skeletal muscle is myosin II. Myosin has two globular heads and a tail.
- It is made of 2 heavy chains and 4 light chains. The light chains and the amino terminals of heavy chains form the head. The rest of the heavy chains are wound on each other to form the tail.
- Each head of the myosin molecule has two binding sites, one for actin and the other is the ATPase site which hydrolyses ATP.
- The myosins are arranged symmetrically in the thick filament and in the center part, on either sides of M line there is a small zone where there is absence of myosin heads and it appears lighter. It is the pseudo-H zone (*refer* **Fig. 2**).
- M line is the site of reversal of polarity of myosin molecules in each of the thick filaments.

Thin Filament

- It is made of actin, troponin and tropomyosin.
- There are 300–400 actin molecules are present in each thin filament. The actin molecule is made of two chains of globular units of G actin. The chain is said to be F-actin. The actin forms a double helix.
- There are 40–60 tropomyosin molecules in each thin filament. It is in the form of strands and lies in the groove between the actin helix. It covers the myosin binding site on actin.
- Troponin molecules are globular units which are present on tropomyosin at intervals. There are 3 subunits—troponin T, I and C.
- Troponin T—attaches other components of troponin to tropomyosin
- Troponin I—inhibits myosin head binding with actin
- Troponin C—binds to calcium ion following which muscle contraction is initiated.

Muscle Contraction

- Sliding theory or ratchet theory had been put forward to explain muscle contraction by AF Huxley and HE Huxley in 1954.
- This theory postulates that the actin filament slide over the myosin filament following the formation of actin-myosin complexes and cross-bridge cycling.
- At rest, the myosin binding site on actin is covered by tropomyosin and inhibits binding of actin and myosin.
- On binding of calcium with troponin C, tropomyosin molecule changes its

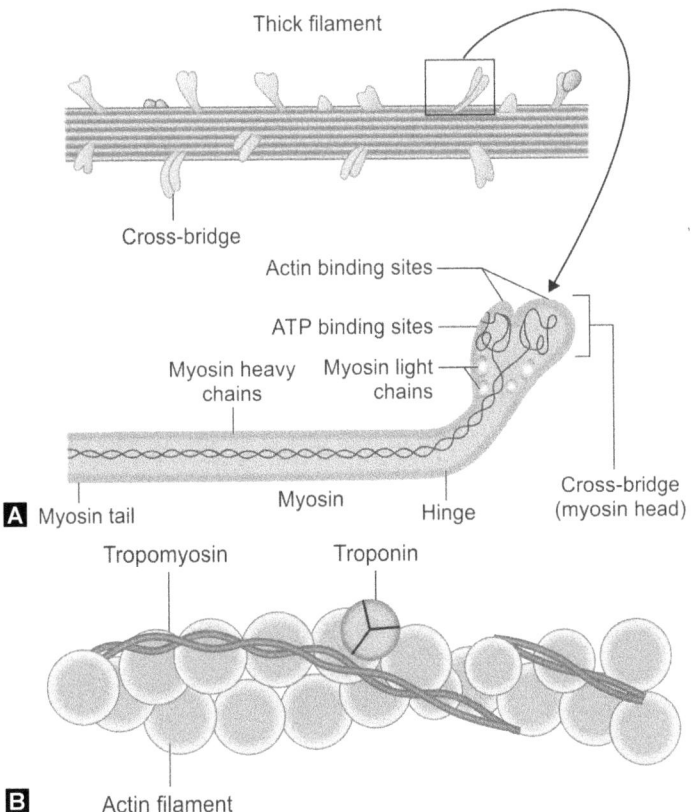

Fig. 2: Structure of myosin in thick filament (A) and structure of actin, tropomyosin and troponin molecules in thin filament (B).

configuration and moves out, exposing myosin binding sites on actin.
- For each tropomyosin molecule moving out, 7 actin molecules are exposed.

Cross-bridge Cycling
- Each myosin head has two binding sites.
- One for binding with actin and other one is an ATPase which hydrolysis ATP.
- On attaching with one ATP, the ATPase hydrolyses the ATP molecule and the energy is stored in the head and thereby it is energized.
- ADP and Pi are also attached to the head.
- The energized head is 90° perpendicular to thin filament.
- **Power stroke:** When the troponin C binds with Ca^{2+}, the actin binding sites for myosin are exposed and the perpendicular energized head binds to actin.
- Immediately after binding, the head flexes from 90° to 45° and ADP and Pi are released. This is said to be the power stroke or cross bridge cycling.
- The bent head is detached from actin molecule when another ATP molecule binds to the myosin head.
- This ATP is again hydrolyzed and the head is re-energized and ready to undergo the next cycle (*refer* **Fig. 3**).
- As a result of repeated cross-bridge cycling, the actin filament from either side is moved towards the center of A band and there is muscle contraction.

---

2. Draw an oxygen dissociation curve and describe how oxygen is transported in the blood. Depict the Bohr effect.

Transport of O_2
- O_2 is transported in blood in 2 forms.
- They are—dissolved form (2%) and as Oxy-Hb (98%)

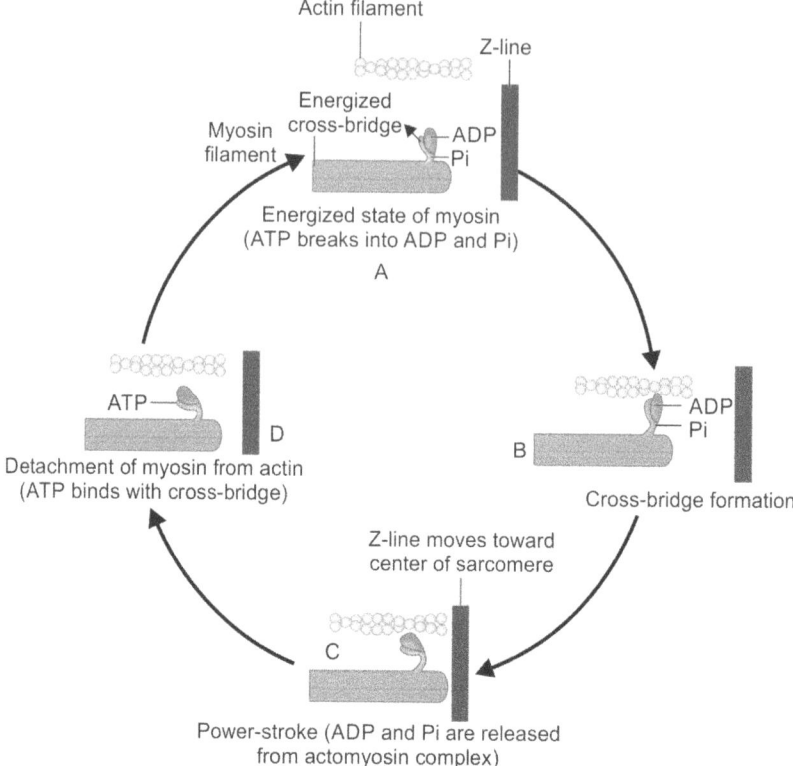

Fig. 3: Cross-bridge cycling in skeletal muscle contraction.

- As O_2 enters the blood, it gets saturated in plasma as dissolved O_2 and then there is a gradient between plasma and RBC → leads to entry of O_2 into RBC → as PO_2 increases inside the RBC, O_2 saturates Hb.

Dissolved O_2

- Dissolved O_2 is measured by the following equation.
- Dissolved O_2 = Solubility of O_2 (0.003 mL/mm Hg) × arterial PO_2 (100 mm Hg) = 0.3 mL/dL
- Partial pressure of O_2 (PO_2) in blood is decided by the dissolved O_2 content of blood.

Oxy-hemoglobin

- Hemoglobin is an O_2 carrying protein in RBC.
- It increases the O_2 carrying capacity of blood by 70 times.
- Iron in the Hb is in ferrous form (Fe^{2+}) and combines with O_2 in appropriate affinity.
- O_2 + Hb ↔ Hb O_2—oxygenation reaction (it is not oxidation reaction)
- If Fe^{2+} gets Oxidized to Fe^{3+} methemoglobin is formed which does not release O_2
- When the binding of O_2 with hemoglobin happens, affinity of Hb for O_2 increases gradually.
- Initially, Hb is in a tense configuration (T), as one molecule of O_2 combines, the Hb changes to relaxed configuration (R) and the affinity to O_2 increases to maximum when the 3rd O_2 molecule has combined.

O_2 Carrying Capacity of Blood

- Each gram of Hb carries 1.34 mL of O_2.
- Maximum amount of O_2 carried by Hb is the **O_2 carrying capacity of blood**.
- In a healthy individual, it is 20 mL/100 mL of blood. (15 × 1.34 mL = 20.1 mL/dL)
- **O_2 content** is the amount actually bound to Hb.
- **% saturation of O_2 (SO_2)** = Hb O_2 content/ HbO_2 capacity × 100.
- Normally in arterial blood % SO_2 is 98%

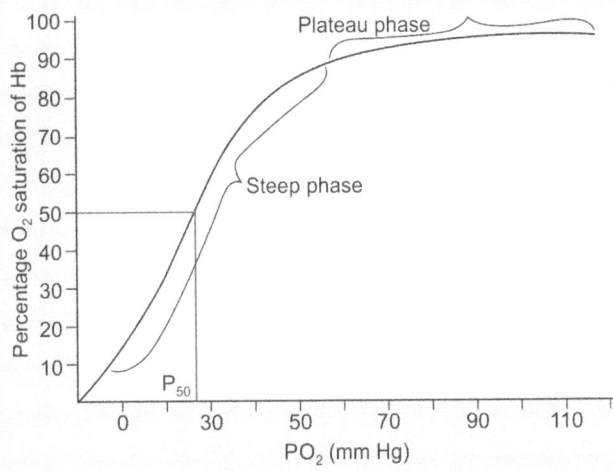

Fig. 4: Oxygen-hemoglobin dissociation curve. P_{50} is the partial pressure of O_2 at which 50% of hemoglobin is saturated with O_2. It is around 27 mm Hg. There are two phases; steep phase and plateau phase.

O_2-Hb Dissociation Curve

- This curve compares the partial pressure of O_2 and % saturation of Hb with O_2.
- It is sigmoid in shape.
- The shape is sigmoid because of the change in configuration of hemoglobin from T to R state and therefore there is gradual increase in affinity for O_2 and then it gets saturated.
- It has a steep and plateau phase.
- About 90% saturation of Hb takes place at a PO_2 of 60 mm Hg.
- P_{50} is the partial pressure at which 50% of the hemoglobin is saturated with oxygen.
- P_{50} is inversely related to the affinity of hemoglobin for oxygen.
- The **steep phase** denotes the unloading zone where even a minimum drop in PO_2 results in unloading of large amounts of oxygen to the tissues.
- The **plateau phase** denotes the loading zone, where O_2 is taken up by hemoglobin in the lungs and once all the four sites in Hb are loaded with O_2 there is no further uptake and thereby a plateau phase is reached (*refer* **Fig. 4**).
- The curve gets shifted to right are left in conditions of decreased or increase in affinity of hemoglobin for O_2 respectively.

Conditions where O_2-Hb Dissociation Curve is Shifted to Right

- Hypoxia
- ↑ PCO_2
- ↑ Temperature
- ↑ 2,3-DPG levels in RBC
- ↑ H^+ concentration (acidosis)

Conditions where O_2-Hb Dissociation Curve is Shifted to Left

- High PO_2
- Low PCO_2
- Low body temperature
- Presence of fetal hemoglobin
- Alkalosis
- Low 2,3-DPG levels in RBC (*refer* **Fig. 5**)
- Carbon monoxide poisoning

3. What are the components of gastric secretion? Explain the regulation of gastric secretion.

Composition of Gastric Juice

- 2–2.5 L/day
- pH 1–2
- Water—99.45%
- Solids—0.55%
- Electrolytes—Na^+, K^+, Mg^{2+}, Cl^-, HCO_3^-, HOP_4^-, SO_4^-
- Enzymes—pepsin, lipase, gelatinase

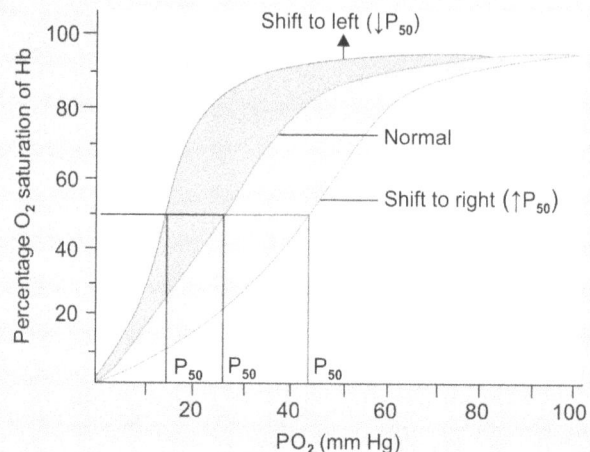

Fig. 5: Right and left shift of O_2-Hb dissociation curve. P_{50}, PO_2 at which hemoglobin is 50% saturated is 27 mm Hg. Right shift denotes decrease in hemoglobin affinity for O_2 and left shift increased affinity for O_2.

- Mucus—insoluble and soluble
- Intrinsic factor

Regulation of Gastric Secretion

Neural, humoral and reflex regulation of secretion

Factors that Stimulate

- Vagus nerve
- Gastrin
- Histamine

Factors that Inhibit

- Low pH in the stomach
- Somatostatin (*refer* **Fig. 6**)
- Prostaglandin E2

Regulation is Discussed in Terms of:

- Cephalic phase
- Gastric phase
- Intestinal phase

Cephalic Phase

- Nearly 500 mL/h (45% of total secretion)
- Initiated by thought, sight, smell, taste of food through stimulation of vagus nerve.
- Emotions also affect secretion (*refer* **Fig. 7**)

Gastric Phase

- About 50% of the total secretion occurs in this phase:
  - Distension of body of stomach (occurs through reflexes—vagal reflex)
  - Distension of antrum (occurs through gastrin secretion)
  - By products of partial digestion of protein (through gastrin secretion)

Intestinal Phase

- It begins when chyme enters the intestine.
- Intestinal influence is inhibitory. By:
  - Enterogastric reflex—by distension, presence of acid and products of digestion—inhibits secretion.
  - Hormonal mechanism—CCK, Secretin, GIP, neurotensin, etc.,—enterogastrone.

---

4. Classify pain. What are the receptors for pain? Describe the dual pathways for pain. What is analgesic system in the brain?

- Pain is an physical adjunct of an imperative protective reflex.
- Pain can be induced by—mechanical, thermal or chemical stimuli.
- **Two types of pain:** Fast pain and slow pain.
- **Receptors:** Free nerve endings of $A\delta$ and unmyelinated C fibers.

Pain Pathway

- Pain sensation is carried by the lateral spinothalamic tract (LSTT).

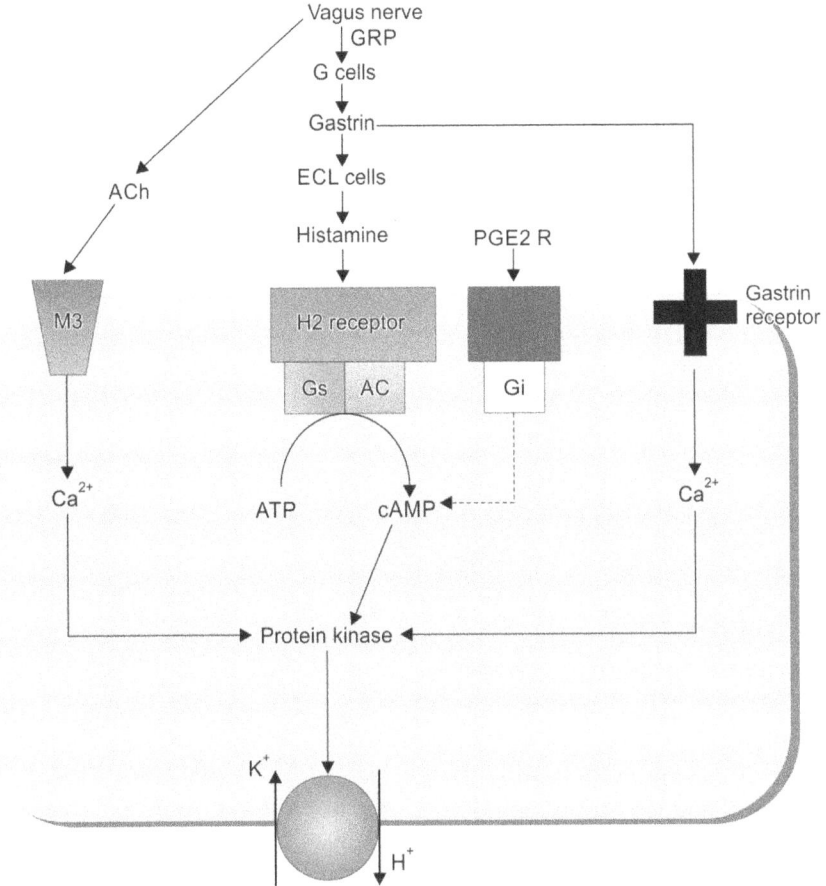

Fig. 6: Parietal cell with the regulating factors for HCl secretion. (PGE2R: prostaglandin E2 receptor; M3: muscrinic receptor)

- There are two types of pain—fast pain and slow pain.
- So, the LSTT has fibers for fast pain and for slow pain. There are separate pathways for fast and slow pain.

Fast Pain

- Fast pain is sensed by the free nerve endings of Aδ fibers.
- The pain sensation from periphery is carried through the Aδ fibers.
- Their cell bodies are present in the dorsal root ganglion.
- The fibers on entering spinal cord terminate on cells in laminae I and V of the dorsal gray horn.
- These are the second order neurons. Neurotransmitter released here is glutamate.
- Second order neurons cross to the opposite side and ascend up as neospinothalamic **tract** in the anterolateral column of spinal cord.
- Neospinothalamic tract reaches thalamus and ends on the ventral posterolateral nucleus of the thalamus (VPLN).
- The tract on its way to thalamus gives a few branches to periaqueductal gray (PAG) in midbrain.
- The third order neurons start from thalamus and reach somatosensory area I.
- This pathway is concerned with localisation and interpretation of pain.

Slow Pain

- Slow pain is sensed by the free nerve endings of unmyelinated C fibers.

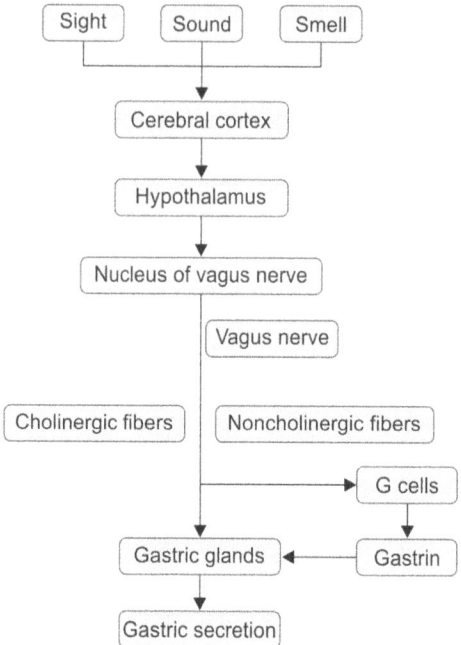

Fig. 7: Cephalic phase of regulation of HCl secretion. This phase of gastric secretion is regulated through vagu nerve.

- Slow pain is carried by the same fibers to spinal cord and they terminate in the laminae II and III of dorsal gray horn.
- This is the first order neuron. The neurotransmitter released here is substance P.
- The second order neuron arises from laminae I and V and the fibers cross to the opposite side and ascends up as **paleospinothalamic tract**.
- It ascends up along with neospinothalamic tract in the anterolateral column of spinal cord (*refer* **Fig. 8**).
- This tract gives many fibers to PAG, reticular formation and tectum.
- It then ends in the non-specific nucleus of thalamus.
- Third order neuron arises from here and is projected to entire cerebral cortex.
- This pathway is concerned with alertness, arousal and perception of pain rather than localization of pain.

Analgesic System in the Brain

Pain modulation takes place in 2 places:
1. At the peripheral nerve endings
2. At the spinal cord level

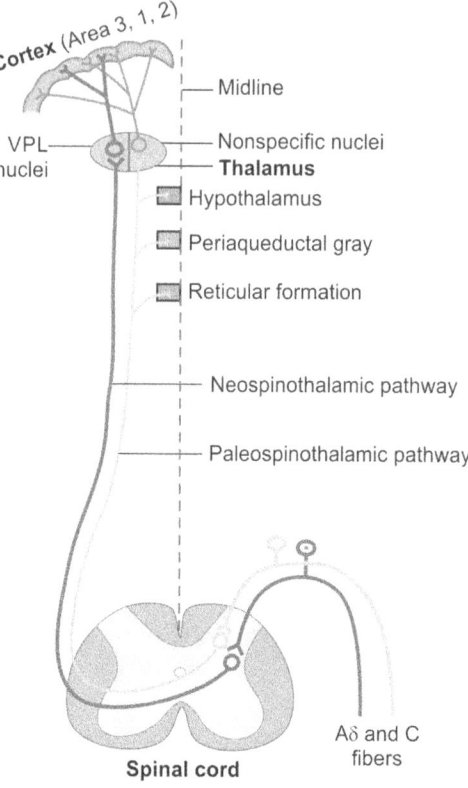

Fig. 8: Neospinothalamic and paleospinothalamic tracts.
(VPLN: ventral posterolateral nucleus of thalamus)

Peripheral Nerve Endings

Endorphins and enkephalins combine with nociceptors and decrease the response to stimuli.

At the Spinal Cord

- **Peripheral mechanism:** By gate control theory—large $A\beta$ fibers (when stimulated by touching or rubbing the painful area) ↓ nociception in C fibers.
- **Central pain suppressing mechanism:** Opioids secreted from areas in brain stem inhibit pain transmission in the spinal cord.

Gate control mechanism:
- Pain sensation is carried by $A\delta$ and unmyelinated C fibers and they ascend up as spinothalamic tract.
- Touch and pressure sensations are carried by large myelinated $A\beta$ fibers and they ascend up as dorsal column tract in spinal cord.

- Dorsal column fibers in the spinal cord give a branch to inhibitory interneurons which secrete enkephalins and which in turn end on the second order neurons in pain pathway.
- So, when there is pain in an area, touching or pressing that region stimulates the large Aβ fibers which in turn inhibit pain pathway and thereby there is decreased pain perception.
- So the large Aβ fibers gate the pain pathway.

Central pain suppressing mechanism:
- Pain pathway, as it ascends up gives branches to periaqueductal gray (PAG) in midbrain.
- There is a pain suppressing descending pathway from PAG to medulla and to spinal cord.

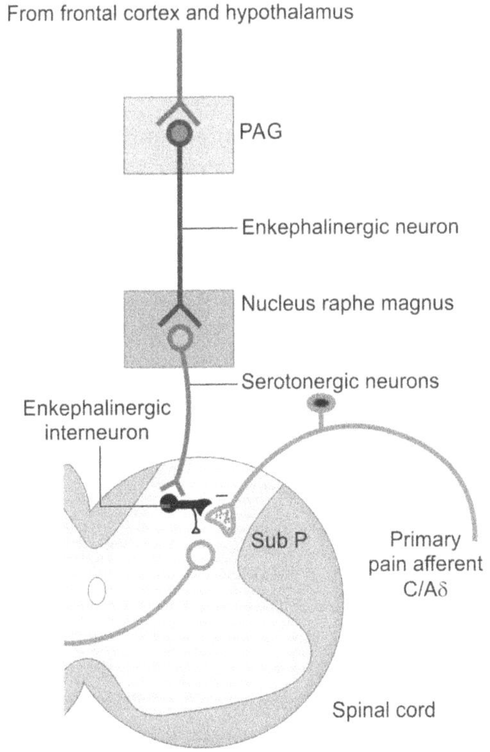

Fig. 9: Endogenous pain inhibition by spinal cord and brainstem structures. PAG—periaqueductal gray. It has enkephalinergic neurons which end on serotonergic neurons of raphe magnus nucleus in medulla. They send out axons which end on Enkephalinergic neurons in spinal cord and decreases pain.

- Axons of the neurons in PAG terminate on serotonergic neurons in raphe magnus nuclei in medulla.
- They secrete enkephalin here.
- Axons of serotonergic neurons in raphe magnus nuclei descend and terminate on the inhibitory interneurons in spinal cord (*refer* **Fig. 9**).
- They secrete serotonin and stimulate internuncial neurons which in turn inhibit second order neurons in the pain pathway by secreting enkephalin.

---

5. What are the normal blood sugar levels? Which hormones regulate the blood sugar level and how? Add a note on diabetes mellitus.

- Normal fasting peripheral venous blood glucose level is 70-90 mg/dL.
- After food intake, it reaches 110-130 mg/dL and after 2 hours it comes back to normal values. Blood glucose levels are 20 mg/dL higher in arterial blood.
- There are hormones which increase blood glucose levels and hormones which decrease blood glucose levels.

Hormones which Increase Blood Glucose Levels are:
- Glucagon
- Glucocorticoids
- Catecholamines
- Growth hormone
- Thyroid hormones

Hormones which Decrease Blood Glucose Levels

Insulin

Mechanisms of Actions of Hormones

Glucagon
- It increases blood glucose levels by various mechanisms, such as glycogenolysis, gluconeogenesis.
- In the liver, it activates the enzyme phosphorylase and breaks down glycogen.
- Glycogenolysis is favored by activating phospholipase C and increase in cytoplasmic Ca^{2+} in the hepatocytes. It has no glycogenolytic action on muscles.

- It increases gluconeogenesis with the help of pyruvate, lactate, glycerol and amino acids.

Glucocorticoids
- Increases gluconeogenesis in liver → increases glycogen stores.
- Antagonizes the action of insulin on muscle and adipose tissue—prevents glucose uptake.
- This spares glucose for the brain.
- Increases glucose output from the liver.
- Induces hyperglycemia

Catecholamines
- Adrenaline acts via β and α-adrenergic receptors.
- Thereby increases hepatic glucose output by activating the enzyme phosphorylase and induces hyperglycemia.
- Phosphorylase is activated in the skeletal muscle also, but glucose-6-phosphate is converted to pyruvate because of the absence of glucose-6-phosphatase.
- Pyruvate is converted to lactate which diffuses into circulation and is oxidized in the liver to pyruvate and then to glycogen.
- Therefore, on stimulation by epinephrine there is initial glycogenolysis followed by glycogen synthesis.
- Stimulates gluconeogenesis
- Epinephrine also decreases peripheral utilization of glucose.
- Stimulates secretion of glucagon

Growth Hormone
- Effects of growth hormone are both direct and indirect (through IGF-1).
- It increases hepatic glucose output by stimulating gluconeogenesis
- It has anti-insulin effect and thereby prevents peripheral utilization of glucose by the tissues.
- It decreases insulin sensitivity

Thyroid Hormone
- It increases blood glucose levels by increasing absorption of glucose from intestines.
- It also for some extent increases hepatic glucose output and thereby depletion of hepatic glycogen.
- Glycogen depletion in hepatocytes induces damage to hepatocytes and decreases glucose uptake.
- It also causes degradation of insulin

Insulin
- Insulin favors glucose storage in the liver. It **enhances glucose entry** into liver cells by stimulating the enzyme glucokinase which phosphorylates glucose to glucose-6-phosphate thereby maintaining a gradient for glucose entry into hepatocytes.
- **Stimulates glycolysis** and conversion of glucose to pyruvic and lactic acids by stimulating the enzymes phosphofructokinase and pyruvate kinase. Since this decreases intracellular glucose concentration, thereby facilitates diffusion of glucose into cells by creating a gradient for glucose.
- **Glycogen synthesis and its storage** are enhanced by stimulation of the enzyme glycogen synthase.
- It inhibits glycogenolysis and prevents glucose output from liver.
- It also **inhibits gluconeogenesis**
- In skeletal muscles and adipose tissues, insulin facilitates glucose entry into muscle cells by inserting the glucose transporter GLUT 4 and it also stimulates the enzyme hexokinase.
- Glucose gets oxidized by the enzyme pyruvate dehydrogenase and also converted to glycogen and stored.
- Glucose in adipose tissue is converted to α-glycerophosphate which in turn esterifies fatty acids.

Glucose Tolerance Test
- It is a test in which an oral dose of glucose is given and series of blood samples are collected to check how quickly the glucose is cleared from blood. It is usually done to test for diabetes, glucose intolerance, etc.
- This test is based on the principle that in diabetics, blood glucose levels rise steeply after food intake. In a diabetic patient, when a glucose load is given, the blood glucose level rises and comes back to baseline level very slowly than in normal individuals.

Methodology
- About 75 g of glucose in 300 mL of water is given to the adults.
- In normal individuals, the fasting venous blood glucose level is less than 115 mg/dL. After 2 hours, the value is less than 140 mg/dL and none of the values is more than 200 mg/dL.
- Impaired glucose tolerance is when the values are above upper normal limit but below the value for diagnosis of diabetes (110-126 mg/dL in fasting and 140-200 mg/dL in peak levels)).
- In diabetics, the glucose tolerance curve is abnormal. Fasting blood glucose is >126 mg/dL and after glucose intake peak value reached is >200 mg/dL and takes nearly 4-6 hours to reach baseline value.

Diabetes Mellitus

Deficiency of insulin is diabetes mellitus.

Causes

Diabetes mellitus occurs due to destruction of β cells of islets in the pancreas or due to decreased sensitivity of receptors for insulin. Based on the causes and features diabetes is classified into two types—type 1 and type 2 diabetes mellitus. **primary diabetes mellitus**.

Secondary diabetes mellitus: Diabetes is secondary to some other diseases, such as Cushing's syndrome, acromegaly, pancreatitis, etc.

Type 1 Diabetes Mellitus
- This is due to autoimmune destruction of β cells and insulin is not secreted.
- Plasma insulin levels are low and undetectable
- This condition is treated with only insulin and therefore also called as insulin-dependent diabetes mellitus (IDDM).
- Antibodies are present against β cell surface antigens.
- It is usually seen in children and adults of <45 years of age.
- They are prone for ketoacidosis and are thin.
- Chance of developing the disease in identical twins is 50%

Type 2 Diabetes Mellitus
- This is due to decreased sensitivity of insulin receptors for insulin.
- Insulin levels are normal or even elevated
- Therefore, it is also called as non-insulin dependent diabetes mellitus (NIDDM).
- The individuals with NIDDM are obese and the disease occurs usually after >45 years of age.
- This is the most common type of DM
- The chance of developing the disease in identical disease is 100%.

Symptoms of DM

DM is characterized by polyphagia, polydipsia, polyuria, weight loss, hyperglycemia and glycosuria. In severe condition, it leads to ketoacidosis and coma.

- **Polyphagia:** Increased food intake. This is due to inability of usage of glucose by the neurons in satiety center of hypothalamus due to absence of insulin. So, the low glucose in these cells leads to stimulation of the feeding center and thereby increased food intake.
- **Polyuria:** Passage of large amounts of urine. As the plasma glucose levels increase, the amount of glucose filtered is also increased. The SGLT transporter in renal tubular cells of PCT gets saturated and is not able to reabsorb glucose from the filtrate and glucose starts appearing in the urine. The glucose when retained in tubule holds back water and other electrolytes in the tubule and results in osmotic diuresis. Other ions, such as Na^+, K^+ and phosphates are also lost in urine.
- **Polydipsia:** When water is lost excessively, thirst mechanism is stimulated because of cellular dehydration and water intake is increased.
- **Weight loss** is due to loss of calories in the urine and mobilization of other stores, such as fats and proteins resulting in weight loss.
- **Hyperglycemia** is due to decreased peripheral utilization of glucose by skeletal

muscles, adipose tissues and liver. There is also increased glucose output from liver.
- **Glycosuria** is excessive loss of glucose in urine. This happens when the renal threshold (>180 mg/dL) is reached. Glycosuria leads to all the symptoms mentioned above.

Physiological Basis of Treatment of DM

- **Sulfonylurea derivatives**, such as tolbutamide, acetohexamide, glipizide, glyburide are hypoglycemic agents and they decrease blood glucose levels by increasing production of insulin. So, they are effective in people with some amount of working b cells. It cannot be used in type 1 DM. They act by inhibiting ATP-inhibited K^+ channels and decrease K^+ efflux thereby depolarizing the membrane and favors Ca^{2+} influx and release of insulin.
- The other groups of drugs are *biguanides*, such as phenformin, metformin which act in the absence of insulin. They decrease the hepatic output of glucose and thereby decreases blood glucose levels. Metformin can be used in combination with sulfonylureas in treatment for Type 2 DM.
- **Thiazolidinediones**, such as troglitazone are hypoglycemic agents which increase the insulin-mediated peripheral utilization of glucose. They act by binding to peroxisome proliferator-activated receptor (PPARγ).
- **Exercise:** Is a very effective strategy to decrease blood glucose levels in type 1 and type 2 DM. Exercise increases glucose entry into skeletal muscle by inserting an insulin independent GLUT 4 glucose transporter in muscle cell membranes. This increases glucose uptake by muscle cells for a prolonged duration after exercise also and therefore regular exercise can increase insulin sensitivity.

---

6. Discuss stages of erythropoiesis and the factors affecting it. Add a note on sickle cell anemia.

- Erythropoiesis is production of RBCs. Life span of RBCs are 120 days.
- Hence continuous destruction and production of RBCs take place at a constant rate.

Site of Erythropoiesis

- **Mesoblastic stage:** In the embryonal stage—yolk sac.
- **Hepatic stage:** Later in the fetal stage up to 5 months—liver, spleen, thymus and lymph nodes.
- **Myeloid stage:** 3 months before birth—red bone marrow of all bones.
- **Adult life:** Red bone marrow of flat bones and epiphysis of long bones.

Changes During Maturation

- Reduction in size of the cell.
- Cytoplasm increases in amount and nucleus decreases in size.
- Cytoplasm changes from basophilic nature to polychromatophilic and then to acidophilic nature due to hemoglobinization of cytoplasm
- Disappearance of RNA
- Loss of nucleoli and then nucleus

Pronormoblast

- Large cell, diameter—20-25 µm.
- Cytoplasm is less.
- High concentration of polyribosomes.
- Large nucleus with multiple nucleoli
- Hemoglobin not formed

Early Normoblast

- Diameter of cell—15-18 µm
- Cell exhibits mitosis
- Cytoplasm is still less, basophilic
- Nucleus large, occupies 3/4th of cell.
- Heterochromatin clumps present.

Intermediate Normoblast

- The cell is smaller in size, 12-15 µm.
- Cytoplasm changes from blue to pink as hemoglobin starts to appear.
- Nucleus small, occupies half the cell. No nucleoli.
- Hemoglobin formation makes the cell acidophilic also—polychromatophilic cytoplasm.
- Mitosis is sluggish.

Late Normoblast
- Cell is smaller in size.
- Cytoplasm is deeply eosinophilic—orthochromatic erythroblast.
- Nucleus is small and pyknotic.
- Cart-wheel arrangement of chromatin.
- Hb synthesis increases

Reticulocyte
- Cell size is 7.8 µm
- Nucleus is extruded
- Hemoglobin present
- Chromatin reticulum seen

Mature RBC
- Cell size is 7.5 µm.
- RBC is biconcave in shape.
- Chromatin reticulum disappears

The whole process of maturation from Pronormoblast to reticulocyte takes 7 days. It takes 2 days for reticulocyte to mature as an RBC (*refer* **Fig. 10**).

Regulation of Erythropoiesis

There are general and special factors regulating erythropoiesis.

General Factor—Hypoxia
- Major function of RBC is to carry oxygen to the tissues.
- So, when there is decrease in tissue oxygen levels, it induces production of RBCs.
- Hypoxia stimulates the interstitial cells of the kidneys to synthesize the hormone **erythropoietin**.
- It acts on bone marrow to stimulate the erythropoietin sensitive stem cells to become proerythroblasts and thereby stimulates formation of RBCs.
- It also increases the release of reticulocytes from the bone marrow.

Factors Increasing Erythropoietin Production
- Hypoxia
- Catecholamines
- Thyroxine
- Testosterone

Special Maturation Factors
Dietary factors:
- Proteins help in globin formation.
- Iron helps in heme formation.
- Copper, cobalt and nickel also helps in heme formation.
- Calcium helps in absorption of iron from GIT.
- Vitamin C also helps in iron absorption.
- Vitamin B12 and folic acid helps in synthesis of nucleic acids and final maturation of RBC.
- Intrinsic factor synthesized in the stomach by the parietal cells help in absorption of vitamin B12.

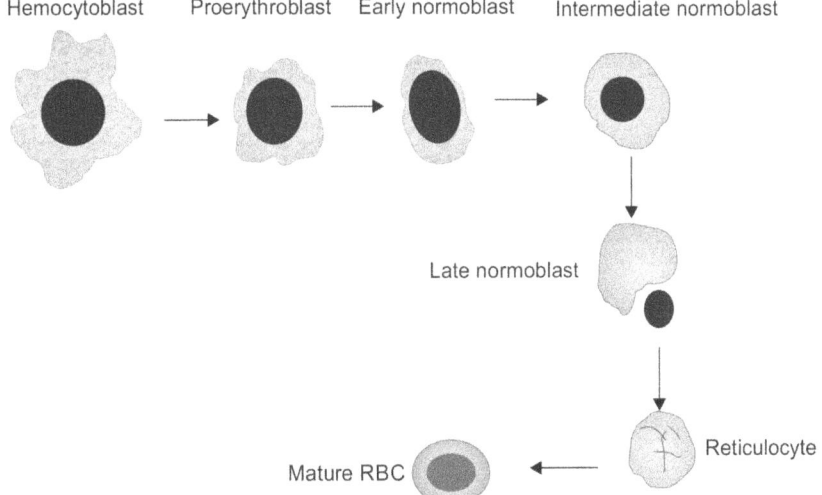

Fig. 10: Stages of erythropoiesis.

Sickle Cell Anemia
- It is a hereditary disorder and the individuals affected have hemoglobin S (HbS).
- In hemoglobin S, the glutamic acid is replaced by valine at the 6th position in beta chain of globulin portion of hemoglobin.
- In conditions of hypoxia, the hemoglobin S crystallizes and normal RBC changes its shape to become sickle shaped and the membrane is rigid and undergoes rapid hemolysis and results in hemolytic anemia.

---

7. Define cardiac output. Discuss the factors affecting cardiac output and any one method of determination. What is the significance of ejection fraction in ventricular functioning?

Cardiac output (CO) is defined as the amount of blood ejected by each ventricle per minute.
- CO = Stroke volume (SV) × heart rate (HR) (*refer* Fig. 11)
- NV = 70 mL/beat × 70/min = 4900 mL/min

Determinants of Cardiac Output
- CO = Stroke volume (SV) × heart rate (HR)
- So factors affecting either of them will alter CO.

I. Factors Affecting SV
1. Preload
2. Contractility
3. After load

II. Factors Affecting HR

HR is affected by nerves supplying heart (sympathetic and parasympathetic nerves) and cardiac centers.

I. Factors affecting SV
1. *Preload:*
   - The initial muscle length is the **preload** (the extent to which the muscle is stretched before contraction).
   - Preload is decided by the **end diastolic volume (EDV).**
   - EDV is decided by the **venous return (VR).**
- Preload affecting stroke volume is based on the Frank-Starling Law.
- It states that within physiological limits, the force of contraction is directly proportional to the initial length of the muscle.

Causes for application of Frank-Starling's law:
- Increase in EDV →↑ stretch of muscle fiber → interaction of thick and thin filament increases →↑ force of contraction.
- Stretch of muscle fibers → opens stretch sensitive Ca^{2+} channels on sarcolemma →↑ Ca^{2+} influx →↑ force of contraction.
- ↑Ca^{2+} influx →↑ Ca^{2+} release from SR (CICR) →↑ force of contraction.
- ↑stretch of muscle fiber →↑ affinity of troponin for Ca^{2+}

EDV is dependent on:
- Venous return, which is dependent on:
  - *Skeletal muscle pump:* Contraction of limb muscles press on the veins and increases forward movement of blood in the veins.
  - *Thoracic pump:* Increase in respiration depresses the diaphragm and decreases intrathoracic pressure and thereby, it acts like a suction force to increase VR.
  - *Abdominal pump:* During respiration compression of abdominal muscles, press on the veins and favors venous emptying.
  - *Cardiac pump:* Vis A Tergo (force from behind), Vis A Fronte (force from front)
  - *Total blood volume:* As the blood volume increases VR increases and vice versa
  - *Capacity of venous system:* Sympathetic stimulation to the veins causes venoconstriction and thereby increases venous emptying
  - *Body position:* On standing, there is venous pooling due to gravity and it may decrease the VR.

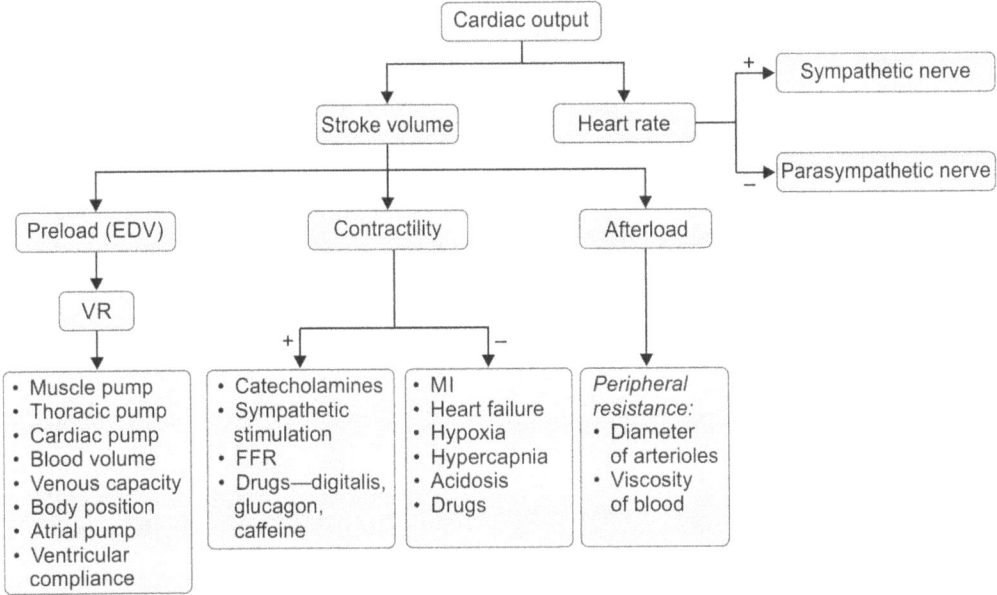

Fig. 11: Regulation of cardiac output.
(FFR: force-frequency relation; MI: myocardial infarction)

- **Atrial pump activity:** Contributes 20% ventricular filling and stimulated by sympathetic stimulation.
- **Ventricular compliance:** Affected by damage to myocardium as in MI, pericardial effusion, cardiac tamponade.

This type of regulation of stroke volume in relation to change in initial length of muscle fiber is said to be **heterometric regulation**.

2. *Contractility:* Contractility is increase in force of contraction and thereby increase in stroke volume without increase in initial muscle length.
   - Ventricles are able to do more work per stroke at a given EDV.
   - Factors which affect contractility—inotropic agents.
   - There are positive and negative inotropic agents.

Contractility is increased by:
- Autonomic activity (sympathetics are positively inotropic)
- **Muscle mass:** Increase in myocardial mass increases contractility as after regular exercise
- Concentration of hormones and chemicals
- **Heart rate:** Force frequency relationship

Factors increasing contractility—positive inotropic agents:
- Sympathetic stimulation
- Circulating catecholamines
- Force frequency relationship
- Digitalis
- Glucagon
- Insulin
- Thyroxine
- Chemicals, such as xanthine, theophylline

Factors decreasing contractility—negative inotropic agents:
- Loss of myocardium as in myocardial infarction
- Hypoxia
- Hypercapnia
- Acidosis
- Acetylcholine

Regulation of stroke volume by affecting contractility of myocardium is **homometric regulation**. Here the force

of contraction is affected without much change in muscle length.
3. **Afterload:**
   - It is the force against which the heart muscle shortens
   - Cardiac output is inversely proportional to After load
   - Cardiac output α 1/after load (anrep effect)
   - It is decided by peripheral resistance
   - **Peripheral resistance is decided by:**
     - Vessel diameter
     - Viscosity of blood
   - This is also included in homometric regulation.

II. **Regulation of heart rate:**
   - Heart rate is also a factor affecting CO.
   - HR is in turn regulated by autonomic nerves.
   - Sympathetics →↑ heart rate
   - Parasympathetics →↓HR
   - Normally ↑ HR →↑CO
   - But in severe tachycardia →↓ duration of diastole →↓ Ventricular filling →↓ CO

Measurement of cardiac output:
Fick's Principle
- Fick's principle is defined as the amount of substance taken up by an organ or the whole body per unit of time and is equal to the arteriovenous difference of the substance times the blood flow.
- Substance taken by an organ = A-V difference X blood flow
- Blood flow = Substance taken by the organ/A-V difference
- Here the substance taken up is oxygen consumed by the whole organ
- Output of left ventricle = O_2 consumption (mL/min)/$A_{(O2)} - V_{(O2)}$
- O_2 consumed is derived with spirometry
- Arterial blood sample is taken from peripheral artery
- Venous sample is collected from pulmonary artery
  = 250 mL/min/200 mL/L-150 mL/L
  = 250 mL/min/50 mL/L
  = 5 L/min

- **Advantage:** Accurate and no chemical is injected
- **Disadvantage:** Needs hospitalization, catheterization, etc.

Ejection fraction
- It is the percentage of end diastolic volume which is ejected per beat.
- Stroke volume is given as the percentage of EDV
- EF = SV/EDV × 100
- Normal value is about 65%
- It is a good indicator of left ventricular functioning.

---

8. List the ascending tracts in the spinal cord and discuss the tracts of posterior column with diagram.

The ascending tracts in the spinal cord are:
☐ Dorsal column—fasciculus gracilis and fasciculus cuneatus
☐ Spinothalamic tracts—lateral and anterior spinothalamic tracts
☐ Spinocerebellar tracts—dorsal and Ventral spinocerebellar tracts
☐ Spinotectal tract
☐ Spino-olivary tract
☐ Spinovestibular tract
☐ Spinoreticular tract

Tracts of Posterior/Dorsal Column
☐ The posterior or dorsal column consists of the tracts of Goll and Burdach
☐ They ascend up in two fasciculi—fasciculus gracilis and fasciculus cuneatus
☐ They are made up of large myelinated fibers which carry sensations, such as touch, pressure, vibration, stereognosis, tactile localization, tactile discrimination and proprioception.
☐ Gracile fasciculus lies medially and carries these sensations from the hind limb and trunk, the cuneate fasciculus lies laterally and carries impulses from the upper half of the body and upper limbs.
☐ It is also called as the lemniscal system (*refer* **Fig. 12**).
☐ First order neurons have their cell bodies in the dorsal root ganglia.

- Medial lemniscus terminate on the ventroposterolateral nucleus (VPLN) of the opposite side thalamus.
- Third order neuron arises from the thalamus and terminates in the somatosensory area 1 (Broadman's are 3, 1, 2) in postcentral gyrus.

II. SHORT NOTES

1. Anticoagulants.

Anticoagulants are chemicals used to prevent clotting of blood. They are classified as in vitro and in vivo anticoagulants.

In vitro anticoagulants: These are chemicals used to prevent clotting of blood while transporting blood to laboratories or while storing blood in blood banks.

They are:
- **Ethylenediaminetetraacetic (EDTA):** This is the anticoagulant of choice in laboratories. It makes Ca^{2+} unavailable for clotting by chelating it. It is used to determine ESR.
- **Trisodium citrate:** This anticoagulant is used for determining clotting disorders and also ESR. This prevents clotting by chelation of Ca^{2+}
- **Double oxalate mixture:** It is a mixture of ammonium oxalate and potassium oxalate. It prevents clotting by forming insoluble calcium oxalate precipitate.
- **Heparin:** A naturally occurring anticoagulant is used as an in vitro and in vivo anticoagulant. It activates antithrombin III and antithrombin III prevents clotting of blood.
- Sodium fluoride is an anticoagulant used in the labs for tests to analyze blood glucose levels.

In vivo anticoagulants: These are drugs taken to prevent clot formation within the blood vessels. They are:
- **Heparin:** It is isolated from the liver, lungs and granules of basophils and mast cells. It facilitates action of antithrombin III and

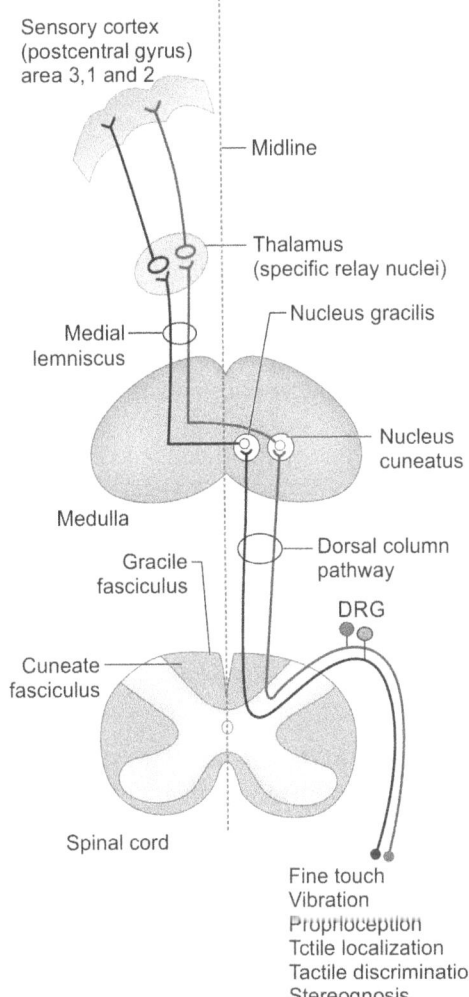

Fig. 12: Pathway of dorsal column tract.

- The peripheral axons of these neurons are nerve fibers from the receptors.
- The central axons from the dorsal root ganglia enter the spinal cord and ascend up in the dorsal column as the dorsal column tract.
- Gracile and cuneate fasciculi reach medulla and synapse with ipsilateral, nucleus gracilis, and nucleus cuneatus respectively.
- From these nuclei, the second order neurons arise and cross to the opposite side and ascend up as the medial lemniscus.

thereby inhibits the active forms of IX, X, XI and XII

☐ **Vitamin K antagonists:**
They are: Coumarin derivatives, such as warfarin, dicoumarol, etc.

They prevent the action of vitamin K by competitively binding with vitamin K receptors.

Vitamin K is a cofactor for the enzyme which catalyzes the conversion of glutamic acid residues to—γ carboxyglutamic acid residues. Six clotting factors require the conversion of glutamic acid to g carboxyglutamic acid. They are factors—II, VII, IX and X, protein C and S.

---

2. G protein.

☐ G proteins are nucleotide regulatory proteins that bind to GTP.
☐ GTP is the guanosine analog of ATP.
☐ There are two types of G proteins—small G proteins and large G proteins.
☐ When signal reaches a G protein, the protein exchanges GDP for GTP and brings about the response. On completion of action, the intrinsic GTPase activity of the protein converts GTP to GDP.

Small G Proteins

These are involved in various cellular functions:
☐ They are members of Rab family—regulate vesicle traffic within a cell.
☐ The Rho/Rac family, which mediates interaction between cytoskeleton and cell membrane.
☐ The Ras family which regulates growth by transmitting signals from cell membrane to nucleus.

Larger Heterotrimeric G Proteins

☐ They couple cell surface receptors to catalytic units on the membrane that catalyzes formation of intracellular second messengers or couple receptors to ion channels.
☐ There are 3 subunits for the G protein—α, β and γ.
☐ Only α subunit is bound to GDP (*refer* **Fig. 13**).
☐ On binding of the ligand to G protein-coupled receptor, GDP is exchanged for GTP and α subunit is separated from β and γ subunits.
☐ The intrinsic GTPase activity of the α subunit converts GTP to GDP and the action is terminated.
☐ There are 5 families of G protein—G_s, G_i, G_t, G_q and G_{13}.

Mechanism of Action Through G Protein-coupled Receptors

☐ Ligand (hormone) binds to the G_s protein coupled receptor
☐ On binding of ligand and receptor, α subunit of G protein seperates from β and γ subunits
☐ On separation of a subunit, the catalytic enzyme—adenylyl cyclase (enzyme) attached to G protein is activated (*refer* **Fig. 14**).
☐ Adenylyl cyclase converts ATP to cAMP.

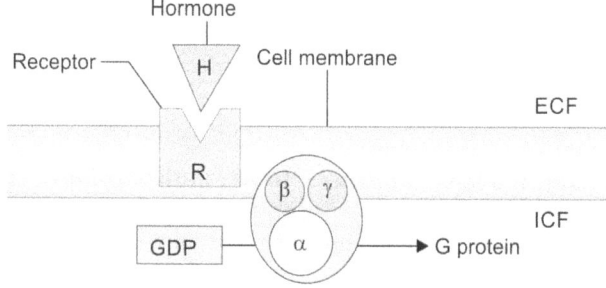

Fig. 13: G protein. Hormone binds to G protein bound receptor on the cell membrane; G protein in inactive form is bound to GDP. There are 3 subunits for G protein-α, β, and γ.

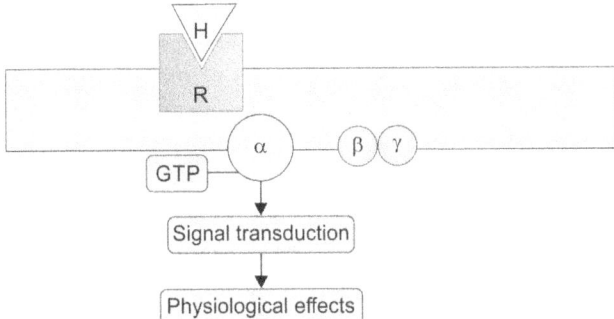

Fig. 14: On binding of hormone to G protein-coupled receptor activates G protein. α-subunit separates and G protein exchanges GDP for GTP. This induces series of actions and is responsible for hormone action.

- cAMP activates the enzyme protein kinase A which phosphorylates proteins and brings about changes.

3. Calcitriol.

Calcitriol is the active form of vitamin D_3 and is also called as 1, 25 dihydroxycholecalciferol.

Synthesis of Calcitriol

Vitamin D_3 is the precursor for synthesis of calcitriol. Vitamin D_3 is got from 2 sources:
- **Dietary intake:** Fish and egg yolk are rich sources of vitamin D_3. The daily requirement in India with good sunlight is 200 IU or 5 µg.
- **From the skin:** Keratinocytes in the skin synthesize vitamin D_3 from 7-dehydrocholesterol, which is an intermediate in synthesis of cholesterol, by the action of sunlight. Previtamin D_3 is formed and is converted to vitamin D_3.
  - Vitamin D_3 is released into blood where it is bound to vitamin D binding protein and reaches the liver.
  - In liver, the next step in synthesis happens. Vitamin D_3 is converted to 25 hydroxycholecalciferol by the enzyme 25 hydroxylase. This next reaches the kidneys in bound form.
  - The last step in synthesis happens in the kidneys. The enzyme 1α hydroxylase converts 25 hydroxycholecalciferol to 1, 25 dihydroxycholecalciferol or calcitriol. 24, 25–dihydroxycholecalciferol, a less active metabolite is also formed.

Regulation of Synthesis of Calcitriol

- **Plasma calcium levels:** Increase in plasma calcium levels decreases parathormone secretion which in turn decreases synthesis of calcitriol. Decrease in blood calcium levels increases PTH levels and calcitriol synthesis increases.
- **Plasma phosphate levels:** Phosphate levels regulate synthesis of calcitriol by negatively inhibiting the enzyme 1, α hydroxylase.
- **Levels of calcitriol:** The calcitriol has a direct negative feedback effect on its synthesis. It also acts on the parathyroid gland and inhibits synthesis of PTH.
- **Other factors,** such as prolactin, estrogen, growth hormone, human chorionic somatomammotropin and calcitonin stimulate synthesis and thyroid hormone excess and acidosis decrease synthesis.

Actions of Calcitriol

- **Action on GIT:** It increases absorption of calcium from the GIT by increasing its permeability of brush border of the enterocytes. It also increases synthesis of calbindin, a calcium binding protein in enterocytes.
- **Actions on bones:** It induces bone resorption and mineralization. In presence of PTH, calcitriol induces bone resorption.
- **Action on kidneys:** It increases reabsorption of calcium and phosphates from the renal tubules.

- **Other actions:** Increases calcium transport into skeletal muscles and bones, stimulation and differentiation of immune cells, it regulates growth and induces formation of growth factors.

Applied Aspects

Rickets

It is metabolic bone disease occurring due to deficiency of vitamin D and there is defective calcification of bone matrix. It is seen in growing children.

Types of rickets:

- **Nutritional rickets:** Due to dietary deficiency of vitamin D, either due to poor intake or poor absorption.
- **Due to inadequate exposure to sunlight:** This happens in cities with less sunlight and children show symptoms by 6 months to 2 years of age.
- **Vitamin D resistant rickets:** Vitamin D deficiency is not there but there is inactivating genetic mutation for renal hydroxylase and calcitriol is not formed.

Symptoms of Rickets

- Weakness and bowing of weight-bearing bones, dental defects, hypocalcemia.
- There could be widening of wrist, collapse of chest wall, kyphosis, pelvic deformities, frontal bossing and rickety rosary—beading of costochondral junction of ribs.

Osteomalacia

This is the adult counter part of rickets. Symptoms are vague, such as muscle pain and weakness, bony tenderness and tetany in few cases.

4. Thyroid function tests.

- Thyroid function tests help us to identify the status of thyroid gland activity.
- It includes, estimation of hormone levels, basal metabolic rate, radioactive iodine uptake, thyroid antibody estimation, thyroid scan, serum cholesterol levels and thyroid biopsy.

Measurement of Thyroid Hormones

- T3 and T4 levels are estimated by ELISA technique.
- More importantly free T3 and free T4 levels are estimated.
- In primary hyperthyroidism, T3 and T4 levels are increased and TSH levels are decreased.
- In primary hypothyroidism, the opposite is seen.

Measurement of Plasma TSH Levels

- It is an important test done to identify thyroid status.
- In primary hypothyroidism, TSH levels are high and T3 and T4 levels are low, but in secondary hypothyroidism TSH, T3 and T4 are all low.
- TSH level is low in primary hyperthyroidism.

TRH Response Test

- Normally on administration of TRH, it increases TSH production and thereby T3 and T4 levels are increased.
- But in primary hyperthyroidism as T3 negatively inhibits TSH production, the levels do not increase.

Radioiodine Uptake Studies

- Iodine is usually taken up by the thyroid gland for formation of T3 and T4.
- So the uptake of radioactive iodine gives an idea about the function of the gland.
- The radioactive forms used are ^{123}I and ^{131}I.
- The RAI is given with water and an X-ray counter is placed on the neck and the thyroid uptake is determined.
- In hyperthyroidism it is increased and in hypothyroidism it is decreased.

Measurement of Basal Metabolic Rate

Normal value is ± 20%, in hyperthyroidism, it is increased up to 100% and in hypothyroidism, it is decreased up to –30 to –40%.

Thyroid Antibody Detection

- This test is done to identify antibodies in Graves' disease and Hashimoto's thyroiditis.
- In Graves' disease, antibodies against TSH receptors are detected and in Hashimoto's disease antibodies against thyroglobulin molecule are detected.

Thyroid Scan

- Ultrasound scanning of the gland gives a clear idea about the nature of lesions in the gland, either cystic or solid lesions.
- CT scan and MRI scan are useful in determining retrosternal and retrotracheal extension of the gland.

Fine Needle Aspiration Biopsy

It is done in patients with nodular goiter to identify malignancies.

---

5. Describe the reflex arcs involved in micturition.

- Urinary bladder is a triangular-shaped sac like structure. The bladder extends down as the urethra.
- The bladder wall is made of detrusor, a smooth muscle and there are two sphincters—internal and external urethral sphincters.
- Internal sphincter is at the neck of the bladder and is made of smooth muscle. It is supplied by sympathetic and parasympathetic nerves.
- External sphincter is made of skeletal muscle and is supplied by somatic motor nerve (pudendal nerve).
- The bladder wall is also supplied by sympathetic and parasympathetic nerves (*refer* **Fig. 15**).
- Parasympathetic nerves (pelvic nerve) have both afferents and efferents to bladder wall and internal sphincter. They arise from S2–S4 segments of spinal cord. When they are stimulated, they cause contraction of bladder wall and relaxation of internal sphincter and therefore emptying of bladder.
- The sympathetic nerves (hypogastric nerve) also have afferents and efferents and they arise from L1–L3 segments of spinal cord. They also supply the bladder wall and internal sphincter. When stimulated, they cause relaxation of bladder wall and contraction of internal sphincter and therefore filling of bladder.
- Somatic nerve (pudendal nerve) to external sphincter arises from S2–S4 segments of spinal cord and have control from higher centers. It is under voluntary control.
- Once urine enters the renal pelvis, it flows through the ureters and enters the bladder, where urine is stored.

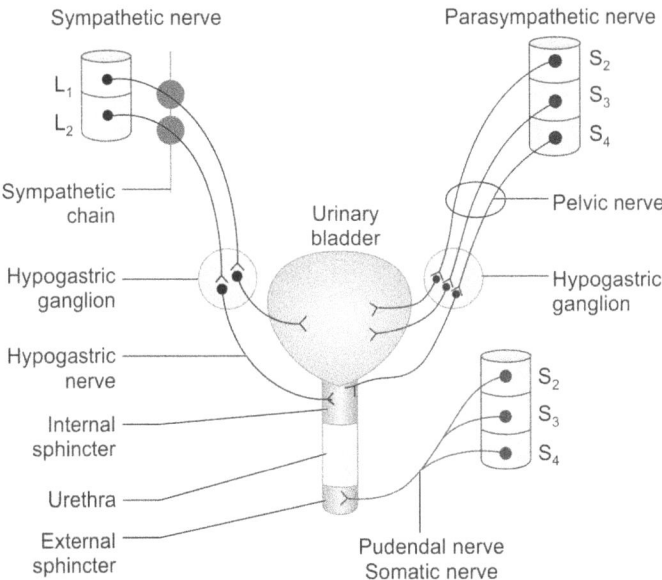

Fig. 15: Nerve supply of urinary bladder.

Micturition Reflex

- Micturition is the process of emptying the urinary bladder.
- **Two processes are involved:**
  1. The bladder fills progressively until the tension in its wall rises above a threshold level, and then
  2. A nervous reflex called the micturition reflex occurs that empties the bladder.

The micturition reflex is an automatic spinal cord reflex; however, it can be inhibited or facilitated by centers in the brainstem and cerebral cortex.

The reflex pathway:
- **Initiation:** Reflex initiated by stimulation of stretch receptors in bladder wall.
- **Stimulus:** Filling of bladder up to 300–400 mL
- **Afferents:** Through pelvic nerves (PS) to reach S2–S4 segments in spinal cord.
- **Efferents:** PS motor fibers from S2–S4 end in the detrusor muscle (excitatory) and internal sphincter (inhibitory) (*refer Fig. 16*).

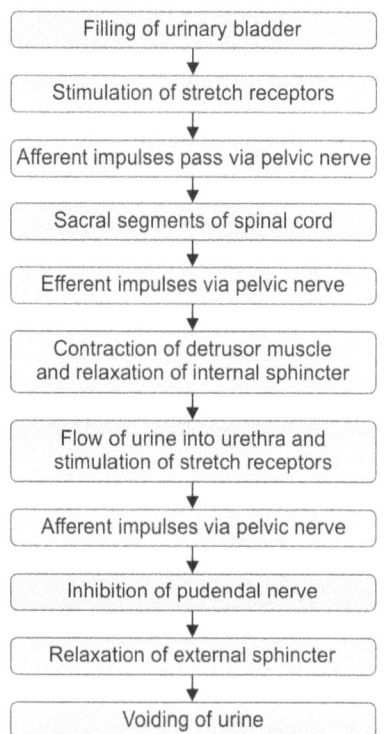

Fig. 16: Micturition reflex.

- **Response:** Causes contraction of bladder wall and relaxation of internal sphincter. Once it becomes powerful another reflex through pudendal nerve relaxes the ES → voiding.

6. Explain the renal contribution to pH control.

- Acids are produced by the body as byproducts of metabolism.
- **They are of two types:**
  1. Volatile acids
  2. Non-volatile acids

Acids are produced by the body as:
- Products of metabolism
- From diets, such as protein
- Strenuous exercise
- Starvation
- Renal tubular generation

Regulation of Acid-base Balance of Kidneys

It is by 3 processes.
1. H^+ secretion in PCT, loop of Henle (LOH) and collecting duct (CD) as Free H^+ (very minimal), as titrable acid and as ammonium.
2. HCO_3^- reabsorption
3. Generation of new HCO_3^- in distal convoluted tubule (DCT) and CD:
   - In most of the segments, H^+ secretion is coupled to HCO_3^- reabsorption as in proximal convoluted tubule (PCT).
   - In PCT and thick ascending limb of loop of Henle (TAL of LOH) it is by Na^+-H^+ exchanger and in I cells of CD it is by ATP driven proton pumps.
   - The renal epithelium secretes nearly 4300 mEq of H^+ daily, of which 85% is from PCT, 10% from DCT and 5% from CD.

H^+ Secretion in PCT
- The filtrate that reaches PCT contains Na^+, HCO_3^-, Cl^-, glucose, amino acids, etc.
- Epithelial cells' lining the PCT secretes H^+ through the secondary active transporter Na^+-H^+ exchanger.
- The epithelial cells lining PCT has the enzyme carbonic anhydrase (CA). It also has many mitochondria.

- CO_2 released following metabolism, combines with water in the presence of CA to form H_2CO_3.
- H_2CO_3 splits into H^+ and HCO_3^-.
- On the luminal membrane, the $Na^+ - H^+$ exchanger secretes H^+ into the lumen in exchange for reabsorption of Na^+.
- As H^+ is being secreted, HCO_3^- is reabsorbed into the interstitium on the basolateral side through an anion exchanger in exchange for Cl^- (refer **Fig. 17**).
- Cl^-, on entering the cell diffuses into the lumen.
- So for every H^+ being secreted into the lumen one bicarbonate is reabsorbed.
- The H^+ which has entered the lumen does not stay as free H^+ and is buffered by the filtered HCO_3^-.
- $H^+ + HCO_3^- \to CO_2 + H_2O$.
- CO_2 enters into the epithelial cells and is recycled to form H^+ and HCO_3^-.
- So the HCO_3^- which is reabsorbed is not the same HCO_3^- which was filtered.
- The H^+ which was added to the tubular fluid does not decrease the pH of the fluid as it is buffered completely by the HCO_3^-.
- So the pH of tubular fluid is not altered much in PCT.
- Mechanism of H^+ secretion in LOH is similar to that of PCT secretion and it happens in the thick ascending limb of LOH.

Secretion of H^+ in DCT and Collecting Duct

- Epithelial cells lining DCT and 'I' cells of CD secrete H^+ through the primary active transporter – H^+ pump or H^+-K^+ pump.
- These cells also contain CA and it catalyzes:
- $CO_2 + H_2O \to H_2CO_3$
- $H_2CO_3 \to H^+ + HCO_3^-$
- H^+ is secreted into the lumen through the pumps.
- HCO_3^- is reabsorbed into the interstitium.
- The H^+ secreted binds to the monobasic phosphate (HPO_4^-) the major buffer present in the tubular fluid in DCT and CD. (By the time the fluid reaches DCT and CD, HCO_3^- is reabsorbed completely and therefore the buffering is done only by HPO_4^- and NH4) (refer **Fig. 18**).
- The H^+ secreted is buffered and results in formation of:
- $HPO_4^- + H^+ \to H_2PO_4$ (Titratable acid)
- $NH_3 + H^+ \to NH_4$ (ammonium)
- Since the H^+ is buffered and stays back in the fluid, pH drops in the tubule and reaches the value 6.
- So this is the site in the renal tubule where maximal acidification of urine happens.
- Here new bicarbonate is also generated.

Generation of New Bicarbonate

It is by two mechanisms:

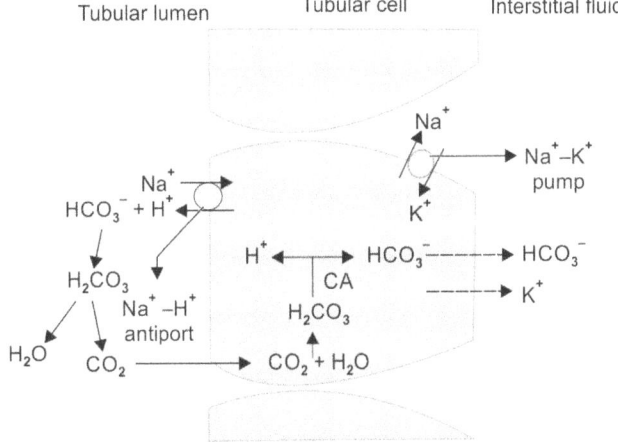

Fig. 17: Secretion of H^+ and reabsorption of HCO_3^- in PCT.

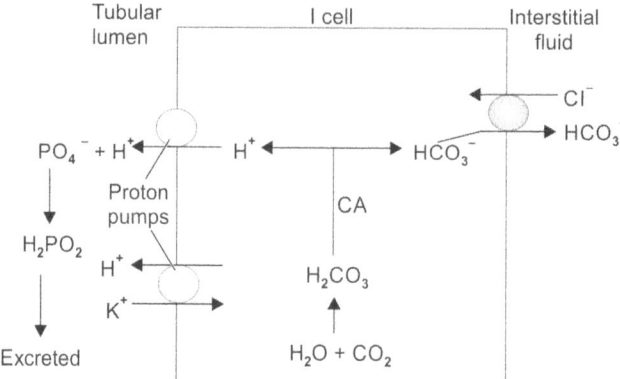

Fig. 18: H^+ secretion in DCT and collecting duct.

1. **Non-bicarbonate buffering:**
   - The H^+ secreted in excess of HCO_3^- reabsorption is buffered in the DCT by HPO_4^{2-} to form the **titrable acid – H_2PO_4**.
   - The amount of H_2PO_4 formed is equal to new HCO_3 formed and re-absorbed.
2. **By glutamine catabolism:**
   - Glutamine → Glutamate + NH_4
   - Glutamate → α-Ketoglutarate + NH_4 + 2 HCO_3
   - $NH_4 \leftrightarrow NH_3 + H^+$
   - Glutamine metabolism happens in the PCT and it generates 2 HCO_3 and NH_3 for buffering H^+.

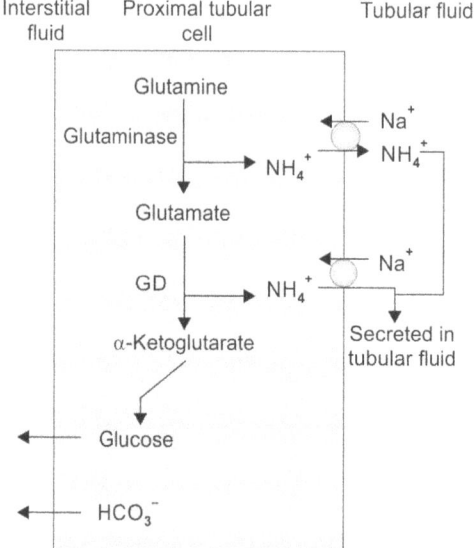

Fig. 19: Formation of ammonium and its excretion.

- NH_3 is easily diffusible across cell membranes whereas NH_4 is not permeable through membranes (refer Fig. 19).
- In TAL of LOH, NH_4 is reabsorbed through Na^+-K^+-2 Cl^- where NH_4 occupies the transporter instead of K^+ and is taken into the interstitium. Here it stays in equilibrium with NH_3. NH_3 diffuses into cells of CD and is secreted into the CD lumen where it binds to H^+ form NH_4. NH_4 cannot diffuse across the cell membrane and therefore stays in the urine to be excreted.
- In metabolic acidosis, the amount of excretion of NH_4 is increased and decreases urinary pH accordingly.

7. Tuguloglomerular feedback mechanism.

- Tubuloglomerular (TG) feedback is an autoregulatory mechanism in the kidneys to regulate the renal blood flow (RBF) and thereby glomerular filtration rate (GFR).
- This feedback mechanism is dependant on the NaCl content in tubular fluid.
- NaCl content in the tubular fluid is sensed by Macula densa cells and signals are sent to the afferent arterioles to regulate RBF and GFR.
- Increased renal arterial pressure increases glomerular capillary pressure and thereby increases filtration.
- Increased GFR leads to increased NaCl content in the tubular fluid. This is

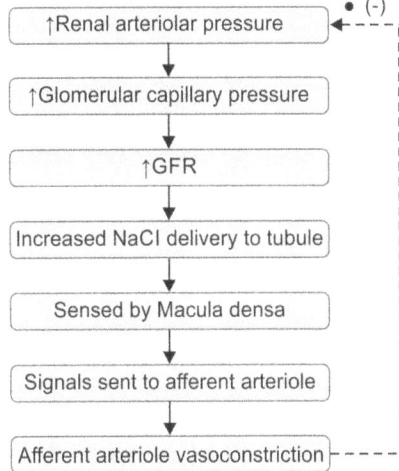

Fig. 20: Tubologlomerular feedback.

sensed by macula densa cells and they send signals to cause vasoconstriction of afferent arterioles and thereby decreases RBF and GFR and NaCl content is brought back to normal.
- **If NaCl content is less, it is sensed by the Macula densa cells and signals are sent to afferent arterioles resulting in vasodilation followed by increased RBF and GFR.**
- The chemicals mediating this feedback may be thromboxane A_2 or adenosine for vasoconstriction and nitric oxide (NO) for vasodilation and they are released by the macula densa cells (*refer* **Fig. 20**).

8. Functions of plasma proteins.

Albumin, globulin and fibrinogen are the plasma proteins.

Functions

- Fibrinogen helps in blood coagulation.
- Albumin helps in maintaining colloidal oncotic pressure which is around 25–30 mm Hg. Oncotic pressure is related inversely to molecular shape, size and directly proportional to concentration of molecules. Therefore, 80% of oncotic pressure is contributed by albumin.
- Maintains acid-base balance in blood. Plasma proteins act as buffers and they are amphoteric in nature. Therefore, they buffer both acids and base and maintain pH at 7.4.
- Maintains the viscosity of blood—since 80% of the total plasma proteins is contributed by albumin, they regulate the viscosity of blood.
- Diastolic blood pressure is regulated by peripheral resistance which in turn is regulated by viscosity of blood and therefore plasma proteins regulate BP.
- Immunoglobulins provide immunity
- Transport function—plasma proteins combine with the following substances and transport them—hormones, drugs, metals, bilirubin, etc.

9. Hemophilia.

- Hemophilia is a bleeding disorder usually seen in the males. In majority of cases, there is deficiency of Factor VIII. This is said to be classical hemophilia or Hemophilia A.
- It is an X-linked recessive disease. Therefore, the males are affected and females are carriers of the disease.
- There are soft tissue hematomas and hemarthrosis which may happen repeatedly resulting in crippling arthropathy.
- Usually, there are no spontaneous hemorrhages but there is excessive bleeding after even a mild injury as in tooth extraction.
- Condition is characterized by prolonged clotting time (normal CT = 3-8 minutes) and normal bleeding time. APTT is prolonged.
- Treatment is done by fresh blood transfusion. Factor VIII can also be prepared from fresh frozen plasma and injected.
- Christmas disease or **Hemophilia** B is due to deficiency of factor IX. It is also a sex-linked recessive disease. Symptoms are similar to hemophilia A. Diagnosis is done by the assay of Factor IX.
- **Hemophilia C** is due to deficiency of Factor XI. It affects both males and females.

10. Counter current blood flow in the villi.

- Counter current flow means flow of fluids, in two closely placed parallel tubes, in opposite directions and there is exchange of substances between the fluids in the tubes.
- This mechanism is present in the kidneys, villi of intestines and in the cutaneous vessels.
- In the intestinal villi, it is between the capillaries and venules and the main arterioles.
- The blood flow in these two vessels is in opposite directions.
- The substance getting exchanged here is oxygen.
- The counter current mechanism favors diffusion of oxygen from ascending arterial limb into the descending venous limb (without going through capillaries).
- So in conditions of slow flow rates, O_2 diffuses out of arterioles and enters the venules at the base of the villus.
- So the cells of the tips of villi suffer from hypoxia and they are prone for necrosis.

11. Frank-Starling's Law of the heart.

It states that within physiological limits, the force of contraction is directly proportional to the initial length of the muscle.

Causes for Application of Frank-starling's Law

- Increase in EDV →↑ stretch of muscle fiber → interaction of thick and thin filament increases →↑ force of contraction.
- Stretch of muscle fibers → opens stretch sensitive Ca^{2+} channels on sarcolemma →↑ Ca^{2+} influx →↑ force of contraction.
- ↑Ca^{2+} influx →↑ Ca^{2+} release from SR (CICR) →↑ force of contraction.
- stretch of muscle fiber →↑ affinity of troponin for Ca^{2+}

12. Cardiac pacemaker potential.

- In the mammalian heart, sinoatrial node is the pace maker. It is said to be the pace maker as it generates impulses by itself without neural input at a faster rate.
- Other tissues of the heart—AV node, atria and ventricle are also capable of generating impulses but SA node generates impulses at a faster rate and therefore said to be the pacemaker of the heart.

Pacemaker Potential

- The ventricular and atrial muscle cells have a resting membrane potential of: –90 mV. On stimulation, the membrane depolarizes and produces an action potential.
- The pacemaker cells are smaller and rounded (P cells) and they do not have a stable resting membrane potential and RMP is around -55 to –60 mV.
- From –60 mV there is a slow depolarization slope which reaches the firing level of –40 mV and there is a rapid depolarization followed by rapid repolarization back to –60 mV and again there is a slow depolarization slope rising to firing level.
- This slope which takes the membrane to firing level is the **pacemaker potential or prepotential**.

Ionic Events Responsible for Pacemaker Potential

- At –60 mV the K^+ channels start closing down thereby preventing K^+ efflux. This is responsible for the first part of prepotential (the slope).
- Next part is due to opening up of 'f' type Na^+ channels (the Na^+ current in this channel is said to be funny current as the channel opens in hyperpolarization).
- Last part of depolarization of the prepotential is due to opening of T-type (Transient) Ca^{2+} channels allowing Ca^{2+} influx (*refer* **Fig. 21**).
- Now as the firing level is reached (-40 mV), the long lasting Ca^{2+} channels (L-Type) open and produces a rapid depolarization and the action potential.
- Then the K^+ channels open and the K^+ efflux bring about rapid repolarization and membrane potential reaches –60 mV. Then the next prepotential starts.
- So in the pacemaker cells, it is a Ca^{2+} dependant depolarization rather than Na^+

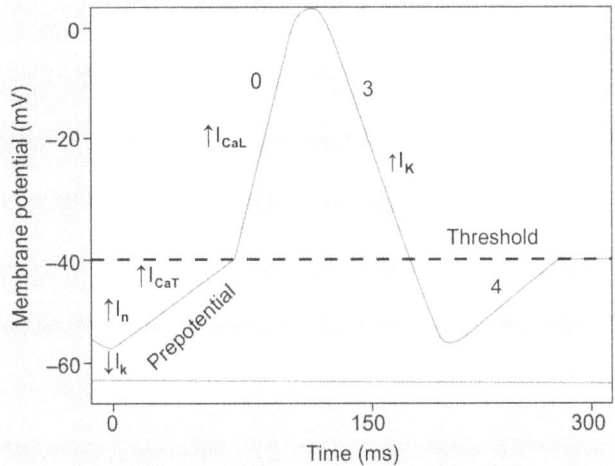

Fig. 21: Pacemaker potential. Slope of pacemaker potential (phase 4), the prepotential is due to 3 events; first part of depolarization is due to closure of K+ channels, 2nd part is due to Na+ influx through sodium channel and last part of depolarization is due to Ca^{2+} influx through T-type Ca^{2+} channels. Rapid depolarization (phase 0) is due to opening of L-type Ca^{2+} channels and repolarization (phase 3) due to opening of K+ channels.

- dependent depolarization as in ventricular muscles.
- The pacemaker cells are supplied by sympathetic and parasympathetic nerves.
- On stimulation by sympathetic nerves, the prepotential slope becomes steeper and the rate of spontaneous discharge increases thereby increasing the heart rate.
- On stimulation by the parasympathetic nerves, the slope of the prepotential decreases and spontaneous firing also decreases thereby heart rate decreases.

13. Draw a labeled diagram of a normal ECG in lead II. Write a brief note on PR interval.

Normal ECG in Lead II

- Lead II is a bipolar limb lead between right arm (negative electrode) and left arm (positive electrode).
- The ECG tracing in lead II shows both negative and positive deflections equally and therefore used as a standard recording.
- There are intervals and segments in the ECG.

ECG Waves

- There are positive and negative waves are deflections in the ECG tracing.
- There are 4 waveforms—P wave, QRS complex, T wave and U wave (*refer* **Fig. 22**).
  a. *P wave:* This is the first positive wave in ECG and is due to atrial depolarization. Duration is 0.1 second.
  b. *QRS complex:* Consists of a negative Q wave, positive R wave and negative S wave. This complex is due to ventricular depolarization. Normal duration is 0.08 seconds.
  c. *T wave* is a positive deflection following QRS complex and is due to

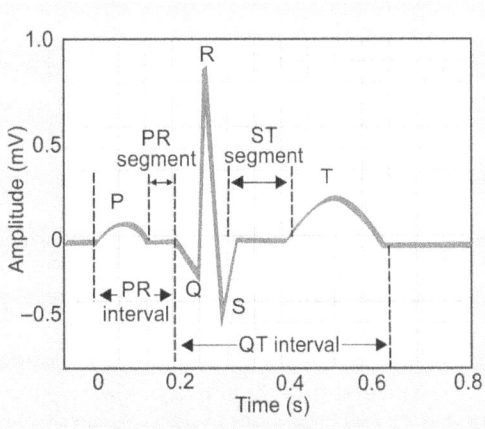

Fig. 22: Normal ECG in lead II with waves, segments and intervals.

ventricular repolarization. Normal duration is 0.27 seconds.

d. *U wave* is also positive deflection and is normally not seen. It is seen in slow depolarization of the papillary muscle. Duration is 0.08 seconds.

PR Interval

- It is between beginning of P wave to beginning of Q wave.
- The normal duration is 0.12–0.2 sec (average 0.18 sec).
- This denotes atrial depolarization and conduction to AV node.
- Prolonged PR interval signifies AV conduction block
- It denotes the diastolic phase of the atria.

14. Non-progressive shock.

- It is a stage in shock where the amount of blood lost is less than 1 L. Various body mechanisms try to compensate the decrease in circulatory volume and try to correct the blood loss and cause full recovery without any treatment.
- It is also called as compensated stage

The following are the compensatory mechanisms:

- Immediate **tachycardia** and increase in pulse rate: Due to decrease in blood volume, baroreceptors are inhibited which results in sympathetic nerve stimulation.
- Sympathetic stimulation causes **vasoconstriction** in all the vessels except cerebral and coronary vasculature.
- Sympathetic nerves also cause **venoconstriction** which results in increased venous return and thereby increased cardiac output and blood pressure.
- Due to loss of RBC and stagnant blood flow, chemoreceptors are stimulated → **Tachypnea** → thoracic pumping → Increases venous return (VR) and thereby cardiac output and BP increase.
- **Restlessness,** due to release of adrenaline → skeletal muscle activity →increase in VR
- Movement of interstitial fluid into capillaries → **increases blood volume**
- Increased **secretion of renin, angiotensin II and aldosterone** → Reabsorption of electrolytes and water from tubules → Increase in blood volume
- Increased secretion of ADH
- Long-term compensations are increase in **erythropoiesis and plasma protein synthesis.**

15. Traveling waves in the ear.

- When sound waves travel in the middle ear and hit on foot plate of stapes and as a result it vibrates.
- This creates pressure waves in the perilymph of scala vestibuli like ripples in water.
- The waves displace the basilar membrane and make the hairs of the hair cells to tilt and thereby stimulate the nerves in the bases of the hair cells.
- Wave of displacement of basilar membrane starts at the base of cochlea near the oval window and gradually moves towards the apex.
- These pressure waves are called as **traveling waves.**
- The site of maximum displacement of the basilar membrane is dependant on the frequency of sound waves.
- Higher frequency sounds creates maximum amplitude of pressure waves and thereby maximum displacement of basilar membrane at the base of cochlea and lower frequency waves induce a wave close to the apex of cochlea.
- So based on place of stimulation of hair cells, the frequency or pitch discrimination of sound is possible.

16. Ventilation-perfusion ratio.

- It is the ratio of ventilation to the lungs to the blood flow through pulmonary circulation.
- Alveolar ventilation (V_a) is 4000 L/min and perfusion (Q) is equal to cardiac output; 5 L/min
- So V_a/Q ratio = 4/5 = 0.8
- Ventilation as well as perfusion increases from apex to the base of lungs due to the effect of gravity.

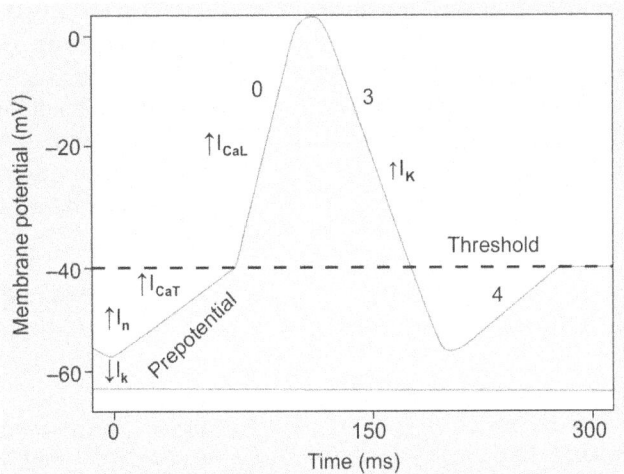

Fig. 21: Pacemaker potential. Slope of pacemaker potential (phase 4), the prepotential is due to 3 events; first part of depolarization is due to closure of K⁺ channels, 2nd part is due to Na⁺ influx through sodium channel and last part of depolarization is due to Ca²⁺ influx through T-type Ca²⁺ channels. Rapid depolarization (phase 0) is due to opening of L-type Ca²⁺ channels and repolarization (phase 3) due to opening of K⁺ channels.

dependent depolarization as in ventricular muscles.
- The pacemaker cells are supplied by sympathetic and parasympathetic nerves.
- On stimulation by sympathetic nerves, the prepotential slope becomes steeper and the rate of spontaneous discharge increases thereby increasing the heart rate.
- On stimulation by the parasympathetic nerves, the slope of the prepotential decreases and spontaneous firing also decreases thereby heart rate decreases.

13. Draw a labeled diagram of a normal ECG in lead II. Write a brief note on PR interval.

Normal ECG in Lead II
- Lead II is a bipolar limb lead between right arm (negative electrode) and left arm (positive electrode).
- The ECG tracing in lead II shows both negative and positive deflections equally and therefore used as a standard recording.
- There are intervals and segments in the ECG.

ECG Waves
- There are positive and negative waves are deflections in the ECG tracing.

- There are 4 waveforms—P wave, QRS complex, T wave and U wave (*refer* **Fig. 22**).
  a. *P wave:* This is the first positive wave in ECG and is due to atrial depolarization. Duration is 0.1 second.
  b. *QRS complex:* Consists of a negative Q wave, positive R wave and negative S wave. This complex is due to ventricular depolarization. Normal duration is 0.08 seconds.
  c. *T wave* is a positive deflection following QRS complex and is due to

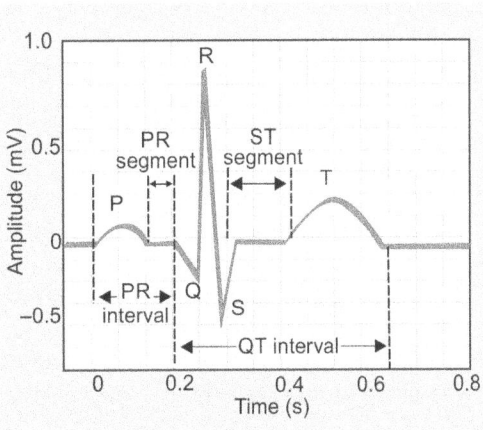

Fig. 22: Normal ECG in lead II with waves, segments and intervals.

ventricular repolarization. Normal duration is 0.27 seconds.

d. *U wave* is also positive deflection and is normally not seen. It is seen in slow depolarization of the papillary muscle. Duration is 0.08 seconds.

PR Interval

- It is between beginning of P wave to beginning of Q wave.
- The normal duration is 0.12–0.2 sec (average 0.18 sec).
- This denotes atrial depolarization and conduction to AV node.
- Prolonged PR interval signifies AV conduction block
- It denotes the diastolic phase of the atria.

14. Non-progressive shock.

- It is a stage in shock where the amount of blood lost is less than 1 L. Various body mechanisms try to compensate the decrease in circulatory volume and try to correct the blood loss and cause full recovery without any treatment.
- It is also called as compensated stage

The following are the compensatory mechanisms:

- Immediate **tachycardia** and increase in pulse rate: Due to decrease in blood volume, baroreceptors are inhibited which results in sympathetic nerve stimulation.
- Sympathetic stimulation causes **vasoconstriction** in all the vessels except cerebral and coronary vasculature.
- Sympathetic nerves also cause **venoconstriction** which results in increased venous return and thereby increased cardiac output and blood pressure.
- Due to loss of RBC and stagnant blood flow, chemoreceptors are stimulated → **Tachypnea** → thoracic pumping → Increases venous return (VR) and thereby cardiac output and BP increase.
- **Restlessness,** due to release of adrenaline → skeletal muscle activity →increase in VR
- Movement of interstitial fluid into capillaries → **increases blood volume**
- Increased **secretion of renin, angiotensin II and aldosterone** → Reabsorption of electrolytes and water from tubules → Increase in blood volume
- Increased secretion of ADH
- Long-term compensations are increase in **erythropoiesis and plasma protein synthesis.**

15. Traveling waves in the ear.

- When sound waves travel in the middle ear and hit on foot plate of stapes and as a result it vibrates.
- This creates pressure waves in the perilymph of scala vestibuli like ripples in water.
- The waves displace the basilar membrane and make the hairs of the hair cells to tilt and thereby stimulate the nerves in the bases of the hair cells.
- Wave of displacement of basilar membrane starts at the base of cochlea near the oval window and gradually moves towards the apex.
- These pressure waves are called as **traveling waves.**
- The site of maximum displacement of the basilar membrane is dependant on the frequency of sound waves.
- Higher frequency sounds creates maximum amplitude of pressure waves and thereby maximum displacement of basilar membrane at the base of cochlea and lower frequency waves induce a wave close to the apex of cochlea.
- So based on place of stimulation of hair cells, the frequency or pitch discrimination of sound is possible.

16. Ventilation-perfusion ratio.

- It is the ratio of ventilation to the lungs to the blood flow through pulmonary circulation.
- Alveolar ventilation (V_a) is 4000 L/min and perfusion (Q) is equal to cardiac output; 5 L/min
- So V_a/Q ratio = 4/5 = 0.8
- Ventilation as well as perfusion increases from apex to the base of lungs due to the effect of gravity.

- But rate of increase of perfusion is more than the rate of increase in ventilation
- So V_a/Q ratio is more in the apex (3.3) than the base (0.63)
- Therefore, there is high oxygen content in apex than base of lungs.

Applied Aspect

- The high O_2 content in the apex favors the growth of TB bacilli there.
- The V_a/Q ratio can get altered in conditions of uneven ventilation and non-uniform blood flow to alveoli as in certain disease conditions.

17. Caisson disease.

- Also called as "dysbarism, the bends, decompression sickness, Diver's palsy".
- This happens when a person breathing compressed air ascends up rapidly.
- At high pressures, N_2 dissolves in body fluids and stays dissolved.
- When the person ascends up to sea level gradually N_2 is converted to air gradually and is blown out.
- But when the ascends up rapidly the dissolved N_2 does not have enough time to be converted to air and to be blown out and therefor it stays in the tissues as N_2 bubbles.
- N_2 dissolved in tissues forms bubbles while escaping from tissues due to rapid ascent.
- Gas bubbles block the blood vessels and stay in tissues to create symptoms.

Symptoms are:
- Pain in joints and muscles of legs or arms.
- Sensation of numbness
- The chokes—shortness of breath, pulmonary edema, etc.
- Paralysis of muscles
- Coronary ischemia
- Neurological symptoms

Treatment: Recompression in pressurized chamber followed by slow decompression.

18. Brown-Séquard syndrome.

Hemi-section of spinal cord is called Brown-Séquard syndrome. It involves lesion of one lateral half of spinal cord.

Following injury to the spinal cord, there are these following stages:
I. Stage of spinal shock
II. Stage of reflex activity
III. Stage of reflex failure

Immediately after the lesion, there is complete loss of function below the level of lesion. This happens because of sudden removal of impulses from higher centers.

The symptoms of Brown-Séquard are seen in the second stage. Symptoms are explained as the features above the level of lesion, at the level and below the level of lesion, on the same side and opposite side of lesion.

	Sensory		Motor	
	Same side	*Opposite side*	*Same side*	*Opposite side*
Above the level of lesion	Small area of hyperesthesia	Normal	Normal	Normal
At the level of lesion	Complete loss of sensation (anesthesia)	Not affected	Lower motor neuron type of paralysis	Not affected
Below the level of lesion	**Damage to dorsal column fibers:** Loss of fine touch, tactile localization, two point discrimination, vibration sense, stereognosis and position sense	**Damage to lateral and anterior spinothalamic tract:** Loss of pain, temperature and crude touch sensations. All other sensations are intact	Upper motor neuron type of paralysis as the inhibition from higher centers is removed. Temporary loss of vasomotor tone	Not usually affected

19. Functions of ascending reticular activating system.

- Reticular formation (RF) is located in the core of brain stem starting from the upper part of spinal cord to the lower part of diencephalon.
- It is like a mesh with many neurons interspersed among bundles of axons.
- Neurons in RF have both sensory and motor functions.
- Ascending reticular activating system (ARAS) is a part of RF consisting of sensory fibers projecting to cerebral cortex (*refer* **Fig. 23**).
- It is an ascending column of fibers.

Functions of ARAS

- It helps to maintain consciousness and also arousal from sleep.
- Controls sleep and wakefulness
- It helps in learning and memory
- Involved in genesis of EEG waves

20. Role of Purkinje cells of cerebellum.

- Purkinje cells are present in the middle layer (Purkinje cell layer) in the cerebellar cortex.
- It is the largest neuron with large amount of dendritic branches
- The dendrites of Purkinje cells project to the outermost layer of the cortex (molecular layer) where they synapse with

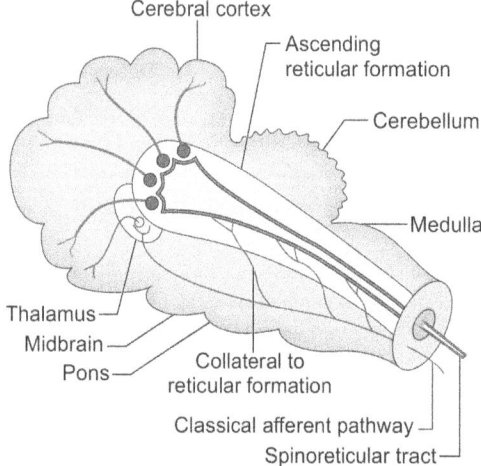

Fig. 23: Ascending reticular activating system.

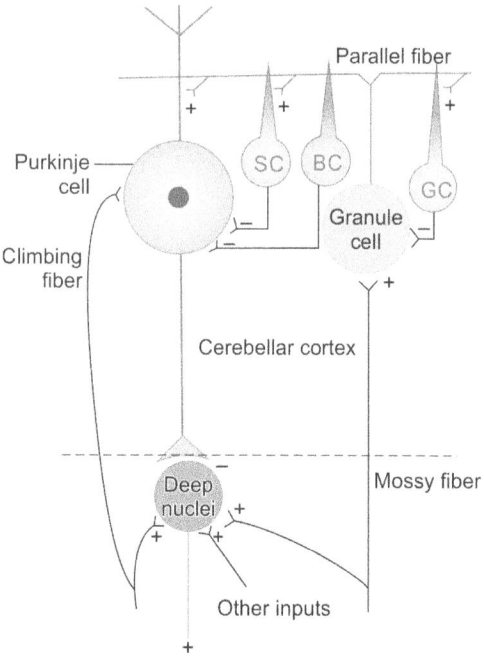

Fig. 24: Purkinje cells in cerebellar cortex. Afferents to cerebellum through climbing fibers end on deep nuclei and Purkinje cell. Mossy fibers end on granule cells. Output of cerebellar cortex is only through Purkinje cell.

axons of the neurons in this layer (*refer* **Fig. 24**).

- The climbing fiber which is one of the afferents coming into the cerebellum ends on the Purkinje cells. Climbing fiber consists of olivocerebellar tract which arises from inferior olivary nucleus in medulla.
- Purkinje cells are the only output from the cerebellar cortex which project to the deep cerebellar nuclei.
- The efferents leave the cerebellum from the deep nuclei.
- Purkinje cells are involved in learning of motor tasks.
- It has been experimentally proved by increased activity in climbing fibers when a motor task is being learnt.

21. Functions of platelets.

- **Role in primary hemostasis or temporary platelet plug formation:** Damage to the endothelial lining of the blood vessels exposes collagen which activates

the platelets and results in adhesion and aggregation of platelets to the injured vessel and thereby seals the injured vessel. Platelets have receptors for collagen, ADP and VWF which favor adhesion of platelets.
- **Role in secondary hemostasis:** Formation of clot is said to be the secondary hemostasis. The platelets release platelet phospholipid and platelet factor II which activates prothrombin to thrombin.
- **Role in clot retraction:** Platelets have contractile proteins actin, myosin and thrombosthenin. Once the platelets and other blood cells are trapped in the fibrin mesh, these contractile proteins contract and the clot shrinks. This squeezes out the serum from the clot. Clot retraction happens only in the presence of functional platelets and it helps in sealing the wound in the blood vessel.
- Platelets store and release serotonin (5HT) which is a potent vasoconstrictor.
- Platelets also stores and release platelet derived growth factor which multiplies endothelial cells and fibroblasts and thereby help in wound healing.
- Platelets are also involved in mild phagocytosis. They ingest carbon particles, immune complexes and viral particles.

22. Composition and functions of gastric Juice.

Composition of Gastric Juice

- 2-2.5 L/day
- pH 1-2
- **Water:** 99.45%
- **Solids:** 0.55%
- **Electrolytes:** Na⁺, K⁺, Mg^{2+}, Cl⁻, HCO_3^-, HPO_4^-, SO_4^-
- **Enzymes:** Pepsin, lipase, gelatinase
- **Mucus:** Insoluble and soluble
- Intrinsic factor

Functions of Gastric Secretion

Role of Enzymes in Stomach

- Pepsin helps in digestion of proteins.
- Rennin causes coagulation of milk and slows the passage of milk from stomach
- Gelatinase liquifies gelatin in connective tissues
- Gastric lipase splits fats

Role of HCl

- It protects against infection from microorganisms entering along with the food.
- It creates a low pH which activates pepsinogen to pepsin.

Role of Mucus

- Soluble mucus secreted by cardiac and pyloric glands provides lubrication for passage of food.
- Viscid mucus secreted by main gastric glands protects the mucosa from digestion of HCl.

Role of Intrinsic Factor

Helps in absorption of vitamin B12.

23. Molecular basis of skeletal muscle contraction.

- Muscle, on excitation by action potential results in contraction.
- So the electrical phenomenon has led to a mechanical response.
- The linking of the electrical event to a mechanical response is given as excitation—contraction coupling.

Excitation—Contraction Coupling

When the motor nerve to the skeletal muscle is excited, the neurotransmitter acetylcholine (ACh) is released at the neuromuscular junction.

The ACh binds to **Nicotinic ACh receptors** in the muscle membrane below the nerve— *the motor end plate*

On binding of ACh with receptor (which by itself is a channel) results in opening of the non-specific cation channels followed by influx of sodium ions and there is a local depolarization of motor end plate—*end plate potential (EPP)*

The EPP excites the neighboring muscle membrane and action potential is generated in the muscle membrane.

↓

The AP spreads to the T-tubule and activates dihydropyridine receptors (DHP) which in turn triggers the calcium release channels called the Ryanodine receptors in SR and calcium ions are released.

↓

Calcium diffuses into the cytoplasm and gets attached to the troponin C. Binding of calcium with troponin C triggers many events resulting in muscle contraction.

Muscle Contraction

- Sliding theory or ratchet theory had been put forward to explain muscle contraction by AF Huxley and HE Huxley in 1954.
- This theory postulates that the actin filament slide over the myosin filament following the formation of actin-myosin complexes and cross-bridge cycling.
- At rest, the myosin binding site on actin is covered by tropomyosin and inhibits binding of actin and myosin.
- On binding of calcium with troponin C, tropomyosin molecule changes its configuration and moves out, exposing myosin binding sites on actin.
- For each tropomyosin molecule moving out, 7 actin molecules are exposed.

Cross-bridge Cycling

- Each myosin head has two binding sites.
- One for binding with actin and other one is an ATPase which hydrolysis ATP.
- On attaching with one ATP, the ATPase hydrolyses the ATP molecule and the energy is stored in the head and thereby it is energized.
- ADP and Pi are also attached to the head.
- The energized head is 90° perpendicular to thin filament.
- **Power stroke:** When the troponin C binds with Ca^{2+}, the actin binding sites for myosin are exposed and the perpendicular energized head binds to actin (*refer* **Fig. 25**).
- Immediately after binding, the head flexes from 90° to 45° and ADP and Pi are released. This is said to be the power stroke or cross bridge cycling.
- The bent head is detached from actin molecule when another ATP molecule binds to the myosin head.
- This ATP is again hydrolyzed and the head is re-energized and ready to undergo the next cycle.
- As a result of repeated cross-bridge cycling, the actin filament from either side is moved towards the center of A band and there is muscle contraction.

24. Sertoli cells.

- These are supporting cells in seminiferous tubules.
- They play a major role in the maturation of spermatozoa. Spermatids mature into spermatozoa in the deep folds of cytoplasm in the Sertoli cells.
- They provide nutrition to the developing spermatozoa and help in spermiation.
- They take part in the formation of blood-testis barrier which selectively allows certain substances to enter seminiferous tubule.
- They phagocytose damaged germ cells.
- They secrete seminal fluid
- Sertoli cells produce substances, such as:
  - Mullerian inhibiting substance (MIS) — causes regression of Mullerian duct and promotes development of structures from the Wolffian duct.
  - Inhibin—inhibits FSH secretion
  - Activin
  - Androgen binding protein (ABP)—this helps to maintain a high concentration of androgens in the seminiferous tubule which is essential for spermatogenesis
  - Estrogen is produced from androgen in the presence of Aromatase which is present in the Sertoli cells.

25. Rh blood group.

Rh System

- Rh system is the 2nd most important blood group system.
- There are 6 antigens of this system—C, D, E, c, d and e.
- But D antigen on the RBC membrane is the most antigenic.

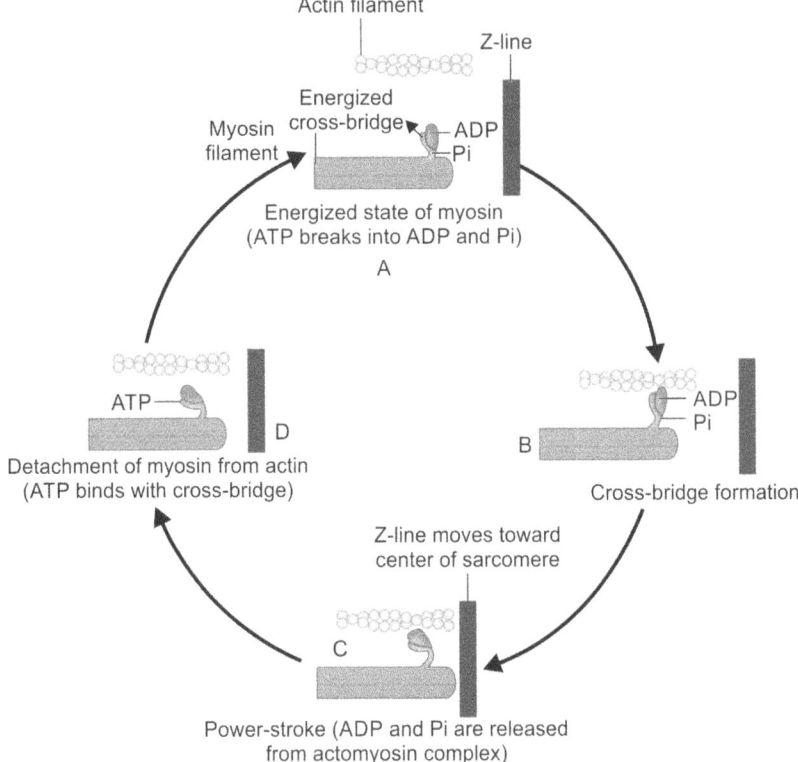

Fig. 25: Cross-bridge cycling in skeletal muscle contraction.

- Therefore individuals with D antigen are Rh-positive and its absence is considered to be Rh-negative.
- About 90–95% of Indian population is Rh-positive.
- Rh system does not follow 2nd law of Landsteiner's, i.e., in an Rh-negative individual the anti-D antibody is not present in plasma.
- But exposure to D antigens for the first time stimulates the immune system to form anti-D antibodies of an Rh-negative person.
- These antibodies can later react on D antigens if they are exposed to it in the second attempt.

Significance of Rh Group

- Rh system is the second most important blood group systems in the body. It was discovered in the rhesus monkey in 1940.
- There are 6 antigens in this system, C, D, E and c, d and e.
- D antigen is highly antigenic and therefore individuals with D antigen on their RBC membrane are Rh-positive and persons without D antigen are Rh-negative.
- Rh antigen is inherited as a dominant gene.
- Therefore, Rh-positive may be homozygous with DD or heterozygous with DD. Rh-negative is homozygous with DD.
- The antibody in Rh system is anti-D antibody.
- There are no naturally occurring antibodies here as in the ABO system.
- But if an Rh-negative person receives Rh-positive blood his immune system recognizes the Rh antigen as foreign and starts producing antibodies.
- So, in first encounter of Rh-positive blood, there is not much complication. On the next exposure, massive antigen antibody reactions happen resulting in agglutination and hemolysis.

- Therefore, the Rh system does not follow the 2nd law of Landsteiner's which states that "If a particular antigen is absent on the RBC membrane the corresponding antibody will be present in the plasma".
- The **most significant aspect** of Rh incompatibility is the mismatch of Rh factor between the mother and the fetus.
- If the mother is Rh-negative and she conceives an Rh-positive fetus, at the time of delivery of the fetus, during the placental separation, a small amount of Rh-positive blood leaks into mother's circulation.
- As the first baby is already born, it is not affected.
- The mother's immune system starts producing anti-D antibodies.
- If she conceives the next time and that fetus is also Rh-positive, the antibodies in the maternal circulation which belongs to IgG type crosses the placenta and attacks the fetal RBCs.
- There is agglutination and hemolysis of fetal RBCs.
- In the subsequent similar pregnancies, the damage to the fetus is severe.
- The child presents with the symptoms of hemolytic disease of the newborn or erythroblastosis fetalis.

The symptoms are:
- **Anemia:** Due to hemolysis the child has anemia.
- **Edema:** The child has generalized edema— hydrops fetalis
- **Jaundice:** Hemolysis releases bilirubin and results in jaundice
- **Kernicterus:** The high bilirubin levels in the neonates damages the basal ganglia. In adults, the blood brain barrier prevents the entry of bilirubin into the brain. But in infants, blood brain barrier is not fully developed, so, the bilirubin easily damages the basal ganglia resulting in motor deficits.
- **Erythroblasts appear in the circulation:** Excessive hemolysis induces erythropoiesis and erythroblasts (the precursors) start appearing in the circulation.

Treatment
- If the hemolysis is mild, no treatment is needed.
- In severe conditions treatment can be given as intrauterine transfusions or after birth, exchange transfusion can be given along with phototherapy.

Prevention
- After the delivery of the Rh-positive fetus by the Rh-negative mother, the mother is immunized with anti-D antibodies.
- These antibodies neutralize the antigens which have entered the mother's circulation and prevent formation of further antibodies.

26. Movements of small intestine.

Five types of movements in the normal state:

Normal Movements
1. **Peristalsis:** Propulsive movement
2. **Mixing movements:** Segmentation contraction and tonic contraction
3. Migrating motor complexes (MMC)
4. Movements of villi
5. Contractions of muscularis mucosa

Abnormal Movements

Peristaltic Rushes
1. *MMC:*
   - Migrating motility complexes are motility present in the interdigestive period.
   - These are bursts of electrical and mechanical activities in GIT
   - It starts in the esophagus and spreads through the stomach and ileum to the ileocecal valve
   - Occurs once in 90 minutes and lasts for 10–20 min.
   - It clears the GIT for the next meal.
   - **Occurs in 3 phases:**
     - **Phase I:** No spike potential, no contractions
     - **Phase II:** Irregular spike potentials and contractions
     - **Phase III:** Regular spike potentials and contractions

2. ***Mixing movements:***
   Segmentation contractions:
   - These are ring like contractions present in short segments of the intestine of 1-2 cm.
   - They are present in regular intervals.
   - Their frequency matches the slow wave frequency.
   - Slow waves are waves generated in the pace maker cells located in the wall of duodenum and it spreads through the muscular wall of the intestines.
   - Strength of the contraction depends on the spike waves superimposed on the slow waves.
   - These ring like contractions appear in one segment and the nearby segment relaxes, this is followed by another set of contractions in the segments between the previous contractions.
   - These contractions appear sausage shaped and they cut into the bolus and move it to and fro and increase their exposure to the absorptive surface of the mucosa.
   - Therefore, these contractions help in mixing the bolus with digestive juices and in digestion and absorption of food.
3. ***Tonic contractions:***
   - These are prolonged contractions of one segment of intestine and the segment appears to be isolated from the rest of the ileum.
   - Segmentation and tonic contractions delay the passage of chyme and thereby allow contact of chyme with enterocytes and favor absorption.
4. ***Peristalsis:***
   - This is a type of propulsive movement which helps to move the chyme forward. It is a reflex initiated by the stretch of the intestinal wall following the entry of food.
   - Stretch of the intestinal wall initiates a ring of constriction behind the bolus and a relaxation in front of the bolus.
   - The ring of contraction behind pushes the bolus to the relaxed segment in front of the bolus.
   - Next ring of contraction now appears in the previous relaxed segment and the bolus is pushed further.
   - These waves always propel the contents from the oral to caudal direction and never in the opposite direction—**law of the Gut**.
   - These waves appear even in the absence of nerve supply but they can be modified by the autonomic nerves, parasympathetic nerves increase the activity and sympathetic nerves decrease the activity.
   - The propelling speed varies from 2-25 cm/s.
   - Sometimes, the peristaltic waves can be very fast and they empty the contents faster—peristaltic rushes, seen in acute diarrhea.
   - Antiperistalsis happens in vomiting.
5. ***Contractions of muscularis mucosa:***
   - Irregular in nature.
   - Occurs at a frequency of 3/min.
   - It helps in mixing the contents and in absorption.
6. ***Contraction of villi:***
   - The type of contraction seen as elongation and shortening of the villi.
   - It helps in emptying of central lacteals of the villi and increases the absorptive surface area.
   - It is stimulated by the hormone villikinin.

Functions of movements of small intestine:
- Mixing the chyme with the digestive juices and helps in digestion
- Propelling the chyme forward
- Presenting the chyme to absorptive surface and helps for absorption

27. Functions of placenta.

Functions of Placenta
- Synthesis of hormones (endocrine function of placenta)
- Transport of substances across the placenta between the mother and fetus
- Protection of fetus

Hormones Synthesized by Placenta

- Human chorionic gonadotropin (hCG)
- Human chorionic somatomammotropin (hCS)
- Placental progesterone
- Placental estrogen
- Relaxin

Human Chorionic Gonadotropin (hCG):

- It is synthesized by syncytiotrophoblasts of placenta
- It is a glycoprotein with a and b subunits
- It starts appearing in the blood of the mother by 6 days after fertilization and reaches a peak by 10-12 weeks.
- Clinically, presence of hCG in urine of a female is "the indicator" of pregnancy.
- It stimulates the corpus luteum to secrete progesterone till the placenta is fully formed.
- hCG helps in sexual differentiation of male fetus.
- It induces hyperemesis in the first trimester.

Human Chorionic Somatomammotropin (hCS)

- It is also secreted from the syncytiotrophoblast of placenta.
- Its secretion starts by 5th week of pregnancy and reaches a peak towards term.
- It is similar to growth hormone and has growth promoting actions, so called as "Maternal growth hormone of pregnancy".
- It stimulates lipolysis, N, K^+ and Ca^{2+} retention and decreases glucose utilization by the mother so that the substrates are diverted to the fetus.
- Amount of hCS secreted is equal to size of placenta and therefore level of hCS indicates placental viability.

Placental Progesterone

- In the early weeks of pregnancy, progesterone is produced by corpus luteum and later the function is taken over by placenta.
- It is produced by coordination between the mother and the fetus—the fetoplacental unit.
- It makes the endometrium secretory and thereby nourishes the fertilized ovum.
- It keeps the myometrium of the pregnant uterus quiescent which is essential for the survival of the fetus.
- It acts on the alveolar system of the maternal breast and facilitates development of maternal breast.
- It has an immunosuppressive role in protecting the fetus.

Placental Estrogen

- The major estrogen in pregnancy is estriol.
- It stimulates development of the ductular system of the maternal breast.
- The levels of estrogen rises during pregnancy but on nearing term estrogen progesterone ratio rises and estrogen makes the myometrium excitable.
- On decrease of levels of estrogen after delivery of fetus, prolactin stimulates milk secretion from the breast.

Relaxin

- Its level in the early pregnancy is high to relax the uterine wall to favor implantation of fetus.
- In later weeks, it causes relaxation of pubic symphysis and pelvic ligaments to facilitate delivery of fetus.

Other hormones secreted are:
CRH, β endorphin, α-MSH, GnRH, inhibin, prolactin, etc.

Transport Functions of Placenta

- **Transport of nutrients:** Placenta transports nutrients from the mother to the fetus. The nutrients transported are glucose, fats, amino acids and Ca^{2+}, inorganic phosphates, K^+, Na^+.
- **Transports of waste products** from the fetus to the mother—substances transported are urea, uric acid and creatinine.
- **Transport of gases:** Dissolved O_2 is transported from maternal side of placenta to the fetus along the pressure gradient. Fetus receives its O_2 from maternal venous sinuses and therefore is living in a hypoxic environment. But the fetal Hb with 2α and

2γ chains have higher affinity for O_2. CO_2 is also eliminated from fetal circulation into maternal blood by diffusion across the placenta.
- **Transport of antibodies:** Maternal antibodies are transferred to the fetus and are responsible for innate immunity.

Protection of Fetus

- It acts as a barrier for prevention of transport of toxic substances from the mother to fetus.
- Progesterone produced by placenta helps to maintain pregnancy.

28. Functions of mitochondria.

- Mitochondria is a sausage-shaped organelle present in almost all the cells.
- It has an outer and an inner membrane. The inner membrane is folded to form the cristae.
- The space between two layers—intracristal space (*refer* **Fig. 26**).
- The space inside the inner membrane—the matrix.
- Mitochondria are the power generating units of the cell and they are present more in cells involved in energy-requiring processes.
- They produce energy rich ATP which is essential for many metabolic activities of the cell.
- The outer membrane is studded with oxidative enzymes and they provide the raw materials for the reactions inside the matrix.
- In the interior, there are enzymes which break down the substrates, such as carbohydrates, fats and proteins into CO_2 and H_2O.

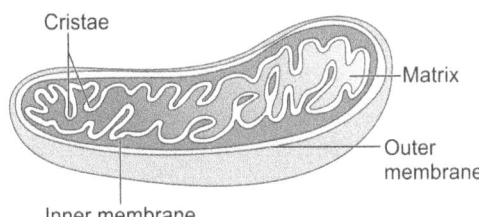

Fig. 26: Structure of mitochondria.

- The enzymes in the inner membrane are NADH dehydrogenase, succinic dehydrogenase, cytochrome C and cytochrome oxidase.
- During these reactions, H^+ are pumped out and a proton gradient is created which will drive the enzyme, ATP synthase to form ATP.
- Mitochondrion has its own genome but the DNA is less when compared to nuclear DNA.
- It is helpful for synthesis of many components of oxidative phosphorylation.
- It has a role in initiation of apoptosis of the cell.

29. Puberty.

- Puberty is defined as the period when the endocrine and gametogenic functions of the gonads have developed to the level of reproduction.
- The age of puberty in females is between 8-13 years and in boys, it is between 9-14 years of age.
- In males, testosterone is secreted in the fetus before birth and another time in the neonatal period. After that, the Leydig cells (which secrete testosterone) remain quiescent.
- Gonads of both sexes reach final maturation at puberty and start secreting sex hormones.

Control of Puberty

Control by GnRH

- Final maturation of the gonads and their hormone secretion are under the control of gonadotropins.
- Gonadotropins from anterior pituitary are under the control of GnRH from hypothalamus.
- At the time of puberty, GnRH starts to secrete in a pulsatile fashion. This pulsatility of GnRH secretion is kept under control by a neural mechanism till the time of puberty.

Control by Leptin

- The other control mechanism is thought to be the body weight of the individual.

A critical body weight has to be reached to attain puberty.
- It is now understood that Leptin, a hormone secreted from adipose tissue is the link between body weight and onset of puberty.

Components of Puberty
- There are two components of puberty—a sudden growth spurt and development of secondary sexual characteristics.
- The changes happening in puberty at various stages are given below in males and females:

Pubertal changes in females:

Stage of puberty	Age in years	Changes in females
Stage 1	Up to 7½	Preadolescent
Stage 2	10½	Thelarche (appearance of breast bud)
Stage 3	11½	• Pubarche (appearance of axillary and pubic hair) Breast enlargement (Elevation) • Growth spurt
Stage 4	13	• Menarche (start of menstrual cycle) • Breast areola elevate and projects
Stage 5	14	• Adult genitalia • Secondary sexual characteristics

Pubertal changes in males:

Stages	Age in years	Characteristics
Stage 1	7½	Preadolescent
Stage 2	12	Enlargement of testis
Stage 3	14	• Enlargement of penis • Appearance of axillary and pubic hair
Satge 4	15	• Further growth of testis, penis and genitalia • Growth spurt
Stage 5	16½	Adult genitalia and secondary sexual characteristics

Hormonal Changes during Puberty
- **FSH and LH** levels are low form birth to childhood. But at the time of puberty, their levels increase following the pulsatile secretion of GnRH.
- **Adrenal androgen** increases towards puberty, 8-10 years in girls and 10-12 years in boys. This called as adrenarche. It is essential for the growth of axillary and pubic hair in both males and females.
- **Growth hormone** levels are intermittent with peaks every day. At the time of puberty, the frequency and amplitude of these peaks are increased and it induces growth spurt in boys and girls.
- **Thyroid hormone** levels also increase at the time of puberty and is needed for the growth hormone to promote growth
- **Sex hormone** levels increase after puberty.

Applied Aspects of Puberty

Precocious puberty: Early onset of puberty below 8 years of age.

It can be:
- True precocious puberty
- Pseudoprecocious puberty

True Precocious Puberty

It is usually due to decreased inhibition of pulsatile secretion of GnRH. Therefore, there is an early otherwise normal puberty. It is more common in girls.

Causes:
- Constitutional (without any cause),
- Cerebral—disorders of posterior hypothalamus, tumors, infections
- Gonadotropin independent precocity

Pseudo-precocious Puberty

This is due to early development of secondary sexual characteristics without gametogenesis due to abnormal exposure of males to androgens and females to estrogens.

Causes:
- **Adrenal:** Congenital virilizing hyperplasia, androgen secreting tumors in males and estrogen secreting tumors in females.
- **Gonadal:** Leydig cell tumors of testis and granulosa cell tumors of ovaries

Delayed Onset of Puberty or Absent Puberty

Puberty is considered to be delayed if in females, the menarche does not appear till 17 years of age and no testicular development till age of 20 in males.

Causes:
- Failure of hypothalamus or anterior pituitary to secrete gonadotropins as in panhypopituitarism.
- Primary gonadal failure as in Klinefelter syndrome or Turner's syndrome.

Symptoms:
- Short stature
- Features of other endocrinal abnormalities
- Delay in puberty

---

30. Functions of glucocorticoids.

Metabolic actions of glucocorticoids are:
- **Effects on carbohydrate metabolism:**
  - Increases gluconeogenesis in liver → increased glycogen stores.
  - Antagonizes the action of insulin on muscle and adipose tissue—prevents glucose uptake.
  - This spares glucose for the brain.
  - Increases glucose output from liver.
  - Results in hyperglycemia
- **Effects on protein metabolism:**
  - It is proteolytic in action
  - Breaks down proteins into AA and inhibits protein synthesis.
  - Amino acids are used for gluconeogenesis
  - Therefore, increased cortisol levels drain the protein stores in the body
- **Effects on lipid metabolism:**
  - Cortisol is permissive for the lipolytic action of catecholamines.
  - But high cortisol levels increase total body fat by 2 mechanisms:
    1. Cortisol stimulates appetite → obesity due to increased caloric consumption.
    2. High cortisol →↑ blood glucose →↑ insulin secretion → lipogenesis.
  - Pattern of fat distribution—**centripetal**-concentrated in trunk, but wasting is seen in arms and legs.

Permissive Action

Cortisol amplifies effects of certain processes of other hormones where it does not act directly.

Example,
1. It does not induce glycogenolysis itself but augments glycogenolysis by glucagon.
2. It also augments vaso responsiveness of blood vessels to catecholamines.

Actions on Bones

Increases bone resorption by:

Cortisol decreases renal and GIT absorption of calcium
↓
Lowers serum calcium levels
↓
Parathyroid hormone secretion stimulated
↓
Mobilizes calcium from bone by resorption and demineralization

Also inhibits action of osteoblasts and suppresses collagen formation. Hence, high cortisol levels result in **osteoporosis**.

Actions on CVS

- Cortisol is permissive for the vasopressor effects of catecholamine and Angiotensin II.
- Hence, it is necessary for maintenance of normal BP.
- Stimulates erythropoietin synthesis and so increases RBC production.

Actions on Connective Tissue

Cortisol inhibits fibroblast proliferation and collagen formation
↓
So excess cortisol levels
↓
Thinning of skin and walls of capillaries
↓
Easy damage to skin and easy bruising of capillaries
↓
Intracutaneous hemorrhage

Action on Kidneys

- Cortisol inhibits ADH secretion and action, so in absence of cortisol a water load leads to water intoxication.

- Cortisol also has a weak mineralocorticoid action →↑ Na^+ and H_2O reabsorption.
- **Increases GFR:**
  - By increasing cardiac output
  - By direct action on kidneys

Action on Muscles
- Cortisol has complex action on muscles.
- Excess cortisol results in muscle weakness due to:
  - Proteolysis
  - Hypokalemia

Actions on GIT
- Cortisol has a trophic action on GIT.
- It also increases appetite → weight gain in hypercortisolism.
- Increased acid secretion → acidity, gastritis

Action on CNS
- Glucocorticoids alters mood and behavior
- REM sleep ↓, but slow wave sleep
- In excess—insomnia, elevated or depressed mood, ↓ memory
- Frank psychosis occurs with excess or reduced cortisol levels.
- Dampens the acuity to olfactory, gustatory, auditory and visual stimuli.

Action in Fetus
- Facilitates maturity of CNS, retina, skin, GIT, and lungs.
- During the last week of pregnancy, the synthesis of surfactant is stimulated by cortisol.
- So, if premature delivery suspected weekly doses of cortisol given to mother till delivery.

Action on Inflammation and Immune System
- Cortisol is frequently used clinically for its anti-inflammatory property.
- It inhibits synthesis of mediators of inflammation.
- Inhibits migration of leukocytes to site of injury.
- Decreases the number of circulating eosinophils.
- Inhibits fibroblast proliferation at inflammatory site which is a defense mechanism in the body to prevent spreading of infection.
- Excess cortisol inhibits normal defense mechanisms of body against infection

Effect on Immune Response
- Cortisol inhibits immune response in the body.
- At high doses, it decreases the number of T lymphocytes (helper t-cells) and their migration to antigenic site.
- B lymphocytes and antibody production are not affected directly.
- Because of these effects, glucocorticoids are used for immunosuppression after organ transplantation.

Effect on Stress
- Protects the body against stress
- During stress, there is increased secretion of CRH from hypothalamus.
- This increases the secretion of ACTH from anterior pituitary
- Therefore, glucocorticoid secretion increases
- Cortisol facilitates lipolysis by catecholamine and increases release of free fatty acids which supplies the energy needed to cope up with stress.
- It is also permissive for the vasoconstriction induced by catecholamines which is needed for maintaining BP during stress.

31. Chemical regulation of respiration.
- Chemical regulation of respiration is also through the modulation of activities of neural centers through chemoreceptors.
- There are 2 sets of chemoreceptors responding to changes in arterial PO_2, PCO_2 and pH.
- They are **peripheral** and **central chemorecptors**.

Peripheral Chemoreceptors
- Carotid and aortic bodies (*refer* **Fig. 27**).
- They have high blood flow (2000 mL/100 g/min) and high metabolic rate.
- Their metabolic needs are met by dissolved O_2.

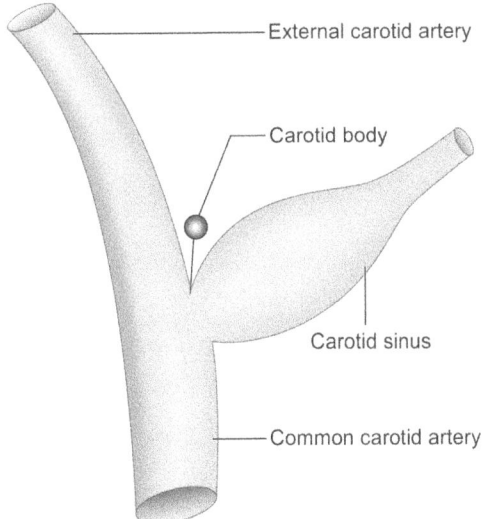

Fig. 27: Location peripheral chemoreceptors at bifurcation of common carotid artery; the carotid body. Carotid sinus is the dilatation in internal carotid artery; the baroreceptor.

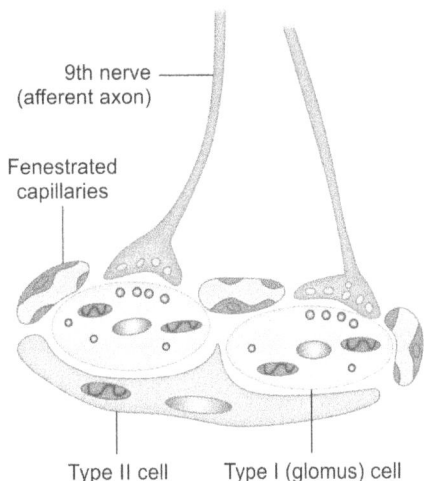

Fig. 28: Cells in carotid body—Type I (glomus cells) and Type II (supporting cells). Glomus cells are supplied by 9th cranial nerve and are close to fenestrated capillaries.

- So, they are highly sensitive to ↓ PO_2, ↑PCO_2 and ↓pH.
- These receptors are not stimulated in anemia or carbon monoxide poisoning.
- They are stimulated in ↓PO_2, vascular stasis, cyanide poisoning
- They have 2 types of cells—glomus and sustentacular cells.

Sensitivity of Peripheral Chemoreceptors (PCR)

- Glomus cells are the sensors (*refer* Fig. 28).
- Hypoxia is the major stimulus. Neurotransmitter is dopamine.
- PCRs also responds to PCO_2 and ⁻pH
- When PO_2 <100 mm Hg, there is firing rate of the nerves supplying them (9th and 10th cranial nerves)
- Response is maximum when PO_2 falls <60 mm Hg
- Effect of hypoxia is less when PO_2 <60 mm Hg because:
  - Hypoxia → Hyperventilation → CO_2 blow out →↓$PaCO_2$ →↓ ventilation
  - Deoxy-Hb has more affinity for H^+ →↓arterial $[H^+]$ →↓ventilation

Mechanism of Hypoxia Stimulating PCR

Hypoxia inhibits K^+ channels by:

- O_2 sensor in the glomus cell is a heme containing protein and is associated with O_2. In hypoxia, the lack of O_2 inhibits the K^+ channels.
- In hypoxia, there is increase in cAMP in glomus cells which inhibits cAMP sensitive K^+ channels (*refer* Fig. 29).

Effect of CO_2 on PCR

Refer Fig. 30.

Integrated Effects of Arterial—PCO_2, PO_2 and pH on Ventilation, by Stimulating PCR

- At low P_{ACO2} level with hypoxia, ventilation is not stimulated till PO_2 <60 mm Hg.
- High P_{ACO2} levels (as in↑metabolic rate/ breathing CO_2 mixtures) →↑ventilation. But if CO_2 content in breathed air is >7% → CNS depression → CO_2 narcosis
- Hypercapnia with hypoxia, shifts the CO_2 curve to left and slope is increased.
- Acidosis by itself (as in diabetic ketoacidosis) can stimulate ventilation by stimulating PCR. (Even in absence of hypoxia or hypercapnia)

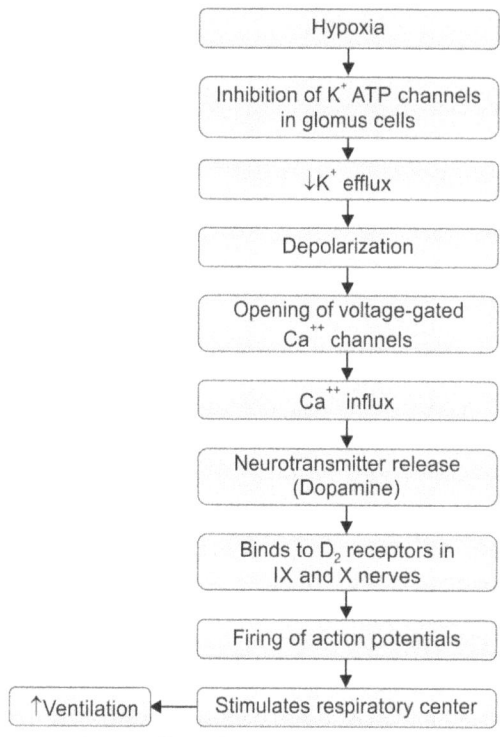

Fig. 29: Effect of hypoxia on peripheral chemoreceptors.

Central Chemoreceptors (CCR)

- Located in the medulla and is different from the other respiratory neurons.
- There are also other such CCR in and around the brain stem nuclei—nucleus tractus solitarius, nucleus ambiguous (*refer* **Fig. 31**).
- They respond maximally to changes in [H^+] in brain CSF and ISF which is in turn decided by P_{ACO_2} and HCO_3^- of CSF.

↑Arterial PCO_2
↓
↑Brain ECF CO_2 level
↓
$CO_2 + H_2O \rightarrow H_2CO_3 \rightarrow H^+ + HCO_3^-$
↓
Increase in brain ECF H^+ level
↓
Stimulation of CCR
↓
Stimulation of medullary inspiratory center
↓

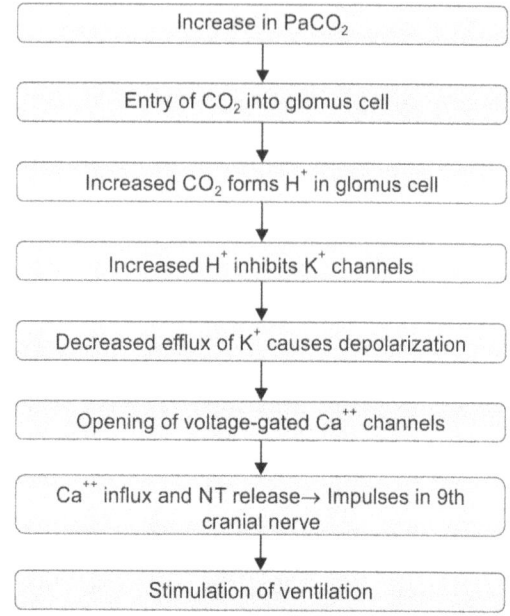

Fig. 30: Effect of hypercapnia on peripheral chemoreceptors.

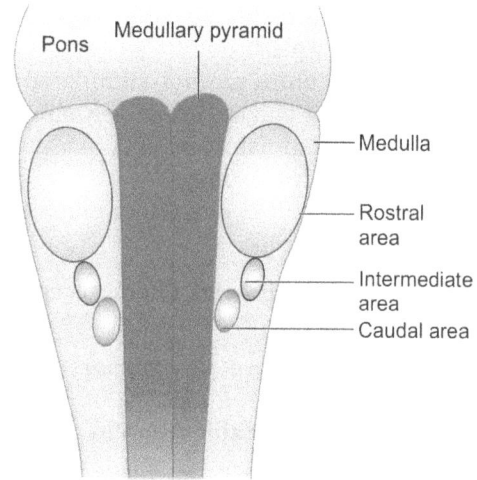

Fig. 31: Location of central chemoreceptors in ventral medulla. There are rostral, intermediate and caudal centers.

Firing of neurons supplying diaphragm and external intercostal muscles
↓
Increase in ventilation

32. Functions of middle ear.

- **Middle ear:** It is an air-filled cavity in temporal bone. It starts at the tympanic membrane and ends at oval window.

- **Contains:** 3 ossicles (malleus, incus and stapes), 2 small muscles (tensor tympani and stapedius), ligaments, nerves, blood vessels, etc.
- **Functions:**
  1. *Tympanic reflex:* It is a protective reflex. When a loud sound is transmitted through the ossicles in middle ear a reflex is initiated with a latent period of 40-80 msec. Contraction of stapedius and tensor tympani pulls the tympanic membrane medially and membrane covering oval window laterally. This makes the ossicular system rigid and there is reduction in transmission of sounds. This reduces the intensity of sound by 30-40 decibels. It is also called as **attenuation reflex**.

     Functions of this reflex:
     - This reflex protects the cochlea from damaging loud sounds.
     - It filters the low frequency sounds
     - It prevents hearing one's own speech
  2. Transmission of sound waves from external ear to internal ear
  3. *Impedance matching:*
     - As the sound waves travel from rarer (air in external and middle ear) to denser medium (fluid in the inner ear) they are dampened (by 30 db).
     - This loss in sound energy is prevented in the middle ear by impedance matching which is by:
       - By area differences
       - By lever action
       - By buckling factor
     a. *Area difference:* Area of tympanic membrane is greater than foot plate of stapes and therefore there is convergence of sound and pressure is increased by 17 times.
     b. *Lever action of the ossicles* increases pressure by 1.32 times
     c. *Buckling factor:* Tympanic membrane is conical in shape and the handle of malleus is attached to the umbo. As the tympanic membrane moves in and out, the buckling of membrane moves the handle of malleus less and this increases the force and decreases the velocity.

33. Hemorrhage shock.

It is a syndrome in which there is inadequate tissue perfusion related with absolute or relative decrease in cardiac output. It is also called as 'cold shock'

Types of shock:
a. Hypovolemic shock
b. Distributive shock
c. Cardiogenic shock
d. Obstructive shock

Causes for hypovolemic shock:
- Trauma
- Hemorrhage
- Surgery
- Burns
- Fluid loss due to vomiting or diarrhea

Stages of shock:
Reversible and irreversible shock

Hypovolemic Shock

Symptoms are:
- Hypotension
- Rapid thready pulse
- Skin is cold and clammy with greyish tinge
- Intense thirst
- Rapid breathing
- Restlessness
- Increased lactic acid production

Stages of shock: Reversible and irreversible shock.

Reversible or non-progressive shock:
It is a stage in shock where the amount of blood lost is less than 1 L and various body mechanisms try to compensate the decrease in circulatory volume and to correct and cause full recovery without any treatment.

It is also called as compensated stage.

The following are the compensatory mechanisms:
- Immediate tachycardia and increase in pulse rate—due to decrease in blood volume baroreceptors are inhibited which results in sympathetic nerves stimulation.

- Sympathetic stimulation causes vasoconstriction in all the vessels except cerebral and coronary vasculature.
- Sympathetic nerves also cause venoconstriction which results in increased venous return and thereby increased cardiac output and blood pressure.
- Due to loss of RBC and stagnant blood flow and acidosis, chemoreceptors are stimulated → Tachypnea → Thoracic pumping → Increase VR and thereby CO and BP.
- Restlessness due to release of adrenaline from adrenal medulla → Acts on reticular formation → skeletal muscle activity → increase in VR
- Movement of interstitial fluid into capillaries → increases blood volume
- Increased secretion of renin, angiotensin II and aldosterone → Reabsorption of electrolytes and water from tubules → increase in blood volume
- Increased secretion of ADH
- Long-term compensations are increase in erythropoiesis and plasma protein synthesis.

Refractory Shock

- Depending upon the amount of blood lost many patients die soon after the blood loss.
- Some recover with the compensatory mechanisms and with appropriate treatment.
- But some patients the shock persists for hours and it progresses to there is no improvement with treatment, cardiac output stays decreased.
- This condition is said to be refractory shock or irreversible shock
- This happens because of operation of various positive feedback mechanisms.
- Severe blood loss → depression of vasomotor center → vasodilatation and decrease in heart rate → further drop in BP → further drop in cerebral blood flow → further depression of VMC and cardiac areas.
- Severe shock → coronary blood flow is decreased due to hypotension and tachycardia → decrease myocardial contractility → further decrease in cardiac output → further decrease in coronary blood flow.
- Acidosis makes the situation worse.

If no treatment advocated it leads to refractory shock resulting in:
- Depletion of ATP
- Tissue damage and necrosis
- Acute tubular necrosis in kidneys
- Respiratory distress—shock lung syndrome.

Treatment

Treatment should aim at correcting the cause and restoring the circulatory volume.

General treatment:
- Patient should be kept at room temperature.
- Raise the foot end of patient's bed to increase venous return.

Treating the cause:
- In hemorrhagic, traumatic and surgical shock the cause is blood loss, so immediately compatible whole blood should be transfused.
- IV fluids can be given temporarily
- In burn shock, plasma is lost and there is hemoconcentration. So plasma should be infused. Plasma expanders which hold the fluid in the capillary can also be given.

34. Ventilation-perfusion ratio.

- It is the ratio of ventilation to the lungs to the blood flow through pulmonary circulation.
- Alveolar ventilation (V_a) is 4000 L/min and perfusion (Q) is equal to cardiac output, 5 L/min
- So V_a/Q ratio = 4/5 = 0.8
- Ventilation as well as perfusion increases from the apex to the base of the lungs due to the effect of gravity.
- But rate of increase of perfusion is more than the increase in ventilation
- So V_a/Q ratio is more in the apex (3.3) than the base (0.63)
- The high O_2 content in the apex favors the growth of tuberculosis bacilli

- The V_a/Q ratio can get altered in conditions of uneven ventilation and non-uniform blood flow to alveoli as in certain disease conditions.

Decreased V_a/Q Ratio

- In conditions where there is inadequate ventilation to the alveoli and normal perfusion, the oxygenation of blood and removal of CO_2 are not normal.
- So, alveolar PO_2 falls and PCO_2 rises.
- So, it is like the deoxygenated blood empties directly into the left atrium.
- So, it is like a physiological shunt (*refer* **Fig. 32**).

Causes

Bronchial asthma, pneumothorax, emphysema, pulmonary fibrosis

Increased Va/Q Ratio

- When perfusion through pulmonary capillary is decreased in relation to alveolar ventilation the ratio increases.
- Alveolar PCO_2 falls and PO_2 increases.
- As the alveolus is underperfused, it is like wasted ventilation and is like increased physiological dead space (*refer* **Fig. 32**).

Causes

- Anatomical shunts in the heart like Fallot's tetralogy
- Decrease in vascular bed as in emphysema
- Pulmonary embolism

35. Parkinson's disease with treatment.

- Also called as paralysis agitans
- Due to destruction of nigrostriatal dopaminergic neurons (fibers to putamen is mostly affected) of basal ganglia.

Characterized by:
- **Hyperkinetic features:**
  - **Rigidity:** Lead pipe or cogwheel
  - **Tremors:** Resting tremors, 6–8 Hz frequency
- **Hypokinesia:**
  - Weakness of movements and lack of initiation of movements—**akinesia**
  - Bradykinesia
- **Lack of automated movements**
- **Mask like face without expression**
- **Festinant or short shuffling gait**

Treatment:
- Treatment with L-Dopa rather than dopamine as it cannot cross the blood brain barrier

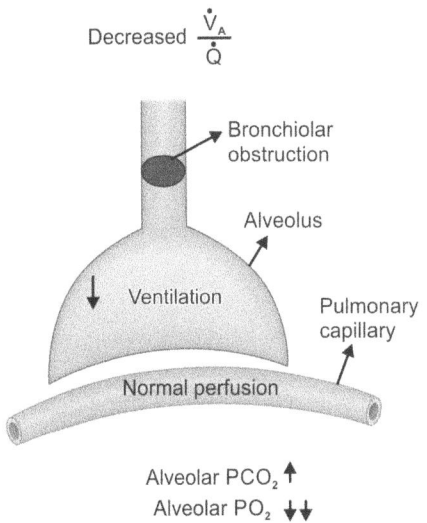
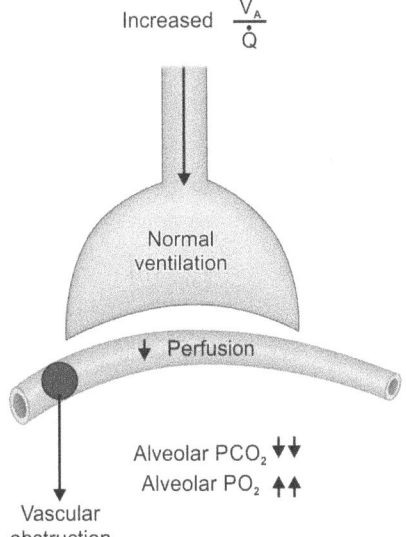

Fig. 32: V_a/Q ratio in complete airway obstruction and complete circulatory obstruction conditions.

- Bromocriptine, a dopamine agonist can also be used
- Anticholinergics, such as atropine, tries to reduce the acetylcholine levels in basal ganglia and regulates the ratio between dopamine and acetylcholine.
- L-deprenyl
- Dopamine agonists, such as bromocriptine.
- Transplantation of adrenal medulla in BG
- Implantation of fetal BG

36. Classification of nerve fibers.

- Nerve fibers are classified based on their functions—sensory and motor nerves
- Based on myelination—myelinated and Unmyelinated nerves
- But the most accepted classification is the Erlanger-Gasser classification.
- It is based on the myelination, thickness of the nerve and its conduction velocity.

Erlanger-Gasser Classification

Fiber type	Functions	Fiber diameter (µm)	Conduction velocity (m/s)	Myelination
Aα	Proprioception, somatic motor	12–20	70–120	Myelinated
Aβ	Touch, pressure	5–12	30–70	"
Aγ	Motor to muscle spindle	3–6	15–30	"
Aδ	Pain, cold, touch	2–5	12–30	"
B	Preganglionic autonomic	<3	3–15	"
C Dorsal root	Pain, temperature, mechanoreception, some reflex response	0.4–1.2	0.5–2	Unmyelinated
Sympathetic	Postganglionic sympathetics	0.3–1.3	0.7–2.3	"

Numerical Classification

Sensory nerves are classified as Ia, Ib, II, III and IV

Number	Origin	Fiber type
Ia	Muscle spindle, annulospiral ending	Aα
Ib	Golgi tendon organ	Aα
II	Muscle spindle, Flower-spray ending touch, pressure	Aβ
III	Pain and cold receptor some touch receptor	Aδ
IV	Pain, temperature and other receptor	Dorsal root C

Classification based on Sensitivity of Nerves to Agents, such as Hypoxia, Pressure and Local Anesthetics:

Susceptibility to	Most susceptible	Intermediate	Least susceptible
Hypoxia	B	A	C
Pressure	A	B	C
Local anesthetics	C	B	A

37. Heart sounds.

Refer Fig. 33.

Heart Sounds can be Recorded by Phonocardiogram

Significance of Heart Sounds

- **1st sound:** Increased in exercise, hyperkinetic states, such as anemia and decreased in shock, MI, pericardial effusion.
- **2nd sound:** Loud in hypertension, low in aortic and pulmonary stenosis. Splitting is common.
- **3rd sound:** Increased in MR. Important sign of heart failure.
- **4th sound:** Always seen in abnormal conditions. Seen in left ventricular hypertrophy.

38. Errors of refraction with correction.

Myopia—short-sightedness

Eyeball may be elongated and therefore parallel rays of light from a distant object are brought to focus in front of the retina. It may be genetic or acquired. It can be corrected by using biconcave lenses. The lens diverges the light rays before they strike the cornea and then they are converged by the lens in the eye, so that the object is focused on the retina. It is the most common error of refraction (*refer* Fig. 34).

Hypermetropia—farsightedness

Here the parallel rays of light from a distant object are brought to focus behind the retina. It occurs due to decrease in anteroposterior diameter of the eye. It can be corrected by using biconvex lenses so that they converge the light rays before they fall on the cornea and therefore the light rays fall on the retina (*refer* Fig. 34).

Astigmatism

The problem here is the corneal surface is not spherical. One meridian of the cornea is different from the other. So, the parallel rays of light are not able to converge to a point of focus as there is unequal refraction from the different meridians. So, a blurred image is seen. It can be corrected using cylindrical lenses

Presbyopia

It is commonly seen in aged people above the age of 40 years.

The near point has receded beyond the normal reading distance due to loss of plasticity of lens. The loss of plasticity results in loss of accommodation property of the lens. It is corrected using convex lens for near work and plain glasses for far work and it is given as the bifocal lenses.

Heart sounds	Events responsible	Duration	Frequency	Others
First sound (S_1)	Due to vibrations set by sudden closure of AV valves at the onset of ventricular systole	0.15 sec	25–45 Hz In PCG recorded as 9–13 waves	Soft and long, heard as "LUBB"
Second sound (S_2)	Associated with closure of aortic and pulmonary valves after the end of ventricular systole	0.12 sec	50 Hz In PCG recorded as 4–6 waves	Normally S2 can be split due to early closure of aortic valve, heard as "Dup"
Third sound (S_3)	Is heard at 1/3rd of diastole due to rapid filling of ventricle due to vibrations set by inrush of blood		0.1 sec In PCG recorded as 1–4 waves	Normally audible only in children and young adults
Fourth sound (S_4)	Heard just before (S_1) Occurs during atrial contraction Due to ventricular filling		20 cyc/sec In PCG recorded as 1–2 waves	Rarely heard in normal adults Heard in vent hypertrophy and CCF

Fig. 33: Heart sounds; their causes and characteristics.

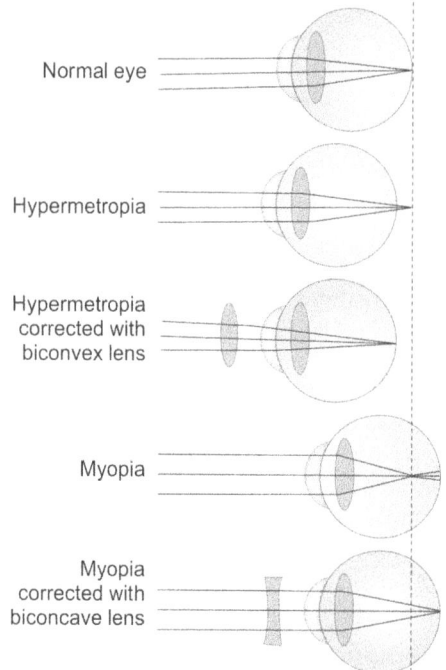

Fig. 34: Refractory errors of with corrections.

39. Transport of oxygen in blood.

Refer answer to essay question 2.

40. Waves of EEG.

Electroencephalogram

- This is a recording of spontaneous electrical activities generated in the cerebral cortex.
- These waves are recorded by placing electrodes on the scalp at various areas and also on the forehead.

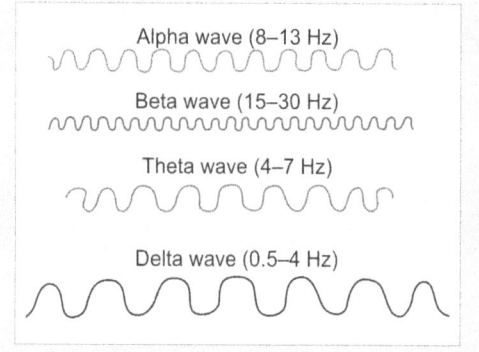

Fig. 35: EEG waves.

- Neurons are known to generate impulses, such as AP and graded potentials—collectively called as brain waves.
- **Waves of EEG:**
  - Alpha waves
  - Beta waves
  - Theta waves
  - Delta waves

Alpha Waves

- Occurs at a frequency of 8–13 per second. Amplitude 50–100 µV
- Present in all normal individuals when they are awake and resting with closed eyes.
- Disappears entirely during sleep.
- It is found in the parieto-occipital region.
- Alpha block—alpha rhythm disappears on opening the eyes.
- Also called as desynchronization.
- Alpha rhythm affected by blood glucose levels, body temperature and glucocorticoids.

Beta Waves

- Frequency between 14–30 Hz.
- Amplitude 5–10 µV
- These waves appear when the nervous system is active.
- These waves appear in frontal regions.

Theta Waves

- At a frequency of 4–7 Hz. Amplitude is larger.
- Occurs normally in children and in adults at time of emotional stress.
- Found over parietal and temporal areas.
- Also occurs in many disorders of brain.

Delta Waves

- Frequency of these waves is 1–5 Hz.
- Amplitude is 20–200 µV
- Delta waves occur in sleep in adults but present in infants during wakefulness.
- When present in an awake adult it indicates brain damage (*refer* **Fig. 35**).

Uses of EEG

- Used to study normal functions of brain.
- To study the changes in brain activity during sleep.

- To diagnose various brain disorders, such as epilepsy, tumors, sites of trauma, degenerative diseases.

III. SHORT ANSWERS

1. Functions of Na⁺-K⁺ pump.

- It pumps out 3 Na⁺ molecules from ICF to ECF and takes in 2 molecules of K⁺. When Na⁺ is pumped out water also move along with it. Thereby, it maintains cell volume and prevents rupture of cell.
- It maintains the resting membrane potential of the cell. This is essential for transmission of impulses in nerves and muscles.
- It is the major energy-using process of the cells in the body and therefore, it is responsible for the basal metabolic rate.
- It maintains a high intracellular K⁺ levels and a high Na⁺ concentration in the ECF.

2. Saltatory conduction.

- In myelinated axons, the action potentials are generated only at the nodes of Ranvier. This part of the axon is exposed to ECF (*refer* **Fig. 36**).
- Voltage-gated Na⁺ channels are concentrated in the nodes of Ranvier and the myelin sheath in the subsequent area acts as an insulator.
- So the current sinks move from one node to another node rather than exciting the neighboring area as in unmyelinated axon.
- This type of impulse conduction is called as saltatory conduction.
- Since the impulses jump across nodes, it can travel faster and impulses are conducted 50–100 times faster than the unmyelinated fibers.

3. Conn's syndrome.

- It is primary hyperaldosteronism.
- It could be due to adenoma of zona glomerulosa, unilateral or bilateral adrenal hyperplasia, adrenal carcinoma or Glucocorticoid-remedial aldosteronism.
- Excess aldosterone secretion results in K⁺ depletion, Na⁺ retention without edema.
- Other symptoms are weakness, hypertension due to volume expansion, tetany (due to alkalosis as excess H⁺ is secreted in the kidneys), polyuria and hypokalemic alkalosis.
- In this condition, renin secretion is decreased.

4. Laron dwarf.

- Laron dwarfism is a type of dwarfism in which the plasma growth hormone levels are normal or even elevated but the growth hormone receptors are insensitive to the hormones.
- The insensitivity is due to a loss-of-mutation of the gene for the receptors.
- The plasma level of IGF-1 is also reduced.

5. Aquaporins.

- Water diffusion across the cell membrane in human beings depends on water channels made of proteins—aquaporins.
- There are 5 types of aquaporins identified.

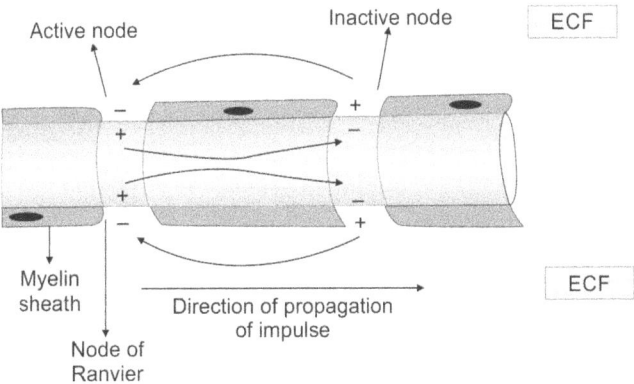

Fig. 36: Saltatory conduction.

- Aquaporins 1, 2 and 3 are found in the kidneys, aquaporin-4 in the brain, 5 in the salivary glands, lacrimal glands and in respiratory tract.
- Aquaporins responding to ADH in the kidneys belong to aquaporin-2.
- They are stored in the collecting duct epithelial cells in endosomes and on activation by ADH, the vesicles translocate to the luminal cell membrane and causes water reabsorption.
- Aquaporin-9 is found in the human leukocytes, liver, lungs and spleen.

6. Anion gap.

- Anion gap refers to the difference in plasma concentration of cations (other than Na^+) and concentration of anions (other than Cl^- and HCO_3^-) and consists mostly of proteins which are anionic, HPO_4^-, SO_4^{2-} and organic acids.
- The normal value is 12 meq/L. It is used to differentiate between types of metabolic acidosis.

Factors which increase anion gap:
- Decrease in plasma concentration of Ca^{2+}, K^+ or Mg^{2+}.
- Increase in concentration of plasma proteins.
- Increase in plasma levels of organic anions, such as lactate or foreign anions.

Factors which decrease anion gap:
- When the above cation levels are increased in the plasma.
- When the plasma albumin levels are decreased.

Anion gap is increased in:
- Diabetic ketoacidosis
- Lactic acidosis
- All forms of acidosis

7. Macula densa.

- It is a component of juxtaglomerular apparatus.
- It is a specialized renal tubular epithelial cell at the junction of thick ascending limb of loop of henle with distal convoluted tubule.
- They are in close contact with Juxtaglomerular cells and lacis cells.
- It is also close to afferent and efferent arterioles.
- They act as chemoreceptors.
- They sense the NaCl content in the tubular fluid.
- By sensing this they are responsible for the tubuloglomerular feedback and regulation of renal blood flow and thereby the GFR.

8. Opsonization.

- Opsonization is a process of coating the bacteria, after it enters the circulation, to make them tasty for the phagocytes and favors phagocytosis.
- Opsonins are—IgG, complement protein C5a, C3b.

9. Immunological memory.

The antibody response to an antigen is of 2 types:
1. **Primary response:** It is the first response when the body encounters the antigen for the first time. The immunological response happens after 4 to 30 days.
2. **Secondary immune response:** This is the body's response to an antigen entering for the second time into the host's system. The response is swift, rapid and abundant. This is because the immune system retains the memory of an antigen exposed previously and responds immediately due to the presence of memory cells (Both T and B cells). This memory is retained for long periods—immunological memory.

It is seen in both humoral and cell-mediated immunities

10. Cholelithiasis.

- **Presence of stones in gallbladder and bile duct is cholelithiasis.**
- **There are two types of stones:**
  1. **Cholesterol stones:** About 85% are cholesterol stones. Bile salts and lecithin solubilizes cholesterol and keeps it in solution.

- But if levels of cholesterol increases or levels of bile salts decrease, cholesterol stones are formed.
- The factors which favor gallstone formation are:
  - Bile stasis, supersaturation of bile with cholesterol and nucleation factors, such as glycoproteins in the mucous favors gallstone formation.
2. **Calcium bilirubinate stones:** About 15% of stones belong to this type.
   - **Symptoms:**
     - Bile stones by themselves do not produce any symptoms but when they are in the bile duct and cause obstruction, they induce severe colicky pain.
     - There may be obstructive jaundice also.
   - It is diagnosed by ultrasound or cholecystography.

11. Enterogastric reflex.

- Entry of acidic chyme into the duodenum inhibits gastric secretion.
- Presence of digested proteins and acid in duodenum inhibits gastric emptying—by enterogastric reflex.

Inhibition of gastric secretion: Presence of food in the intestine initiates a reflex through myenteric nervous system and extrinsic sympathetic and vagus nerves and thereby inhibits gastric acid secretion. The presence of acids and protein break down products in upper intestine and its distension inhibits gastric secretion.

Inhibition of gastric emptying: The food when it enters the duodenum initiates a nervous reflex and inhibits gastric emptying through—enteric nerves, extrinsic inhibitory sympathetic nerves and through inhibition of vagus nerve to stomach.

The factors in duodenum which initiate enterogastric reflex and inhibit gastric emptying are:
- Distension of duodenum
- Irritation of duodenal mucosa
- Degree of acidity of chyme in duodenum
- Hyper- and hypo-osmolality of chyme in duodenum
- Presence of protein break down products in the duodenal chyme

12. Peristaltic rush.

- Normally peristaltic waves are weak.
- But in conditions of severe intestinal irritation as in intestinal infections there is intense rapid, powerful peristalsis—peristaltic rushes.
- It is mediated through autonomic nerves and brain stem and also by intrinsic enhancement of myenteric plexuses.
- These strong peristaltic waves move chyme for longer distances within minutes and thereby sweep the contents of intestine into colon and thereby relieve the intestine of its irritating chyme and distension.

13. Progeria.

- Progeria is called as Hutchinson-Gilford progeria syndrome.
- It is an extremely rare, progressive genetic disorder that causes children to age rapidly, beginning in their first two years of life.
- Children with progeria appear normal at birth.
- During the first year, signs and symptoms, such as slow growth and hair loss, begin to appear.

Signs and Symptoms
- Slow somatic growth, with below-average height and weight
- Narrowed face, small lower jaw, thin lips and beaked nose
- Head disproportionately large for face
- Prominent eyes and incomplete closure of the eyelids
- Hair loss, including eyelashes and eyebrows
- Thinning, spotty, wrinkled skin
- Visible veins
- High-pitched voice
- Heart problems or strokes are the eventual cause of death in most children with progeria.

- The average life expectancy for a child with progeria is about 13 years, but some with the disease die younger and some live 20 years or longer.

Cause of Progeria

- Researchers have discovered a single gene mutation responsible for progeria.
- The gene, known as lamin A (LMNA), makes a protein, necessary for holding the center (nucleus) of a cell together.
- When this gene has a defect, researchers believe the genetic mutation makes cells unstable, which appears to lead to progeria's aging process.

14. Pills.

By pills we mean the oral contraceptive pills used for contraception. In females, they are usually synthetic preparation of estrogen, progesterone or combination of both.

The pills can be of different types:
1. Combined pill or classical pill
2. Sequential pill
3. Minipill
4. Post-coital pill

Combined pill: It is a combination of estrogen and progesterone. It contains a strip of 21 tablets and is consumed for 21 days from 5th day of menstrual cycle. After 21 days, on stopping the tablets, withdrawal bleeding happens. Again from 5th day the next cycle is started.

It acts by:
- Prevents ovulation, as the high estrogen levels disorganize the LH and FSH secretions.
- Prevents implantation of fertilized ovum as the endometrial changes are disorganized.
- Progesterone makes the cervical mucus thick and prevents sperm penetration

Sequential pill: It has high dose of estrogen and minimal amounts of progesterone. It is not used nowadays as the high estrogen levels may induce endometrial cancer or breast cancer.

Minipill: It is progesterone only pill. It does not affect ovulation but makes the cervical mucus thick and prevents sperm penetration.

Postcoital pill: It is used within 72 hours of unprotected intercourse. It has high doses of estrogen and is given for 4-6 days. In this condition, the high estrogen prevents implantation of the fertilized ovum rather than inducing changes in gonadotropin secretion.

Depot preparation: These are implants of progesterone and they are subdermally implanted and prevent pregnancy for 5 years. The only problem is, it can cause amenorrhea.

There are also male contarceptive pills:
- **Gossypol:** A phenolic derivative of cottonseed oil. It induces azoospermia.
- **Testosterone:** High testosterone levels induce azoospermia.

15. Permissive action.

The presence of glucocorticoids is essential for the physiological actions of other hormones—permissive action of glucocorticoids.

The permissive actions of cortisol are:
- Vasoconstrictive action of catecholamines require the presence of glucocorticoids
- Lipolytic actions of catecholamines need the presence of glucocorticoids
- For bronchodilator action of catecholamines
- For calorigenic action of glucagon and catecholamines
- Synthesis of surfactant by fetal lung and for the lung maturation

16. Astigmatism.

Refer answer to short note 38.

17. Ocular dominance columns.

- Ocular dominance columns are a feature of the visual cortex.
- The cells in lateral geniculate body (in thalamus) and the layer 4 cells of visual cortex receive inputs only from one eye.
- The cells receiving inputs from one eye alternate with cells receiving input from the other eye.
- If radioactive amino acids are injected in one eye, they are incorporated into

proteins and by way of axoplasmic flow go out of the eye through axons of ganglion cells, to geniculate body and via geniculocalcarine fibers to visual cortex.
- So in layer 4 of visual cortex, the radioactive labeled endings from the injected eye alternate with unlabeled endings from uninjected eye.
- As a result when viewed from above a vivid pattern of alternating dark and light stripes are seen.
- These are said to be the ocular dominance columns.

18. Dicrotic notch.

- The blood forced into the aorta during systole not only moves the blood forward but also sets up a pressure wave that travels along the arteries.
- The pressure wave expands the arterial walls as it travels and the expansion is palpable as the **pulse**.
- The arterial tracing shows two waves and one notch.
- The upstroke is the percussion wave (p wave) and it is due to the ejection of blood in systole.
- The downstroke is the dicrotic wave (d wave) and is due to rebound of blood against the closed aortic valve.
- The dicrotic notch (n) is due to the closure of the aortic valve (*refer* **Fig. 37**).

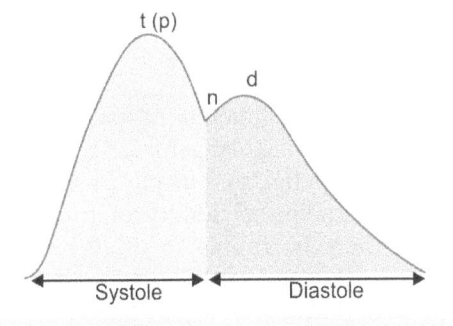

Fig. 37: Arterial pulse tracing from a peripheral artery. 't' is the tidal wave, 'd' dicrotic wave, 'n' is dicrotic notch.

19. Cardiac reserve.

- It is the amount of blood that can be pumped out of each ventricle in excess of the normal cardiac output.
- Normal value is 15–25 L/min

20. Reynolds number.

- The blood flow in a straight vessel is laminar or streamline. The velocity of blood flow in the center of the stream is greatest and lowest immediately below the vessel wall.
- Laminar flow occurs at velocities up to a level called as the **critical velocity**.
- At or above this velocity, the flow becomes turbulent.
- Laminar flow is silent but turbulent flow creates sounds.
- The probability of turbulence is also related to diameter of vessel and viscosity of blood.
- **This is given as the Reynolds number (Re)**
  $Re = \rho DV/\eta$
  ρ = Density of fluid
  D = Diameter of tube
  V = Velocity of flow
  η = Viscosity of fluid
- Higher the value of Re greater is the turbulence
- When D is in cm, V is in cm/s^{-1}, η is in poises, flow is not turbulent if Re is <2000. When Re >3000, there is always turbulent flow.

21. J point.

- It is the point in ECG where the S wave meets the isoelectric line (*refer* **Fig. 38**).
- This is an indicator of end of ventricular depolarization and start of ventricular repolarization.

22. Extrasystole.

- Extrasystole is a premature beat originating from an ectopic focus either in the atrium or the ventricle.
- If it is from atria, it is atrial extrasystole and if it is from ventricle it is a ventricular extrasystole.

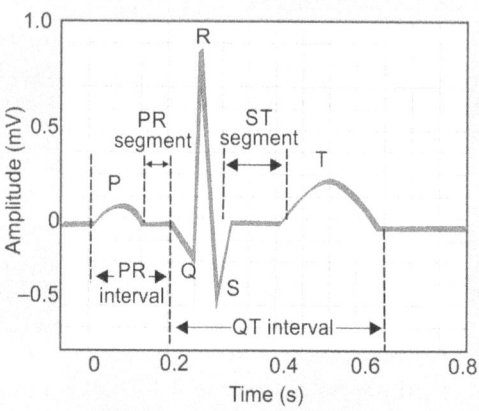

Fig. 38: Normal ECG in lead II. J point is marked with arrow.

- If it is from atria, it is atrial extrasystole and if it is from ventricle, it is a ventricular extrasystole.
- The electrical activity from the ectopic focus is called as an **ectopic wave**
- Configurations of the ectopic waves are **abnormal** (P wave or QRS complex).
- Atrial extrasystole can be benign and are seen in conditions, such as anxiety, excess consumption of coffee, tea.
- QRS complex of the ventricular ectopics are bizzarre in shape and appears earlier than expected.
- There is a compensatory pause following the extrasystole.
- Ventricular extrasystole is also seen in both normal and abnormal conditions.

23. Bell-Magendie law.

Bell-Magendie law states that in the spinal cord the dorsal nerve roots are sensory and ventral nerve roots are motor.

24. Cogwheel rigidity.

- It is a type of rigidity seen in Parkinson's disease.
- Here resistance to passive movement disappears intermittently.
- It is like series of catches during passive movement

25. Betz cells.

- The cerebral cortex is histologically divided into 6 layers.
  1. Layer 1—molecular layer or plexiform layer
  2. Layer 2—external granular layer
  3. Layer 3—external pyramidal layer
  4. Layer 4—internal granular layer
  5. Layer 5—internal pyramidal layer
  6. Layer 6—fusiform layer.
- Layer 5 contains the large pyramidal cells called as the giant cells of Betz.
- These are usually seen in the primary motor area (area 4)
- Their dendrites reach the outer layer and their axons project to the brain stem and spinal cord and terminate there.

26. Homunculus.

- Representation of the whole body in the somatosensory area 1 and primary motor cortex are called as sensory homunculus and motor homunculus respectively.
- The whole body is represented upside down in the homunculus (*refer* **Fig. 39**).
- In sensory homunculus, the body parts with more number of receptors have a larger representation. For example, the lips, fingers which have more numbers of receptors have a larger area of representation than the trunk and lower limbs.
- In motor homunculus, the parts with fine, skilled movements have large areas of representation, for example, hand, thumb, etc.

27. Anomic aphasia.

- It is a type of difficulty in speech due to lesion in the angular gyrus (area 39).
- The person has no difficulty in speech or understanding of auditory information.
- But there is trouble in understanding written language and pictures because the visual information is not processed and transmitted to Wernicke's area.
- It is also called as word blindness.

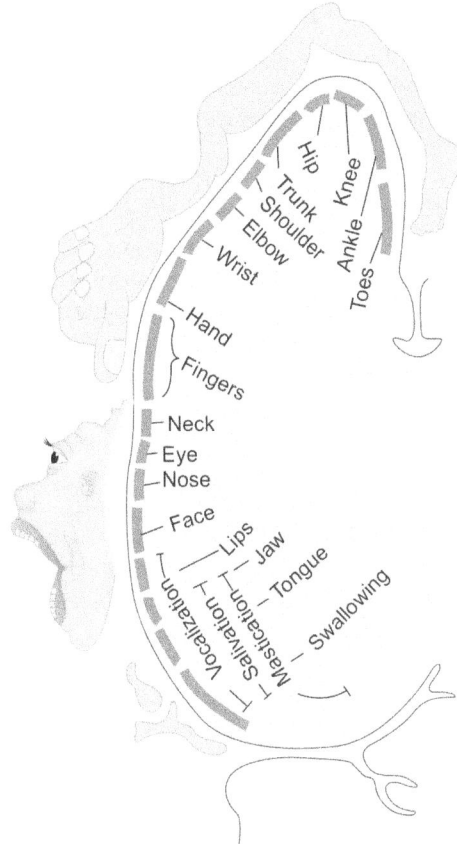

Fig. 39: Homunculus.

28. Timed vital capacity.

- When vital capacity is related to time, it is said to be timed vital capacity.
- **It is defined as the percentage of vital capacity that is expired in a unit of time**.
- It is also called as forced vital capacity or forced expiratory volume (FEV) as the person exhales rapidly and forcibly in a unit of time.
- **FEV1:** Volume expelled in the 1st second—80% of VC
- **FEV2:** Volume expelled in the 2nd second—90% of VC
- **FEV3:** Volume expelled in 3rd second—100% of VC
- FEV1/FVC ratio is a good indicator to diagnose obstructive and restrictive pulmonary diseases.
- In obstructive disease, FEV1/FVC ratio is decreased.
- In restrictive disorders, it may be normal or increased.

29. Pneumotaxic center.

- It is the respiratory center in the pons.
- Located in nucleus parabrachialis and Kolliker-fuse N in the rostral medulla.
- It is active during both inspiration and expiration.
- It coordinates switching between inspiration and expiration.
- Normally, it inhibits apneustic center

30. Asphyxia.

- It is a condition produced by occlusion of airways.
- There is acute hypoxia and hypercapnia
- There is pronounced stimulation of respiration with violent efforts
- BP and heart rate rise and there is sympathetic stimulation
- Eventually BP and HR falls
- Artificial respiration should be started immediately; if not cardiac arrest happens in 4–5 minutes.
- It is seen in conditions, such as strangulation, foreign body in trachea or larynx, drowning and traumatic compression of chest.

31. Inulin clearance.

- Clearance is defined as the quantity of plasma cleared of a particular substance per unit time.
- Clearance of various substances are used to assess the functions of the kidneys.
- Clearance of a substance, which is excreted from the body by only filtration and is neither reabsorbed or secreted or metabolized, is used to measure GFR.
- It should be also non-toxic
- Inulin is a polymer of fructose and meets the above criteria.

Methodology

- A loading dose of inulin is administered intravenously followed by a continuous infusion to maintain its plasma arterial levels.

- After equilibration of inulin in plasma, a timed sample of urine and a sample of plasma are collected half way through.
- Plasma and urine concentrations of inulin are calculated.
- Clearance of inulin is calculated by the formula:

$$C_{IN} = U_{IN} \cdot V/P_{IN}$$

- U_{IN} = Urinary concentration of inulin
- V = Volume of urine excreted
- P_{IN} = Plasma concentration of inulin

32. Oxytocin.

- Oxytocin is an oligopeptide with 9 amino acids and is secreted from posterior pituitary.
- It is synthesized from magnocellular neurons of paraventricular nucleus of hypothalamus and is secreted into circulation from posterior pituitary.

Functions of Oxytocin

- It stimulates milk ejection reflex.
- It induces parturition reflex.
- It also acts on non-pregnant uterus to facilitate sperm transport.
- In males, it is secreted during ejaculation and causes contraction of smooth muscles of vas deferens to propel the sperm towards urethra.

33. Fever.

- Fever is the increase in body temperature above normal range. It is a symptom of infection.
- Fever can be induced by infections, such as bacterial or viral infections.
- It can be non-infectious as in inflammations, such as rheumatoid arthritis, injuries, malignancies, etc.
- It is induced by chemicals called as pyrogens. They can be exogenous or endogenous pyrogens.
- **Exogenous pyrogens** enter the body from outside through microorganisms. For example, endotoxin of gram-negative bacteria is an exogenous pyrogen.

Endogenous Pyrogen

- Endogenous pyrogens are substances produced by monocytes, macrophages and Kupffer cells by action of endotoxins from bacteria.
- Cytokines, such as IL-1β, IL–6, β-IFN, γ-IFN and TNF-α can individually induce fever by modulating the activity of hypothalamic thermoregulatory areas.
- These cytokines are polypeptides and therefore they cannot penetrate the blood brain barrier.
- But they act on organum vasculosum of lamina terminalis (OVLT), one of the circumventricular organs.
- This will in turn activate the preoptic area of hypothalamus.
- On activation, prostaglandins are released in the hypothalamus which induces fever.
- PGE_2 is one of the prostaglandins which induce fever.
- PGE_2 acts on EP_1, EP_2, EP_3 and EP_4 receptors in hypothalamus and alters the firing rate of thermoregulatory control center raising its set point.

Fever is a defense mechanism against the disease. It eliminates the disease by:

- The high temperature kills the microorganisms
- Fever stimulates enzymatic activity and kills the pathogen
- Fever stimulates production of antibodies.

34. Second messengers.

- Second messengers are intracellular signaling molecules formed as a result of series of reactions following the binding of peptide/protein hormones with their cell membrane receptors.
- Hormone binding with the receptor is the first messenger.

The major second messengers are:
- Cyclic AMP (cAMP)
- Diacylglycerol (DAG)
- Inositol triphosphate (IP3)
- Cyclic GMP (cGMP)
- Ca^{2+}

Second messengers formed depends on the hormone signaling of the effector cells.

The signal transduction pathways are activated depending on G protein activation of membrane enzymes.

35. Functions of bile salts.

- **Digestion and absorption of fats:** Bile salts have detergent action and emulsifies fats into smaller molecules on which the pancreatic lipase acts and aids in digestion of fats.
- **Absorption of fats:** The bile salts along with lecithin forms micelles because of their amphipathic nature. The lipids are kept in the core of the micelles and are made water-soluble and carried to the enterocytes. They micelle move to the brush border of the enterocytes and the lipids diffuse out of the micelle and is absorbed into the brush border.
- **Choleretic action:** Bile salts are present in the bile and they stimulate further secretion of bile from the liver.
- Bile salts on entering the intestine are converted into bile acids and are added to the bile acid pool of the body.
- Bile salts also help in *absorption of fat-soluble vitamins*.
- Bile salts along with lecithin solubilize cholesterol and *prevent formation of gallstones*.
- Bile salts are synthesized from cholesterol and when its excretion is increased more cholesterol is lost from the circulation.

36. ESR.

- Erythrocyte sedimentation rate is the rate at which the RBCs get settled down when anticoagulated blood is allowed to stand in a narrow tube.
- This happens because the RBCs have the property of piling on each other—rouleaux formation.
- The piled up RBCs get heavy and they settle down.

The stages of ESR are:
1. Stage of aggregation
2. Stage of falling
3. Stage of settling down

The normal value is 3-7 mm/h in males and 5-9 mm/h in females.

Factors affecting ESR:
It depends on the shape and number of RBCs and plasma factors, such as fibrinogen and globulin.

RBC:
Biconcave shape favors rouleaux formation, spherical and sickle cells inhibit rouleaux formation.

Anemia increases ESR and polycythemia decreases ESR.

Plasma factors:
- Fibrinogen and globulin neutralize the negative charges on RBC and attract them and favors rouleaux formation.
- Acute phase reactive proteins secreted during acute infections and inflammations will also neutralize the negative charges on RBC and increase ESR.

Other factors are body temperature and plasma viscosity.

Significance of ESR:
- ESR is increased in many diseases and therefore does not have any diagnostic value.
- It is elevated in chronic inflammatory conditions, such as rheumatoid arthritis.
- It is used to assess the prognosis of a disease when the patient is getting treated.

Variations in ESR:
- **Physiological variations:** Increased in pregnancy, is more in females and new borns.
- **Pathological variations:**
  Increased in—
  - Acute and chronic inflammations
  - Tuberculosis
  - Malignancies
  - All anemias except hereditary spherocytosis and sickle cell anemia

  Decreased in—
  - Polycythemia
  - Sickle cell anemia
  - Hereditary spherocytosis

37. Hypocalcemic tetany.

Tetany

- Tetany is neuromuscular hyperexcitability due to hypocalcemia.
- The decrease in calcium ions in plasma results in reduction in the amount of depolarization needed to excite the nerves.

The signs and symptoms are:

- **Carpopedal spasm:** There is flexion at metacarpophalangeal joints, extension at interphalangeal joints and opposition of thumb (*refer* **Fig. 40**). In the legs, the toes are plantarflexed and feet are drawn up.
- **Trousseau's sign:** It is seen in latent tetany. On inflation of the sphygmomanometer cuff to the arm and occlusion of blood vessels results in appearance of the carpal spasm.
- **Chvostek's sign:** On tapping the facial nerve at the angle of the jaw, there is twitching of facial muscles.
- **Laryngeal stridor:** Spasm of laryngeal muscles results in constriction of larynx and it may result in asphyxia.
- **Paresthesia:** Tingling sensation in peripheral parts of limbs

Tetany is treated with infusion of ionized calcium and parathormone replacement.

38. Placental hormones.

Hormones Synthesized by Placenta

- Human chorionic gonadotropin (hCG)
- Human chorionic somatomammotropin (hCS)
- Placental progesterone
- Placental estrogen
- Relaxin

Human Chorionic Gonadotropin (hCG)

- It is synthesized by syncytiotrophoblasts of placenta.
- It is a glycoprotein with α and β subunits.
- It starts appearing in the blood of mother by 6 days after fertilization and reaches a peak by 10–12 weeks.
- Clinically, presence of hCG in urine of a female is "the indicator" of pregnancy.
- It stimulates the corpus luteum to secrete progesterone till the placenta is fully formed.
- hCG helps in sexual differentiation of male fetus.
- It induces hyperemesis in the first trimester.

Human Chorionic Somatomammotropin (hCS)

- It is also secreted from the syncytiotrophoblast of placenta.
- Its secretion starts by 5th week of pregnancy and reaches a peak towards term.
- It is similar to growth hormone and has growth promoting actions, so called as "Maternal growth hormone of pregnancy"
- It stimulates lipolysis, N_2, K^+ and Ca^{2+} retention and decreases glucose utilization by the mother so that the substrates are diverted to the fetus.
- Amount of hCS secreted is equal to size of placenta and level of hCS indicates placental viability.

Placental Progesterone

- In the early weeks of pregnancy, progesterone is produced by corpus luteum and later the function is taken over by placenta.
- It is produced by coordination between the mother and the fetus—the fetoplacental unit.

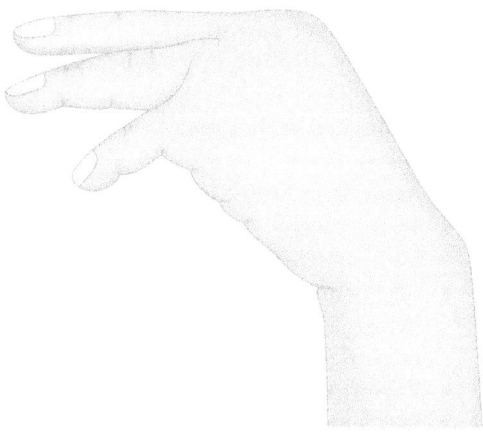

Fig. 40: Trousseau's sign.

- It makes the endometrium secretory and thereby nourishes the fertilized ovum.
- It keeps the myometrium quiescent which is essential for the survival of the fetus.
- It acts on the alveolar system of the maternal breast and facilitates the development of breast.
- It has an immunosuppressive role in protecting the fetus.

Placental Estrogen

- The major estrogen in pregnancy is estriol.
- It stimulates development of the ductular system of the maternal breast.
- The levels of estrogen rises during pregnancy but on nearing term, estrogen—progesterone ratio rises and estrogen makes the myometrium excitable.
- On decrease of levels of estrogen, after delivery of fetus, prolactin stimulates milk secretion from the breast.

Relaxin

- Its level in the early pregnancy is high to relax the uterine wall to favor implantation of fetus.
- In later weeks, it causes relaxation of pubic symphysis and pelvic ligaments to facilitate delivery of fetus.

The other hormones secreted are:
CRH, β endorphin, α-MSH, GnRH, inhibin, prolactin, etc.

39. Myasthenia gravis.

- It is an autoimmune disease.
- Antibodies are formed against the nicotinic ACh receptors in neuromuscular junction.
- There is weakness, fatigue and the muscles become weak with repeated use and therefore symptoms worsen towards the evening.
- The antibodies not only combine with ACh for the receptors but they also flatten the post-synaptic membrane and cause endocytosis of ACh into presynaptic membrane.
- Because of these effects, the muscle response to repeated stimulation gradually decreases.
- Symptoms improve after rest and are better on getting up in the morning.
- The extraocular and facial muscles are the first to be affected and ptosis and diplopia are present.

Treatment

- Acetylcholine esterase (ACh E) inhibitors—ACh E inhibitors increase the amount of ACh in the NMJ and they can displace the antibodies and improve functions.
- **Thymectomy:** Decreases the immune response by inhibiting T cell activation.
- Immunosuppressants
- Plasmapheresis

40. Immunoglobulins.

- Immunoglobulins (Ig) or antibodies are of 5 types.
- The structure of IgG forms the basic structure of all other types of Igs.
- IgG is "Y"-shaped and made of 4 polypeptide chains—2 heavy chains and 2 light chains.
- The chains are held together by disulfide bonds.
- The two heavy chains are long and light chains are short.
- There are 2 types of light chains κ (kappa) and λ (lambda) and there are 8 types of heavy chains.
- Each heavy chain has a variable segment (v) in which the amino acid sequence are highly variable and is the binding site of antigen (*refer* **Fig. 41**).
- There is a diversity segment (D) and the amino acid segments are also variable.
- The adjoining region is the hinge or joining segment (J) and the amino acids are moderately variable.
- The remaining region is said to be the constant region (C) and is common to all the Igs of the particular type of immunoglobulin.
- Each light chain also has a V, a J and a C segment.
- The V segment of both the chains (Fab portion) is the antigen binding sites and the Fc portion of the molecule is the effector portion which mediates the reactions of antibodies.

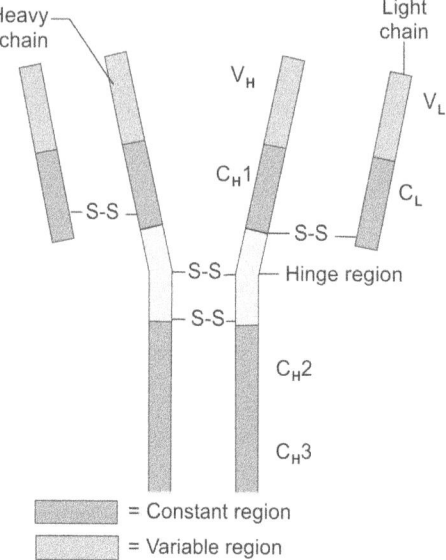

Fig. 41: Structure of immunoglobulin.

Types of Immunoglobin

- **IgG:** It is a monomer and it has the function of complement activation and is an opsonin.
- **IgA:** It is a monomer or dimer. It is present in the secretions of the body, such as the tears, breast milk, etc., therefore, it is called as 'secretory immunoglobulin'.
- **IgM:** Complement fixation, ABO antibodies belong to this category
- **IgD:** Antigen recognition by B cells.
- **IgE:** Reagin activation, releases histamine from basophils and mast cells.

Functions of Immunoglobulins

Immunoglobulins attack the antigens in two ways:
1. Direct attack on the antigens
2. Complement activation and thereby inactivation of antigens

Direct inactivation of antigens is by:
- Agglutination of antigens, by binding to antibodies making them a large clump which favors phagocytosis by the phagocytes.
- Precipitation of antigen-antibody complexes.
- Antibodies cover the antigen and neutralize it.
- Directly attacks the membrane of the pathogen and lyses it.

Activation of complement system and thereby destroying the antigens:
- Opsonization and phagocytosis by neutrophils and macrophages
- Lysis by forming a lytic complex which gets inserted on the pathogen and destroying it
- Agglutination
- Neutralization of antigen
- Chemotaxis
- Activation of basophils and mast cells

41. Summation.

- Summation means adding up of impulses.
- In the synapse, following release of neurotransmitters there could be depolarization or hyperpolarization of the membrane.
- These are called as postsynaptic potentials and they belong to the category of graded potentials.
- So, these individual potentials from many synapses can summate and excite the membrane and take it to the firing level.
- There are two types of summations—spatial and temporal summation.
- Temporal summation—the same input stimulates the postsynaptic neuron repeatedly and thereby excites it.
- Spatial summation—here many inputs stimulate simultaneously to excite it.

42. Hering-Breuer inflation reflex.

- Hering and Breuer found that over inflation of the lungs results in decreased output through the phrenic nerves to the diaphragm and thereby stimulates expiration.
- This reflex is a protective reflex to prevent over inflation of the lungs.
- The receptors are slowly adapting nerve endings of the myelinated vagus nerves in the airways of the lungs.
- This reflex is stimulated by steady increase in lung volume resulting in immediate and prolonged expiration.
- It is more useful in infants than adults and it regulates the tidal volume in infants.

43. Taste receptor.

- Taste receptors are epithelial cells and are located in the taste buds.
- Cells in taste buds are of three types:
  1. Type 1 and 2—are supporting cells.
  2. Type 3 cells—receptor epithelial cells which have microvilli projecting into the taste pore on the dorsum of the tongue and they respond to the tastants
- Type 3 cells extend to full length of the taste buds
- They are replaced constantly in 10 days.
- Each taste bud has 50-150 receptor cells
- Each bud is innervated by 50 nerves at bases of receptor cells.
- Each nerve innervates 5 taste buds.
- On sectioning the nerve taste bud degenerates.
- Taste buds are located in—fungiform, filiform and vallate papillae.

44. PR interval in ECG.

- It is between beginning of P wave to beginning of Q wave.
- The normal duration is 0.12-0.2 Sec (average 0.18 sec).
- This denotes atrial depolarization and conduction to AV node.
- Prolonged PR interval signifies AV conduction block

45. Chronaxie.

The time duration for which double the strength of rheobase current should be given to excite a tissue is said to be the **chronaxie**. Chronaxie is an indicator of tissue excitability. Shorter the chronaxie for a tissue, excitability is better. Smooth muscles have the longer chronaxie.

Rheobase is the minimum strength of a stimulus given for a particular time and is able to excite a tissue.

46. CSF formation.

- CSF is formed from the **choroid plexus** in the walls of all the ventricles.
- Rate of formation is 0.35 mL/min or 20 mL/hr or 500 mL/D.
- Normal volume of CSF at any time is 70-150 mL.
- Formation is by passive diffusion, active transport and facilitated diffusion.
- There are 2 steps—ultrafiltration and active secretion.
- The choroid plexus are network of capillaries which are covered by ependymal cells of the ventricles.
- These cells form CSF from blood by filtration and secretion.
- The cells are joined by tight junctions to prevent leakage between the cells.

47. Phasic changes in coronary circulation.

- There are phasic changes in blood flow through coronaries.
- In systole as the myocardium contracts, the blood vessels are compressed and there is no blood flow through the coronaries.
- In diastole as the myocardium relaxes, the vessels dilate and blood flow increases through the vessels.
- The endocardial vessels show the maximum phasic variation in blood flow. Therefore, these areas suffer from hypoxia and are prone for ischemia in compromised states.

48. FEV1.

- When vital capacity is related to time, it is said to be timed vital capacity.
- It is defined as the percentage of vital capacity that is expired in a unit of time.
- It is also called as forced vital capacity or forced expiratory volume (FEV) as the person exhales rapidly and forcibly in a unit of time.
- FEV_1—volume expelled in the 1st second—80% of VC
- FEV_2—volume expelled in the 2nd second—90% of VC
- FEV_3—volume expelled in 3rd second—100% of VC
- FEV_1/FVC ratio is a good indicator to diagnose obstructive and restrictive pulmonary diseases.
- In obstructive disease FEV_1/FVC ratio is decreased

- In restrictive disorders, it may be normal or increased.

49. Dopamine.

- It is secreted by small intensely fluorescent cells (SIF) in the autonomic ganglia and in the brain.
- In basal ganglia, it is secreted by the nigrostriatal pathway and is very important clinically as the deficiency of dopamine in this pathway results in Parkinson's disease.
- It is synthesized from the amino acid tyrosine.
- It is metabolized to inactive compounds by monoamine oxidase (MAO) and catechol-O-methyltransferase (COMT) pathways.
- There are 5 different types of receptors for dopamine—D1, D2, D3, D4, and D5.
- Most of the receptors act through G proteins
- D2 and D4 receptors are increased in schizophrenia and blockers of these receptors help to treat schizophrenia.

Answers to 2013 Question Paper

ANSWER ALL QUESTIONS

I. Essay Questions (15 Marks each)

1. Define hemostasis. Describe in detail about extrinsic and intrinsic mechanism of clotting.
2. Give an account of composition and functions of pancreatic juice. How is the secretion regulated?
3. Define cardiac cycle. Describe in detail the pressure volume changes that occur during a cardiac cycle with suitable diagram.
4. Describe the connections and functions of hypothalamus.
5. What are blood groups? Discuss their importance.
6. Describe the hormonal regulation of human menstrual cycle.
7. Describe the process of transport of carbon dioxide from tissues to lungs.
8. Describe in detail the photochemical mechanism of vision and mechanism of dark adaptation.
9. Describe digestion and absorption of fat in the digestive tract. Write a note on steatorrhea.
10. What do you understand by the terms innate and acquired immunity? Describe the phenomenon of cell-mediated immunity.
11. Define the term blood pressure. Discuss the determinants and regulation of blood pressure.
12. Trace the pathway for perception of pain. Discuss the descending pain modulatory pathways. Discuss the terms 'gating of pain' and 'referred pain'.

II. Short Notes (5 Marks each)

1. Erythroblastosis fetalis.
2. Isotonic and isometric contraction.
3. Facilitated diffusion.
4. Enterohepatic circulation.
5. Juxtaglomerular apparatus.
6. Counter current exchanger.
7. Transport maximum (TM).
8. Acromegaly.
9. Steps in thyroxine synthesis.
10. Stages of spermatogenesis.
11. Functional residual capacity and its significance.
12. Types of hypoxia and its cause.
13. Respiratory membrane.
14. Neural centers for regulation of respiration.
15. Dead space.
16. Pacemaker potential.
17. Cardiac index.
18. Dark adaptation.
19. Functions of basal ganglia.
20. Vestibulocerebellum.
21. Tests for ovulation.
22. Contraceptives.
23. Thyroxine synthesis.
24. Tetany.
25. Juxtaglomerular apparatus.
26. Dialysis.
27. Gastric emptying.
28. Enterohepatic circulation.
29. Functions of saliva.
30. Autoimmune disease.
31. Decompression sickness.
32. Middle ear functions.
33. Define cardiac output. What are the methods to measure the cardiac output?

34. Heart sounds.
35. Define synapse and describe its properties.
36. Describe the functions of thalamus.
37. What are the functions of basal ganglia?
38. Describe the physiology of speech.
39. Decerebrate rigidity.
40. Functions of prefrontal lobe.
41. G-Protein coupled receptors.
42. Primary active transport.
43. Autoregulation of GFR.
44. Renal glycosuria.
45. Mechanism of bicarbonate generation in distal tubule.
46. Stimuli for secretion of aldosterone and actions of aldosterone.
47. Pancreatic C-peptide and its significance as a laboratory test.
48. Cretinism—its cause, features and strategy to prevent it.
49. What is the function of corpus luteum of pregnancy? How is it supported?
50. Parturition.
51. Ionic basis of the pace-maker potential.
52. Windkessel effect of aorta.
53. Illustrate with a diagram, the left ventricular volume and pressure changes during a cardiac cycle.
54. Role of myelin sheath in conduction of nerve impulse.
55. Functions of hypothalamus.
56. Clinical features of cerebellar lesions.
57. Physiological roles of muscle spindle.
58. Chemical regulation of respiration.
59. Hamburger's chloride shift.
60. Role of surfactant in pulmonary function.

III. Short Answers (2 Marks each)

1. Chronaxie
2. Motor unit.
3. Apoptosis.
4. Osmotic diuresis.
5. LH surge.
6. Somatomedins.
7. Hormones of adrenal cortex.
8. Types of diabetes.
9. Action of parathormone on bone.
10. Menarche.
11. Muscles of inspiration.
12. P50.
13. End diastolic volume.
14. Attenuation reflex.
15. Perimetry.
16. Summation.
17. Referred pain.
18. Types of memory.
19. Thalamic syndrome.
20. Klüver-Bucy syndrome.
21. Functions of sodium potassium ATPase pump.
22. Mention the normal value of GFR and substance used to measure GFR.
23. Enumerate heat loss mechanism.
24. Peristalsis.
25. What is the role of vitamin K in the body?
26. What is the normal blood calcium level?
27. Name the hormones of adrenal cortex.
28. Name the hormones of placenta.
29. Cryptorchidism.
30. Why are ovarian cycles suppressed during lactation?
31. What is P50?
32. What are the types of hypoxia?
33. Mention common refractory errors of the eye.
34. SA node as pacemaker.
35. PR interval.
36. Reflex arc.
37. Functions of cerebrospinal fluid.
38. What is righting reflex?
39. Name the nuclei responsible for hunger and satiety in human being.
40. What is referred pain?
41. Extracellular fluid volume and blood volume in an adult male weighing 70 kg.
42. Calcium transporters on the membrane of sarcoplasmic reticulum.
43. Mechanism of edema in congestive cardiac failure.
44. State a manifestation of hypocalcemic tetany. Give one cause leading to this condition.
45. List the vitamin K-dependent coagulation factors.
46. Rh status of mother, father and child for occurrence of Rh incompatibility.

47. Role of tropomyosin in muscle contraction.
48. Type of acetylcholine receptor on skeletal muscle and its function.
49. Hormones secreted by hypothalamus.
50. Hormonal defect in (a) Addison's disease (b) Conn's syndrome.
51. List the calcium transporters on the sarcoplasmic reticular membrane in the ventricular muscle.
52. State Starling's law of the heart.
53. What is the effect of 2,3 diphosphoglycerate on the oxygen-hemoglobin dissociation curve? Does it help in loading or unloading of oxygen?
54. What are the types of hypoxia?
55. Region of the cochlea which vibrates most for the highest sound frequency in the audible range.
56. Visual field defect when the optic chiasma is cut in the center.
57. State the refractive error in astigmatism. How is it corrected?
58. What is 'Blind spot'?
59. Receptors for vestibular sensation.
60. Name of tracts made up by second order neurons in the pathway for (a) fine touch, (b) pain.

I. ESSAY QUESTIONS

1. Define hemostasis. Describe in detail about extrinsic and intrinsic mechanism of clotting.

- Blood while flowing in the vessels is fluid in nature, but when the vessel wall is injured or the blood is removed from the body and collected in a test tube it becomes a jelly like mass—The Clot.
- Clotting or coagulation of blood involves a series of cascade of events in which many clotting factors (proteins in the plasma) are activated in a serial manner. There are many such clotting factors.

They are:
- **Factor I:** Fibrinogen
- **Factor II:** Prothrombin
- **Factor III:** Thromboplastin
- **Factor IV:** Calcium
- **Factor V:** Labile factor or proaccelerin
- **Factor VI:** Non-existent
- **Factor VII:** Stable factor or proconvertin
- **Factor VIII:** Antihemophilic factor
- **Factor IX:** Christmas factor or plasma thromboplastic component (PTC) or antihemophilic factor B
- **Factor X:** Stuart-Prower factor
- **Factor XI:** Plasma thromboplastin antecedent (PTA) or antihemophilic factor C.
- **Factor XII:** Hageman factor or glass factor or contact factor
- **Factor XIII:** Laki-Lorand factor or fibrin stabilizing factor
- **HMW: K**—High molecular weight kininogen or Fitzgerald factor
- **Pre-Ka** (Prekallikrein or fletcher factor)
- **Kallikrein:** Ka
- **PL:** Platelet phospholipid

The coagulation process involves three major steps:
1. Formation of prothrombin activator
2. Conversion of prothrombin to thrombin
3. Conversion of fibrinogen to fibrin

Formation of Prothrombin Activator is by 2 Mechanisms
- Extrinsic pathway
- Intrinsic pathway

Intrinsic Pathway

This pathway is activated when there is injury to vessel wall and exposure of collagen or blood itself.

Steps involved are:
- Injury to vessel wall exposes collagen activates factor XII to XIIa
- Factor XIIa activates factor XI to XIa
- Factor XIa activates factor IX to IXa
- Factor IXa in the presence of VIII, Ca^{2+} and platelet phospholipids (PPL) activates factor X to Xa.
- The activated factor Xa, platelet phospholipids, factor Va and Ca^{2+} forms the prothrombin activator (*refer* **Fig. 1**).

The *extrinsic pathway* is triggered when the injury involves damage to the blood vessels and the surrounding tissues.

The damaged tissue releases tissue thromboplastin, a protein-phospholipid

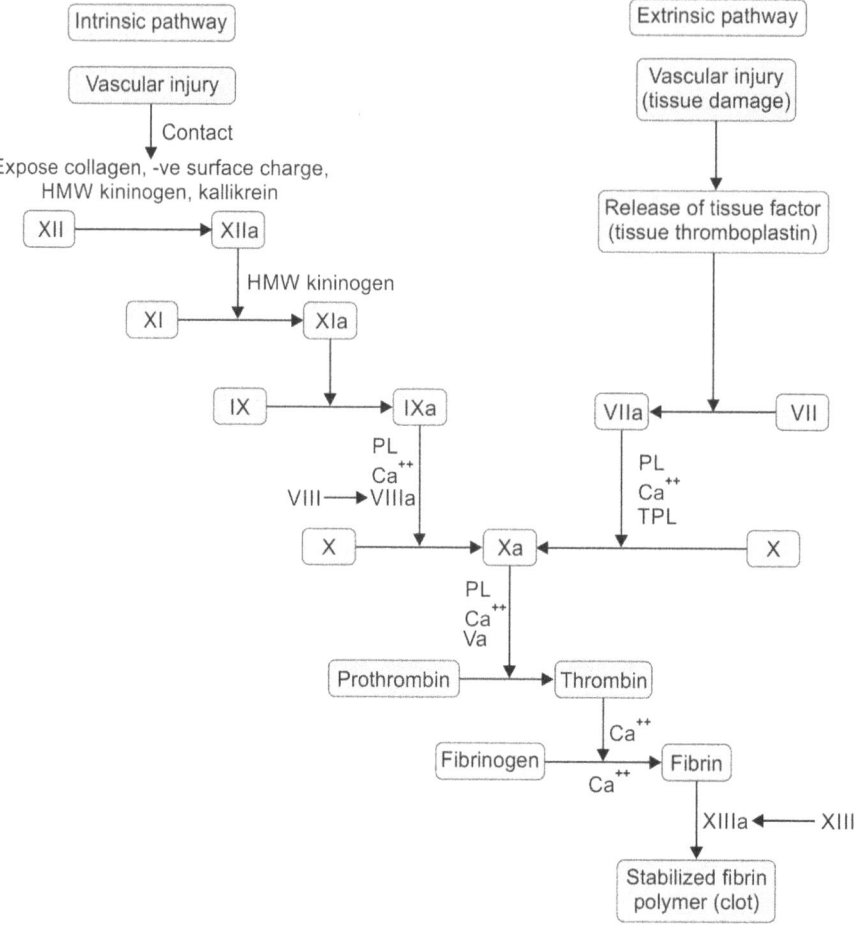

Fig. 1: Mechanism of clotting.
(TPL: tissue phospholipid, PL: platelet phospholipid)

mixture which activates factor VII. This triggers the extrinsic pathway.
- Inactive factor VII is activated to active factor VIIa.
- VIIa in the presence of Ca^{2+}, platelet phospholipid (PL) and tissue thromboplastin, activates factors IX and X.
- Active factor Xa, Va, Ca^{2+} and PL, forms the Prothrombin activator.
- Prothrombin activator converts prothrombin to thrombin.
- Thrombin catalyzes the conversion of fibrinogen to fibrin
  - Fibrinogen a soluble glycoprotein in plasma is converted to insoluble fibrin.
  - Fibrin forms a mesh and traps the blood cells.
- This is facilitated by the fibrin stabilizing factor (factor XIII).
- The stabilized fibrin mesh with entrapped blood cells forms the clot. This pathway involves fewer steps in the clot formation and therefore is a faster pathway than the intrinsic pathway.

Conversion of Prothrombin to Thrombin

Prothrombin activator in the presence of Ca^{2+} converts Prothrombin to thrombin. This happens at the surface of platelets. Thrombin is a proteolytic enzyme.

Conversion of Fibrinogen to Fibrin

- Thrombin, a proteolytic enzyme removes two pairs of polypeptide chains from each

fibrinogen molecule and converts it to fibrin monomer.
- The fibrin monomers now polymerize to form long fibrin threads. The fibrin is initially a loose mesh of interlacing strands. This meshwork traps the blood cells
- It is later converted to a dense tight aggregate by formation of covalent cross-linkages. This is catalyzed by factor XIII and Ca^{2+}. The stabilized fibrin mesh with the trapped blood cells forms the CLOT.

2. Give an account of composition and functions of pancreatic juice. How is the secretion regulated?

Composition of Pancreatic Juice

- Rate of secretion—1200–1500 mL/day
- Specific gravity—1.010–1.018
- pH—7.8–8.4, due to high concentration of HCO_3^-
- About 99.5% is water and 0.5% solids
- **Organic constituents:** Contains enzymes, such as amylase, lipase, protease, trypsin inhibitor and traces of albumin and globulin.
- **Inorganic constituents:**
  - Cations, such as: Na^+, K^+, Ca^{++}, Mg^{++} and Zn^{2+}
  - Anions, such as: HCO_3^-, Cl^-, SO_4^{2-} and HPO_4^{2-}

Fuctions of Pancreatic Juice

Digestive Function of Pancreatic Juice

- **Digestion of lipids:**
  - Pancreatic lipase is the major fat digesting enzyme. It digests triglycerides into monoglycerides and fatty acids
  - **Colipase:** It exposes active sites of pancreatic lipase and facilitates its action
  - **Phopholipase A_2:** It acts on phospholipids and converts it to fatty acids and lysophospholipids.
  - Cholesterol ester hydrolase acts on cholesterol esters and splits it into cholesterol and fatty acids.

- **Digestion of proteins:**
  - Proteolytic enzymes are secreted in the inactive forms—trypsinogen, chymotrypsinogen,
  - Proelastase and procarboxypeptidase A and B.
  - Trypsinogen on secretion into duodenum is activated to trypsin by the enzyme enterokinase in the intestine.
  - Trypsinogen → Trypsin, happens in presence of enterokinase
  - Chymotrypsinogen → Chymotrypsin, in presence of trypsin
  - Proelastase and procarboxylase → Elastase and carboxylase, in presence of trypsin
  - ***Trypsin and chymotrypsin*** act on proteins and polypeptides and cleaves the peptide bonds in basic and aromatic amino acids.
  - Elastase acts on elastin and some other proteins.
  - Carboxypeptidases also act on proteins and polypeptides
  - Nucleases split ribose and deoxyribose nucleotides
  - Collagenase digests collagen
- **Digestion of carbohydrates:** Pancreatic α amylase—It is secreted in active form and just like salivary amylase it hydrolysis glycogen, starch and other complex carbohydrates to form disaccharides.
- **Trypsin inhibitor** secreted from pancreas inhibits activation of trypsinogen and thereby prevents autodigestion of pancreas by trypsin.

  Trypsin if activated initiates a chain of reaction and activates other proteolytic enzymes and can digest the pancreas.

Regulation of Intestinal pH

- Pancreatic juice is rich in HCO_3^- and therefore alkaline in nature.
- HCO_3^- is secreted by the ductal cells.
- The alkalinity created by HCO_3^- neutralizes the HCl derived from gastric juice as it enters the intestine.

Regulation of Pancreatic Secretion

- Pancreatic secretion is regulated by neural and humoral mechanisms.
- Neural regulation is by vagal efferents supplying exocrine pancreas.
- Hormonal regulation is by the hormones—secretin, cholecystokinin (CCK), gastrin and somatostatin
- Regulation is discussed under the headings—cephalic phase, gastric phase and intestinal phase.

Regulation in Cephalic Phase

- This phase is under the reflex vagal stimulation
- Regulation of this phase starts even before the food enters stomach.
- It happens by unconditioned reflex (presence of food in mouth and actions of mastication and
- Swallowing) and conditioned reflexes (by sight, smell and thought of food).

Regulation in Gastric Phase

- This phase starts when food enters the stomach.
- It is stimulated by distension of stomach.
- It is under the influence of vagus stimulation and by the hormone gastrin.

Regulation in Intestinal Phase

- This phase starts when the food enters duodenum and jejunum.
- It stimulates secretion of pancreatic juice rich in bicarbonate.
- It is under the control of intestinal hormones—secretin and CCK.

Role of secretin:

- Secretin is secreted by the 'S' cells of duodenum and jejunum.
- Its secretion is stimulated by presence of acid in the intestine.
- It acts on the pancreatic ductal cells and stimulates secretion of large volume of watery bicarbonate rich pancreatic juice.
- It also stimulates bicarbonate rich bile secretion from hepatocytes in liver.

Role of cholecystokinin:

- It is secreted from 'I' cells of the duodenum and jejunum.
- Its secretion is stimulated by presence of products of amino acids and fatty acids in the intestine.
- CCK is secreted into blood and it acts on the pancreatic acini and stimulates secretion of enzyme rich pancreatic juice.

---

3. Define cardiac cycle. Describe in detail the pressure volume changes that occur during a cardiac cycle with suitable diagram.

Definition

- Cardiac cycle is defined as the cycle of mechanical and electrical events taking place from beginning of one beat to the beginning of next beat.
- It is given as the changes in volume, pressure and flow in different cardiac chambers, the electrical activities occurring (recorded through ECG) and coinciding heart sounds (using PCG) in various phases of cardiac cycle.
- Duration of a cardiac cycle is 0.8 s when heart rate is 75/min.

Phases of Cardiac Cycle and their Duration

- Atrial systole—0.1 s
- Atrial diastole—0.7 s
- Ventricular systole—0.3 s
- Ventricular diastole—0.5 s
  - Atrial diastole merges with ventricular systole.
  - So the phases described here are atrial systole, ventricular systole and diastole.
- **Ventricular systole: 2 phases—0.3 sec**
  - **Isovolumetric contraction phase—0.05 s**
  - **Phase of ejection 0.25 s**
    - Phase of rapid ejection—0.1 s
    - Phase of reduced ejection—0.15 s
- **Ventricular diastole: 0.5 s**
  - Protodiastole—0.04 s
  - Isovolumetric relaxation phase—0.06 s
  - Rapid ventricular filling—0.11 s
  - Diastasis—0.19 s
- **Atrial systole: 0.1 s**

Atrial Systole

- Duration is 0.1 sec
- This follows the phase of diastasis

- Begins from peak of "P" wave in ECG to peak of "QRS" complex
- Atria contracts and increases intra-atrial pressure. Blood is pumped into ventricles.
- Final filling of ventricle takes place here (last 25-30%).
- Already the ventricles are in diastole and 75% of filling is complete.
- 4th heart sound is recorded in phonocardiogram.

Ventricular Systole

Isovolumic Contraction Phase

- Starts at peak of 'QRS' complex. Duration is 0.05 sec.
- Rise in ventricular pressure closes the AV valves and semilunar valves have not yet opened.
- 1st heart sound (S1) is heard, due to closure of AV valves.
- Ventricular pressure rises (>80 mm Hg) steeply and ventricular volume remains same.
- There is bulging of AV valves into the atria due to ventricular contraction. This creates 'C' wave in JVP curve.
- Phase ends with opening of semilunar valves and ejection of blood (*refer* **Fig. 2**).

Ventricular Ejection

- **Rapid ejection phase:** (0.1s)
  - Semilunar valves open and blood is rapidly ejected (2/3rd of stroke volume) into aorta/pulmonary artery.
  - Steep fall in ventricular volume and steep increase in aortic flow
  - Ventricular pressure increases to a peak (120 mm Hg in the left and 25 mm Hg in the right)
  - Aortic pressure also increases.
  - Corresponds to ST segment in ECG
- **Reduced ejection phase:** (0.15s)
  - Duration is 0.15 sec
  - Ventricular and aortic pressure decreases but aortic pressure is greater.
  - Aortic blood flow decreases. Only 1/3rd of stroke volume is ejected here.
  - Ventricular volume further decreases.
  - Momentum keeps blood flowing into aorta.
  - 'T' wave appears in ECG

Ventricular Diastole—0.5 s

- Protodiastole—0.04 s
- Isovolumetric relaxation—0.06 s
- Phase of rapid ventricular filling—0.11 s
- Phase of reduced filling or diastasis—0.19 s
- Phase of second rapid filling—0.1 s

Protodiastole

- Duration is 0.04 sec
- As the reduced filling phase ends, the ventricles start relaxing.
- Intraventricular pressure drops.
- This phase ends when aortic valve closes.

Isovolumetric Relaxation Phase

- Duration is 0.06 sec
- This phase is between closure of semilunar valves and opening of AV valves.
- Second heart sound (S2) appears due to closure of semilunar valves.
- Closure of semilunar valves creates '**dicrotic notch**' in aortic pressure curve
- Ventricular volume remains the same and pressure drops steeply as the ventricles relax (2-3 mm Hg)
- When intraventricular pressure drops below atrial pressure, AV valves open.

Rapid Ventricular Filling

- Duration is 0.11 sec
- As the AV valves open there is rapid inrush of blood into ventricles.
- This is because the atria are filled with venous return and pressure is high here.
- This vibration of ventricular wall creates the 3rd (S3) heart sound (*refer* **Fig. 3**).
- Major filling takes place here.

Diastasis

- Duration 0.19 sec.
- This is a slow filling phase.
- Ventricular volume rises slowly.
- Ventricular and atrial pressures reduce and remain same (Little >0 mm Hg).
- Nearly 75% of filling has occurred.

Last Rapid Filling

- Duration 0.1 sec.
- Atria contracts and pumps the last 25% of blood into ventricles.
- At rest, this volume is not essential.

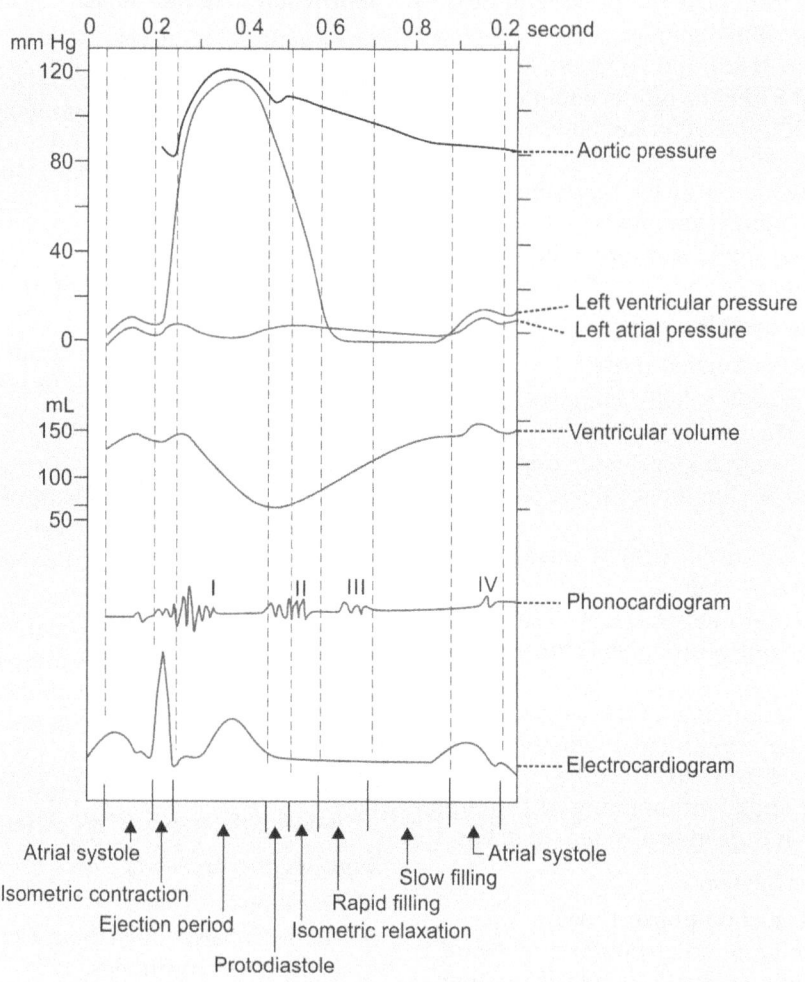

Fig. 2: Cardiac cycle with pressure volume changes in aorta, left ventricle, left atrium, ECG and phonocardiogram.

- But in tachycardia (as in exercise) when the duration of diastole decreases this volume assumes importance

4. Describe the connections and functions of hypothalamus.

- It is a small part located inferior to thalamus, composed of dozen nuclei.
- It is divided into four major areas.
  a. **Preoptic region:** Medial and lateral preoptic N
  b. **Supraoptic region:** Supraoptic, supra-chiasmatic, paraventricular and anterior nuclei
  c. **Tuberal region:** Ventromedial, dorsomedial, arcuate, lateral and posterior nuclei
  d. **Mammillary region:** Medial and lateral mammillary nuclei, pre- and supramammillary nuclei (*refer* **Fig. 4**).

Connections

- **Fornix:** Through fornix, it is connected to limbic system.
- **Medial forebrain bundle:** Extensively and reciprocally connected to brain stem.
- **Periventricular system:** Reciprocally connects midbrain and sensory pathways to hypothalamus

Heart sounds	Events responsible	Duration	Frequency	Others
First sound (S_1)	Due to vibrations set by sudden closure of AV valves at the onset of ventricular systole	0.15 sec	25–45 Hz In PCG recorded as 9–13 waves	Soft and long, heard as "LUBB"
Second sound (S_2)	Associated with closure of aortic and pulmonary valves after the end of ventricular systole	0.12 sec	50 Hz In PCG recorded as 4–6 waves	Normally S2 can be split due to early closure of aortic valve, heard as "Dup"
Third sound (S_3)	Is heard at 1/3rd of diastole due to rapid filling of ventricle due to vibrations set by inrush of blood		0.1 sec In PCG recorded as 1–4 waves	Normally audible only in children and young adults
Fourth sound (S_4)	Heard just before (S_1) Occurs during atrial contraction Due to ventricular filling		20 cyc/sec In PCG recorded as 1–2 waves	Rarely heard in normal adults Heard in vent hypertrophy and CCF

Fig. 3: Heart sounds.

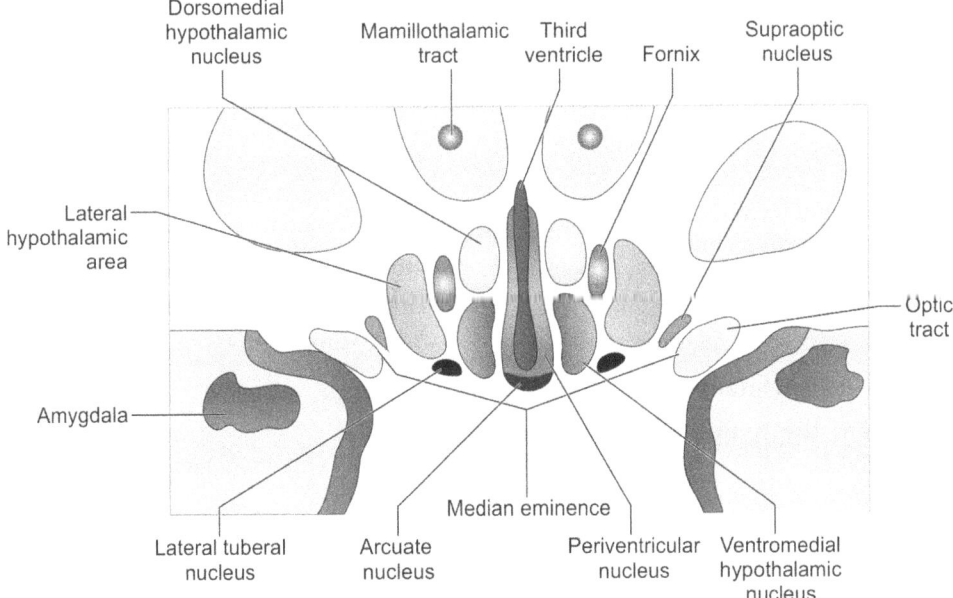

Fig. 4: Nuclei in hypothalamus.

- **Mammillothalamic tract:** Connects mammillary body to anterior thalamic N
- **Retinohypothalamic fibers:** Connects retina with suprachiasmatic nucleus of hypothalamus and is responsible for regulation of circadian rhythm.
- **Mammillotegmental tract:** Mamillary body to Tegmental N in brain stem.
- **Hypothalamo-hypophyseal tract:** Connections with anterior and posterior pituitary glands and regulates their secretions

- **Tuberoinfundibular tract:** Connects arcuate and ventromedial N of hypothalamus and infundibulum.
- **Dorsal nor-adrenergic bundle:** Connects locus ceruleus to dorsal HT.
- Serotonergic neurons
- Cortico-hypothalamic fibers (*refer* **Fig. 5**).

Functions

- Regulation of food intake
- Regulation of body temperature
- Regulation of thirst
- Regulation of anterior pituitary hormones
- Regulation of posterior pituitary hormones
- Regulation of sleep wake cycle
- Control of autonomic nervous system
- Control of reproduction
- Control of emotions
- Control of circadian rhythm
- Role in stress
- Role in visceral and somatic function
- Role in reward and punishment

Regulation of Food Intake

There are 2 groups of neurons involved in food intake:
1. **Ventromedial N (Satiety center)**
2. **Lateral N (Feeding center)**

Feeding center stimulates appetite and increases food intake and satiety center inhibits feeding center and brings satiety.

Regulation of Food Intake

- **These are the hypothesis regulating food-intake:**
  - *Glucostatic hypothesis*: Activity of satiety center is regulated by glucose utilization of the neurons. When the glucose utilization is low their activity is less and vice versa. When satiety center activity is less the feeding center's activity is unchecked and the person feels hungry. When utilization is high, the glucostats activity is unchecked and there is inhibition of feeding center and the person feels sated. Hypoglycemia is an appetite stimulant and the decrease in plasma glucose decreases the utilization of glucose by the cells.
  - *Lipostatic hypothesis:* This hypothesis is based on the fact that the adipose tissues send humoral signals like Leptin, a hormone secreted by adipose tissue. When fat depots are more, the leptin levels increase and it decreases food intake and increases energy output.
  - *Gut-peptide theory:* After food intake, there are hormones released from the GIT which act on the hypothalamus and thereby inhibits food intake
  - *Thermostatic theory:* Food intake is increased in cold weather and decreased in warm weather.

Hormones and NT Regulating Food Intake

- **Hormones increasing food intake:**
  - Neuropeptide Y
  - Orexins
  - Ghrelin
  - MCH
  - AGRP (Agouti-related peptide)
  - Galanin
  - GHRH

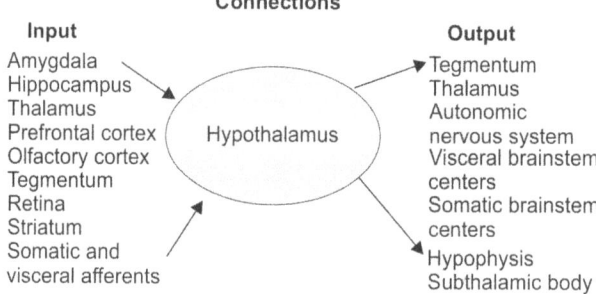

Fig. 5: Connections of hypothalamus.

- **Hormones decreasing food intake:**
  - Estrogen
  - Dopamine
  - α MSH
  - Cocaine- and amphetamine-regulated transcript (CART)
  - Corticotropin-releasing hormone (CRH)
  - Gut hormones
  - Cholecystokinin
  - Leptin

Temperature Regulation

- Humans need to maintain body temperature at 37°C.
- Preoptic region of anterior hypothalamus has a role in regulation of body temperature in warmth. When body temperature goes above set point it stimulates heat dissipating mechanisms, such as vasodilation and sweating.
- Posterior hypothalamus acts in cool temperature and involved in heat conserving mechanisms, such as vasoconstriction, pilo- erection and sympathetic stimulation.

Regulation of Thirst

- Thirst center is located in the hypothalamus.
- It is located in the lateral hypothalamus.
- It is stimulated by osmoreceptors in increase in tonicity of body fluids.
- A decrease in ECF volume also stimulates thirst center.

Regulation of ECF Volume

Achieved by regulation of ADH, Aldosterone and thirst mechanism.

Regulation of Endocrine Functions

- Hypothalamus controls anterior pituitary and through anterior pituitary it regulates secretion of other endocrine glands.
- It secretes posterior pituitary hormones.
- Hypothalamus is considered to be the master of endocrine orchestra.
- It is a part of the brain and therefore is the link between neural and endocrine systems.

Control of Reproduction

- Hypothalamus releases GnRH which regulates the release of FSH and LH from anterior pituitary gland.
- They in turn control reproductive function in males and females.
- They regulate spermatogenesis, development of accessory sex organs in males and menstrual cycle and secondary sexual characteristics in females.
- Also the sexual behavior are influenced by hypothalamus (preoptic and anterior hypothalamus)

Regulation of Sleep Wake Cycle

- Hypothalamus regulates sleep wake cycle.
- There are 2 sleep centers:
  1. Diencephalic sleep zone
  2. Basal forebrain sleep zone
- Stimulation of these areas at the frequency of 8 Hz induces slow wave sleep

Control of ANS

- Hypothalamus controls and integrates the activities of ANS.
- Through ANS, it is a major regulator of visceral activities.
- Stimulation of posterior hypothalamus results in increase in HR, BP, pupillary dilatation, piloerection (sympathetic system stimulated).
- Stimulation of anterior hypothalamus results in decreased HR, increased HCl secretion, urination, etc., (parasympathetic system stimulated).

Regulation of Emotional and Behavioral Patterns

- With the limbic system it participates in the expressions of emotions.
- The circuit given below is responsible for emotions (*refer* **Fig. 6**).

Regulation of Circadian Rhythm

- The suprachiasmatic nucleus establishes patterns of awakening and sleep that occur on a circadian (daily) schedule.
- This is mediated through retinohypothalamic tract.

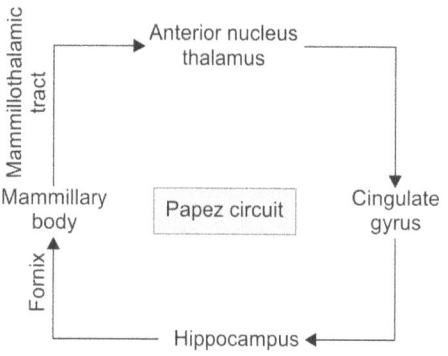

Fig. 6: Papez circuit.

□ **Example,**
  • Cortisol secretion
  • Body temperature
  • ACTH secretion
  • Melatonin secretion
  • Sleep-wakefulness

Regulation of Reward and Punishment Areas

□ Hypothalamus along with LS and cortex integrate and bring about smooth responses for reward and punishment.
□ VM nucleus is associated with reward and posterior and lateral N of hypothalamus with punishment.

---

5. What are blood groups? Discuss their importance.

□ The blood groups are classified based on the presence of antigens or agglutinogens on the membranes of RBCs.
□ An individual with a particular antigen on RBC membrane will not possess the corresponding antibody or agglutinin in his plasma.
□ This forms the basis of blood grouping.
□ There are more than 30 blood group systems based on the presence of nearly 400 antigens.
□ The blood group systems are: ABO system, Rh system, MNS, Lutheran, P, Kell, Kidd, Duffy, Lewis, etc.
□ Most of the antigens are cold antigens and therefore they do not react in body temperature.
□ The ABO and Rh systems are the major blood group systems as they react in body temperature and when they react with their corresponding agglutinins, they produce major reactions.
□ Since the above two systems of blood groups are more important, it is discussed in detail.
□ Karl Landsteiner has framed two laws based on the presence and absence of agglutinogens and agglutinins.
  a. If a particular agglutinogen (antigen) is present on the RBC membrane, the corresponding agglutinin (Antibody) will be absent in the plasma.
  b. If a particular agglutinogen is absent on the RBC membrane then the corresponding agglutinin will be present in the plasma.

ABO system follows both the laws whereas Rh system follows only the first law.

ABO System

□ This blood group system is based on the presence of the antigens A and B or both or none on RBC membrane.
□ There are 4 types of blood groups—A group, B group, AB group and O groups.
  • A has two subtypes—A_1 and A_2.
  • AB has A_1B and A_2B subtypes.
□ Antigens are present on the RBC membrane and also in secretions, such as saliva, semen, amniotic fluid and other tissues, such as salivary glands, testis, pancreas, etc.
□ These antigens are basically oligosaccharides and they differ among each other in their terminal sugars.
□ Agglutinogen A has N-acetylgalactosamine as the terminal sugar and B antigen has galactose as the terminal sugar and O does not have any terminal sugars.
□ Antigens start appearing since fetal age of 6 weeks.
□ Agglutinins of ABO systems are anti-A and anti-B antibodies and they belong to IgM type of antibodies and therefore they do not cross the placenta.
□ Antibodies are not present since fetal life and they start appearing in the 2nd week of neonatal life and reach a peak level by 10 years of age.

The blood types, antigens and antibodies in the ABO system are:

Blood groups	Agglutinogen present	Agglutinin present
A	A	Anti-B
B	B	Anti-B
AB	A and B	Nil
O	Nil	Anti-A and Anti-B

Rh System

- Rh system is the 2nd most important blood group system.
- There are 6 antigens of this system—C, D, E, c, d and e.
- But D antigen on the RBC membrane is the most antigenic.
- Therefore, individuals with D antigen are Rh positive and its absence is considered to be Rh negative.
- About 90–95% of Indian population is Rh positive.
- Rh system does not follow 2nd law of Landsteiner's, i.e., in an Rh negative individual the anti-D antibody is not present in plasma.
- But exposure to D antigens for the first time stimulates the immune system to form anti-D antibodies of a Rh-negative person.
- These antibodies can later react on D antigens if they are exposed to it in the second attempt.

Importance of Doing Blood Grouping

- The knowledge of the blood group of an individual helps in compatible blood transfusions in emergency situations of blood loss, such as surgery, trauma, etc.
- Blood grouping helps us to identify Rh incompatibility between mother and fetus and prevention of hemolytic disease of the newborn.
- The basis of antigens on RBC has given us an understanding about other hemolytic diseases.
- Certain blood group antigens are susceptible to certain diseases, such as malaria, viral infections and it also provides resistance to certain diseases.
- It is also useful for organ transplantation.
- ABO and Rh blood grouping is useful to settle paternity disputes.

Procedure for Determining the Blood Group

- To determine the blood group of an individual, a suspension of RBC is made by diluting a drop of blood in one mL normal saline.
- On a porcelain tile, drops of antisera A, B and D are put.
- To the antisera, a drop of RBC suspension is added and mixed with separate sticks for each antisera and left aside for 10 minutes.
- After 10 minutes, look for agglutination reactions in each of the antisera.
- Agglutinated RBCs look like clumps.
- If there is agglutination in antisera A the person's blood group is A and agglutination in antisera B it is B group and in anti-D the person is Rh positive.
- Agglutination is present because of the presence of a particular antigen on RBC membrane and is agglutinated when mixed with its corresponding antisera.

Blood group	Agglutination in antisera A	Agglutination in antisera B	Agglutination in antisera D
A Positive	+	-	+
A negative	-	-	-
B Positive	-	+	+
B Negative	-	+	-
AB Positive	+	+	+
AB Negative	+	+	-
O Positive	-	-	+
O Negative	-	-	-

Erythroblastosis Fetalis (EBF)

- It is also called as hemolytic disease of the newborn (HDN).
- This is due to Rh incompatibility between the mother and fetus.
- It happens if the mother is Rh negative and the fetus is Rh positive.
- Since Rh system does not follow the 2nd law of Landsteiner's, there are no

preformed antibodies in the Rh-negative mother's blood.
- So in first pregnancy, there are no complications.
- At the time of parturition, few fetal RBCs enter the mother's circulation.
- Mother's immune system recognizes the Rh antigen in the fetal RBCs as foreign antigens and starts producing antibodies for D antigen on fetal RBCs.
- These anti-D antibodies belong to IgG type and therefore can cross the placenta.
- If the mother conceives for the second time and if that fetus happens to Rh positive, the anti-D antibodies from mother crosses the placenta and destroys the fetal RBCs resulting in HDN/EBF.
- As the number of conceptions increase antibody titer increases and causes more damage to the fetus.
- **The symptoms are:**
  - *Anemia:* Due to massive hemolysis anemia sets in following agglutination
  - *Hemolytic jaundice:* The released hemoglobin, following hemolysis, is converted to bilirubin and the levels may rise very high resulting in jaundice.
  - *Hydrops fetalis:* Generalized edema due to anemia and hypoproteinemia
  - Erythroblasts start appearing in the circulation due to exaggerated erythropoiesis following severe anemia.
  - *Kernicterus:* It happens due to hemolysis and formation of excess bilirubin, and the bilirubin crosses the blood brain barrier (BBB) since the BBB is not fully developed in the fetus. Basal ganglia in the brain, has great affinity for bilirubin and therefore it gets deposited in the basal ganglia. There are motor dysfunctions due to this.

Prevention of EBF

EBF is prevented by administering the mother with anti-D antibodies after delivery of the fetus. Injected antibodies neutralize the antigens which had entered the mother's body and no further antibody production is prevented.

Treatment of EBF
- **Exchange transfusion:** The newborns with the above symptoms are treated with exchange transfusion after birth. This removes sensitized Rh-positive RBCs from the blood and is replaced with Rh-negative blood. This is continued till the antibodies are removed from the fetal circulation. The transfused blood should be ABO negative and Rh-negative.
- **Phototherapy** can also be given to reduce bilirubin levels.

6. Describe the hormonal regulation of human menstrual cycle.

- Menstrual cycle is the female sexual cycle and it happens once in 28–30 days. It is associated with uterine bleeding—menstruation.
- It is a preparatory cycle for fertilization and implantation of the fertilized ovum
- Therefore, cyclic changes happen in the uterus, ovaries, cervix and vagina.
- All these changes are under the control of various hormones.
- The hormones regulating menstrual cycle are hypothalamic hormones (GnRH), anterior pituitary hormones (FSH and LH) and ovarian hormones (Estrogen and progesterone).
- GnRH from hypothalamus is the key controller of gonadotropin released from anterior pituitary.
- GnRH is secreted in pulsatile fashion and the pulsatility of GnRH is very important in regulating secretions of LH and FSH.
- GnRH pulsatility is in turn kept in check by levels of estrogen and progesterone. Just before LH surge, pulsatility of GnRH is increased by high levels of estrogen.
- We will be now discussing the hormonal regulation for ovarian changes and endometrial changes separately.

Regulation of Ovarian Changes

Ovarian changes happen in 3 phases:
1. Follicular phase
2. Ovulatory phase
3. Luteal phase

Follicular phase:
- This phase starts from day 1 of menstruation to the day of ovulation (usually 14th day).
- Day 1 onwards the FSH and LH levels start increasing. Due to the actions of FSH, 10–20 follicles start to grow in size (*refer* **Figs. 7A to D**).
- The granulosa cells of the follicles acquire FSH receptors and start secreting estrogen. Only one follicle continues to grow and become the dominant follicle and this is the follicle which secretes estrogen maximally. Other follicles become atretic.
- The estrogen levels start increasing. Estrogen along with FSH induces LH receptors on granulosa cells and theca cells.
- LH acts on theca cells to increase androgen synthesis and this androgen is diverted to granulosa cells for synthesis of estrogen.
- Now the rising estrogen levels have a **positive feedback** effect on LH secretion

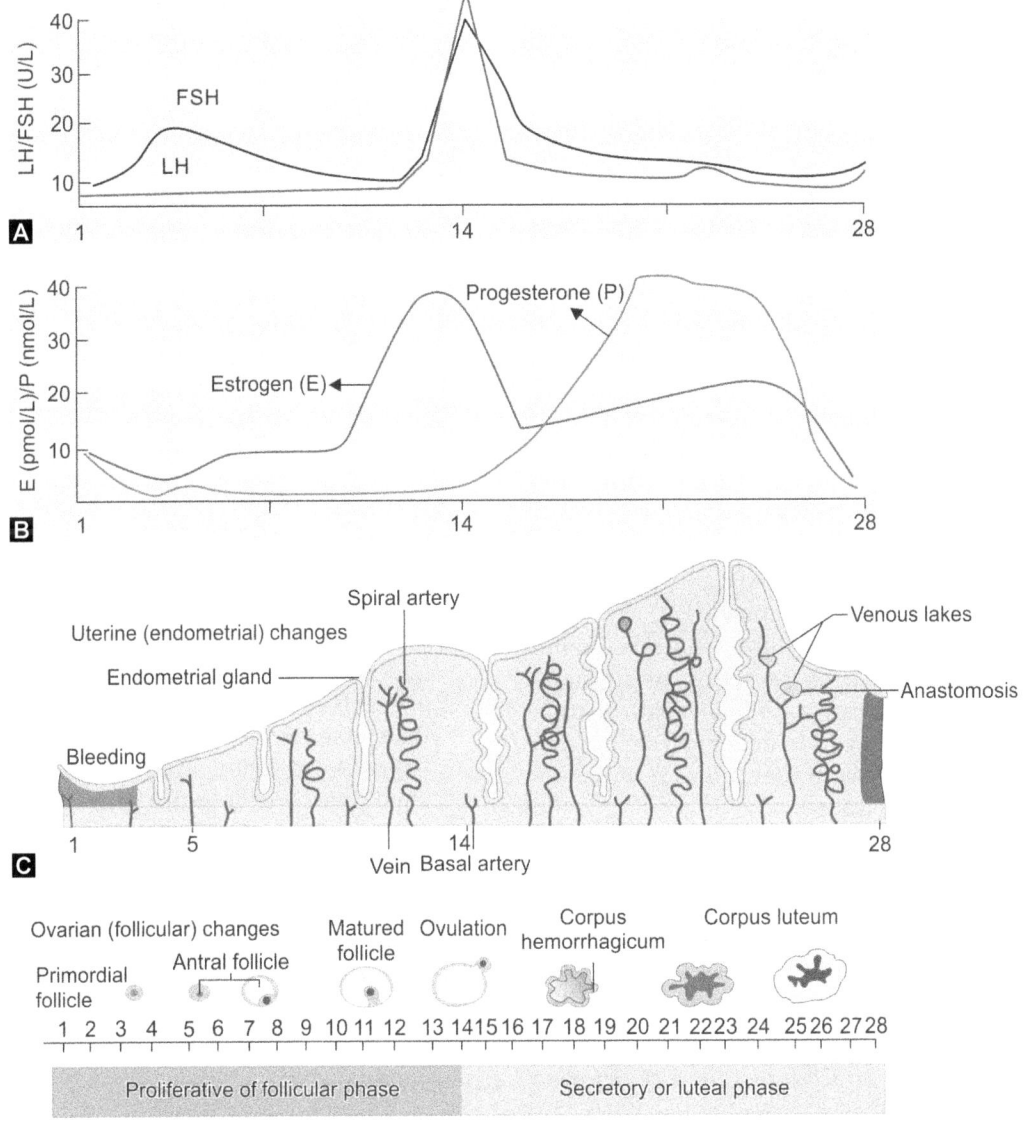

Figs. 7A to D: Menstrual cycle. Hormonal changes, changes in endometrium and changes in ovary.

from the anterior pituitary resulting in LH peak or LH surge. LH stimulates granulosa cells to synthesize progesterone.
- 9 hours after the LH surge, ovulation happens on the 14th day.
- As LH increases, progesterone levels increase and the proteolytic enzyme activity (Plasmin) is enhanced resulting in distension of follicle and the rupture of follicle is stimulated by prostaglandins and leukotrienes. This results in ovulation.

Luteal phase:
- This phase starts after the ovulation and lasts for 14 days. This time period is a constant one.
- Following ovulation, the follicle is filled with blood and is called as corpus hemorrhagicum.
- Soon after the release of ovum, granulosa and theca cells of the follicle proliferate and become lipid laden and are now yellow in color and are called as luteal cells. Now the follicle is called as—corpus luteum.
- Corpus luteum, under the influence of LH, starts secreting progesterone, estrogen and inhibin. High levels of these hormones negatively inhibit the secretion of FSH and LH.
- The maintenance of corpus luteum function is by the action of LH.
- If ovum is not fertilized, corpus luteum reaches a peak secretion of steroidal hormones by 7 days following ovulation and then begins to undergo degeneration and luteolytic and becomes a scar tissue—corpus albicans.
- Now the hormone production of corpus luteum drops and progesterone, estrogen and inhibin levels decrease.
- The inhibition over FSH and LH is lifted and there is a rise in FSH levels which induces the next cycle with the development of new set of follicles.

Regulation of Changes in the Uterine Endometrium

The uterine changes are given in 3 phases:
1. Proliferative phase
2. Secretory phase
3. Menstrual phase

1. **Proliferative phase:**
   - This phase correlates with the follicular phase of ovarian cycle.
   - Estrogen secreted from the follicle stimulates growth of uterine endometrium and therefore it thickens.
   - Glands in the endometrium and the blood vessels in endometrium also grows.
   - This phase is from day 5 till the day of ovulation.

2. **Secretory phase:**
   - This phase is from the day of ovulation to 25th day of the cycle.
   - It correlates with the luteal phase in the ovarian cycle.
   - Progesterone levels are high and they make the endometrium secretory by acting on the glands. Maximum action is 5–7 days after ovulation.
   - The secretion from the endometrial glands is rich in glycogen and can nourish the fertilized ovum.
   - The secretory endometrium is favorable for implantation of fertilized ovum.
   - If fertilization does not happen, corpus luteum starts to regress and the progesterone and estrogen levels decrease.
   - Withdrawal of hormonal support of the endometrium and release of prostaglandins result in vasoconstriction of the spiral arteries → uterine ischemia happens and endometrial necrosis and shedding of endometrium happens resulting in bleeding.

3. **Menstrual phase:** It starts with the menstrual bleeding with the shedding of outer 2/3rd of endometrium, unfertilized ovum and continues for 5 days.

7. Describe the process of transport of carbon dioxide from tissues to lungs.

CO_2 is transported in 4 forms:
1. As dissolved form in plasma
2. As carbamino-compound—combination with plasma proteins.

3. As bicarbonate
4. As carbamino-hemoglobin—combination with hemoglobin

As Dissolved Form

- CO_2 in dissolved form in plasma is proportional to the partial pressure of CO_2.
- It has 20 times more solubility than O_2 in blood.
- Some amount of CO_2 combines with plasma proteins to form carbamino-protein complex.

As Bicarbonate

- The major form by which CO_2 is transported is as bicarbonate. Nearly 70% is transported as HCO_3^-
- As the CO_2 enters the blood, it saturates the plasma and quickly diffuses into the RBCs.
- In the RBC, the enzyme carbonic anhydrase catalyzes the reaction of CO_2 combining with water to form H_2CO_3.
- $H_2CO_3 \rightarrow H^+ + HCO_3^-$
- As the HCO_3^- levels increase within the RBC, it starts leaving the RBC in exchange for Cl^-.
- This exchange happens through the band 3 protein which is an anion exchanger. It is present on the membrane of RBC (*refer* **Fig. 8**).
- This is called as the "chloride shift" or "hamburger shift".
- So in the venous blood the RBCs have more osmotically active particles which causes water retention in the RBC and increases its size.
- Therefore, hematocrit of venous blood is 3% more than the arterial blood.

- The H^+ is buffered by hemoglobin within the RBC.
- As Hb binds with H^+ the Oxy-Hb curve shifts to the right and O_2 is released to the tissues.
- As the venous blood reaches the lungs, the reverse process of all the above happens and CO_2 is released and blown out.
- High O_2 levels in the lungs helps in unloading of CO_2.

As Carbamino Compound

- CO_2 in RBC binds to hemoglobin to form carbamino hemoglobin.
- About 23% of CO_2 is transported in this form.

---

8. Describe in detail the photochemical mechanism of vision and mechanism of dark adaptation.

Structure of Rods and Cones

- Rods are named because of their structure.
- They have 4 parts—outer segment, inner segment, nucleus and synaptic terminal.
- The cones also have similar parts but the outer segment differs.
- In the rods, outer segments contain membranous disks arranged in stacks.
- They contain the photopigments (Rods—**Rhodopsin**).
- They are constantly renewed.
- In cones the outer segment is broader at the base and tapers above and there are no stacks of disks, but there are infoldings of membrane.
- Cone pigments are present in the membrane of infoldings.

Photopigments

- The photopigments are made up of two parts—opsin and retinal.
- Opsin is a glycoprotein and there are 4 types in the eye, one for rods and 3 for three different cones.
- Retinal is derived from vitamin A and exists as *cis*-retinal form.
- Photosensitive pigments are present in the rods and cones.
- In the rods, it is—Rhodopsin—Retinene 1 + Scotopsin.

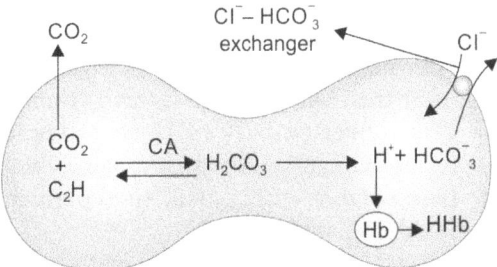

Fig. 8: Chloride shift.

- In cones also, there is retinene 1 but 3 different types of opsins in the 3 types of cones.
- The 3 cone pigments are—red-sensitive pigment (560 nm), green-sensitive pigment (530 nm) and Blue-sensitive pigment (420 nm)

Phototransduction

- When light strikes the eye there are potential changes which results in generation of action potential in ganglion cells and is transmitted via optic nerves.
- This conversion of light energy to electrical action potential is called as phototransduction.
- Before seeing what happens when light strikes the eye, we should know what happens in the eye in dark.

In Darkness

- There are Na^+ channels in the outer segments of the rods and cones. And they are open in dark. There is a gradient for Na^+ movement from inner to outer segment and also to the terminals of the rod.
- These Na^+ channels are cGMP dependent and in darkness, guanylyl cyclase hydrolyses GTP to cGMP and cGMP keeps the channel open (*refer* **Fig. 9**).
- This results in decrease in potential in the synaptic terminal which results in opening of Voltage-gated Ca^{2+} channels.
- There is Ca^{2+} influx followed by exocytosis of neurotransmitter vesicles (Glutamate).
- So the photoreceptor is depolarized in dark or rest.

In Presence of Light

- In the dark, the retinene 1 in rhodopsin is in 11-*cis* configuration.
- When light strikes the eye the only action of eye is to change the shape of retinene to all-*trans* configuration.
- After the conversion, retinene separates from Opsin which is called as "Bleaching" effect
- This in turn activates the configuration of Opsin and the changed Opsin will activate the associated G-protein, transducin.

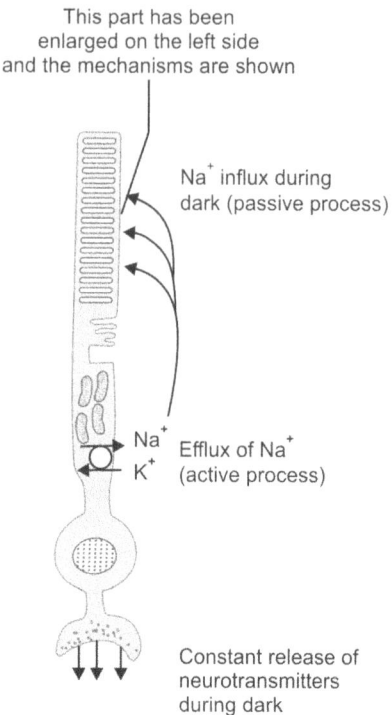

Fig. 9: Structure of rod and the flow of Na^+ current from inner segment to outer segment in darkness results depolarization and release of neurotransmitters.

- The G-protein exchanges GDP for GTP and the α subunit separates and remains active till the intrinsic activity of GTPase hydrolysis the GTP.
- The activated α subunit activates cGMP phosphodiesterase which converts cGMP to 5'GMP.
- Decline in cytoplasmic levels of cGMP causes closure of Na^+ channels and there is hyperpolarization of the rods.
- On activation of the receptors, there is hyperpolarization of rods, which finally results in depolarization of ganglion cells and propagation of action potentials in optic nerves.
- After this, some of the all-*trans* retinal gets converted back to 11-*cis* retinene by the enzyme retinal isomerase then reassociates with opsin, to replenish Rhodopsin (*refer* **Fig. 10**).
- Some 11-*cis* retinene is also synthesized from vitamin A.

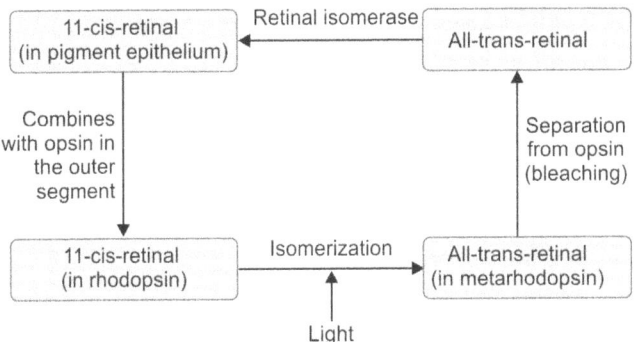

Fig. 10: Effect of light on conversion of retinene 1.

Light strikes the eye
↓
Change in configuration of retinene 1 of rhodopsin
↓
Change in confirmation of photopigment
↓
Activation of transducin
↓
Activation of phosphodiesterase
↓
Decrease in level of cytoplasmic cGMP levels
↓
Closure of cGMP dependent Na$^+$ channels
↓
Hyperpolarization of rods
↓
Decreased release of neurotransmitter
↓
Response in bipolar and other cells
↓
Action potential in ganglion cells and impulse transmission in optic nerve

9. Describe digestion and absorption of fat in the digestive tract. Write a note on steatorrhea.

Dietary fat consists of neutral fats—triglycerides and also phospholipids, cholesterol, free fatty acids and lecithin. It also has fat-soluble vitamins.

Digestion of Fats

- There are fat-digesting enzymes in the mouth, stomach and pancreatic juice.
- Lingual lipase is secreted by the Ebner's gland on the dorsal surface of tongue.
- Lingual lipase starts its action while in the stomach and digests 30% of triglycerides. Gastric lipase is of little importance in digestion of fats except in conditions of pancreatic insufficiency.
- Most of the digestion of fats begin in the duodenum by the action of pancreatic lipase.
- It acts on the fats emulsified by bile salts.
- Action of lipase is potentiated by the action of colipase, an enzyme which is also present in the pancreatic juice.

Emulsification of Fats by Bile Salts

- Emulsification means breaking down of large fat molecules into smaller molecules by the detergent action (lowering of surface tension) of bile salts.
- The bile salts are amphipathic and their hydrophobic tails face the center (where fat droplets are placed) and the heads are hydrophilic and they face the water in the lumen.
- This property along with the intestinal movements break the fat droplets to smaller molecules.
- The breaking down of fats into smaller molecules is essential as it increases the surface area on which the pancreatic lipase can act.
- Pancreatic lipase is water-soluble and it can act only on lipid-water interface of the fats.

Digestion of Fats by Lipolytic Enzymes

- Fat digestion begins mostly in duodenum by the action of pancreatic lipase.
- Pancreatic lipase is rich in enzymes and HCO_3^- and thereby it changes the pH of chyme from 6 to 7. This is the optimal pH for the action of lipases.
- Colipase is an enzyme secreted by pancreas which opens up a lid like structure in the amphipathic helix so that Lipase can act on triglycerides.
- Lipase acts on 1- and 3-bonds of triglycerides and on 2-bond at a low rate and the products of digestion are free fatty acids and 2-monoglycerides.
- The other lipase present in pancreatic juice is bile salt- activated lipase and it hydrolyses the cholesterol esters, esters of fat-soluble vitamins, phospholipids and triglycerides.
- Cholesteryl ester hydrolase in pancreatic juice hydrolyses cholesterol esters.
- Phospholipase A2 hydrolyses phospholipids and separates fatty acids from them.
- There are similar brush border lipases which act on the lipids in a similar way.

Absorption of Fats

- It starts in the duodenum and is completely absorbed by the time the fats reach jejunum.
- Absorption of fats is favored by formation of micelles by the bile salts and lecithin.
- The lumen of intestine contains water and therefore movement of digested fats is favored only by micelle formation.
- On reaching enterocytes, fats move out of micelles and enter enterocytes by passive diffusion.
- The rate-limiting step in absorption of fats is formation and movement of micelles from the chyme in the lumen to the brush border.
- The bile salts forming the micelles, are absorbed in the terminal ileum.
- Fate of fats, entering the enterocytes is dependent on their size.
- Fats containing 10–12 carbon atoms, easily pass through the basal side of the enterocytes and enter the portal blood vessels as free fatty acids and are transported.
- Fatty acids with more than 12 carbon atoms are esterified to triglycerides and the absorbed cholesterol is also esterified and they are coated with protein (β lipoprotein), cholesterol and phospholipids to form **chylomicrons.**
- The chylomicrons now exocytose through the basal side of the enterocytes to enter the lymphatics in the villus, the **lacteal**.
- They are transported in the lymphatics and are drained into the thoracic duct and finally they enter the blood circulation.
- Absorption of large chain fatty acids are more in the upper parts of the intestine and some amount of absorption happens in terminal parts also.
- In moderate fat intake, nearly 95% of ingested fats are absorbed.

Steatorrhea

- Steatorrhea is malabsorption of fats resulting in excretion of fat in stools.
- The indigested fats appear in stools and the stools are fatty, bulky and clay-colored. This is said to be steatorrhea.
- The fecal fat content is more than 40–50 g/day.
- It happens due to either destruction of exocrine pancreas, lipase deficiency or absence of bicarbonate in pancreatic juice which results in acidic environment in the intestine precipitating the bile salts.
- Acids also inhibit pancreatic lipase and therefore patients with gastrin-secreting tumor have steatorrhea.
- It is also seen in conditions with defective absorption of bile salts in terminal ileum.

10. What do you understand by the terms innate and acquired immunity? Describe the phenomenon of cell-mediated immunity.

- **Innate or non-specific immunity** is present since birth and offer protection against wide variety of pathogens and foreign substances. Non-specific means there is no specific response for specific invaders; protective mechanisms function the same way regardless of the type of invaders.

- **Acquired immunity or specific immunity,** the ability of the body to defend against specific invading agents, such as bacteria, toxins, viruses and foreign tissues, is called as specific resistance or immunity and it develops after exposure to the antigen.
- It has two properties—specificity and memory.
- Specificity for particular antigen which involves distinguishing self from non-self molecules.
- Memory for previously encountered antigen is present and when a second encounter happens there is a swift and rapid response.
- It includes two types—**cell-mediated and humoral immunity.**

Cell-mediated Immunity

- It is mediated by T lymphocytes.
- T Lymphocytes are formed in the bone marrow and they are processed in the thymus.

Stages of Cell-mediated Immunity

1. **Antigen presentation:** Cells, such as macrophages, mast cells and dendritic cells act as antigen presenting cells (APCs). Macrophages phagocytose the antigens entering the body and breaks it down to peptide fragments. The antigenic fragment forms a complex with the MHC II protein formed by the macrophages. The antigen and MHC II complex are expressed on the membrane of macrophage.
2. **Antigen recognition by lymphocytes:** The APC with the antigen-MHC II complex is recognized by the T lymphocytes with the receptors for the antigen. T cells become activated if it binds to the antigen and is co-stimulated with cytokines like IL-2. Once 2 stimulations have happened, the lymphocyte is activated. The activated T cells enlarge and begin to proliferate and differentiate to form a clone of similar T cells. This happens in the secondary lymphoid organs like the lymph nodes.
3. **Types of T cells:** There are 3 main types of T cells—helper T cells (CD4 cells), cytotoxic T cells (CD8 cells) and memory T cells.
    a. *Helper T cells:* Helper T cells or CD4 cells recognize the antigen presented along with MHC II and cytotoxic or CD8 cells recognize the antigens presented with MHC I. After co-stimulation of helper T cells, they secrete many cytokines. The most important cytokine is IL-2 which is needed for all the immune responses and is the major stimulator for T cell proliferation. IL-2 is also the co-stimulator for resting Helper T cells and cytotoxic T cells. It also enhances activation and proliferation of B cells and natural killer cells.
    b. *Cytotoxic T cells:* The T cells that express CD8 develop into cytotoxic T cells. They recognize foreign antigens expressed along with MHC I on the membranes of body cells infected by viruses, tumor cells and cells of tissue transplant. But to get activated into a killer cell it needs co-stimulation by IL-2 produced by helper cells. Therefore, for maximal activation of cytotoxic T cells it needs antigen presentation with MHC I and II.
    c. *Memory T cells:* The T cells for a specific antigen which remain in the lymph organ after the immune response is over are termed as memory T cells. If the same pathogen is encountered for the second time, these cells get activated and they initiate a swift and fast immune response. The second response is faster and vigorous and the pathogen is eliminated even before any symptom develops (*refer* **Fig. 11**).

Elimination of the Pathogens

The killing of the pathogen is done by the cytotoxic T cells.

- The activated CD8 cells synthesize and secrete proteins called "**perforins**" which are inserted into the membrane of the pathogen. The perforins are water channels which allow influx of water and thereby swelling of the microbe and cause its lysis.

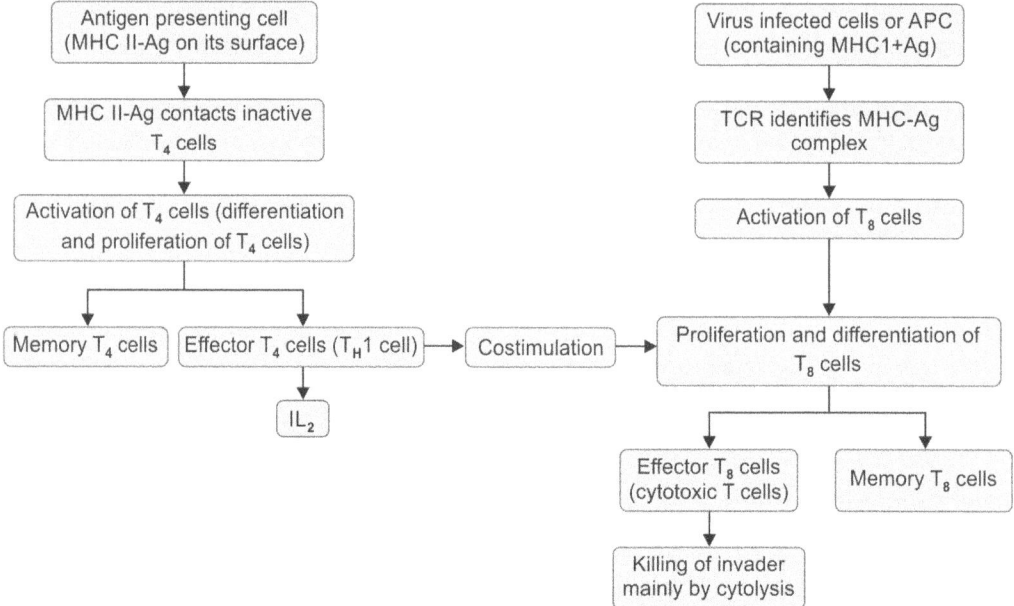

Fig. 11: Mechanism of cell-mediated immunity.

- Release of lymphotoxins by activated T cells. These cytokines destroy the microbes.
- Cytotoxic T cells secrete interferons which will favor the phagocytic activity of the neutrophils and macrophages by promoting opsonization.

Role of Cell-mediated Immunity

- It is activated against intracellular pathogens, such as viral infections and bacterial infections, such as *Mycobacterium tuberculosis*.
- It removes the tumor cells.
- It is responsible for rejection of transplanted tissues.
- It is responsible for hypersensitivity reactions.

---

11. Define the term blood pressure. Discuss the determinants and regulation of blood pressure.

BP is defined as the lateral pressure exerted by the moving column of blood on the vessel wall. Normal value = 120/80 mm Hg.

Components of BP

- Systolic BP
- Diastolic BP
- Pulse pressure
- Mean arterial pressure

Determinants of BP

- Blood pressure is determined by **cardiac output** and **peripheral resistance**.
- Cardiac output is determined by **stroke volume** and **heart rate**.
- Stroke volume is determined by **cardiac contractility** and **end diastolic volume (EDV)**
- EDV is determined by **venous return**. Venous return is determined by **skeletal muscle pump, cardiac pump, blood volume, respiratory pump, sympathetic stimulation.**
- **Contractility** is determined by **sympathetic stimulation, hypoxia, acidosis,** etc.
- **Heart rate** is modulated by **sympathetic and parasympathetic** nerves.
- **Peripheral resistance** is determined by afterload, which in turn is determined by **caliber of arterioles and viscosity of blood.**
- **Systolic BP** is determined by **cardiac output** and **diastolic BP** is determined by **peripheral resistance.**

Regulation of BP

Neural Regulation of BP

- Regulation by autonomic nerves
- Regulation by medullary control centers
- Regulation by reflexes
  - Baroreceptor reflex
  - Chemoreceptor reflex
  - CNS ischemic response

Regulation by autonomic nerves:

- Blood vessels are supplied by sympathetic nerves.
- **They are of two types:** Sympathetic vasoconstrictor and vasodilator fibers.
- **Sympathetic VC fibers:** In all blood vessels
- **Sympathetic VD or cholinergic fibers:** Blood vessels of skeletal muscles, sweat glands and they originate from frontal cortex to hypothalamus, midbrain medulla and end in the IML of SC.
- **Sympathetic stimulation results in:** vaso- and venoconstriction, ↑in HR and contractility and therefore the BP is increased.

Regulation by medullary control centers:

- There are two areas in the medulla which control the CVS.
- They are—vasomotor center (VMC) and Cardiac vagal center (CVC).
- CVC—nucleus tractus solitarius, nucleus ambiguus
- Vagal center—dorsal motor nucleus of vagus.
- Stimulation of VMC—↑HR, contractility, vaso- and venoconstriction—BP and on inhibition vice versa.
- The final pathway from VMC is through sympathetic nerves to heart (*refer* **Fig. 12**).

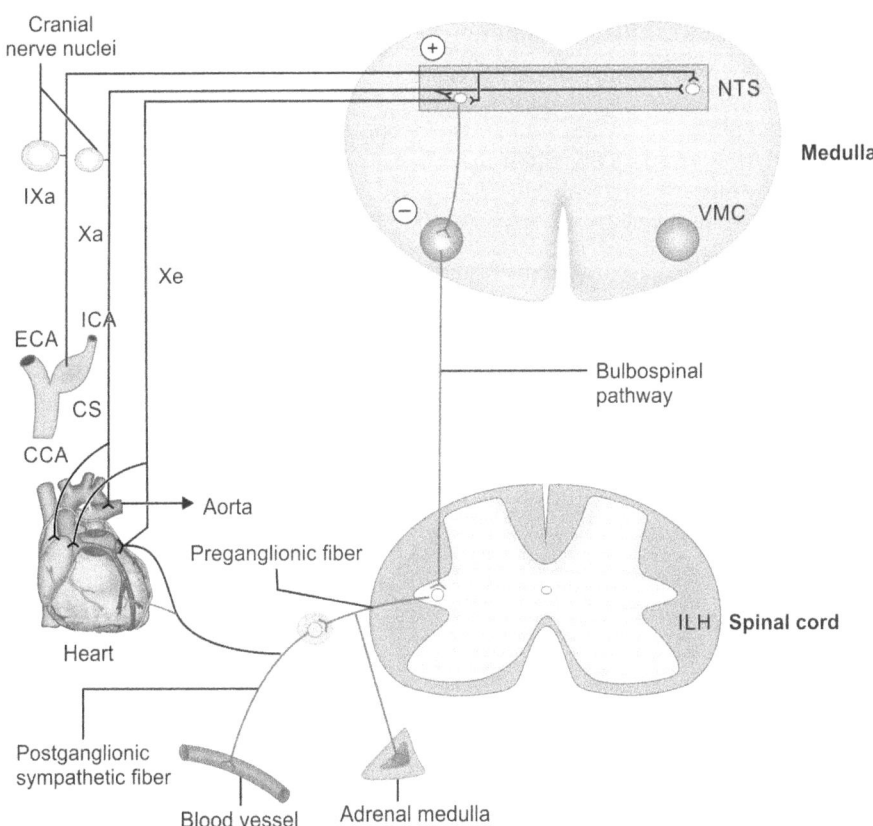

Fig. 12: Medullary cardiovascular centers and baroreceptor reflex pathway.
(CS: carotid sinus; CCA: common carotid artery; ECA: externa carotid artery; Xa: afferents of vagus nerve; Xe: efferents of vagus nerve, IX a: afferents of glossopharyngeal nerve; VMC: Vasomotor center; NTS: Nucleus tractus solitarius; ILH: Intermediolateral horn of spinal cord)

- Stimulation of CVC—↓HR, decreased vasoconstriction—↓BP.
- Final pathway is through vagus nerve to heart.
- There are inputs to VMC, from limbic centers through hypothalamus which are responsible for BP modulation in emotional states, such as anxiety (increase in BP and heart rate).

Reflex regulation of BP:
- **Baroreceptor reflex:**
  Baroreceptors:
  - There are two types of baroreceptors (BRs). High pressure and low pressure baroreceptors.
  - High pressure BRs are present in the Carotid and aortic sinuses (*refer* **Fig. 13**).
  - Low pressure BRs are present in the great veins, right and left atria.
  - High pressure BRs are there to monitor and correct the day to day change in BP as in change of posture from supine to standing position.
  - They regulate BP maximally when the MAP is between 70-110 mm Hg and stops firing when MAP falls <40 or rises above 150 mm Hg.

  The reflex:
  - Most important reflex to regulate BP
  - Also called as sino-aortic reflex
  - Receptor—carotid and aortic sinuses
  - Stimulus—stretch of baroreceptors (as in increased BP)
  - Afferents—IXth (supplies carotid sinus) and Xth cranial nerves (aortic sinus)
  - Efferents—sympathetic nerves and vagus nerve
  - Effector—heart and blood vessels
  - Response—decrease in BP (*refer* **Fig. 14**)

- **Chemoreceptor reflex:**
  - Chemoreceptors are located in the carotid and aortic bodies.
  - They sense the change in pO_2, pH and pCO_2 in arterial blood and stimulate respiration.
  - They are supplied by IX and X cranial nerves.
  - They usually project to respiratory centers and also to cardiovascular centers in medulla.
  - They also send inputs to VMC and CVC and regulate BP
  - They are active within a range of 40-100 mm Hg MAP.

Decrease in BP MAP 40-100 mm Hg)
↓
Decreased blood flow to chemoreceptors
↓
Stimulation of chemoreceptors
↓
Impulses carried through IXth and Xth cranial nerves to medulla
↓   ↓   ↓
Respiratory   VMC   Cardiac vagal
center   center (CVC)
↓   ↓   ↓
Hyper-   Vasoconstriction, Bradycardia
ventilation,   TC, release of   (BC)
TC   catecholamines

- The net effect is mild tachycardia and vasoconstriction → Increase in BP

- **CNS ischemic response:**
  - It is activated when MAP falls below 40 mm Hg. It is said to be the "last ditch stand", the last effort put up by the body to try to correct the fall in BP.

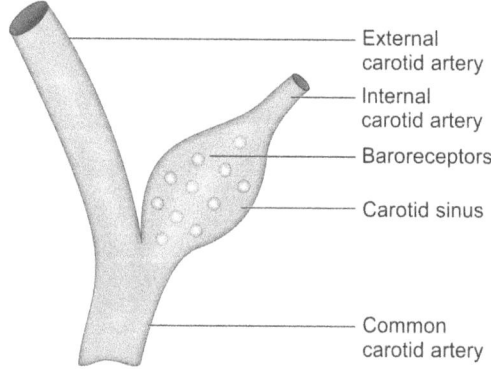

Fig. 13: Baroreceptor—carotid sinus.

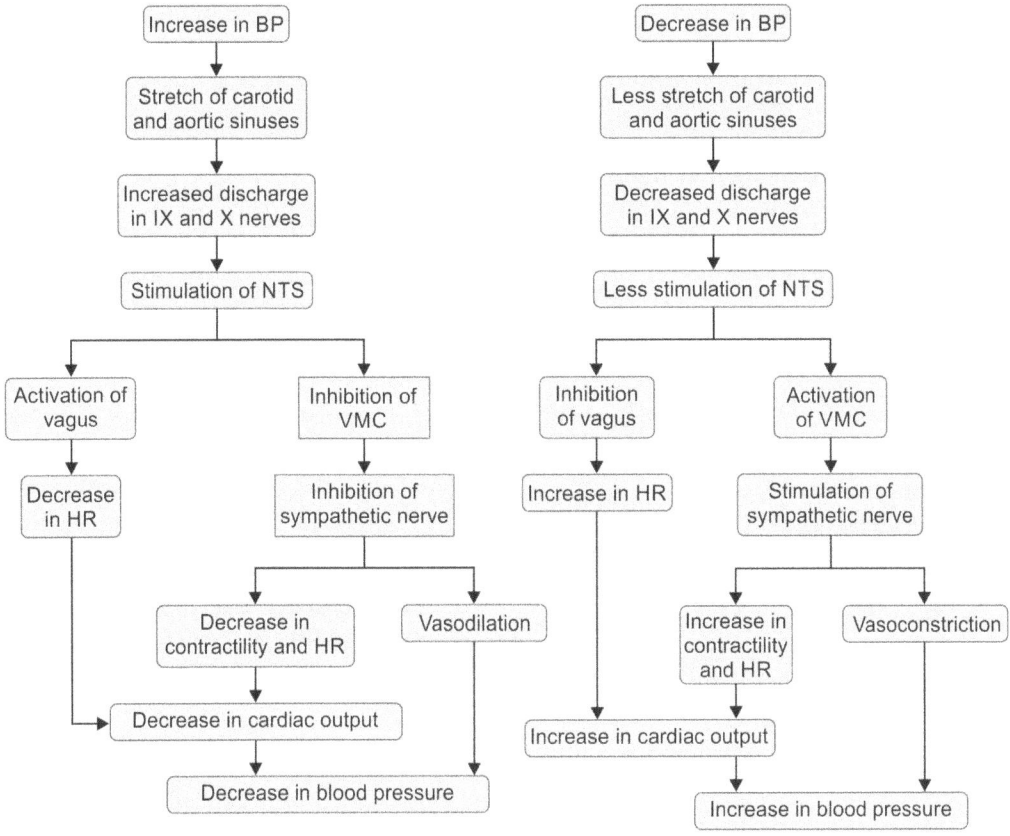

Fig. 14: Regulation of BP by baroreceptors.

Severe hypotension
↓
Decreased cerebral blood flow
↓
Hypoxia and hypercapnia at VMC
↓
Strong stimulation of VMC
↓
Intense vasoconstriction
↓
↑BP

Intermediate Regulation of BP

- They come into play after several minutes and reach full effect in few hours.
- They act for few days.
- They alter the blood volume and try to correct BP.

They are:

- **Capillary fluid shift mechanism:** Capillary hydrostatic pressure is dependent on arterial blood pressure and therefore when BP increases the capillary hydrostatic pressure increases and there is filtration of fluid into the interstitium resulting in decrease in ECF volume and thereby the decrease in BP. It is more effective than short-term regulatory mechanisms but it takes longer time to bring BP back to normal.
- **Stress-relaxation mechanism:** When there is increase in ECF volume as in IV infusion of fluids, the blood flow to visceral organs like spleen, liver and lungs increase, resulting in relaxation of blood vessels of the viscera by local mechanisms

and blood is pooled here. The blood volume decreases and BP decreases.
- **Reverse stress relaxation mechanism:** It is the opposite of stress-relaxation process. In conditions of fall in BP, the vessels in the visceral organs tighten and push the stored blood back into circulation. By this ECF volume and BP increase.

Long-term Regulation of BP
- These mechanisms are slow to begin and last for a longer duration. It continues for years to months.
- They bring the BP back to normal. It is done by the kidneys.

It is by 2 mechanisms:
1. **Direct mechanism:**
   - Kidneys directly control the blood volume and thereby regulate the BP.
   - Also called as the renal fluid mechanism or ECF volume mechanism

   Decrease in BP
   ↓
   ↓Blood flow to kidneys
   ↓
   ↓GFR
   ↓
   ↑Reabsorption of water and electrolyte reabsorption
   ↓
   Water and electrolyte retention
   ↓
   ↑ECF volume
   ↓
   ↑Blood volume
   ↓
   ↑Cardiac output
   ↓
   ↑BP

2. **Indirect mechanism:**
   - Here hormones are secreted which in turn acts through the kidneys to regulate BP.
   - It is by the Renin-Angiotensin-Aldosterone mechanism.

   Decreased blood pressure
   ↓
   Renal ischemia
   ↓
   Renin from JG cells
   ↓
   Angiotensinogen → Angiotensin I
   ↓ACE
   Angiotensin II
   ↓

- Increases reabsorption of water and electrolytes from PCT
- Induces potent vasoconstriction
- Stimulates adrenal cortex to secrete aldosterone

Aldosterone
- It acts on the DCT and collecting duct to increase water and salt reabsorption.
- Thereby increases ECF volume and increases BP.

---

12. Trace the pathway for perception of pain. Discuss the descending pain modulatory pathways. Discuss the terms 'gating of pain' and 'referred pain'.

Pain Pathway
- Pain sensation is carried by the Lateral spinothalamic tract (LSTT).
- There are two types of pain—fast pain and slow pain.
- So the LSTT has fibers for fast pain and for slow pain. There are separate pathways for fast and slow pain.

Fast Pain
- Fast pain is sensed by the free nerve endings of Aδ fibers.
- The pain sensation from periphery is carried through the Aδ fibers.
- Their cell bodies are present in the dorsal root ganglion.
- The fibers on entering spinal cord terminate on cells in laminae I and V of the dorsal gray horn.
- These are the second order neurons. Neurotransmitter released here is Glutamate.
- Second order neurons cross to the opposite side and ascend up as **neospinothalamic tract** in the anterolateral column of spinal cord.

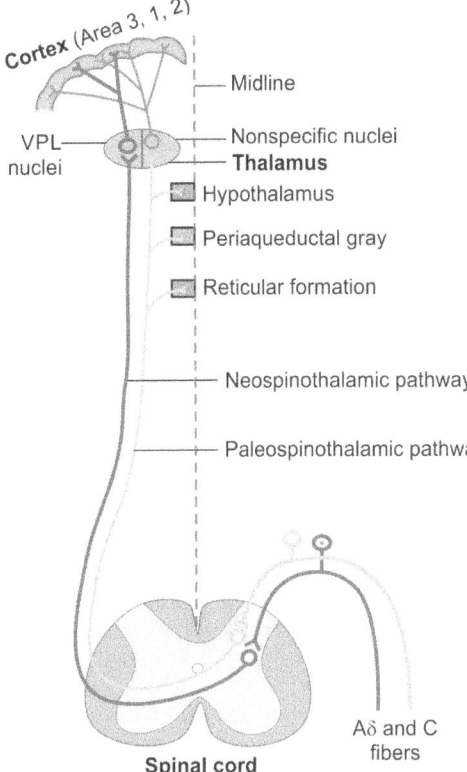

Fig. 15: Neospinothalamic and paleospinothalamic tracts.
(VPLN: ventral posterolateral nucleus of thalamus)

- Neospinothalamic tract reaches thalamus and ends on the Ventral posterolateral nucleus of the thalamus (VPLN) (*refer* **Fig. 15**).
- The tract on its way to thalamus gives a few branches to periaqueductal gray (PAG) in midbrain.
- The third order neurons start from thalamus and reach somatosensory area I.
- This pathway is concerned with localization and interpretation of pain.

Slow Pain
- Slow pain is sensed by the free nerve endings of unmyelinated C fibers.
- Slow pain is carried by the same fibers to spinal cord and they terminate in the laminae II and III of dorsal gray horn.
- This is the first order neuron. The neurotransmitter released here is Substance P.

- The second order neuron arises from laminae I and V and the fibers cross to the opposite side and ascends up as **paleospinothalamic tract**.
- It ascends up along with neospinothalamic tract in the anterolateral column of spinal cord.
- This tract gives many fibers to PAG, Reticular formation and tectum.
- It then ends in the non-specific nucleus of thalamus.
- Third order neuron arises from here and is projected to entire cerebral cortex.
- This pathway is concerned with alertness, arousal and perception of pain rather than localization of pain.

Analgesic System in the Brain

- **Pain modulation takes place in 2 places:**
  1. At the peripheral nerve endings
  2. At the spinal cord level

Peripheral Nerve Endings

Endorphins and enkephalins combine with nociceptors and decrease the response to stimuli

At the Spinal cord
- **Peripheral mechanism:** By gate control theory—large Ab fibers (when stimulated by touching or rubbing the painful area) ↓ nociception in C fibers.
- **Central pain suppressing mechanism:** Opioids secreted from areas in brain stem inhibit pain transmission in the spinal cord.

Gate Control Mechanism
- Pain sensation is carried by Ad and unmyelinated C fibers and they ascend up as spinothalamic tract.
- Touch and pressure sensations are carried by large myelinated Ab fibers and they ascend up as dorsal column tract in spinal cord.
- Dorsal column fibers in the spinal cord give a branch to inhibitory interneurons which secrete enkephalins and which in turn end on the second order neurons in pain pathway.

- So, when there is pain in an area, touching or pressing that region stimulates the large Aβ fibers which in turn inhibit pain pathway and thereby there is decreased pain perception.
- So, the large Aβ fibers gate the pain pathway.

Central Pain Suppressing Mechanism

- Pain pathway, as it ascends up gives branches to periaqueductal gray (PAG) in midbrain.
- There is a pain suppressing descending pathway from PAG to medulla and to spinal cord.
- Axons of the neurons in PAG terminate on serotonergic neurons in raphe magnus nuclei in medulla.
- They secrete enkephalin here.
- Axons of serotonergic neurons in raphe magnus nuclei descend and terminate on the inhibitory interneurons in spinal cord (*refer* **Fig. 16**).
- They secrete serotonin and stimulate internuncial neurons which in turn inhibit second order neurons in the pain pathway by secreting enkephalin.

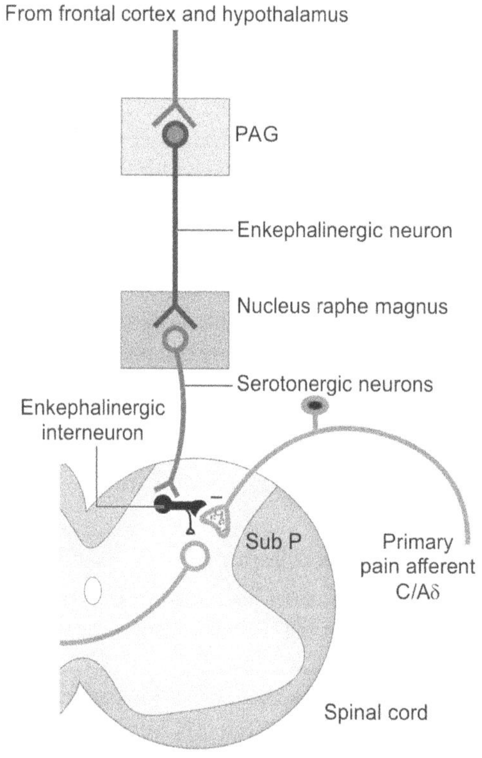

II. SHORT NOTES

1. Erythroblastosis fetalis.

- It is also called as hemolytic disease of the newborn (HDN).
- This is due to Rh incompatibility between the mother and fetus.
- It happens if the mother is Rh negative and the fetus is Rh positive.
- Since Rh system does not follow the 2nd law of Landsteiner's, there are no preformed antibodies in the Rh-negative mother's blood.
- So, in first pregnancy, there are no complications.
- At the time of parturition, few fetal RBCs enter the mother's circulation.
- Mother's immune system recognizes the Rh antigen in the fetal RBCs as foreign antigens and starts producing antibodies for D antigen on fetal RBCs.
- These Anti-D antibodies belong to IgG type and therefore can cross the placenta.
- If the mother conceives for the second time and if that fetus happens to Rh positive, the anti-D antibodies from mother crosses the placenta and destroys the fetal RBCs resulting in HDN/EBF.
- As the number of conceptions increase antibody titer increases and causes more damage to the fetus.
- **The symptoms are:**
  - **Anemia:** Due to massive hemolysis anemia sets in following agglutination
  - **Hemolytic jaundice:** The released hemoglobin, following hemolysis, is converted to bilirubin and the levels may rise very high resulting in jaundice.
  - **Hydrops fetalis:** Generalized edema due to anemia and hypoproteinemia

Fig. 16: Endogenous pain inhibition by spinal cord and brainstem structures. PAG—periaqueductal gray. It has enkephalinergic neurons which end on serotonergic neurons of raphe magnus nucleus in medulla. They send out axons which end on enkephalinergic neurons in spinal cord and decreases pain.

- Erythroblasts start appearing in the circulation due to exaggerated erythropoiesis following severe anemia.
- **Kernicterus:** It happens due to hemolysis and formation of excess bilirubin, and the bilirubin crosses the blood brain barrier (BBB) since the BBB is not fully developed in the fetus. Basal ganglia in the brain, has great affinity for bilirubin and therefore it gets deposited in the basal ganglia. There are motor dysfunctions due to this.

Prevention of EBF

EBF is prevented by administering the mother with anti-D antibodies after delivery of the fetus. Injected antibodies neutralize the antigens which had entered the mother's body and no further antibody production is prevented.

Treatment of EBF

- ❏ **Exchange transfusion:** The newborns with the above symptoms are treated with exchange transfusion after birth. This removes sensitized Rh-positive RBCs from the blood and is replaced with Rh negative blood. This is continued till the antibodies are removed from the fetal circulation. The transfused blood should be ABO negative and Rh negative.
- ❏ **Phototherapy** can also be given to reduce bilirubin levels.

2. Isotonic and isometric contraction.

- ❏ Muscle contains both elastic and viscous elements.
- ❏ Elastic elements are the connective tissue in the muscle fibers and there are series and parallel elastic elements.
- ❏ The parallel ones are in between the muscle fibers and the series are at the ends of the muscles connecting the muscle to the bones.
- ❏ The viscous elements are the contractile component of the muscle.
- ❏ So when a muscle contracts there can be differences in the response of the elastic and viscous elements.
- ❏ Based on that the muscle contraction is classified as—isometric and Isotonic contractions.

Isometric Contraction

- ❏ As the name implies, in this type of contraction length of the muscle remains same but tension developed in the muscle is increased.
- ❏ The muscle length remains the same because as the contractile components are shortening the series elastic elements are stretched and thereby the tension increases but length remains the same.
- ❏ There is no shortening and therefore no movement is happening here (*refer* **Fig. 17**).
- ❏ Work done = Force X Distance and since no distance is changed here, there is no actual work done in isometric contraction.

Examples of Isometric Contraction

- ❏ Contraction of arm muscle while pushing against the wall
- ❏ Contraction of anti-gravity muscles of the body

Isotonic Contraction

- ❏ In this type of contraction, the muscle length shortens but the tension developed in the muscle remains the same.
- ❏ Here the contractile component and parallel elastic elements shorten and series elastic components are not stretched.
- ❏ Since the muscle shortens, there is work being done in this type of contractions.

Examples are:

- ❏ Contraction of upper limb muscles while lifting an object

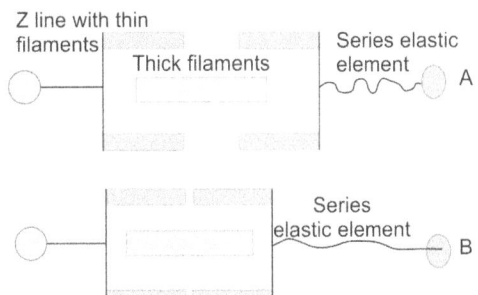

Fig. 17: Isometric contraction: (A) Relaxed state; (B) Contracted state.

- Walking
- Swimming

3. Facilitated diffusion.

- Large water-soluble substances (e.g., glucose) are carried by a protein which changes configuration on binding (*refer* **Fig. 18**).
- This change in configuration shifts the molecule in or out.
- Highly selective and specific
- **Types:**
  - Uniport
  - Symport
  - Antiport

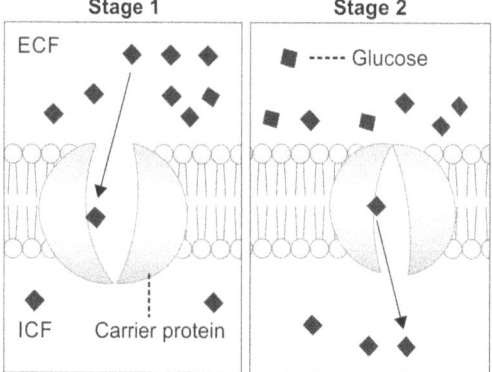

Fig. 18: Facilitated diffusion. A uniport transporting glucose molecules.

- **Characteristics:**
  - Specificity
  - Saturation
  - Competition

4. Enterohepatic circulation.

- Bile acids and salts present in the bile on entering the intestine are absorbed from the terminal part of the ileum and re-enter the portal vein to be secreted back into the bile from hepatocytes.
- This process repeats many times—enterohepatic circulation.
- The conjugated bile salts are absorbed and recirculated in the above manner.
- Also, bile salts are unconjugated and some of it is also absorbed.
- Colonic bacteria act on free bile acids and are converted to secondary bile acids and a part of it is also absorbed back into the portal vein (*refer* **Fig. 19**).
- About 95% of secreted bile salts are absorbed by the enterohepatic circulation and only 200–500 mg/day are excreted.

Significance of enterohepatic circulation:

- Only the amount of bile salts which are excreted, are synthesized and replaced daily, to maintain the pool of bile salts in

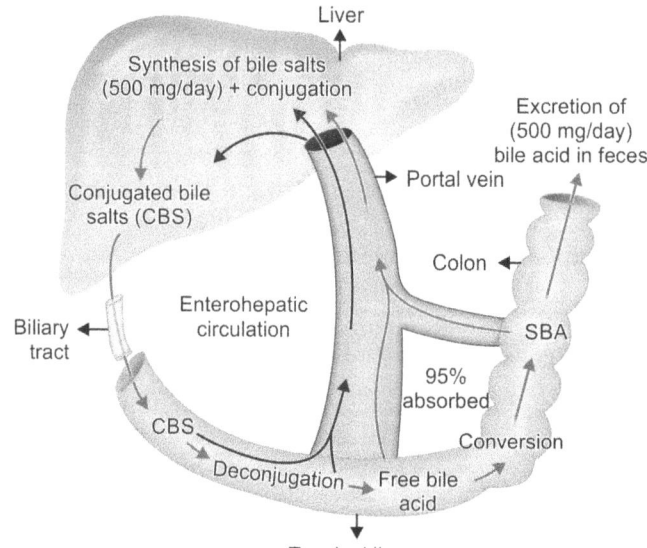

Fig. 19: Enterohepatic circulation. It is the circulation of bile salts following its synthesis from liver in bile and its secretion into duodenum and its reabsorption in terminal ileum and recirculation through portal veins.

the body which are essential for digestion and absorption of fats.
- The total amount of bile salts is 2–4 g.
- This amount is circulated daily many times to digest and absorb fats in the diet taken.

5. Juxtaglomerular apparatus.

- Juxtaglomerular apparatus is a combination of tubular cells and vascular cells.
- It is located near the glomerulus where the afferent arteriole enters and efferent arteriole leaves the glomerulus.

It is made up of the following components:
- Juxtaglomerular cells
- Macula densa cells
- Lacis cells

Juxtaglomerular Cells
- These are myoepithelial cells lining the afferent arteriole just before it enters the glomerulus.
- These cells are rich in endoplasmic reticulum and they secrete the hormone Renin.
- They act as baroreceptors and they sense the change in the renal arterial pressure and respond to the pressure gradient between the afferent arteriole and the interstitium (*refer* **Fig. 20**).
- When the renal arterial pressure drops JG cells release renin.
- These cells also sense the ECF volume and respond to hypovolemia by secreting renin.
- They are also supplied by sympathetic nerves and when the sympathetic stimulation is there it releases renin.

Macula Densa Cells
- They are present in the renal tubules at the junction of thick ascending limb of loop of Henle and the distal convoluted tubule.
- These cells are modified; they are more columnar and densely packed.
- They are in close contact with the mesangial cells and the JG cells.
- They act as chemoreceptors and they sense the NaCl content in the tubular fluid.
- They act through tubuloglomerular feedback and regulate the Renal blood flow and GFR.

Mesangial Cells or Lacis Cells
- These are present in between the afferent and efferent arterioles and are in close contact with the JG cells and macula densa cells.
- They are contractile in nature and therefore they regulate GFR.
- They also secrete some amount of renin.

6. Counter current exchanger.

- Counter-current mechanism in general is a mechanism in which fluids flow in opposite directions in closely placed structures.

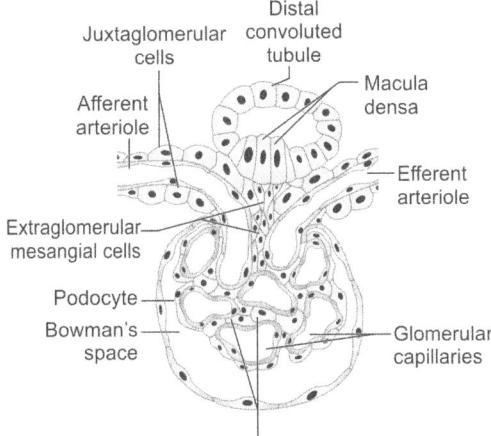

Fig. 20: Juxtaglomerular apparatus. It includes juxtaglomerular cells, macula densa and Lacis cells.

- In kidneys, the counter-current mechanism is used to generate and maintain a hyperosmolar gradient from the outer to inner region of the medulla, the highest osmolality is at the tip of the renal papillae.
- Hyperosmolar medullary interstitium is essential for the process of concentration of urine.
- Only in the presence of this hyperosmolar interstitium ADH can reabsorb water from the collecting ducts.
- The counter-current system in the kidneys has two components—the counter-current multiplier and the counter-current exchanger.
- The descending and ascending loops of Henle act as the counter-current multiplier. Flow of fluid in descending loop is towards the deeper parts of medulla and is highly permeable to water and in the ascending limb the flow of fluid is towards the cortex and it is totally impermeable to water and permeable to solutes. This selective permeability of the loops of Henle helps in generating a hyperosmolar gradient in the medulla.
- Vasa recta acts as the counter-current exchanger. The flow of blood in the ascending and descending limbs of the vasa recta helps in maintaining the hyperosmolar environment created by the counter-current multiplier (*refer* **Fig. 21**).
- The ascending and descending limbs of vasa recta are also selectively permeable to water and solutes.
- Solutes come out of the ascending limb and enters descending limb and water enters the ascending limb and moves out into the general circulation. Solutes get circulated in the deeper parts of the medulla and thereby the vasa recta prevents the dilution of solutes in the medullary interstitium.
- This is the mechanism by which the counter-current exchanger is able to maintain the hyperosmolar medullary gradient generated by the counter-current multiplier.

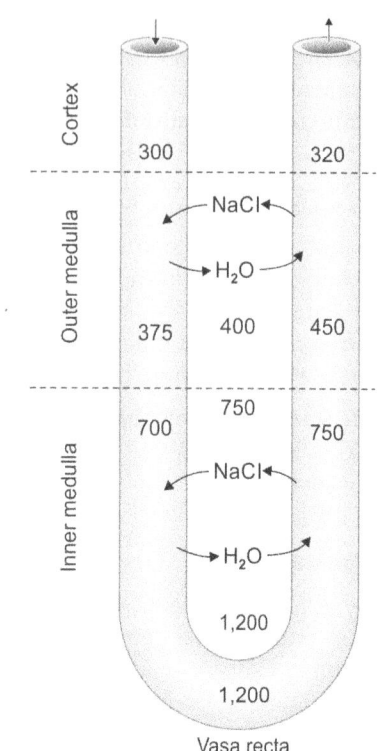

Fig. 21: Vasa recta (counter-current exchanger).

7. Transport maximum (TM).

- Transport maximum or tubular maximum (TM) is the maximum amount of the solute that can be actively transported (reabsorbed or secreted) per minute by the renal tubules.
- TM is the level at which the carrier, transporting the substance, gets saturated and beyond this level, the substances are no more reabsorbed or secreted.
- Therefore, the amount of substance transported depends on the amount of the solute present in the tubular fluid up to the TM for the solute.
- Therefore, TM is the amount of substance delivered to the tubule per minute and is given as the **tubular load**.
- **Tubular load** is the quantity of a solute filtered by the glomerulus and presented to the tubule.
- TM depends on plasma concentration of the solute and the rate of filtration of the

substance, so it is given as **TM = plasma concentration X GFR**

- For example, if it is a transporter used for reabsorption of glucose, after the TM is reached, glucose is no more reabsorbed and starts appearing in the urine.
- TM for glucose in males is 375 mg/min and 300 mg/min in females.
- Therefore, plasma levels of glucose up to 300 g% can transport glucose from tubular fluid (300 mg/100 mL X 125 mL/ min) into plasma.
- But glucose starts appearing in urine if a plasma concentration reaches 200 mg/dL. This is because of differences in the TM of the tubules of various nephrons for reabsorption of glucose.
- **Renal threshold** is the concentration of a solute in plasma at or above which the substance starts appearing in the urine.
- TM is applicable only for substances which are actively transported and not for substances which are passively transported.
- Substances having a TM are—glucose, amino acids, uric acid, PAH, etc.
- Substances which do not have a TM are—Na^+, HCO_3^-

8. Acromegaly.

- Acromegaly is a clinical condition due to excess secretion of growth hormone (GH) in the adults (after the fusion of the epiphyseal plates in the long bones).
- It is usually due to a tumor of the growth hormone producing cells (somatotrophs) in the anterior pituitary gland.
- Rarely, it can also be due to hypothalamic tumors secreting GRH.
- There is no increase in height of the individual.
- But because of the excess levels of GH, there is thickening of bones and proliferation of soft tissues, such as connective tissue and skin.
- This leads to coarse disfigured appearance. "Acro" means extremity and "megaly" is large.

Clinical features are:
Effect of excess GH levels leads to:
- **Acromegalic face:** Jaw and cheek bones become more prominent, lips are thickened, nose is broad and thick, enlarged brows and coarse skin.
- **Prognathism:** Protrusion of the lower jaw due to elongation and thickening of mandible.
- Enlarged spade, such as hands, broad fingers and large feet.
- Body hair is increased
- **Kyphosis:** Since the vertebral bones continue to grow person has kyphosis.
- They develop osteoarthritis
- **Organomegaly:** Internal organs, such as heart, liver, spleen and kidneys are enlarged.
- High levels of GH decrease insulin sensitivity in the tissues and the patient has hyperglycemia and are prone to develop diabetes mellitus.

Effect of tumor on neighboring structures:
- The tumor in the anterior pituitary compresses the optic chiasma resulting in visual disturbances.
- There will be enlargement of sella turcica and headache.

9. Steps in thyroxine synthesis.

- Synthesis takes place in the follicular cells and the hormone is stored in follicular lumen as colloid.
- Structure of follicles change in relation to activity of the gland (*refer* **Fig. 22**).
- Thyroid hormones are iodothyronines, formed by coupling of iodinated tyrosine molecules by ether linkages.

Following are the steps in synthesis of thyroid hormones:
1. Iodide trapping
2. Thyroglobulin synthesis
3. Oxidation of iodide
4. Organification
5. Coupling
6. Storage
7. Release

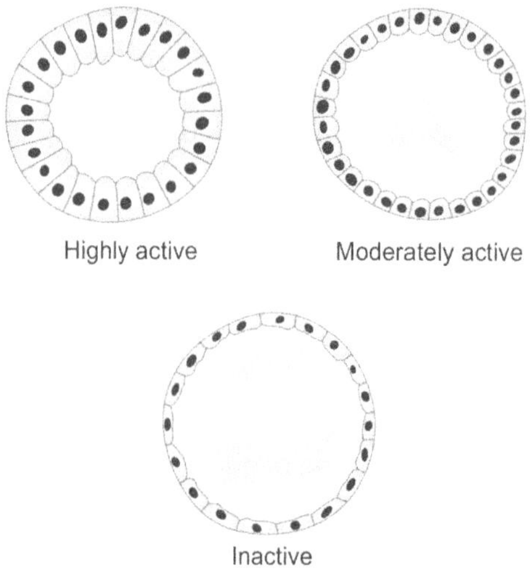

Fig. 22: Thyroid follicle—active follicle, moderately active follicle and inactive follicle with colloid content. Inactive follicle is lined by flattened epithelial cells and the colloid content is more. In an active follicle, the cells are columnar and colloid content is less.

Iodide Trapping

- Iodide is transported from the blood in thyroid capillaries to the follicular cell through **sodium-iodide symporter** (NIS).
- NIS transports I⁻ against electrochemical gradient.
- TSH stimulates I⁻ trapping and concentration in the gland.
- Iodide immediately moves towards the apical membrane of the follicular cell.

Thyroglobulin Synthesis

- As iodide is being trapped, thyroglobulin is also synthesized in the endoplasmic reticulum of follicular cells and transferred to colloid.
- TG is a glycoprotein. Has ^{131}I tyrosine amino acids.

Oxidation of Iodide

- Iodide on reaching the colloid—apical membrane interface is oxidized to iodine.
- This reaction is catalyzed by thyroid peroxidase enzyme (TPO) present in the colloid-membrane interface.
- $2I^- + H_2O_2 I_2 + 2 HO^-$

Organification

- The tyrosine molecules of thyroglobulin get iodinated in the colloid to form iodotyrosines.
- This is organification and is catalyzed by TPO.
- It forms either monoiodotyrosine (MIT) or diiodotyrosine (DIT) depending on the number of iodine attached to tyrosines (refer **Fig. 23**).

Coupling Reaction

Two DIT molecules couple to form Tetraiodotyrosine (T_4) or Thyroxine.

or

One molecule of MIT and DIT couple to form Triiodothyronine (T_3)

or

One molecule of DIT and MIT couple to form reverse T_3 (RT_3), an inactive component formed in the follicular cells (refer **Fig. 24**).

This is coupling reaction and is catalyzed by TPO.

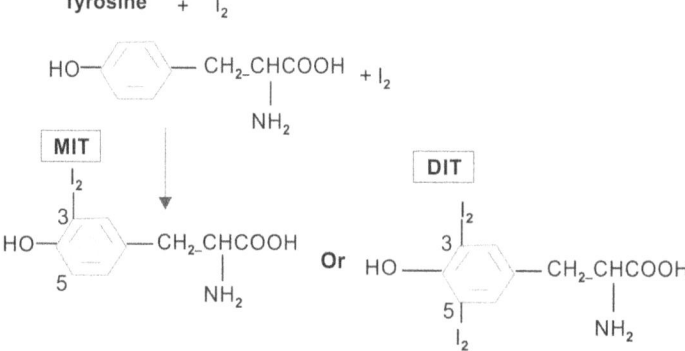

Fig. 23: Organification reaction—I_2 molecule is bound to tyrosine molecules. If it is bound in one position (3) then MIT (monoiodotyrosine is formed). If I_2 is bound in two positions (3 and 5), it is DIT (diiodotyrosine).

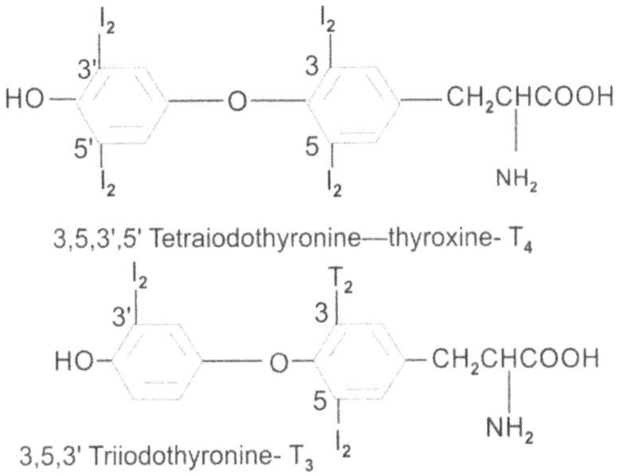

3,5,3',5' Tetraiodothyronine—thyroxine- T_4

3,5,3' Triiodothyronine- T_3

Fig. 24: Coupling reaction. Two MITs couple to form T_4 (Thyroxine) and one MIT and one DIT binds T_3 (Triiodothyronine) is formed.

Storage

- TG after iodination is stored in the colloid until release.
- In each molecule of thyroglobulin (TG): MIT-7, DIT-6, T_4- 2, T_3- 0.2 molecules are present.
- The gland is capable of storing secretions needed for 100 days.

Release of the Hormone

- On stimulation by TSH, colloid droplets (with TG and T3 and T4) are endocytosed through megalin into the cell.
- The droplet gets attached to a lysosome and forms a phagosome.
- Proteolytic enzymes of the phagosome break the peptide bonds between thyroid hormone (TH) and TG.
- This releases T_3, T_4, MIT and DIT.
- Released thyroid hormones enter into the capillaries by diffusion.
- MIT and DIT are deiodinated by the enzyme, thyroid deiodinases, which are selective for iodotyrosines and not for iodothyronines.
- Small amounts of TG are also released (*refer* **Fig. 25**).

10. Stages of spermatogenesis.

- The process of formation of mature sperm is called spermatogenesis.
- It takes place in the seminiferous tubule. It happens in the wall of the tubule from basal lamina towards the lumen.
- The immature cells are present in the basal aspect of the tubule and the maturing cells move toward the adluminal compartment.
- Spermatogenesis involves both mitotic and meiotic divisions and spermiogenesis.

Mitotic Division

- The primitive germ cell, spermatogonia, in the basal lamina of the seminiferous tubule undergoes mitotic divisions to form primary spermatocytes.
- Each spermatogonium divides 5 times to produce 32 spermatogonia.
- 32 spermatogonia (44+X+Y) reach the adluminal side of the tubule and undergo mitosis to become 64 primary spermatocytes (44+X+Y).
- Primary spermatocytes are large cells with diploid number of chromosomes (2n)

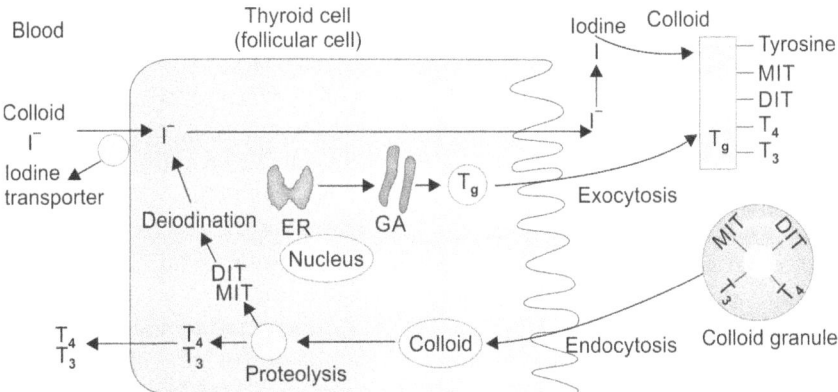

Fig. 25: Synthesis of thyroid hormone in follicular cell.
(DIT: diiodotyrosine; MIT: monoiodotyrosine; ER: endoplasmic reticulum; GA: Golgi apparatus; Tg: thyroglobulin; T4: thyroxine; T3: triiodothyronine)

Meiotic Divisions

- The primary spermatocytes with diploid number of chromosomes undergo the first meiotic division to form the secondary spermatocyte which is haploid in nature.
- The second meiotic division results in formation of spermatids (22+X or Y).
- A total of 512 spermatids are derived from single spermatogonia.

Spermiogenesis

- The spermatids do not undergo further divisions but structural changes take place as the spermatids mature into sperm—spermiogenesis.
- This process happens in the deep folds of Sertoli cells.

The changes taking place are:
- The amount of cytoplasm is reduced in spermatids
- The nucleus elongates to become the head of sperm
- The acrosomal cap is formed
- The tail and middle piece are formed.

Spermiation

- After the maturation, the sperms stay attached to the Sertoli cells.
- The release of sperms into the tubule is called spermiation.

Factors Regulating Spermatogenesis

Hormones regulating spermatogenesis are—androgens, gonadotropins and estrogen
- **Androgens:** A high concentration of testosterone in the tubular fluid is essential for spermatogenesis. LH stimulates Leydig cells to secrete testosterone. Sertoli cells secrete androgen binding protein (ABP) to which testosterone binds and its levels are kept elevated.
Spermiogenesis is androgen dependent.
- **LH:** It stimulates Leydig cells to secrete testosterone and thereby is needed for spermatogenesis.
- **FSH:** Stimulates Sertoli cells and Sertoli cells help in conversion of spermatids to sperms, secretion of ABP and secretion of inhibin. It also increases LH receptors in Leydig cells. It maintains gametogenic function of testis.
- **Estrogen** content is high in the fluid in rete testis and estrogen acts to increase fluid reabsorption and spermatozoa is concentrated. This is essential for fertility of an individual.
- **Body temperature:** Spermatogenesis takes place in a temperature less than the inner body temperature. The testes are kept at a temperature of 32°C. If the testes are exposed to higher temperatures the tubular walls degenerate and sterility results.

---

11. Functional residual capacity and its significance.

- It is the volume of air remaining in the lung at the end of tidal expiration.
- It is equal to residual volume + expiratory reserve volume
- Normal value is 2.5 L

Measurement of FRC

It can be measured by two methods:
1. Nitrogen washout method
2. Helium dilution method

1. **Nitrogen washout method:**
   - It is based on the fact that alveoli contain 80% N_2 (Got from breathing atmospheric air which has 80% N_2).
   - The subject is asked to breathe 100% O_2 for 5 minutes.
   - Then he is asked to expire into the Douglas bag (Which is washed with 100% O_2)
   - The volume of air expired and the concentration of N_2 in the expired air is measured and with these values FRC is calculated.

For example:
The volume of air expired into the bag = 40 L
N_2 concentration is 5%
So, 100 mL of air contains 5 mL of N_2 and therefore 40,000 mL of air will contain
= 5 × 40,000/100
= 2000 mL of N_2

The 2000 mL of N_2 has been washed out from the alveoli and there is 80% N_2 in the air, i.e., 80 mL of N_2 in 100 mL of air.
So 2000 mL would have been present in = 2000 × 100/80 = 2500 mL
2500 mL is the FRC.

2. **Helium dilution technique:**
   - Here the subject is made to breathe from the spirometer containing a mixture of air and helium.
   - He is asked to exhale, till the tidal expiration and then he breathes in and out of the spirometer continuously till the amount of helium in spirometer and lungs are equilibrated.
   Then FRC is calculated by using the formula:
   - Initial volume (V_1) × Initial concentration of helium (He_i) = Final volume (V_1+FRC) × Final concentration of helium (He_f)
   - Therefore FRC = $V_1 (He_i - He_f)/He_f$
   - If V_1 = 2000 mL
   - He_i = 12%
   - He_f = 5%
   - Then FRC = 2000 (12–5)/5 = 2000 X 7/5 = 2800 mL
   - FRC = 2800 mL

Significance of FRC

- FRC acts as a buffer and allows continuous exchange of gases in inspiration as well as expiration.
- Without FRC, the pO_2 in alveoli will increase to 150 mm Hg during inspiration and in expiration it may reach even zero.
- Presence of FRC maintains pO_2 at 100 mm Hg.
- FRC dilutes the toxic gases, as the FRC (2300 mL) is always present in lungs
- Helps in breath holding
- Work of breathing is minimized by the FRC as the presence of this volume of air in lungs prevent the collapse of the alveoli
- FRC prevents collapse and thereby decreases pulmonary vascular resistance.

12. Types of hypoxia and its cause.

- Hypoxia is defined as deficiency of O_2 at tissue level.
- **Types:**
  - Hypoxic hypoxia
  - Anemic hypoxia
  - Stagnant hypoxia
  - Histotoxic hypoxia

Hypoxic Hypoxia

Arterial pO_2 is low, therefore tissue pO_2 is less.

Mechanism of Hypoxia

- pO_2 of arterial blood is low due to either ↓O_2 in inspired air or disease of respiratory apparatus.

Conditions

- Low pO_2 in inspired air (as in high altitude)
- Hypoventilation as in airway obstruction, paralysis of respiratory muscles
- Diffusion defects as in pulmonary edema
- Ventilation/perfusion mismatch
- A-V shunt as in congenital cyanotic heart disease

Anemic Hypoxia

- It is due to decreased O_2 carrying capacity of blood and so ↓O_2 content in blood. pO_2 is normal.
- **Conditions:** Anemia, CO poisoning, Presence of altered Hb (methemoglobin), etc.
- In mild conditions, the 2,3-DPG levels increase in the RBC → Easy dissociation of O_2.

Stagnant Hypoxia

- Hypoxia due to decreased blood flow to tissues. Also called as ischemic hypoxia.
- **Mechanism:** O_2 content and pO_2 are normal in arterial blood. Hypoxia is due to stagnation of blood → circulatory hypoxia.
- **Seen in:**
  - Heart failure
  - Shock
  - Vascular obstruction
  - Hemorrhage

Histotoxic Hypoxia

- Tissues cannot utilize O_2 in spite of normal O_2 supply as in cyanide poisoning.
- Venous pO_2 is high (>46 mm Hg)
- Cyanide poisoning is treated with methylene blue or nitrites → forms methemoglobin → reacts with cyanide → cyanmethemoglobin. It is less poisonous.
- Hyperbaric O_2 is also used for treatment.
- **Features of types of hypoxia:**

Features	Hypoxic hypoxia	Anemic hypoxia	Stagnant hypoxia	Histotoxic hypoxia
Arterial PO_2	Decreased	Normal	Normal	Normal
% O_2 saturation of hemoglobin	Decreased	Decreased	Normal	Normal
Arterial O_2 content (mL/dL)	Decreased	Markedly decreased	Normal	Normal
A-V PO_2 difference	Decreased	Normal	More than normal	Less than normal
Peripheral chemoreceptor stimulation	Present	Absent	Present	Present
Cyanosis	Present	Absent	Present	Absent

13. Respiratory membrane.

- The alveolocapillary membrane is also called as the respiratory membrane.
- It separates the blood in the capillaries and the air in the alveoli.
- The gases which have to move from alveoli to capillary or in the opposite direction they have to diffuse across this membrane.
- It is made up of alveolar epithelial lining, basement membrane and the capillary endothelial lining (*refer* **Fig. 26**).
- The thickness of the membrane is 0.2 to 0.5 μm.

14. Neural centers for regulation of respiration.

- Breathing is an automatic process occurring throughout life without conscious effort.

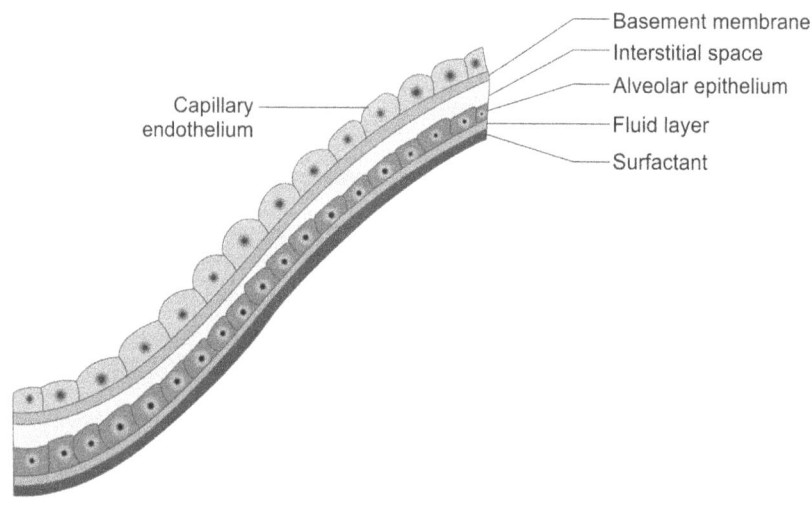

Fig. 26: Respiratory membrane.

- Respiration is a process which is highly regulated.
- Spontaneous respiration is due to rhythmic discharge of neurons from respiratory centers supplying the inspiratory muscles.
- This is under cortical (voluntary) and medullary and pontine control (automatic).
- These centers in turn are regulated by alterations in the PCO_2, PO_2 and pH of arterial blood and other non-chemical influences.

Cortical Control or Voluntary Control of Respiration

Impulses from cerebral cortex
↓
Corticospinal tract
↓
Motor neurons supplying the inspiratory muscles

- Impulses also reach the innervation of expiratory muscles.
- There is a reciprocal inhibition between the motor neurons supplying the
- I and E neurons.
- There is an exception for this at the start of expiration were the "I" neurons are active.
- The inspiratory muscles are active for some time during expiration to brake the elastic recoil of lungs and make expiration smooth.

Automatic Control of Respiration

Impulses from brainstem respiratory centers in pons and medulla → supplies neurons in intermediolateral horn cells of cervical and thoracic segments → supplies inspiratory muscles.

Medullary Respiratory Centers
- **Dorsal respiratory group of neurons (DRG):** Has 'I' neurons
- **Ventral respiratory group of neurons (VRG):** Has 'I' and 'E' neurons (*refer* **Fig. 27**)
- Central pattern generator (CPG): Prebotzinger complex (*refer* **Fig. 28**)

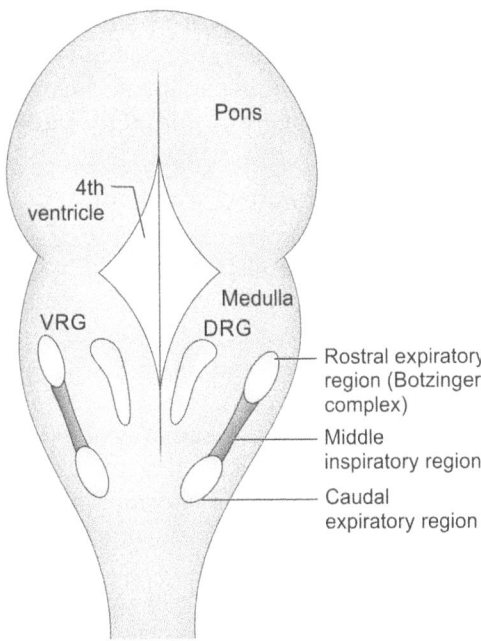

Fig. 27: Respiratory centers in medulla.
[DRG: dorsal respiratory group of neurons (has only inspiratory neurons); VRG: ventral respiratory group of neurons (has both inspiratory and expiratory neurons)]

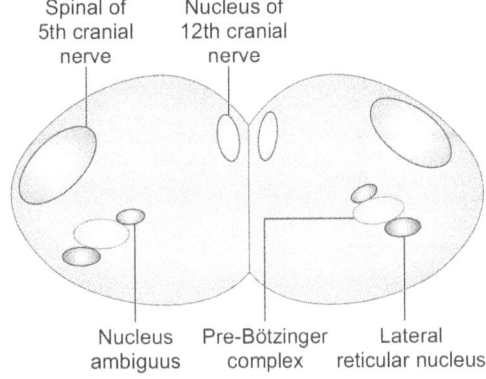

Fig. 28: Location of pacemaker (pre-Botzinger complex) for rhythm generation in medulla.

Dorsal Respiratory Group of Neurons
- Located near nucleus tractus solitarius (NTS)
- Contains only inspiratory neurons
- They project to cell bodies of phrenic nerves in spinal cord.
- Its activity is weaker to start with and gradually increases in a ramp fashion for 2 seconds and abruptly stops for 3 seconds.

- The ramp signal helps in steady increase in lung volume during inspiration
- Receives input from peripheral chemoreceptors through 9th and 10th cranial nerves.

Ventral Respiratory Group of Neurons
- Located in ventrolateral medulla in region of nucleus ambiguus (NA)
- Contains both inspiratory and expiratory group of neurons
- Three regions—rostral, middle and caudal inspiratory regions
- Middle region—has inspiratory neurons
- Rostral and caudal—has expiratory neurons—supply expiratory muscles.
- They are active only during forceful respiration.
- I and E neurons reciprocally inhibit each other

Pacemaker Cells for Respiration
- Located close to DRG and VRG neurons
- Present in the pre-Botzinger complex between nucleus ambiguus and lateral reticular nucleus.
- They are pace-maker cells and are responsible for generating respiratory rhythm → rhythmically activate phrenic nerves.
- It receives input from higher centers

Pontine Centers

There are two centers:
1. **Pneumotaxic center:**
   - Located in nucleus parabrachialis and Kolliker-Fuse N in the upper part of pons (*refer* **Fig. 29**)
   - Active during both inspiration and expiration.
   - On stimulation, it shortens the duration of inspiration. When its activity is less, the duration of inspiration is longer.
   - Its major function is to limit inspiration, by inhibiting apneustic center
   - It coordinates switching between inspiration and expiration.
2. **Apneustic center:**
   - Present in lower part of pons (*refer* **Fig. 29**)

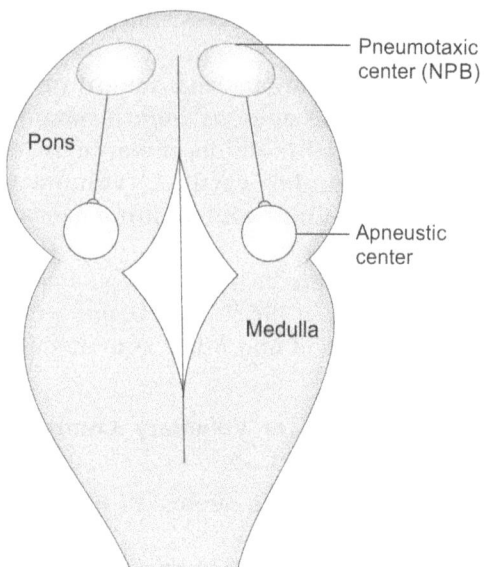

Fig. 29: Respiratory centers in pons, pneumotaxic and apneustic centers.

- On stimulation → Leads to prolonged inspiratory spasms—apneusis
- It sends inputs to DRG to cause a prolonged inspiration
- It is constantly stimulating DRG.
- But its actions are kept in check by inputs from pneumotaxic center and vagal afferents from airways.

Mechanism of Breathing
- The neurons in DRG discharge steadily and spontaneously in a ramp like fashion for 2–3 seconds.
- Muscles of inspiration contract steadily resulting in expansion of the lung and chest wall resulting in inspiration.
- As the inspiration happens, the stretch receptors in lungs and airways are stimulated and impulses from here travel through vagus nerve to stop the firing of DRG neurons.
- Impulses from pneumotaxic center through inhibition of apneustic center stops the firing of DRG.
- Inspiratory muscles relax and the lung and chest wall recoils and induces expiration.
- At the end of expiration, the next cycle starts.

15. Dead space.

- Dead space is the space in the airways in which the volume of air present does not take part in gaseous exchange.
- There are 3 types of dead spaces—anatomical dead space, alveolar dead space and physiological or total dead space.
    1. **Anatomical dead space** is the conducting zone of the respiratory pathway in which the gaseous exchange does not take place and the volume of air is said to be the dead space air.
    2. **Alveolar dead space** is the alveoli which do not have blood supply and the volume of air in these alveoli do not take part in gas exchange and is considered to be wasted ventilation.
    3. **Physiological dead space** is the sum of the above two dead spaces.
- Since in normal conditions, there are no alveolar dead spaces, physiological dead space is equal to anatomical dead space.
- In a normal adult, of the 500 mL of tidal volume inhaled, 150 mL remains in the anatomical dead space, which is also the physiological dead space.

Measurement of Physiological Dead Space

It is by using the Bohr's equation or single breath CO_2 technique:
- Bohr's equation is used to measure physiological dead space by measuring the CO_2 levels in the alveolar and arterial blood and the tidal volume.
- CO_2 gas is used as it is very less in inspired air and all the CO_2 in expired air is got from the alveoli.

Bohr's Equation

$P_{ECO2} \times V_T = P_{aCO2} \times (V_T - V_D) + P_{ICO2} \times V_D$
$(V_T - V_D) \times P_{aCO2} + P_{ICO2} \times V_D = P_{ECO2} \times VT$
Since inspired CO_2 is negligible, $P_{ICO2} \times V_D = 0$,
So:
$V_T - V_D = P_{ECO2} \times V_T / P_{aCO2}$
$V_D = V_T - [P_{ECO2} \times V_T / P_{aCO2}]$
V_T = tidal volume
V_D = physiological dead space

P_{ECO2} = CO_2 in expired air
P_{ICO2} = CO_2 in inspired air
P_{aCO2} = CO_2 in alveolar air

16. Pacemaker potential.

- In the mammalian heart, sinoatrial node is the pace maker. It is said to be the pace maker as it generates impulses by itself without neural input at a faster rate.
- Other tissues of the heart—AV node, atria and ventricle are also capable of generating impulses but SA node generates impulses at a faster rate and therefore said to be the pacemaker of the heart.

Pacemaker Potential

- The ventricular and atrial muscle cells have a resting membrane potential of –90 mV. On stimulation, the membrane depolarizes and produces an action potential.
- The pacemaker cells are smaller and rounded (P cells) and they do not have a stable resting membrane potential and RMP is around –55 to –60 mV (*refer* **Fig. 30**).
- From –60 mV there is a slow depolarization slope which reaches the firing level of –40 mV and there is a rapid depolarization followed by rapid repolarization back to –60 mV and again there is a slow depolarization slope rising to firing level.
- This slope which takes the membrane to firing level is the **pacemaker potential or prepotential**.

Ionic Events Responsible for Pacemaker Potential

- At –60 mV, the K^+ channels start closing down thereby preventing K^+ efflux. This is responsible for the first part of pre-potential (the slope).
- Next part is due to opening up of **'f'** type Na^+ channels (The Na^+ current in this channel is said to be funny current as the channel opens in hyperpolarization)
- Last part of depolarization of the pre-potential is due to opening of T-type

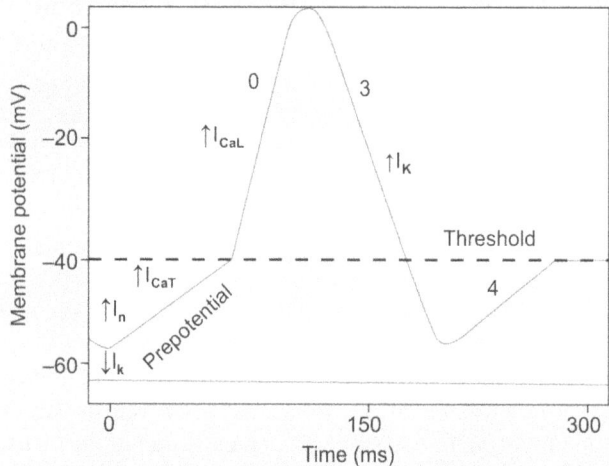

Fig. 30: Pacemaker potential. Slope of pacemaker potential (Phase 4), the prepotential is due to 3 events; first part of depolarization is due to closure of K⁺ channels, 2nd part is due to Na⁺ influx through sodium channel and last part of depolarization is due to Ca^{2+} influx through T-type Ca^{2+} channels. Rapid depolarization (Phase 0) is due to opening of L-type Ca^{2+} channels and repolarization (Phase 3) due to opening of K⁺ channels.

- (Transient) Ca^{2+} channels allowing Ca^{2+} influx.
- Now as the firing level is reached (–40 mV), the long lasting Ca^{2+} channels (L-Type) open and produces a rapid depolarization and the action potential.
- Then the K⁺ channels open and the K⁺ efflux bring about rapid repolarization and membrane potential reaches –60 mV. Then the next prepotential starts.
- So in the pacemaker cells, it is a Ca^{2+} dependent depolarization rather than Na⁺ dependent depolarization as in ventricular muscles.
- The pacemaker cells are supplied by sympathetic and parasympathetic nerves.
- On stimulation by sympathetic nerves, the prepotential slope becomes steeper and the rate of spontaneous discharge increases thereby increasing the heart rate.
- On stimulation by the parasympathetic nerves, the slope of the prepotential decreases and spontaneous firing also decreases thereby heart rate decreases.

17. Cardiac index.

- Cardiac output per minute per square meter of body surface area is cardiac index.
- Cardiac index = cardiac output at rest/body surface area
- 5 L/min/1.7 m² = 3L/min/mm²
- Normal average value = 3.2 L/min/mm²
- Cardiac index is used to standardize cardiac output for the different body surface areas.

18. Dark adaptation.

- When a person moves from a brightly illuminated place to a dark environment, he is not able to see anything. But gradually the eyes get accommodated to the darkness and his vision improves. This is said to be dark adaptation. Complete adaptation happens in 20 minutes.
- The changes happening in the eye in darkness are—dilatation of pupil, shifting of cone vision to rod vision and regeneration of rhodopsin in darkness.
- The changes happening are discussed under neural adaptation and chemical adaptation.

Neural Adaptation

- The dark adaptation happens in two phases.
- The first phase is due to cone adaptation and it happens in the first 5–10 minutes (*refer* **Fig. 31**).

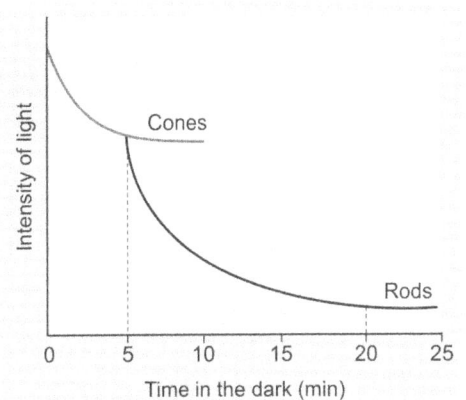

Fig. 31: Dark adaptation curve. There are two curves, red curve shows cone adaptation and violet curve shows rod adaptation.

- This increases the retinal sensitivity to light 100 times.
- In the second phase of adaptation, the rod sensitivity to light increases and the retinal sensitivity increases by 1000–10,000 times.
- Once rod adaptation has happened even a single photon of light is visible to the eye.

Chemical Adaptation

- When a person stays in bright light, the rod pigment rhodopsin is bleached and is converted to all-trans-retinal and opsin.
- Therefore, rods are insensitive to light and do not respond to light.
- The rod sensitivity can increase only when the rhodopsin is re-synthesized and this takes several minutes to happen.
- That is why the dark adaptation by rods takes 20 minutes (*refer* **Fig. 31**).
- The rods are present in the retina 15–20 degrees away from the fovea. That is the reason there is dilatation of the pupil to expose the retina rich in rods to light.
- The time taken for dark adaptation depends on the degree of brightness of light to which the eye is exposed and for how long it is being exposed.
- Brighter the light and longer the duration later it takes for dark adaptation.

19. Functions of Basal Ganglia.

- Basal ganglia is involved in planning and programming of voluntary movement.
- Controls muscle tone through inhibition of motor cortex and inhibitory medullary RF.
- Controls the limb movements. In diseases of BG unpurposeful limb movements appear.
- Controls automated associative limb movements, such as swinging of arms while walking.
- Caudate nucleus plays a role in cognition because of its connections with associative cortex.
- Somatic movements associated with emotions are controlled by BG
- Functions in motivated behavior

20. Vestibulocerebellum.

Functional Divisions of Cerebellum

1. **Vestibulocerebellum:** It includes the flocculonodular lobe
2. **Spinocerebellum:** Includes the paleocerebellum
3. **Cerebrocerebellum:** Includes the neocerebellum (*refer* **Fig. 32**)

Vestibulocerebellum

Connections:
- **Afferents:** Receive input from vestibular nuclei and primary vestibular apparatus
- **Efferents:** Projects to the vestibular nucleus → vestibulospinal tract and medial longitudinal fasciculus → motor neurons of anterior horn

Functions

1. Modulate muscular activity to achieve postural equilibrium or posture.
2. Coordinate movements of eye with movements of head.
3. Involved in eye movements and maintain balance

21. Tests for ovulation.

- **Rise of basal body temperature:** There is a rise in 0.5°C in basal body temperature after ovulation. The rise is due to the thermogenic effect of progesterone which is secreted by corpus luteum. It is recorded first thing in the morning, orally, before

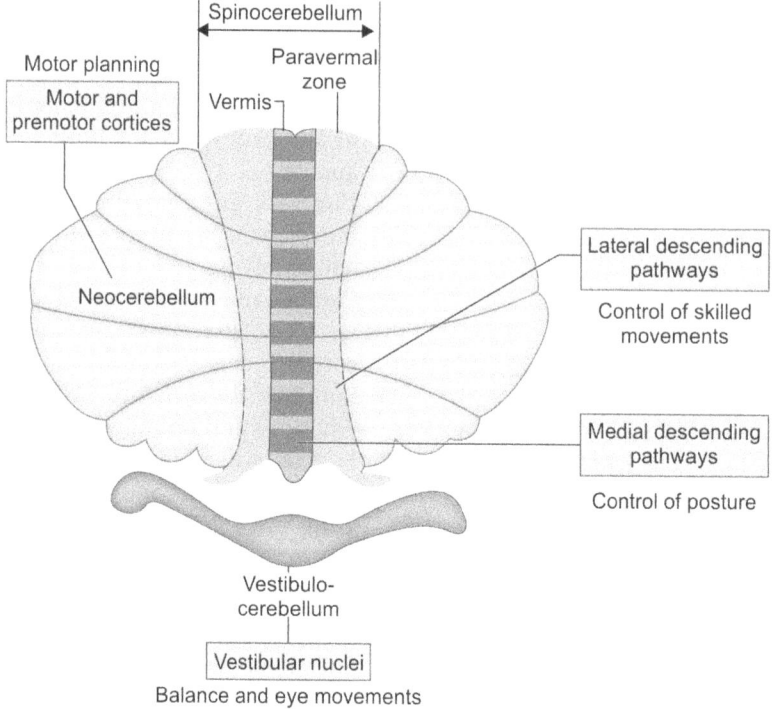

Fig. 32: Functional divisions of cerebellum with their connections and functions.

getting up from bed, before eating or drinking anything.

- **Mittelschmerz:** After ovulation, bleeding into the ruptured follicle happens, some amount of blood is also spilt into the abdominal cavity close to the ovary and results in fleeting abdominal pain.
- **Spinnbarkeit:** During proliferative phase, under the influence of estrogen, cervical mucus is very thin and at the time of ovulation, it is the thinnest and a drop of mucus between the thumb and index finger can be stretched to 10 cm, this is spinnbarkeit.
- Sometimes following ovulation **mild spotting** can also be present
- **Fern test:** At the time of ovulation, under the effect of estrogen, the cervical mucous is thin and when spread on a slide and viewed under the microscope gives a fern shape. In the luteal phase when progesterone is present, this fern pattern is absent.
- **Demonstration of LH peak:** LH surge is seen just before ovulation and therefore regular estimation of LH levels can give us an idea about ovulation.
- Laparoscopic examination
- Ultrasound scanning of pelvis

22. Contraceptives.

Contraception is prevention of pregnancy.

The needs for prevention of pregnancy are:
- To control population explosion
- To prevent pregnancy in mothers with heart diseases

Certain methods prevent transmission of sexually transmitted diseases, such as AIDS

The methods can be:
- Temporary or spacing methods
- Terminal or permanent methods

The methods are described as contraceptive methods in males and females.

Contraceptive Methods in Males

Temporary Methods
1. Natural method
2. Barrier method
3. Pills

1. **Natural method or coitus interruptus:** Withdrawal of penis before ejaculation prevents deposition of semen in the vagina. This method needs practice and timing is very important. The disadvantages are that the precoital secretions may contain sperms and it can lead to pregnancy.
2. **Barrier method:** Condoms are the widely used barrier method in males. It is made of fine latex sheet. It prevents deposition of semen in the vagina and prevents fertilization of ovum. It can be used to prevent transmission of sexually transmitted diseases.
3. **Pills:**
   - Drugs are used to inhibit spermatogenesis.
   - Gossypol and testosterone are used.
   - Gossypol—it is derived from cottonseed oil. It decreases sperm count.
   - Testosterone—high testosterone levels inhibit sperm production.

Permanent Methods

Vasectomy: A small portion of vas deferens is removed after clamping. Both the open ends are ligated and sutured.

Contraceptive Methods in Females

Temporary Methods
- Rhythm method
- Barrier method
- Oral contraceptive pills
- Intrauterine contraceptive device

Rhythm Method
- This method can be followed in females with regular menstrual cycles of 28-30 days.
- During a normal menstrual cycle, ovulation happens on 14th day of the cycle.
- The ovum stays viable for 48-72 hours after ovulation.
- After ejaculation, sperm stays viable in female reproductive tract for 24-48 hours.
- So, pregnancy can happen if intercourse happens within this period.
- This is said to be the "dangerous period".
- So, the days are calculated from first day of menstrual cycle and intercourse should be avoided in the dangerous period.
- 5-6 days after the bleeding phase and 5-6 days before the next menstruation is considered to be the "safe period".
- It can be utilized by females with regular cycles and who can keep a record of their time of ovulation by checking basal body temperature.

Barrier Method
- Barriers can be mechanical or chemical barriers. They basically prevent the meeting of sperm and ovum.
- **Mechanical barrier:** Diaphragm and cervical caps
- **Chemical barriers:** Spermicidal agents, such as nonoxynol, ricinoleic acid in the form of jelly or foam is placed in the female reproductory tract before coitus.

Oral Contraceptive Pills
- By pills we mean the oral contraceptive pills used for female contraception.
- They are usually synthetic preparation of estrogen, progesterone or combination of both.
- **The pills can be of different types:**
  a. Combined pill or classical pill
  b. Sequential pill
  c. Minipill
  d. Post-coital pill

  a. *Combined pill:*
     - It is a combination of estrogen and progesterone pill.
     - It contains a strip of 21 tablets and is consumed for 21 days from 5th day of menstrual cycle.
     - After 21 days, on stopping the tablets, withdrawal bleeding happens.
     - Again from 5th day, next cycle is started.
     It acts by:
     - Prevents ovulation, as the high estrogen levels disorganize the LH and FSH secretions.
     - Prevents implantation of fertilized ovum.

- Progesterone makes the cervical mucus thick and prevents sperm penetration

b. *Sequential pill:*
- It has high dose of estrogen and minimal amounts of progesterone.
- It is not used nowadays as the high estrogen may induce endometrial cancer or breast cancer.

c. *Minipill:*
- It is progesterone only pill.
- It does not affect ovulation but makes the cervical mucus thick and prevents sperm penetration.

d. *Post-coital pill:*
- It is used within 72 hours of unprotected intercourse.
- It has high doses of estrogen and is given for 4–6 days.
- High estrogen prevents implantation of the fertilized ovum.

Depot preparation
- These are implants of progesterone and they are subdermally implanted and prevent pregnancy for 5 years.
- The only problem is it can cause amenorrhea and irregular cycles.

Intrauterine Contraceptive Devices

These are small devices made of plastic or copper and placed in the uterus to prevent implantation of fertilized ovum.

Lippe's loop
- It is a simple 'S' shaped plastic device with nylon threads.
- Under aseptic precautions, the loop is inserted into the uterus and the thread is present in the vagina.
- The loop is also impregnated with a small amount of barium sulfate for checking its presence by radiographs.

Copper 'T'
- It is a 'T' shaped device made of copper with nylon threads.
- They are inserted during the first 10 days of menstrual cycle.
- Copper prevents implantation of fertilized ovum by stimulating an aseptic inflammation of the endometrium.

Permanent Method

Tubectomy
- It can be done by an open surgery or by laparoscopic surgery.
- Here the fallopian tubes are cut and ligated and buried.

23. Thyroxine synthesis.

Refer short note 9.

24. Tetany.

- Tetany is neuromuscular hyperexcitability due to hypocalcemia.
- The decrease in calcium ions in plasma results in reduction in the amount of depolarization needed to excite the nerves.

The signs and symptoms are:
- **Carpopedal spasm:** There is flexion at metacarpophalangeal joints, extension at interphalangeal joints and opposition of thumb. In the legs, the toes are plantarflexed and feet are drawn up (*refer* Fig. 33).
- **Trousseau's sign:** It is seen in latent tetany. On inflation of the sphygmomanometer cuff to the arm and occlusion of blood vessels results in appearance of the carpal spasm.

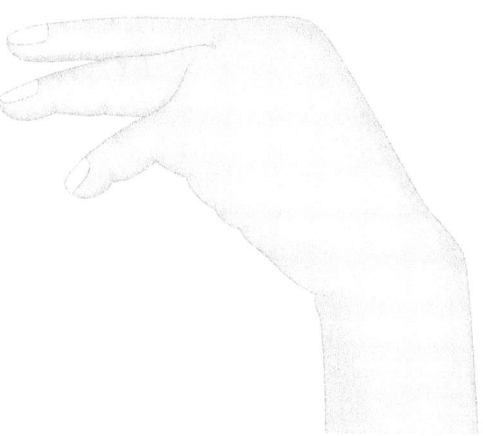

Fig. 33: Trousseau's sign.

- **Chvostek's sign:** On tapping the facial nerve at the angle of the jaw, there is twitching of facial muscles.
- **Laryngeal stridor:** Spasm of laryngeal muscles results in constriction of larynx and it may result in asphyxia.
- **Paresthesia:** Tingling sensation in peripheral parts of limbs

Tetany is treated with infusion of ionized calcium and parathormone replacement.

25. Juxtaglomerular apparatus.

Refer short note 5.

26. Dialysis.

- Acute and chronic renal failure is treated with **artificial kidney or dialysis**.
- It helps to remove the toxic substances from the body and restores body fluid volume and composition to normal.
- There are two types of dialysis—**hemodialysis and peritoneal dialysis.**
- Basic principle of dialysis is diffusion of solutes from higher to lower concentration across a semi-permeable membrane (*refer* **Fig. 34**).
- Blood which is needed to be purified is passed through minute blood channels bounded by a thin semi-permeable membrane.
- The other side of the membrane contains the dialyzing fluid with which exchange of substances happen.

Peritoneal Dialysis

- It can be done by the patient 4–5 times/day in his/her place.
- The peritoneal membrane is used as the semi-permeable membrane across which movement of substances happen between plasma and the dialyzing fluid.
- A catheter is inserted into the peritoneal cavity and is connected to a bag with 2 Liters of dialyzing fluid.
- There is an outlet tube through which the fluid containing the waste products are removed and measured.
- The exchange takes place for 20 minutes.

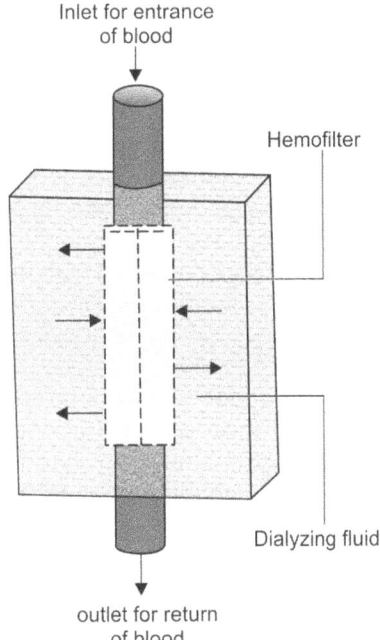

Fig. 34: Basic principle of dialysis. The blood to be dialyzed passes through small coiled cellophane tubes which is separated from the dialyzing fluid in the machine. Solutes diffuse from their higher to lower concentrations between blood and the dialyzing fluid through the semipermeable cellophane membrane.

- The input and output measurements are made.
- This can be done with the patient ambulatory.

Hemodialysis or Artificial Kidney

- Here the blood which has to be purified is passed through a machine.
- It is usually done in a hospitalized patient by an expert.
- The radial artery of the patient is connected to the machine and at a time 500 mL of blood enters the machine and passes through a coiled cellophane tube which is surrounded by the dialyzing fluid.
- The fluid contains less amount of sodium, potassium and more amounts of glucose, bicarbonate and calcium ions.
- The fluid is devoid of waste products, such as urea, uric acid, etc., and therefore they move out of the blood into the fluid by the gradient.

- This favors removal of excess of unwanted ions and addition of solutes which are necessary.
- By this process, the wastes are removed and electrolytes are restored in the blood and the purified blood is returned back into the patient's body through a peripheral vein.
- The blood is anticoagulated with heparin when it passes through the machine.

---

27. Gastric emptying.

- Gastric emptying is a slow process in which food from stomach is gradually emptied into the duodenum and jejunum.
- **There are 3 mechanisms in gastric emptying:**
  a. *Peristaltic contractions:* These are ring like contractions starting in the body of stomach and gradually push the contents towards the antrum. The waves in the proximal part are weak and as it reaches the antrum the waves become stronger and dig into the chyme. So adequate mixing and breaking down of food particles happen in the antrum. (*refer* **Fig. 35A**)
  b. *Contractions of antrum:* Antral contractions are very strong and they help in proper mixing of gastric juice with food contents. Not only mixing of food and gastric juice happens but also the force of contraction forces the food towards the pylorus. But the pyloric sphincter ahead is strongly contracted. (*refer* **Fig. 35B**)
  c. *Retropulsion:* Forceful contraction of antrum and closure of pyloric sphincter pushes the food back into the proximal part of the antrum and this continues for few times. The retropulsion helps in mixing and grinding the food particles. The pyloric sphincter opens partially allowing small quantities of chyme at a time to be squirted into the duodenum. (*refer* **Figs. 35C and D**)

Regulation of Gastric Emptying

Regulation is done by neural and humoral mechanisms. Factors which affect emptying are—pH of contents in duodenum, osmotic pressure, products of fat and protein digestion.

- **Low pH:** Acidic content in the duodenum is sensed by receptors in the duodenum

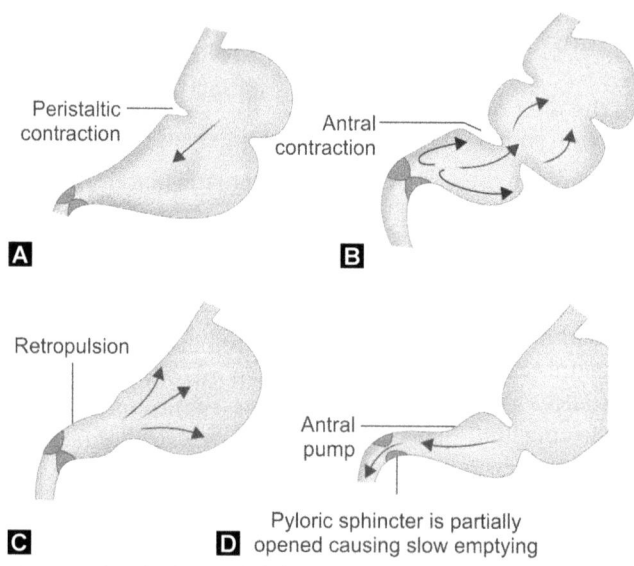

Figs. 35A to D: Gastric emptying; In A, B and C the pyloric sphincter is closed. The contractions in antrum digest the food and is converted to chyme; (C) There is forward movement of chyme and as the sphincter is closed there is retropulsion of chyme which further breaks food particles; (D) Sphincter is partially open allowing small amounts of chyme to be emptied.

and gastric emptying is delayed by secretin released from small intestines.
- **Osmolality of contents:** If the osmolality of the contents entering the duodenum is high, it is sensed by osmoreceptors here and hormones are released which inhibit gastric emptying.
- **Products of digestion of fat:** Presence of digested fats and fatty acids are sensed by the duodenum and CCK is released which causes delay in gastric emptying.
- **Products of protein digestion:** Protein products, such as peptides and amino acids in duodenum cause release of gastrin which in turn causes antral contraction and closure of pyloric sphincter resulting in delaying the gastric emptying.
- **Volume and type of meal:** When volume of meal is more there is delayed emptying. Watery meal hastens the emptying. Carbohydrate emptying is faster and fat emptying is the slowest.
- **Stretch of duodenum:** When duodenal wall is stretched, it induces enterogastric reflex which inhibits gastric emptying.
- **Neural factors:** Vagus stimulation promotes emptying and sympathetic stimulation delays emptying.

28. Enterohepatic circulation.

- Bile acids and salts present in the bile on entering the intestine are absorbed from the terminal part of the ileum and re-enter the portal vein to be secreted back into the bile from hepatocytes (*refer* **Fig. 36**).
- This process repeats many times—enterohepatic circulation.
- The conjugated bile salts are absorbed and recirculated in the above manner.
- Also, bile salts are unconjugated and some of it is also absorbed.
- Colonic bacteria act on free bile acids and are converted to secondary bile acids and a part of it is also absorbed back into the portal vein.
- About 95% of secreted bile salts are absorbed by the enterohepatic circulation and only 200–500 mg/day are excreted.

Significance of Enterohepatic Circulation

- Only the amount of bile salts which are excreted, are synthesized and replaced daily, to maintain the pool of bile salts in the body which are essential for digestion and absorption of fats.
- The total amount of bile salts is 2–4 g.

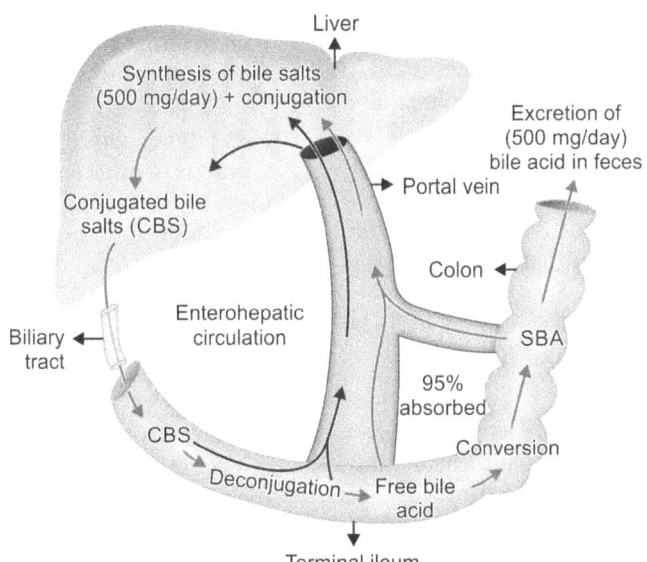

Fig. 36: Enterohepatic circulation. It is the circulation of bile salts following its synthesis from liver in bile and its secretion into duodenum and its reabsorption in terminal ileum and recirculation through portal veins.

- This amount is circulated daily many times to digest and absorb fats in the diet taken.

29. Functions of saliva.

- Ptyalin (α-amylase) in saliva splits starches. Action of amylase is maximum at a pH of 6.8. Digestion continues in stomach for some time till the pH becomes less than 4.
- **Protective function:** Saliva cleans the mouth after a meal and prevents growth of harmful bacteria.
- Saliva contains lysozyme, IgA and lactoferrin for protection. Lysozymes are bactericidal and lactoferrin is bacteriostatic in action.
- Saliva facilitates speech.
- It helps in taste of food.
- Mucus in saliva helps in lubrication of food, mastication and swallowing
- It buffers the gastric juice in stomach.
- Proline rich proteins in the saliva protect the enamel of tooth.
- Saliva dilutes hot and irritant foods and protects buccal mucosa. It also dilutes regurgitated bile and Hcl
- In animals it helps in temperature regulation.
- Helps in excretion of heavy metals, alcohol, morphine, thiocyanate, etc.

30. Autoimmune disease.

- During the processing of development of immunity, the lymphocytes are presented with self and nonself-antigens and the cells and antibodies responding to self-antigens are eliminated—**tolerance**.
- Sometimes antibodies against self-antigens are not eliminated and it results in **autoimmune diseases**.
- It can be B cell or T cell mediated, it can be organ-specific or systemic in nature.

Examples are:
- **Type 1 diabetes mellitus:** Antibodies against B cells in Islet of pancreas.
- **Myasthenia gravis:** Antibodies for nicotinic acetylcholine receptors in NMJ
- **Multiple sclerosis:** Antibodies against myelin basic protein and several other components of myelin

- **Grave's disease:** Antibodies for TSH receptors and the receptors are activated resulting in hyperthyroidism.
- **Molecular mimicry:** Antibodies against certain bacteria will cross-react with body constituents, as in rheumatic fever where antibodies against *Streptococcus* attacks the cardiac myosin induces damage to heart.

31. Decompression sickness.

- Also called as "Dysbarism, The bends, Caisson's disease, Diver's palsy".
- This happens when a person breathing compressed air ascends up rapidly.
- At high pressures, N_2 dissolves in body fluids and stays dissolved.
- When the person ascends up to sea level gradually N_2 is converted to air gradually and is blown out.
- But when he ascends up rapidly the dissolved N_2 does not have enough time to be converted to air and to be blown out and therefor it stays in the tissues as N_2 bubbles.
- N_2 dissolved in tissues forms bubbles while escaping from tissues due to rapid ascent.
- Gas bubbles block the blood vessels and stay in tissues to create symptoms.

Symptoms are:
- Pain in joints and muscles of legs or arms.
- Sensation of numbness
- The chokes—shortness of breath, pulmonary edema, etc.
- Paralysis of muscles
- Coronary ischemia
- Neurological symptoms

Treatment:
Recompression in pressurized chamber followed by slow decompression

32. Middle ear functions.

- **Middle ear:** It is an air-filled cavity in temporal bone. It starts at the tympanic membrane and ends at oval window.
- **Contains:** 3 ossicles (malleus, incus and stapes), 2 small muscles (tensor tympani and stapedius), ligaments, nerves, blood vessels, etc.

Functions

1. **Tympanic reflex:** It is a protective reflex. When a loud sound is transmitted through the ossicles in middle ear a reflex is initiated with a latent period of 40-80 msec. Contraction of stapedius and tensor tympani pulls the tympanic membrane medially and membrane covering oval window laterally. This makes the ossicular system rigid and there is reduction in transmission of sounds. This reduces the intensity of sound by 30-40 decibels. It is also called as attenuation reflex.

   Functions of this reflex:
   - This reflex protects the cochlea from damaging loud sounds.
   - It filters the low frequency sounds
   - It prevents hearing one's own speech
2. **Transmission of sound waves from external ear to internal ear**
3. **Impedance matching:**
   - As the sound waves travel from rarer (air in external and middle ear) to denser medium (Fluid in the inner ear) they are dampened (by 30db).
   - This loss in sound energy is prevented in the middle ear by impedance matching which is by:
     a. By area differences
     b. By lever action
     c. By buckling factor

     a. **Area difference:** Area of tympanic membrane is greater than foot plate of stapes and therefore there is convergence of sound and pressure is increased by 17 times.
     b. **Lever action of the ossicles** increases pressure by 1.32 times
     c. **Buckling factor:** Tympanic membrane is conical in shape and the handle of malleus is attached to the umbo. As the tympanic membrane moves in and out, the buckling of membrane moves the handle of malleus less and this increases the force and decreases the velocity.

33. Define cardiac output. What are the methods to measure the cardiac output?

Cardiac output (CO) is defined as the amount of blood ejected by each ventricle per minute.
- CO = stroke volume (SV) × hear rate (HR)
- NV = 70 mL/beat × 70/min = 4900 mL/min

Measurement of Cardiac Output

Fick's Principle
- Fick's principle is defined as the amount of substance taken up by an organ or the whole body per unit of time and is equal to the arteriovenous difference of the substance times the blood flow.
- Substance taken by an organ = A-V difference X blood flow
- Blood flow = substance taken by the organ/ A-V difference
- Here the substance taken up is oxygen consumed by the whole organ
- Output of left ventricle = O_2 consumption (mL/min)/$A_{(O2)} - V_{(O2)}$
- O_2 Consumed is derived with spirometry
- Arterial blood sample is taken from peripheral artery
- Venous sample is collected from pulmonary artery
  = 250 mL/min/200 mL/L - 150 mL/L
  = 250 mL/min/50 mL/L
  = 5 L/min
- **Advantage:** Accurate and no chemical is injected
- **Disadvantage:** Needs hospitalization, catheterization, etc.

Other methods used are:
- **Indicator dye dilution method:** In this method, a known amount of a dye is injected into a vein and serial sampled of arterial blood is analyzed for concentration of the dye. The cardiac output is then calculated by dividing the amount of the dye injected by the average of the concentration of the dye in the samples after a single circulation through the heart.
- **Thermodilution method:** In this method, cold saline is injected into the right atrium

through one side of a double-lumen catheter and the temperature change in the blood is recorded in the pulmonary artery using a thermistor in the other side of the catheter. The temperature change is inversely proportional to the blood flowing through the pulmonary artery.
- **Advantages:** Saline is completely innocuous and the cold is dissipated into tissues.

34. Heart sounds.

Refer **Fig. 37**.

Heart sounds can be recorded by phonocardiogram.

Significance of Heart Sounds

- **1st sound:** Increased in exercise, hyperkinetic states, such as anemia and decreased in shock, MI, pericardial effusion.
- **2nd sound:** Loud in hypertension, low in aortic and pulmonary stenosis. Splitting is common.
- **3rd sound:** Increased in MR. Important sign of heart failure.
- **4th sound:** Always seen in abnormal conditions. Seen in left ventricular hypertrophy.

35. Define synapse and describe its properties.

- Junction between two neurons is said to be the synapse.
- Neurons communicate with each other through synapse.

Properties of Synapse

- Summation—spatial or temporal
- Convergence and divergence
- One way conduction of impulses
- Synaptic delay
- Facilitation
- Subliminal fringe
- Occlusion
- Synaptic plasticity and learning
- Synaptic fatigue

Summation

- Summation means adding up of impulses. In the synapse following release of neurotransmitters, there could be depolarization or hyperpolarization of the membrane. These are called as postsynaptic potentials and they belong to the category of graded potentials.
- So these individual potentials from many synapses can summate and excite the membrane and take it to the firing level.

Heart sounds	Events responsible	Duration	Frequency	Others
First sound (S_1)	Due to vibrations set by sudden closure of AV valves at the onset of ventricular systole	0.15 sec	25–45 Hz In PCG recorded as 9–13 waves	Soft and long, heard as "LUBB"
Second sound (S_2)	Associated with closure of aortic and pulmonary valves after the end of ventricular systole	0.12 sec	50 Hz In PCG recorded as 4–6 waves	Normally S2 can be split due to early closure of aortic valve, heard as "Dup"
Third sound (S_3)	Is heard at 1/3rd of diastole due to rapid filling of ventricle due to vibrations set by inrush of blood		0.1 sec In PCG recorded as 1–4 waves	Normally audible only in children and young adults
Fourth sound (S_4)	Heard just before (S_1) Occurs during atrial contraction Due to ventricular filling		20 cyc/sec In PCG recorded as 1–2 waves	Rarely heard in normal adults Heard in vent hypertrophy and CCF

Fig. 37: Heart sounds; their causes and characteristics.

- There are two types of summations—spatial and temporal summation.
- Temporal summation—the same input stimulates the postsynaptic neuron repeatedly and thereby excites it.
- Spatial summation—here many inputs stimulate simultaneously to excite it.

Convergence and Divergence

When many presynaptic neurons end one postsynaptic neuron it is convergence and on presynaptic terminal divides and ends on many postsynaptic neurons—Divergence.

One Way Conduction

Impulse transmission always happen from presynaptic to postsynaptic neurons as the receptors for the neurotransmitter released from presynaptic terminal is present on the postsynaptic membrane.

Synaptic Delay

There are many steps involved in the impulse transmission from the presynaptic neuron to postsynaptic neuron so there is a delay of 0.5 msec in each synapse.

Facilitation

- When a single stimulus is applied to the neuron some response is obtained but if repeated stimuli are given the response is better than the single stimulus response.
- So the previous stimulus has been facilitatory for the second and third one.

Subliminal Fringe

- It is a partially excited stage of the neuron.
- If two neurons are stimulated simultaneously the response obtained is more than the sum of stimulation of each neuron individually.
- This is because some neurons are in a subliminal fringe.

Occlusion

- The response obtained by stimulating two presynaptic neurons together is less than the response obtained by stimulating each one individually.
- This is because of common neurons in both the groups.

Synaptic Plasticity

The changes that occur in a synapse after repeated stimulation is called as synaptic plasticity.

Synaptic Fatigue

On repeated stimulation, the synapse goes in for fatigue due to exhaustion of neurotransmitters.

36. Describe the functions of thalamus.

- Thalamus functions as a major relay station for most sensory impulses reaching the cortex.
- Thalamus acts as a crude center for sense perception, such as crude touch, pain, crude form of temperature sensation.
- It also contributes to motor function by relaying impulses from cerebellum and basal ganglia to motor cortex.
- Relays impulse between different areas of cortex.
- Contributes to regulation of autonomic activities and maintenance of consciousness.
- Due to the intimate connections of thalamus with frontal cortex and hypothalamus, it is involved in various emotions.
- It is an integrating center for sleep, intralaminar nuclei for NREM sleep and lateral geniculate body for REM sleep.
- Concerned with recent memory and emotions due to its involvement in Papez circuit.
- Concerned with language.
- Important role in genesis of synchronization of EEG waves and alertness of the individual. Induces alertness due to its connections with RAS.

37. What are the functions of basal ganglia?

- Basal ganglia is involved in planning and programming of voluntary movement. The neurons of basal ganglia fire impulses even before the movements starts. Caudate loop is involved in planning of movements (direct pathway through caudate nucleus).

- Controls muscle tone through inhibition of motor cortex and inhibitory medullary RF. The pathway involved is cortex—striatum—GP—SN—medullary RF—spinal cord via reticulospinal tract. In lesion of BG, there is hypertonia.
- Controls the limb movements. In diseases of BG unpurposeful limb movements appear.
- Controls automated associative limb movements like swinging of arms while walking. Putamen circuit (direct pathway through putamen nucleus) is involved in control of subconscious movements.
- Timing the movements is also a role of BG.
- BG exerts an inhibitory effect on spinal reflexes which help to regulate posture
- Somatic movements associated with emotions are controlled by BG.
- Provides muscle tone for skilled movements
- Functions in motivated behavior
- Caudate nucleus plays a role in cognition because of its connections with associative cortex. Lesion leads to deficits of performance-based learning
- Because of its connections with RF, GP has a role in arousal mechanism

Lesion of head of left caudate nucleus leads to dysarthric aphasia

---

38. Describe the physiology of speech.

- Understanding spoken and written words and to express ideas in speech and writing is language.
- It is a role of the dominant or categorical hemisphere.
- It is one of the higher functions of cerebral cortex.
- Speech is thought to be a mode of communication between human beings.
- There are two forms of speech—written words and spoken words.
- Speech involves coordinated activities of central and peripheral speech apparatus.

Areas Involved in Language

All areas for language are around the sylvian fissure. They are:
- **Wernicke's area (Area 22):** Comprehension of auditory and visual information.
- **Broca's area (Area 44):** Processes the information comprehended by Wernicke's area into a coordinated pattern for vocalization.
- **Arcuate fasciculus:** Transmits information from Area 22 to 44 (refer **Fig. 38**).
- **Angular gyrus (area 39):** Processes information from that are read and converted to auditory form of words in Area 22.
- Motor area

Mechanism of Speech

- Speaking and understanding are complex behavior handled by various areas.
- Two important areas are—**Broca's** area and **Wernicke's** area.
- Broca's area is said to be the motor speech area.
- Wernicke's area is responsible to recognize and understand spoken words.

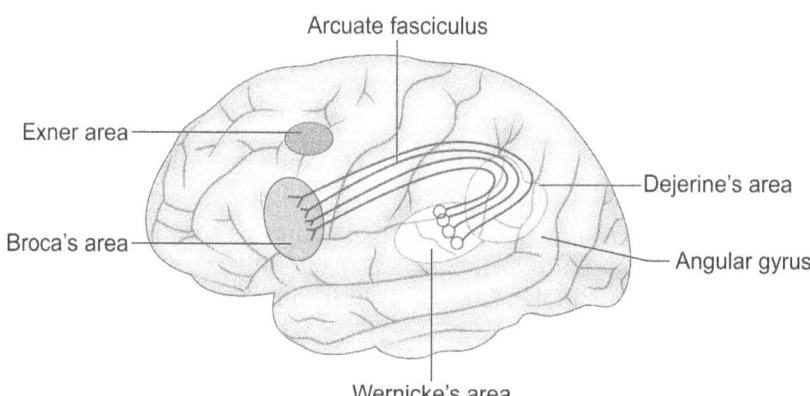

Fig. 38: Speech areas in cerebral cortex.

Example: When a person asks a question orally how do you answer?

The question is received in area 41 (primary auditory area).
↓
Wernicke's area (interprets and understands the question)
↓
Sends information to Broca's area and it fires
↓
Broca's area sends information to area 4 and muscles of speech contract and the answer is given
- The same thing happens when a person starts reading a book.
- The impulse is received in area 17 → area 18 → angular gyrus → Wernicke's area → Broca's area (if he wants to read it aloud).

Mechanism of Written Speech

- Perception of written words is due to the presence of an intact visual cortex.
- Area 17 receives impulses from both retinae through optic nerves. And perceives visual impulses.
- From here impulses reach the visual association area (area 18 and 19)—interpretation happens here.
- Generation of new ideas/thought in response to written words—angular gyrus (area 39—visual speech center).
- Impulses reach Broca's area for coordination and to form a pattern for vocalization or writing.
- Finally reaches Exner's area in middle frontal gyrus.
- Along with motor cortex initiates appropriate movement of hand and fingers to form written speech.

39. Decerebrate rigidity.

- Decerebration is a procedure where the medulla is separated from the brainstem by making a mid-collicular transection (between superior and inferior colliculi). It is done experimentally in animals to study the role of medulla in posture regulation.
- Muscle tone is exaggerated in the decerebrate animal.
- Righting reflexes are lost.
- There are no features of shock immediately after the transection.
- Immediately after transection, there is marked rigidity in the muscles especially in the extensor group of muscles and the back muscles.
- So, limbs and spine are hyperextended.
- The rigidity is due to hyperactive stretch reflex in the extensor groups of muscles.

It happens by two mechanisms:
1. Increased excitability of alpha motor neurons supplying the muscles
2. Increased activity in gamma motor neurons supplying the muscle spindles of extensors.
   - For understanding the cause of increase in activity of the above two groups of neurons we need to understand the higher centers controlling the stretch reflex.
   - There are two major areas in the brain stem controlling the excitability of anterior horn cells in the spinal cord:
     a. A large facilitatory area in the pontine reticular formation which gives rise to the pontine reticulospinal tract.
     b. A small inhibitory area in the medullary reticular formation, giving rise to the medullary reticulospinal tract.
   - The facilitatory area discharges spontaneously whereas the inhibitory medullary area is under the control of higher centers—cerebral cortex, basal ganglia and cerebellum (*refer* **Fig. 39**).
   - The basal ganglia act through cerebral cortex and from the cortex the cortical fibers control the medullary inhibitory area.
   - So, the net effect of stimulation of 3 inhibitory areas and one facilitatory area is overall inhibition of stretch reflex in normal condition.
   - In midcollicular section, two of the inhibitions are removed and the facilitation continues resulting in rigidity and hypertonia.

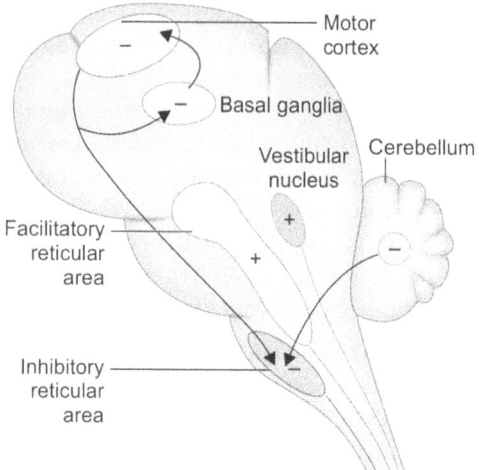

Fig. 39: Higher control of muscle tone; inhibitory areas—cerebral cortex, basal ganglia, cerebellum and inhibitory medullary reticular area. Facilitatory area—pontine facilitatory reticular formation.

40. Functions of prefrontal lobe.

- In animals, it is considered to be the seat of intelligence but in humans, it is the seat of mind.
- It controls the mood and feelings of the subject.
- It is involved in higher functions, such as emotions, learning and memory.
- It controls various intellectual activities, such as planning of future, concentration on actions, solving mathematical problems, etc.
- It helps in appreciation and discrimination of odors.
- It initiates movements in relation to emotions.
- It plans the sequence of movements for an action along with motor cortex for actions.

41. G-protein coupled receptors.

- Many hormones (peptide hormones), neuromodulators and other regulatory molecules act through signal transduction pathways that involve heteromeric GTP binding proteins called G-proteins.
- G-protein exists in two states—active and inactive states.
- In active state, G-protein has higher affinity for GTP and in inactive state it prefers GDP.
- When agonist molecules (hormones) bind to their G-protein-coupled receptors, the receptors interact with G-proteins and convert it to active state and G-protein binds to GTP.
- The activated G-protein in turn interacts with many membrane-bound proteins and enzymes or ion channels to alter their activities.
- The activated G-protein has intrinsic GTPase activity, thereby GTP is hydrolyzed to GDP and the activity is terminated.
- Activated G-proteins acts on enzymes to increase the intracellular concentrations of second messengers cyclic AMP, cyclic GMP, IP3, Ca^{2+} and diacylglycerol.
- G-protein mediated cAMP mechanisms are powerful modulators of adenylyl cyclase and cGMP of phosphodiesterase, the enzymes responsible for the synthesis of cAMP and break down of cGMP respectively.
- Ca^{2+} channel activities may be modulated directly by G-proteins or indirectly by second messengers.
- G-proteins also regulate K^+ channels, phospholipase, etc.

The G-protein-protein kinase-mediated signal transduction pathway includes:
- Peptide hormone binds to membrane receptor
- The ligand bound receptor interacts with G-protein and activates it (*refer* **Fig. 40**)
- Activated G-protein binds to GTP.

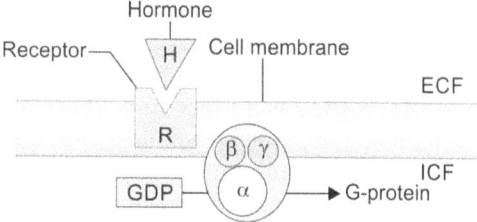

Fig. 40: G-protein coupled receptor; G-protein has 3 subunits—α, β, and γ subunits. In inactive state, G-protein is bound to GDP.

- Activated G-protein interacts with one or more of the following—adenylyl cyclase, cGMP phosphodiesterase, Ca^{2+} or K^+ channels or phospholipases.
- The cellular levels of the following second messengers may increase or decrease—cAMP, cGMP, Ca^{2+}, IP_3 or diacylglycerol.
- The increase or decrease of second messengers changes the activities of one or more second-messenger-dependent protein kinase, cGMP dependent kinase, etc.
- The level of phosphorylation of an enzyme or an ion channel is altered or an ion channel activity changes and brings about the final result.

42. Primary active transport.

Active Transport

- It is also carrier mediated
- Moves substances uphill against concentration gradient.
- So associated with energy expenditure. Energy is derived from ATP, either directly or indirectly
- **Types:**
  - Primary active transport
  - Secondary active transport

Primary Active Transport

Here substances are moved uphill across the cell membrane with the help of energy-driven pumps. It involves energy expenditure which is directly derived from break down of ATP.

Example,
- Na^+-K^+ Pump
- H^+-K^+ Pump
- Ca^{2+} ATPase

Na^+-K^+ Pump
- Sodium potassium ATPase is a ubiquitous pump.
- It pumps out 3 Na^+ molecules from the cell in exchange for 2 K^+ molecules into the cell.
- Na^+ concentration is more in the ECF and K^+ concentration is more in the ICF.
- So both the ions are pumped against their concentration gradients out and in of the cell respectively.
- The pump is present in all the cells to maintain the cell volume and to maintain the membrane potential.
- It is an electrogenic pump as it pumps 3 Na^+ out of the cell and 2 K^+ into the cell.
- It catalyzes hydrolysis of ATP and uses the energy to move the ions.
- Its activity is inhibited by Ouabain and digitalis used for heart failure.
- It has α and β subunits. Na^+ and K^+ are transported through α subunit (*refer* **Fig. 41**).
- α subunit is larger and has intracellular Na^+ and ATP binding sites and a phosphorylation site. When Na^+ binds to α subunit, ATP also binds and is converted to ADP and the P is added to phosphorylation site. This changes the configuration and extrudes Na^+ into ECF. K^+ then binds extracellularly.

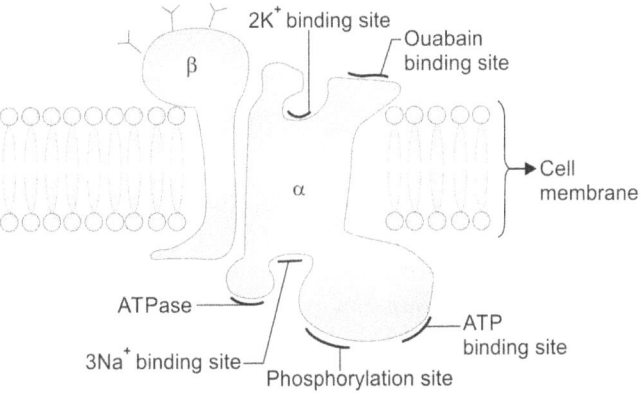

Fig. 41: Sodium-potassium pump; primary active transporter.

- Dephosphorylating α subunit and comes back to original configuration and releases K^+ intracellularly. β subunit is a glycoprotein and has no transport action but its presence is needed for pump activity.
- Extracellularly, there are binding sites for K^+ and Ouabain.
- Pump activity is regulated by 2nd messengers and hormones. Thyroid hormone, aldosterone and insulin increase the pump activity, whereas dopamine decreases the pump activity.

Other Primary Active Transports
- **Ca^{2+} ATPase:** It is present on the cell membranes, endoplasmic reticulum and sarcoplasmic reticulum of muscles. These pumps help in maintaining a lower concentration of Ca^{2+} in the cytoplasm by pumping it either into ECF or into the SR in muscles.
- **H^+-K^+ ATPase:** These pumps are present on the apical membrane of parietal cells in the gastric mucosa and the luminal side of the 'I' cells of the collecting tubule in the nephron. In the stomach the pump is the primary mechanism of secreting H^+ into the lumen. In nephron, the pump helps in secreting H^+ into the tubule and thereby acidification of urine.
- **H^+ ATPase:** It is present in the luminal membrane of parietal cells of gastric mucosa and also in the 'I' cells of collecting tubule of nephrons. It is also present in the membrane of lysosomes and endoplasmic reticulum. The acidic nature of the lysosomes is essential for its degenerative actions.

43. Autoregulation of GFR.

- The autoregulatory mechanism of GFR is similar to autoregulation of renal blood flow.
- Autoregulation of GFR maintains a constant rate of filtration in spite of change in arterial pressure within the range of 80–180 mm Hg.
- There are two autoregulatory mechanisms of GFR—Myogenic mechanism and Tubuloglomerular feedback.

- **Myogenic mechanism:** As the renal blood pressure increases the afferent arteriole is stretched and the stretch induces reflex contraction smooth muscles of the afferent arteriole. This result in vasoconstriction of afferent arteriole and thereby decreases renal blood flow and thereby decreases GFR.
- **Tubuloglomerular feedback:**
  - TG feedback is an autorgulatory mechanism in the kidneys to regulate the renal blood flow (RBF) and thereby the GFR. This feedback mechanism is dependant on the NaCl content in the Tubular fluid. The NaCl content in the tubular fluid is sensed by the macula densa cells and signals are sent to the afferent arterioles to regulate the RBF and GFR.
  - Increased renal arterial pressure increases glomerular capillary pressure and thereby increases filtration. The increased GFR leads to increased NaCl content in the tubular fluid. This is sensed by the macula densa cells and they send signals to cause vasoconstriction of the afferent arterioles and thereby decrease RBF and GFR and NaCl content is brought back to normal.
  - If NaCl content is less, it is sensed by the Macula densa cells and signals are sent to the afferent arterioles resulting in vasodilation followed by increased RBF and GFR.
  - The mediating chemicals may be Thromboxane A2 or Adenosine for vasoconstriction and NO for vasodilation and they are released by the Macula densa cells.

44. Renal glycosuria.

- Renal glucosuria is the excretion of glucose in urine in detectable amounts at normal blood glucose concentrations in the absence of any signs of generalized proximal renal tubular dysfunction due to a reduction in the renal tubular reabsorption of glucose.

- The inherited form of this disorder is called familial renal glycosuria (FRG).
- FRG is a rare disorder due mainly to mutations in the sodium-glucose co-transporter 2 gene (*SGLT2*) that are responsible for the majority of cases.
- Over seventy mutations have been identified including missense mutations, nonsense mutations, small deletions and splicing mutations.
- Glucosuria in these patients can range from <1 to >150 g/1.73 m² per day (normal value: range 0.03 to 0.3 g/d).
- In general, renal glucosuria is a benign condition and does not require any specific therapy. Glucosuria may also be associated with tubular disorders, such as Fanconi-de Toni-Debre syndrome, cystinosis, Wilson disease, hereditary tyrosinemia, or oculocerebrorenal osteodystrophy (Lowe syndrome).
- Renal glucosuria has also been reported in patients with acute pyelonephritis in the presence of a normal blood glucose level. Glucose loss in the urine may vary from a few grams to more than 100 g (556 mmol) per day.

45. Mechanism of bicarbonate generation in distal tubule.

Renal regulation of acid-base balance is by 3 processes:
- Secretion of H^+ by renal tubules
- Reabsorption of HCO_3^-
- Generation of new HCO_3^-

H^+ secretion in the tubules is coupled to reabsorption of HCO_3^-.

Generation of new HCO_3^-
- This happens in the distal convoluted tubule.
- It happens during the formation of titrable acid and NH4.
- New bicarbonate is generated during metabolism of glutamine to glutamate.
- For every glutamine metabolized to glutamate in the tubular cells, 2 molecules of NH_4^+ and two molecules of bicarbonate.

46. Stimuli for secretion of aldosterone and actions of aldosterone.

Actions of Aldosterone

Physiological Actions of Aldosterone
- Promotes Na^+ and water reabsorption and K^+ and H^+ excretion from collecting duct (CD) and DCT.
- It acts mainly on the P cells of CD and DCT, sweat and salivary glands and colon.
- Controls only 3% of total Na^+ reabsorption.
- This is done by:
  - Insertion of ENaCs on apical membrane of P cells of collecting duct
  - Stimulates Na^+-K^+ pumps on basolateral side of P cells
  - Stimulates ATP generation to activate the pump.
  - As Na^+ is reabsorbed, Cl^- follows and water is reabsorbed by osmosis.

It is Classified as Rapid and Slow Effect

Rapid Effect
- Increased insertion of ENaC on the luminal membrane of cells from a cytoplasmic pool.
- It also binds to cell membrane and increases Na^+-K^+ exchanger.
- On the basilar membrane Na^+-K^+ pump activity is also increased.

Slower Effect
- Increases synthesis of ENaCs
- As a result of this, Na^+ reabsorption increases with K^+ and H^+ secretion into urine.
- Along with Na^+, Cl^- and H_2O is also reabsorbed.

Regulation of Secretion

Stimuli that Increase Aldosterone Secretion
- High potassium intake
- Angiotensin II
- ACTH
- Low sodium intake
- Constriction of IVC in thorax
- Standing

- Secondary hyperaldosteronism
- Hemorrhage
- Surgery
- Physical trauma
- Anxiety

Stimuli that Decrease Secretion
- Expansion of ECF volume
- Hypernatremia
- Hypokalemia
- ANP

47. Pancreatic C-peptide and its significance as a laboratory test.

- Insulin is a peptide hormone and is synthesized in the endoplasmic reticulum (ER) and transferred to Golgi apparatus and is packaged to membrane bound vesicles.
- Like other Polypeptide hormones insulin is synthesized as a large Preprohormone.
- Preproinsulin has 23 amino acid signal peptide which is removed as it enters the ER.
- The rest of the molecule is folded to form the Proinsulin.
- The peptide segment connecting the A and B chains is said to be the C-Peptide (*refer* Fig. 42).
- It facilitates the folding and then gets separated and is stored inside the granules before secretion.
- The C-peptide is separated by converting enzymes in the secretory granules.
- C-peptide has no physiological actions.

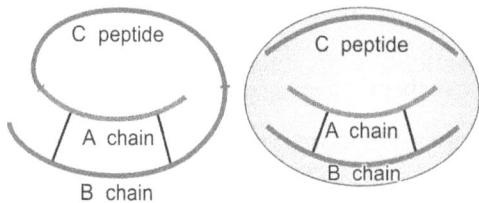

Fig. 42: Structure of insulin with C-peptide. Insulin is a polypeptide hormone with 51 amino acids. It is formed as preproinsulin and proinsulin (86 AA). A and B chains of proinsulin are connected by the C chain. There are disulfide bridges between C peptide chain B chain. On cleavage of C peptide chain, insulin is formed and stored in secretory vesicle along with C-peptide.

Significance of C-peptide
- Normally, 90–97% of the products released from B cells is insulin along with equimolar amounts of C-peptide.
- The rest is mostly proinsulin.
- C-peptide can be measured by radioimmunoassay and its levels give an index of B cell function in patients receiving exogenous insulin.

48. Cretinism—its cause, features and strategy to prevent it.

Hypothyroid children from birth or from in utero are called cretins and the disease is said to be cretinism.

The main causes for cretinism are:
- Maternal iodine deficiency
- Fetal thyroid dysgenesis
- Inborn error of thyroid hormone synthesis
- Maternal antithyroid antibodies that cross the placenta and damage fetal thyroid
- Fetal hypopituitary hypothyroidism.

If the mother's thyroid status is normal, mother's T4 can cross the placenta and thereby the fetal growth and development are normal till birth.

The child with cretinism has the following symptoms:
- Stunted growth
- Mental retardation
- Potbelly
- Enlarged and protruding tongue
- Hoarse cry
- Poor feeding
- Umbilical hernia
- Retarded bone age
- Deaf mutism and rigidity
- Respiratory distress syndrome

Prevention of cretinism:
- Worldwide congenital hypothyroidism is the most common cause of preventable mental retardation.
- So if the thyroid screening is done immediately after birth and thyroid hormone replacement is done early, the prognosis for normal growth and development is good and mental retardation can be prevented.

- If the mother is hypothyroid as in iodine deficiency, mental development is further affected and response to treatment is less after birth.
- This can be prevented by using iodized salts by the mothers.

49. What is the function of corpus luteum of pregnancy? How is it supported?

- Corpus luteum in early pregnancy is "the Source" of progesterone.
- Progesterone is essential for the maintenance of pregnancy and survival of fetus.
- It also secretes the hormone relaxin.
- In pregnancy, relaxin relaxes the pubic symphysis and other pelvic joints and softens the cervix. It also inhibits uterine contractions and aids in development of mammary glands.

Maintenance of Corpus Luteum

- Human chorionic gonadotropin (hCG) secreted by syncytiotrophoblasts in pregnancy is luteinizing and autotrophic in nature.
- hCG is detected in maternal blood as early as 6 days after conception and starts increasing and reaches a peak by 3 months after which it starts decreasing.
- The major role of hCG is to maintain/support corpus luteum and thereby maintains the secretion of progesterone and thereby maintains pregnancy.
- After 3 months, hCG levels decline and corpus luteum seizes to function and after that phase, progesterone synthesis is taken over by placenta.

50. Parturition.

- The duration of normal pregnancy is 40 weeks from 1st day of last menstrual cycle.
- Delivery of the fetus at term is said to be parturition.

Parturition Reflex

- Towards the term of pregnancy, estrogen levels in blood rise and increases the sensitivity of oxytocin receptors in the uterine myometrium to oxytocin.

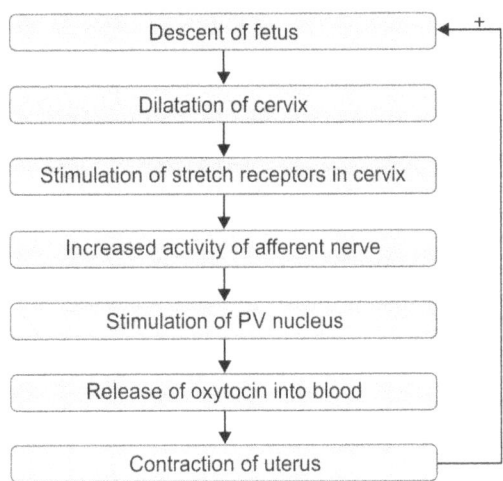

Fig. 43: Parturition reflex.

- As a result of action of oxytocin, the uterus contracts and the fetal head is pushed down stretching the cervix. There are stretch receptors in the cervix.
- As the cervix is stretched, the stretch receptors are stimulated and impulses are transmitted through sensory afferent fibers to supraoptic and paraventricular nuclei of hypothalamus.
- These nuclei synthesize oxytocin and secretes it from posterior pituitary gland.
- Oxytocin binds to the receptors in the uterine myometrium and induces further contractions. This further pushes the fetal head down, further stretching the cervix and more oxytocin is released (*refer* Fig. 43).
- This continues as a positive feedback mechanism till the fetus is born.

51. Ionic basis of the pace-maker potential.

Refer answers to short note 16.

52. Windkessel effect of aorta.

- The distal portion of aorta and large arteries contain large amount of elastin in the tunica media of the vessel wall.
- During systole when the blood is pumped into the vessels, they distend with blood and are stretched because of the large amount of elastin present in the vessel wall.

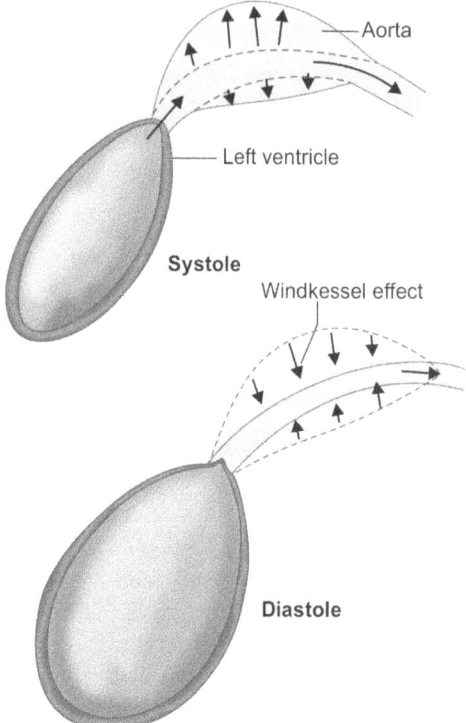

Fig. 44: Windkessel effect in aorta in systolic and diastolic phase of cardiac cycle.

- Following systole, the stretched vessel walls recoil and convert the blood flow into a continuous one.
- This recoiling effect also contributes to the diastolic BP (*refer* **Fig. 44**).
- This is said to be the **Windkessel effect** and the large arteries and aorta are the **Windkessel vessels**.

---

53. Illustrate with a diagram, the left ventricular volume and pressure changes during a cardiac cycle.

- Cardiac cycle is defined as the cycle of mechanical and electrical events taking place from beginning of one beat to the beginning of next beat.
- It is given as the changes in volume, pressure and flow in different cardiac chambers, the electrical activities occurring (through ECG) and coinciding heart sounds (using PCG) in various phases of cardiac cycle.
- Duration of a cardiac cycle is 0.8 s when heart rate is 75/min.

Phases of cardiac cycle and their duration:
- Atrial systole—0.1 s
- Atrial diastole—0.7 s
- Ventricular systole—0.3 s
- Ventricular diastole—0.5 s
  Atrial diastole merges with ventricular systole.
  So the phases described here are atrial systole, ventricular systole and diastole.
- **Ventricular systole:** 2 phases—0.3 sec
  - **Isovolumetric contraction phase—0.05 s**
  - **Phase of ejection 0.25 s**
    - Phase of rapid ejection—0.1 s
    - Phase of reduced ejection—0.15 s
- **Ventricular diastole: 0.5 s**
  - Protodiastole—0.04 s
  - Isovolumetric relaxation phase—0.06 s
  - Rapid ventricular filling—0.11 s
  - Diastasis—0.19 s
- **Atrial systole: 0.1 s**

Atrial Systole

- Duration is 0.1 sec
- This follows the phase of diastasis
- Begins from peak of "P" wave in ECG to peak of "QRS" complex
- Atria contracts and increases intra-atrial pressure. Blood is pumped into ventricles.
- Final filling of ventricle takes place here (Last 25-30%).
- Already the ventricles are in diastole and 75% of filling is complete.
- 4th heart sound is recorded in phonocardiogram.

Ventricular Systole

Isovolumic Contraction Phase
- Starts at peak of 'QRS' complex. Duration is 0.05 sec.
- Rise in ventricular pressure closes the AV valves and semilunar valves have not yet opened.
- 1st heart sound (S1) is heard, due to closure of AV valves.
- Ventricular pressure rises (>80 mm Hg) steeply and ventricular volume remains same.

- There is bulging of AV valves into the atria due to ventricular contraction. This creates 'C' wave in JVP curve.
- Phase ends with opening of semilunar valves and ejection of blood (*refer* **Fig. 45**).

Ventricular Ejection
- **Rapid ejection phase:** (0.1 s)
  - Semilunar valves open and blood is rapidly ejected (2/3rd of stroke volume) into aorta/pulmonary artery.
  - Steep fall in ventricular volume and steep increase in aortic flow
  - Ventricular pressure increases to a peak (120 mm Hg in the left and 25 mm Hg in the right)
  - Aortic pressure also increases.
  - Corresponds to ST segment in ECG
- **Reduced ejection phase:** (0.15 s)
  - Duration is 0.15 sec
  - Ventricular and aortic pressure decreases but aortic pressure is greater.
  - Aortic blood flow decreases. Only 1/3rd of stroke volume is ejected here.
  - Ventricular volume further decreases.
  - Momentum keeps blood flowing into aorta.
  - 'T' wave appears in ECG

Ventricular Diastole—0.5 s
- Protodiastole—0.04 s
- Isovolumetric relaxation—0.06 s
- Phase of rapid ventricular filling—0.11 s
- Phase of reduced filling or diastasis—0.19 s
- Phase of second rapid filling—0.1 s

Protodiastole
- Duration is 0.04 sec
- As the reduced filling phase ends, the ventricles start relaxing.
- Intraventricular pressure drops.
- This phase ends when aortic valve closes.

Isovolumetric Relaxation Phase
- Duration is 0.06 sec
- This phase is between closure of semilunar valves and opening of AV valves.
- Second heart sound (S2) appears due to closure of semilunar valves.
- Closure of semilunar valves creates 'dicrotic notch' in aortic pressure curve

- Ventricular volume remains the same and pressure drops steeply as the ventricles relax (2–3 mm Hg) (*refer* **Fig. 45**)
- When intraventricular pressure drops below atrial pressure, AV valves open.

Rapid Ventricular Filling
- Duration is 0.11 sec
- As the AV valves open there is rapid inrush of blood into ventricles.
- This is because the atria are filled with venous return and pressure is high here.
- This vibration of ventricular wall creates the 3rd (S3) heart sound.
- Major filling takes place here and ventricular volume increases.
- Ventricular pressure is less than atrial pressure

Diastasis
- Duration 0.19 sec.
- This is a slow filling phase.
- Ventricular volume rises slowly.
- Ventricular and atrial pressures reduce and remain same (Little >0 mm Hg).
- Nearly 75% of filling has occurred.

Last Rapid Filling
- Duration 0.1 sec.
- Atria contracts and pumps the last 25% of blood into ventricles.
- At rest, this volume is not essential.
- But in tachycardia (as in exercise) when the duration of diastole decreases this volume assumes importance

54. Role of myelin sheath in conduction of nerve impulse.

- Myelin sheath is present outside axolemma
- In Peripheral nervous system it is formed by Schwann cells.
- In CNS by oligodendrocytes
- Initially axons near the Schwann cells invaginate into its membrane.
- This forms mesaxon. This winds around many times with lipids in between—myelin sheath.
- Outside this a thin layer of Schwann cell cytoplasm—neurilemma is present.
- Along the axon Schwann cells surround for 1 mm.

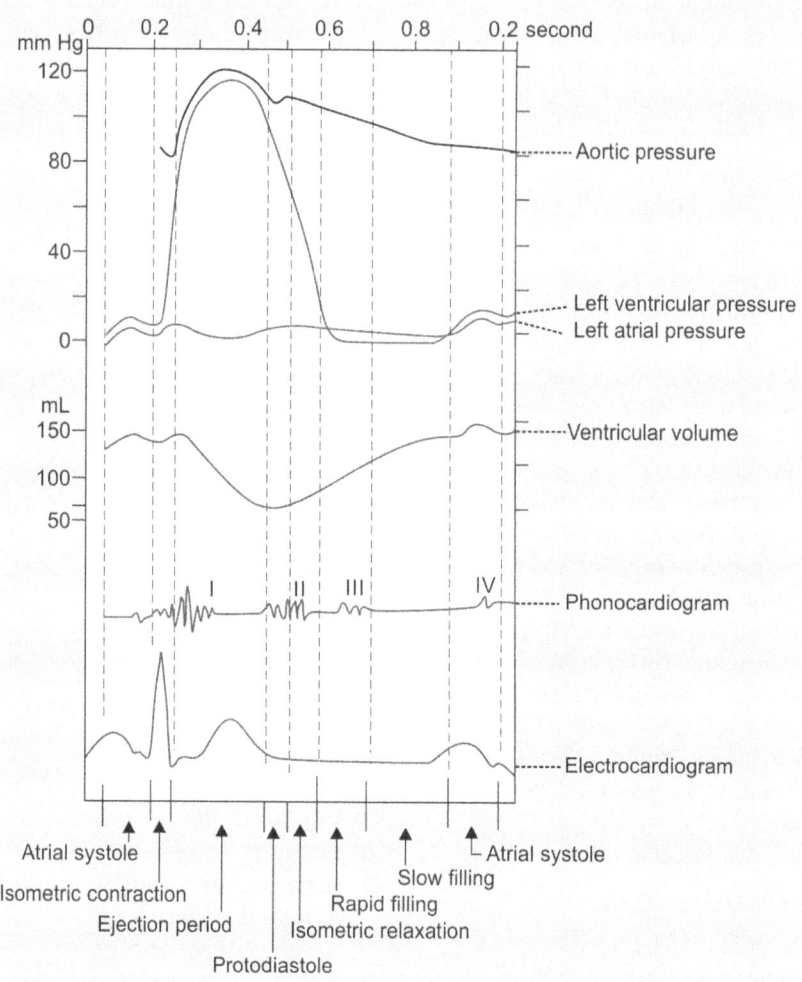

Fig. 45: Cardiac cycle with pressure volume changes in aorta, left ventricle, left atrium, ECG and phonocardiogram.

- In between two wrappings of Schwann cells is the nodes of Ranvier
- The myelin sheath acts as an insulator and prevents transmission of impulse across it
- But in the nodes of Ranvier the voltage-gated sodium channels are concentrated more in number (2000–12000 per square micrometer of the membrane)
- Conduction of action potentials happens in the form of circular currents (current sinks).
- In unmyelinated neurons this currents sinks happen in the neighboring parts of the membrane and therefore the conduction of impulse is slower.
- In the myelinated neurons since the myelin sheath acts as an insulator and the Nodes of Ranvier are concentrated with voltage-gated sodium channels are concentrated the impulses jumps from one node to the other node. This type of conduction is said to be saltatory conduction (refer **Figs. 46A and B**).
- It is a faster conduction and myelinated nerves conduct impulses 50 times faster than the unmyelinated nerve fibers.
- The other factors which affect the conduction of impulses are the thickness or the diameter of the nerve and the temperature.

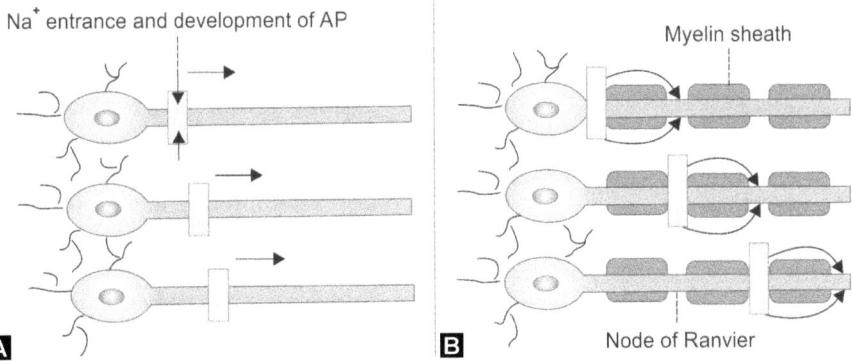

Figs. 46A and B: Impulse transmission in unmyelinated (A) and myelinated axons (B). In myelinated, axons impulses travel from one node to another node—saltatory conduction. In unmyelinated, axons impulses travel in neighboring regions of membrane and are a slow transport.

- As the diameter increases, the resistance to flow of axoplasmic current is less and therefore impulse transmission is faster in large diameter nerves.
- Temperature is directly proportional to conduction velocity.

55. Functions of hypothalamus.

Refer answer to essay 4.

56. Clinical features of cerebellar lesions.

- Patients with cerebellar lesion do not show much abnormalities when they are at rest.
- The symptoms are well established when they move.
- There is **no paralysis or sensory defects**.
- The effect of lesion is manifested on the same side of lesion.
- But there is marked incoordination of movements—ataxia.
- This is due to errors in rate, range, force and direction of movement.
- There is hypotonia.

Ataxia is expressed as:
- Instability during walking which is expressed as **drunken gait or wide-based gait**.
- There are also defects in skilled movements, such as **scanning of speech**.
- **Past pointing or dysmetria:** Attempting to touch an object with one finger results in overshooting to one side or the other. This is followed by correction of the overshoot which results in overshooting to the other side.
- Therefore, the finger oscillates back and forth resulting in **intention tremors**.
- It is called so as it is seen when the person attempts to do an action.
- The person with cerebellar lesion is unable to brake a movement or stop a movement. For example, in a normal person flexion of the forearm against resistance is kept in check when the resistance is suddenly released. But in a person with cerebellar lesion the patient is unable to brake the movement and the forearm flies backward in an arc—**rebound phenomenon**.
- They also show the feature of **adiadochokinesia**—inability to do rapid alternating opposite movements, such as repeated supination and pronation of the hands.
- They show **decomposition of movement**—The movements are dissected into individual components and carried out in each joint at a time.
- Defects in flocculonodular lobe (Vestibulocerebellum) results in **vertigo, nystagmus and motion sickness**.

57. Physiological roles of muscle spindle.

- Muscle spindle is also called as the intrafusal fibers.
- They are placed parallel to the extrafusal fibers.
- They are the receptors for stretch reflex.

- They are of two types—nuclear bag (NB) and nuclear chain (NC) fibers (*refer* Fig. 47).

They are supplied by:
Afferents:
- Type **Ia fibers—Aα (also known as annulospiral fibers)**
- **Type II fibers - Aβ nerves**.
- Type Ia fibers are stimulated on stretch of extrafusal and intrafusal fibers.
- Ia fibers supply both NB and NC fibers. Type II supplies only NC fibers.

Efferents:
- γ **Motor neurons**
- β **Efferents**
- Stimulation of γ efferents, increases sensitivity of Ia fibers to stretch. (They get stimulated when the muscle contracts)
- β efferents supply both intra and extrafusal fibers. Their role is not known.

Stretch Reflex
- When a muscle is stretched, the intrafusal fibers in parallel, also stretch → stimulates Ia fibers—afferent impulse reaches a motor neuron supplying the same muscle → contraction of muscle—**monosynaptic stretch reflex.**
- When the a motor neurons discharge (to contract a muscle) the spindles shorten and stop firing. Information to CNS comes to a halt. But for posture maintenance, this should not happen.
- Therefore when a motor neurons fire they also send impulse to γ motor neurons → Impulses are sent to the ends of NB fibers → they contract (as there are contractile proteins only in the ends of NB fibers)—there is maintained stretch in the center of NB fibers (sensitivity increased). Therefore, spindles respond not only in stretch of a muscle but also during contraction of a muscle—α-γ linkage.
- Muscle spindles respond in both conditions (stretching and contraction of the extrafusal fibers). It is essential to maintain posture in a steady state.
- **Two types of response:** Dynamic and static.
  1. **Dynamic response:** The nerves from nuclear bag region discharge most rapidly while being stretched and less rapidly during sustained stretch.
  2. **Static response:** The nerves from the nuclear chain fibers discharge at an increased rate during sustained stretch.

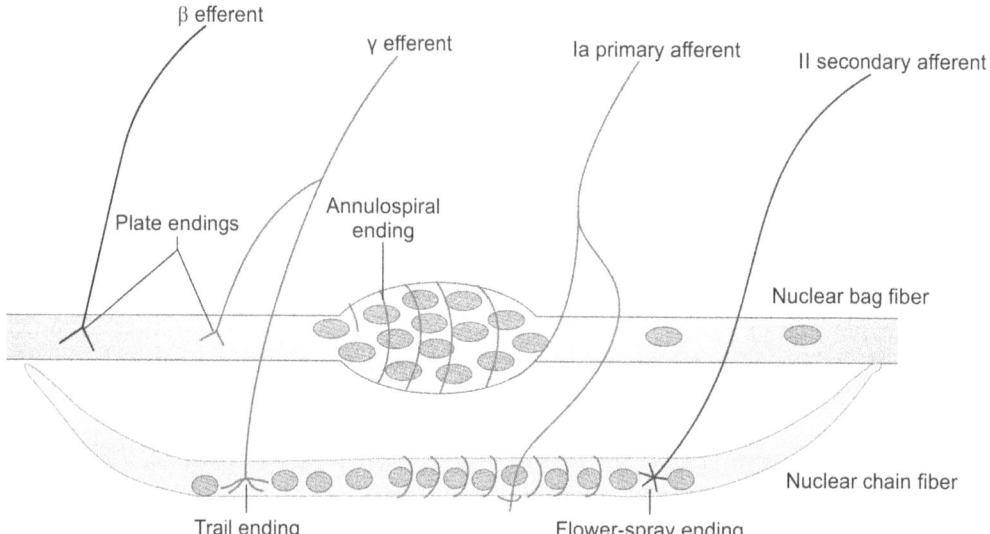

Fig. 47: Muscle spindle with its nerve supply. Nuclear bag and nuclear chain fibers are present in the muscle spindle. Afferents to muscle spindles are Ia primary afferents and II secondary afferents. γ-efferents supply the contractile ends of the fibers.

- Thus, the primary endings respond to both changes in length and changes in the rate of stretch.

Functions of Muscle Spindle
- It is the receptor for stretch reflex and therefore it is responsible for stretch reflex.
- It helps in regulation of muscle length.
- Stretch reflex in antigravity muscles regulates muscle tone and therefore posture and therefore muscle spindles are responsible for regulation of tone and posture.
- Monitors velocity of muscle contraction
- Concerned with conscious perception of joint position and movement

This is in turn essential for:
- Maintenance of posture
- Facilitates locomotion
- Smoothens voluntary activity

58. Chemical regulation of respiration.

- Chemical regulation of respiration is also through the modulation of activities of neural centers through chemoreceptors.
- There are 2 sets of chemoreceptors responding to changes in arterial PO_2, PCO_2 and pH
- They are peripheral and central chemoreceptors.

Peripheral Chemoreceptors
- Carotid and aortic bodies (refer **Fig. 48**).
- They have high blood flow (2000 mL/100 g/min) and high metabolic rate.
- Their metabolic needs are met by dissolved O_2
- So they are highly sensitive to ↓ PO_2, ↑PCO_2 and ↓pH.
- These receptors are not stimulated in anemia or carbon monoxide poisoning.
- They are stimulated in ↓PO_2, vascular stasis, Cyanide poisoning
- They have 2 types of cells—glomus and sustentacular cells (refer **Fig. 49**).

Sensitivity of Peripheral Chemoreceptors (PCR)
- Glomus cells are the sensors.
- Hypoxia is the major stimulus. Neurotransmitter is dopamine

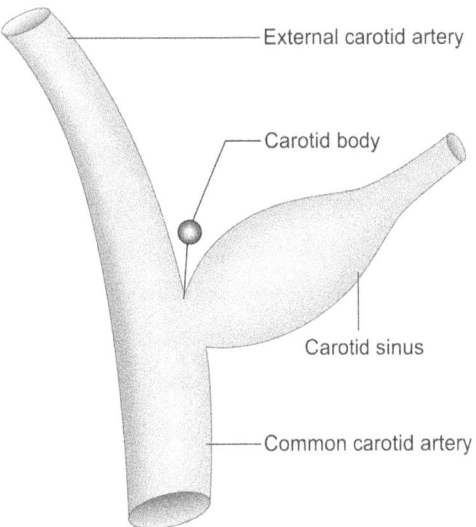

Fig. 48: Location peripheral chemoreceptors at bifurcation of common carotid artery; the carotid body. Carotid sinus is the dilatation in internal carotid artery; the baroreceptor.

- PCRs also responds to ↑PCO_2 and ↓pH
- When PO_2 <100 mm Hg, there is firing rate of the nerves supplying them (9th and 10th cranial nerves)
- Response is maximum when PO_2 falls <60 mm Hg
- Effect of hypoxia is less when PO_2 <60 mm Hg because:
  - Hypoxia → Hyperventilation → CO_2 blow out →↓$PaCO_2$ →↓ventilation
  - Deoxy-Hb has more affinity for H^+ →↓arterial $[H^+]$ →↓ventilation (refer **Fig. 50**).

Mechanism of Hypoxia Stimulating PCR

Hypoxia inhibits K^+ channels by:
- O_2 sensor in the glomus cell is a heme containing protein and is associated with O_2. In hypoxia, the lack of O_2 inhibits the K^+ channels.
- In hypoxia, there is increase in cAMP in glomus cells which inhibits cAMP sensitive K^+ channels.

Effect of CO_2 On PCR

Integrated effects of arterial—PCO_2, PO_2 and pH on ventilation, by stimulating PCR
- At low P_{ACO2} level with hypoxia, ventilation is not stimulated till PO_2 <60 mm Hg.

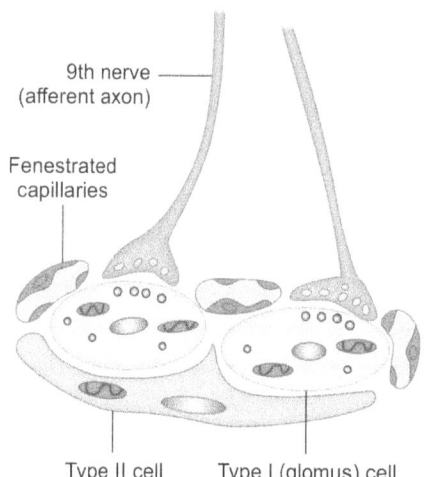

Fig. 49: Cells in carotid body—Type I (glomus cells) and Type II (supporting cells). Glomus cells are supplied by 9th cranial nerve and are close to fenestrated capillaries

- High P_{ACO2} levels (as in ↑metabolic rate/ breathing CO_2 mixtures) →↑ventilation. But if CO_2 content in breathed air is >7% → CNS depression → CO_2 narcosis

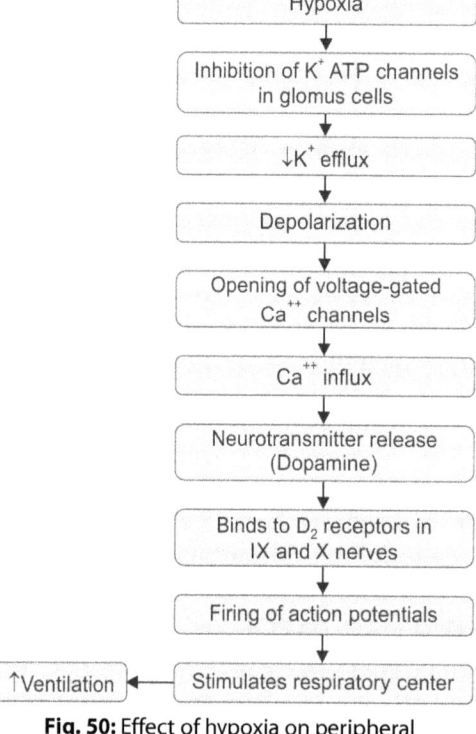

Fig. 50: Effect of hypoxia on peripheral chemoreceptors.

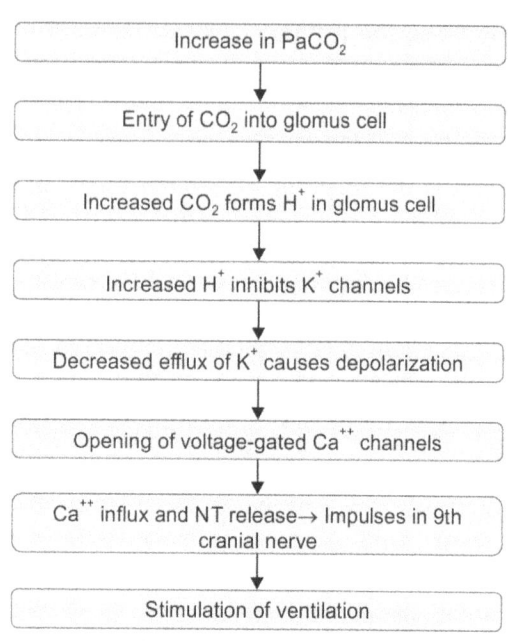

Fig. 51: Effect of hypercapnia on peripheral chemoreceptors.

- Hypercapnia with hypoxia, shifts the CO_2 curve to left and slope is increased.
- Acidosis by itself (as in diabetic ketoacidosis) can stimulate ventilation by stimulating PCR. (Even in absence of hypoxia or hypercapnia) (*refer* **Fig. 51**)

Central Chemoreceptors (CCR)

- Located in the medulla and is different from the other respiratory neurons.
- There are also other such CCR in and around the brain stem nuclei—nucleus tractus solitarius, nucleus ambiguous (*refer* **Fig. 52**).
- They respond maximally to changes in [H⁺] in brain CSF and ISF which is in turn decided by P_{ACO2} and HCO_3^- of CSF.

↑Arterial PCO_2
↓
↑Brain ECF CO_2 level
$CO_2 + H_2O \rightarrow H_2CO_3 \rightarrow H^+ + HCO_3^-$
Increase in brain ECF H⁺ level
↓
Stimulation of CCR
↓

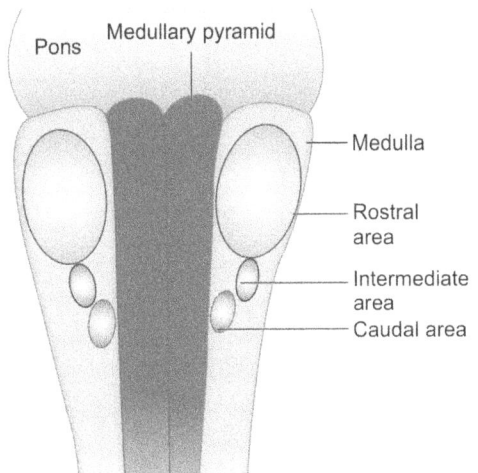

Fig. 52: Location of central chemoreceptors in ventral medulla. There are rostral, intermediate and caudal centers.

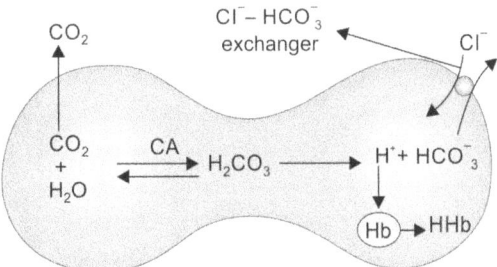

Fig. 53: Chloride shift in RBC.

Stimulation of medullary inspiratory center
↓
Firing of neurons supplying diaphragm and external intercostal muscles
↓
Increase in ventilation

59. Hamburger's chloride shift.

- The major part of CO_2 (70%) is transported as HCO_3^- in plasma. CO_2 diffuses from the tissues and enters the interstitial tissue and from there it enters the RBC due to the pressure gradient in these areas.
- Inside the RBC the enzyme carbonic anhydrase (CA) is present.
- CO_2 enters RBC and combines with H_2O in presence of CA to form H_2CO_3
- H_2CO_3 dissociates immediately and splits into H^+ and HCO_3^-.
- HCO_3^- levels increase within the RBC and the excess of HCO_3^- leaves the cell in exchange for an anion, Cl^- through the anion exchanger, Band 3 protein.
- This exchange is called **chloride shift or Hamburger shift.**
- For each molecule of CO_2 added to a red cell there is an increase of one osmotically active particle in the cell—either Cl^- or HCO_3^- (*refer* **Fig. 53**).
- Therefore, the RBC takes up water and swells up and increases in size.
- This increases the hematocrit of venous blood by 3% than the arterial blood.

60. Role of surfactant in pulmonary function.

- It is a protein-lipid complex secreted by the Type II alveolar epithelial cells lining the alveoli (*refer* **Fig. 54**).
- Surfactant is a mixture of Dipalmitoyl-phosphatidylcholine (DPPC), other lipids and proteins—SP-A, SP-B, SP-C and SP-D.
- It acts as a detergent to reduce the surface tension of the fluid lining the alveoli and prevent its collapse during expiration.
- The phospholipids have hydrophobic tails and a hydrophilic head. They arrange themselves with the tails facing the alveolar lumen and intersperse between water molecules.
- So during inspiration as the alveoli enlarge the surfactant molecules move apart and surface tension of water increases and during expiration they come closer and the surface tension is lowered.
- Surfactant is important at birth. After birth, the infant tries to breathe and makes inspiratory movements and the lungs expand after which the lung tends to recoil and the presence of surfactant prevents the collapse of the alveoli.
- Surfactant deficiency results in alveolar collapse, which results in infant respiratory distress syndrome (IRDS)
- Maturation of surfactant in the lungs is enhanced by glucocorticoids. During term the fetal and maternal cortisol increases and favors maturation of surfactant.

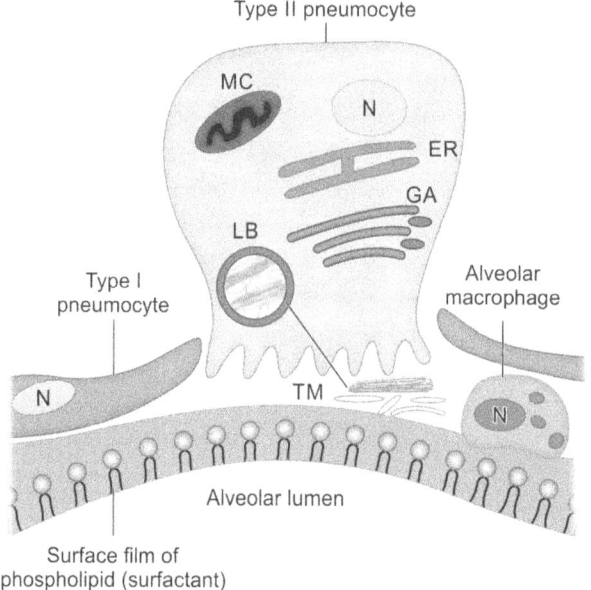

Fig. 54: Arrangement of surfactant molecules in alveolar lumen.

Other Functions of Surfactant

- Stabilizes the lung alveoli
- It also decreases the effect of surface tension, which if not countered will increase the pulmonary capillary hydrostatic pressure and thereby fluid accumulation in the alveolus. So surfactant prevents pulmonary edema.
- As it prevents alveolar collapse, it decreases the work of breathing
- They help in immunity

III. SHORT ANSWERS

1. Chronaxie.

- Chronaxie is the time required for stimulus of double the strength of rheobase current to excite a tissue. It is an indicator of excitability of tissues.
- Rheobase is the minimum strength of current given for a particular duration which is able to excite a tissue.
- Chronaxie and excitability are inversely related.
- Nerve has a shorter chronaxie and smooth muscles have a longer chronaxie.

2. Motor unit.

- Motor unit is a single motor neuron with all its branches and all the muscle fibers supplied by it.
- The size of the motor unit is decided by the muscle fibers supplied by it (refer Fig. 55).

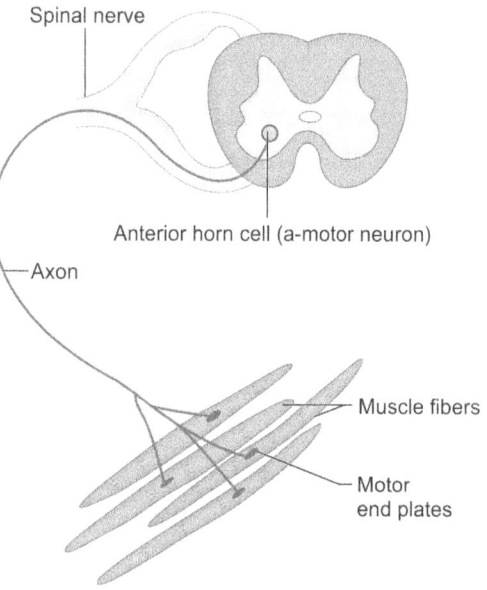

Fig. 55: Motor unit.

- The ones which supply the intrinsic muscles of the hand supply only less than 10 fibers and produce less tension but the ones which supply back muscles are large motor units and have hundreds of fibers.
- All the muscle fibers in a single motor unit are of the same type, i.e., either oxidative type or glycolytic type.
- Based on this, the motor units may be classified as either oxidative or slow and glycolytic or fast motor units.

3. Apoptosis.

- Apoptosis is "Programmed cell death".
- It is also said to be "Cell suicide' as the cell's own genes program the cell death.
- It is a common happening in the growth and development and also in adulthood.

Examples are:

- In the nervous system development, many neurons are removed by apoptosis while remodeling and formation of synapse.
- In immune system development, apoptosis removes the inappropriate clones of immunocytes and is responsible for the destruction of lymphocytes by glucocorticoids.
- It is responsible for removal of webs between fingers in developmental period of fetal life.
- It is responsible for regression of duct system in development of sexual organs.
- In adults cyclical breakdown of endometrium and menstruation is also an example of apoptosis:
  - Apoptosis is triggered by Fas ligand in the membrane of natural killer cells and T lymphocytes and tumor necrosis factor.
  - Fas ligand binds with its receptors triggering apoptosis and it activates an important pathway through the mitochondria which releases cytochrome C and it in turn activates caspases, a cysteine protease.
  - It results in DNA fragmentation, cytoplasmic and chromatin condensation and membrane bleb formation and cell break up and removal of debris by phagocytosis.

4. Osmotic diuresis.

- The presence of large quantities of unreabsorbed solutes in the tubular fluid results in increased volume of urine—**osmotic diuresis**.
- This usually happens when solutes are not reabsorbed in the PCT. So the solutes exert an osmotic effect as the volume of tubular fluid decreases and concentration of solute increases.
- They start holding back water in the tubules.
- This decreases the gradient across which Na^+ has to be reabsorbed. Na^+ reabsorption requires a particular gradient and when water stays back in tubule with unreabsorbed solutes this gradient reaches a limiting level—the limiting gradient.
- So now, sodium also stays in the tubule and water also stays along with it.
- Now this isotonic fluid reaches the loop of Henle. Here the decreased concentration of solutes in medullary interstitium prevents further reabsorption of Na^+ and water.
- There is decreased medullary osmolarity because the reabsorption of Na^+, K^+ and Cl^- is decreased in ascending limb as the limiting gradient is reached.
- Fluid passes through DCT and collecting duct and because of medullary gradient for water reabsorption, water stays back in tubule.
- This results in marked increase in urine volume and excretion of Na^+ and other electrolytes.
- Solutes which can cause such osmotic diuresis are mannitol and similar polysaccharides.
- In diabetes mellitus, when there is high plasma glucose levels, it leads to appearance of glucose in tubular fluid and all the above effects and osmotic diuresis is produced.
- In osmotic diuresis, in contrast to water diuresis, solutes and water are not

reabsorbed in PCT and urinary volumes are very high and urine is isotonic in nature.

5. LH surge.

- Just before ovulation, there is an LH surge and it triggers the ovulation.
- The surge happens 9 hours before the ovulation.
- High LH level is necessary for the final maturation and rupture of Graafian follicle.
- The estrogen levels are also rising in the preovulatory phase.
- It is a unique pattern here, the high estrogen levels positively stimulates further secretion of LH and LH stimulates estrogen secretion and it reaches a peak level (6-10 times baseline value) 9 hours before ovulation.
- The FSH levels also increase (2-3 times).
- LH acts on the granulosa and theca cells and make them secrete progesterone.
- Now progesterone levels rise just before ovulation and estrogen levels decrease.
- All the above hormonal changes results in ovulation.
- So without the LH surge ovulation does not happen.

6. Somatomedins.

- Somatomedins are polypeptide growth factors secreted by the liver and other tissues.
- They resemble insulin, except for the C-peptide, they are called as insulin, such as growth factors (IGF).
- There are two types; somatomedin C (IGF-I) and Insulin, such as growth factor II (IGF-II).

IGF-I

- The secretion of IGF-I is independent of GH in fetal period and is dependent on GH after birth.
- It is low during childhood, reaches a peak in puberty and declines thereafter.
- Receptors of IGF-I are similar to insulin receptor.
- They induce skeletal and cartilage growth and protein metabolism.
- They stimulate collagen formation.

IGF-II

- Its secretion is independent of GH levels and is always constant.
- Receptors of IGF-II are mannose 6-phosphate receptors
- IGF-II plays a major role in fetal growth.

7. Hormones of adrenal cortex.

- The adrenal cortex is in 3 layers and each layer secretes different hormones (*refer* **Fig. 56**).
- **The outermost layer is the zona glomerulosa:** It secretes the mineralocorticoid—aldosterone and 11-deoxycorticosterone.
- **The middle layer is the zona fasciculata:** It secretes glucocorticoids—corticosterone and cortisol.
- **The innermost layer the zona reticularis secretes adrenal androgens:** Dehydroepiandrosterone (DHEA) and androstenedione.
- The middle and inner layer secrete both glucocorticoids and androgens but more of glucocorticoids from zona fasciculata and more of androgens from zona reticularis.

8. Types of diabetes.

- The term "Diabetes" in Greek and Roman denotes the passing of large volumes of urine.
- There are two types—diabetes mellitus and diabetes insipidus.
- In diabetes mellitus, urine tastes sweet and in diabetes insipidus it has no taste.
  a. **Diabetes mellitus** is due to deficiency of the hormone insulin and **Diabetes insipidus** is due to deficiency of antidiuretic hormone.
     - **Diabetes mellitus** is of two types—type 1 diabetes mellitus or insulin dependent diabetes and type 2 diabetes mellitus or non-insulin dependent diabetes mellitus.
       1. **Type 1 DM:** There is autoimmune destruction of beta cells in

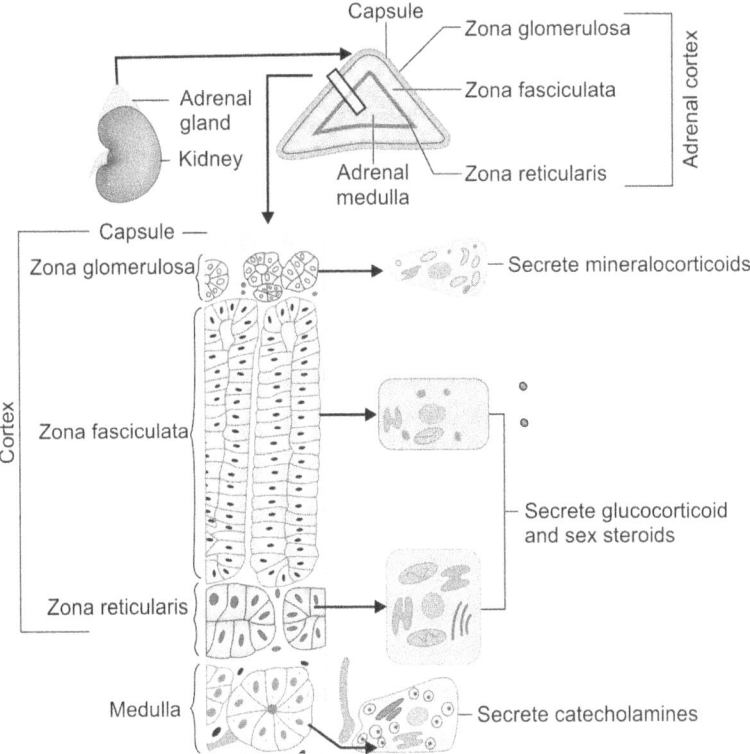

Fig. 56: Layers of adrenal cortex and the hormones they secrete. Zona glomerulosa secretes aldosterone, zona fasciculata secretes glucocorticoids and some amount of androgens, zona reticularis secretes androgens and some amount of glucocorticoids.

islets of Langerhans and the insulin secretion is less or even completely absent. The patient is treated with insulin injections.

2. **Type 2 DM:** Here the insulin secretion is normal but the insulin receptors are insensitive to insulin. It occurs after the age of 40 years and is treated with anti-hyperglycemic agents.

   The symptoms are polyuria, polydipsia, polyphagia, hyperglycemia, weight loss, glycosuria, ketosis, acidosis and coma.

b. **Diabetes insipidus** is of two types—neurogenic or central diabetes insipidus and nephrogenic diabetes insipidus.

   1. **Neurogenic DI:** There is defect in synthesis of ADH from hypothalamus.

   2. **Nephrogenic DI:** Here the synthesis and secretion of ADH is normal but there could be congenital defects of receptors to ADH or mutations of genes for aquaporins and defects in aquaporins, the water channels on the luminal side of principal cells of collecting duct.

❏ Symptoms of DI are polyuria, polydipsia. They pass a large volume (up to 23 L/day) of hypotonic urine (30 mosm/kg H_2O).

9. Action of parathormone on bone.

❏ It increases activity of both osteoclasts and osteoblasts.

❏ But the osteoclastic activity is the major effect resulting in resorption of bone and release of calcium and phosphates into the ECF.

❏ PTH stimulates the differentiation of precursors into osteoclasts, increases

their numbers and size. The products of resorption are present in blood and are excreted in urine.
- PTH increases calcium resorption from the bones in 2 phases—rapid phase and slow phase.
- **Action on osteoclasts:** This effect comes into action after a few days of exposure to PTH. The number and activity of osteoclasts are increased. Osteoclasts increase bone resorption and thereby increases calcium and phosphate levels in the blood. Also, levels of hydroxyproline and hydroxylysine are increased.
- **Action on osteoblasts:** At low doses PTH increases osteoblastic activity but in high doses it inhibits action of osteoblasts.

10. Menarche.

- Menarche is the first menstrual period at the time of puberty.
- It is the last stage of puberty.
- It occurs by 11-14 years of age.
- The initial periods are anovulatory and regular ovulation happens after 1 year.

11. Muscles of inspiration.

- **Primary muscles** of inspiration are diaphragm and external intercostals.
- **Accessory muscles** are—scalene, sternocleidomastoid, neck and back muscles and muscles of upper respiratory tract.

12. P50.

- It is the partial pressure of oxygen in the arterial blood at which 50% of the hemoglobin is saturated with oxygen.
- Normal value is 27 mm Hg.
- P_{50} is inversely related to hemoglobin affinity for oxygen.

13. End diastolic volume.

- It is the volume of blood in the ventricle at the end of diastole.
- Normal value is 130 mL.
- It is decided by the venous return.
- It is the preload for the ventricular muscle.

14. Attenuation reflex.

It is a protective reflex. When a loud sound is transmitted through the ossicles in middle ear a reflex is initiated with a latent period of 40-80 msec. Contraction of stapedius and tensor tympani pulls the tympanic membrane medially and membrane covering oval window laterally. This makes the ossicular system rigid and there is reduction in transmission of sounds. This reduces the intensity of sound by 30-40 decibels. It is also called as **tympanic reflex**.

15. Perimetry.

- It is an instrumental method to map the peripheral field of vision.
- Each eye is mapped separately.
- The instrument used is perimeter.
- Lister's perimeter is used.
- The chart for recording the field of vision has circles—**isopters**, drawn at 10° intervals and radial line—**meridians**, drawn at 10° intervals.
- The field of vision of each eye is mapped in the isopters and meridians.
- One eye is checked at a time.
- One eye is covered and the other eye is fixed on a central point.
- A small target is moved towards the central point along selected meridians and along each meridian the site where the object is first visible is plotted in degrees of arc away from the central point.
- These points are joined to form the eye's visual field.
- Field of vision of each eye is not circular as it is cut off medially by the nose and superiorly by the roof of orbit

16. Summation.

- Summation means adding up of impulses.
- In the synapse, following release of neurotransmitters there could be depolarization or hyperpolarization of the membrane.
- These are called as postsynaptic potentials and they belong to the category of graded potentials.

- So these individual potentials from many synapses can summate and excite the membrane and take it to the firing level.
- There are two types of summations—spatial and temporal summation.
- **Temporal summation:** The same input stimulates the postsynaptic neuron repeatedly and thereby excites it.
- **Spatial summation:** Here many inputs stimulate simultaneously to excite it.

17. Referred pain.

Irritation of a vicus or viscera usually produces pain which is not usually felt in the location of the viscus but in a somatic structure that is in a distance from the viscus. This is **referred pain**.

For example:
- Cardiac pain is usually referred to the inner aspect of the left arm or to the neck.
- When there is an irritation of central region of diaphragm, there is pain in the tip of the shoulder.
- Pain in the testicle due to distension of ureter as in ureteric calculus.

Theories of Referred Pain

The pain in viscera is usually referred to a somatic structure that has developed from the same embryonic segment or dermatome as the structure in which the pain originates—**dermatomal rule**.

Theories of referred pain are—convergence theory and facilitation theory.

Convergence Theory
- Peripheral nerve fibers from the somatic and visceral structures converge on the same second order neuron present in lamina V of dorsal gray horn.
- The second order neuron is common for impulses from somatic and visceral structures.
- So the tract carrying pain sensation from somatic structures also carry pain fibers from visceral structures (*refer* **Fig. 57**).
- Cortex sometimes cannot differentiate from somatic and visceral inputs and so pain from visceral structure is referred to the somatic structure.

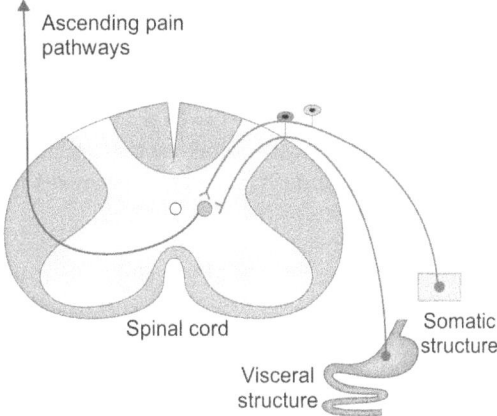

Fig. 57: Convergence theory of referred pain. Note the afferents from somatic and visceral structures converge on the same second order neuron.

Facilitation Theory
- The visceral afferent fibers on entering spinal cord give collaterals to afferents coming from the somatic structures.
- So impulses coming from the visceral afferents facilitate and strengthen the impulses coming from the somatic structure (*refer* **Fig. 58**)
- So a minor activity in the somatic afferents is facilitated by the visceral afferents and therefore pain is referred to the somatic structure.

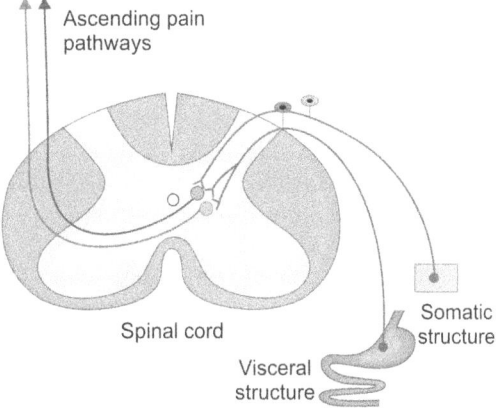

Fig. 58: Facilitation theory of referred pain. Note the visceral afferents give a collateral to second order neurons of somatic structure.

18. Types of memory.

- **Memory** is the process by which acquired information is stored and and can be retrieved.
- **Memory is classified based on how long it is stored and retrieved—short-term or long-term memory.**
  - *Short-term memory:* Ability to recall ongoing experiences for a few seconds.
  - *Long-term memory:* If the information is repeatedly used, it results in reinforcement of the synaptic pathway and results in long term memory.
- **Another classification is based on how the learned details are retrieved—either with conscious awareness or without conscious awareness:**
  - *Explicit or declarative memory:* Memory for events, facts and names. Here conscious awareness of the subject is needed.
  - *Implicit memory or procedural memory:* Ability to learn and remember motor skills. There is no need of conscious awareness.

19. Thalamic syndrome.

- Thrombosis of the artery supplying thalamus leads to dysfunction of thalamus.
- **Signs and symptoms:**
  - Alteration of various sense perception
  - Emotional disturbances
  - Ataxia, weakness and tremor
- **Loss of sensations:**
  - Most of the sensations relay in thalamus and therefore in thalamic syndrome there is loss of sensations in contralateral side of body.
  - Loss of tactile localization, tactile discrimination and stereognosis.
  - Loss of kinesthetic sensations → Thalamic phantom limb, ameliognosia, sensory ataxia.
  - Hyper-reactivity to pain
- **Damage to motor system:**
  - Hypotonia
  - Choreoathetosis
  - Thalamic hand—moderate flexion of the wrist with hyperextension of fingers.
- **Disturbances in sleep-wakefulness cycle.**

20. Kluver-Bucy syndrome.

Lesions of the temporal lobe, especially the amygdala leads to temporal lobe syndrome or Kluver-Bucy syndrome.

Features of Kluver-Bucy syndrome are:
- Inability to identify objects visually, in spite of normal vision—visual agnosia
- Loss of hearing since the auditory area is in the temporal lobe
- Tends to examine any object orally (oral tendencies)
- Hyperphagia
- Hypersexuality
- Tends to show attention to all peripheral stimuli—hypermetamorphosis
- Change in eating habits, monkeys start eating meat
- Absence of fear, monkeys tend to handle the snakes
- Loss of recent memory

21. Functions of sodium potassium ATPase pump.

- It is present in all cells of the body.
- It is an electrogenic pump as it pumps 3 Na^+ out of the cell and 2 K^+ into the cell. It catalyzes hydrolysis of ATP and uses the energy to move the ions.
- It regulates intracellular Na^+ concentration and thereby the cell volume is maintained.
- It is essential for maintenance of resting membrane potential.
- It is needed for regaining the membrane potential following generation of action potential.
- Its activity is inhibited by Ouabain and digitalis used for heart failure.

22. Mention the normal value of GFR and substance used to measure GFR.

- GFR is defined as the rate at which the filtrate is formed in all the nephrons of both the kidneys per unit of time.
- **The normal values are:** 125 mL/min, 90–140 mL/min or 180L/day.

Measurement of GFR

It is done by measuring renal clearance of inulin, creatinine and urea.

23. Enumerate heat loss mechanism.

- **Cutaneous vasodilatation:** Warm blood flows to the periphery and heat is lost to the environment
- **Heat is lost from the body to the environment by:**
  - *Conduction:* Heat is exchanged between objects (of different temperatures) in contact with each other
  - *Radiation:* It is transfer of heat by infrared electromagnetic radiations from one object to another object which are not in contact with each other.
- **Vaporization of sweat**
- **Increased respiration (panting in animals)**
- **Urination and defecation.**

24. Peristalsis.

- It is a type of propulsive movement which helps to move the chyme forward. It is a reflex initiated by the stretch of the intestinal wall following the entry of food.
- Stretch of the intestinal wall initiates a ring of constriction behind the bolus and a relaxation in front of the bolus.
- The ring of contraction behind pushes the bolus to the relaxed segment in front of the bolus.
- Next ring of contraction now appears in the previous relaxed segment and the bolus is pushed further.
- These waves always propel the contents from the oral to caudal direction and never in the opposite direction—law of the gut.
- These waves appear even in the absence of nerve supply but they can be modified by the autonomic nerves, parasympathetic nerves increase the activity and sympathetic nerves decrease the activity.
- The propelling speed varies from 2–25 cm/S.
- Sometimes the peristaltic waves can be very fast and they empty the contents faster—peristaltic rushes, seen in acute diarrhea.
- Antiperistalsis happens in vomiting.

25. What is the role of vitamin K in the body?

- Vitamin K is a cofactor for the enzyme which catalyzes the conversion of glutamic acid residues to— γ carboxyglutamic acid residues in the liver.
- Six clotting factors, synthesized in the liver, require the conversion of glutamic acid to γ carboxyglutamic acid. They are factors— II, VII, IX and X, and protein C and S.
- **Vitamin K antagonists:** Coumarin derivatives, such as warfarin, dicoumarol, etc.
- They prevent the action of vitamin K by competitively binding with vitamin K receptors.

26. What is the normal blood calcium level?

- The normal plasma calcium level is 10 mg/dL (5 meq/L, 2.5 mmol/L).
- It is partly protein-bound and partly diffusible.

Diffusible calcium—6 mg/dL (1.5 mmol/L)
- Ionized calcium (50% of total plasma calcium)—5 mg/dL (1.25 mmol/L)
- Complexed to HCO_3^-, citrate, etc.—1 mg/dL (0.25 mmol/L)

Non-diffusible calcium—4 mg/dL

27. Name the hormones of adrenal cortex.

The hormones of adrenal cortex are:
- Mineralocorticoids—C_{21} steroids
  - Aldosterone
  - Deoxycorticosterone
- Glucocorticoids—C_{21} steroids
  - Cortisol
  - Cortisone
  - Corticosterone
- Adrenal androgens—C_{19} steroids
  - Dehydroepiandrosterone
  - Androstenedione

28. Name the hormones of placenta.

- Human chorionic gonadotropin (hCG)
- Human chorionic somatomammotropin (hCS)

- Estrogen
- Progesterone
- Relaxin
- Prolactin
- CRH
- β-Endorphin
- α-MSH
- GnRH
- Inhibin

29. Cryptorchidism.

- The testis develops in the abdomen and descends to the scrotum during fetal development.
- The descent of the testes is under the control of Mullerian inhibiting substance and gonadotropins.
- Undescended testis is called as cryptorchidism.
- It is seen in 2% in less than 1-year-old children and is less than 0.3% after puberty.
- It is treated with gonadotropins.
- The treatment has to be started early as the incidence of malignancy in undescended testis is high than when it is present in the scrotum.

30. Why are ovarian cycles suppressed during lactation?

- The nursing mother does not have regular menstrual cycle.
- The menstrual cycles are absent for 6 months in women who do not nurse their infants.
- Mothers who nurse regularly have amenorrhea for 25 to 30 weeks.
- This is because; nursing stimulates prolactin secretion and prolactin—inhibits GnRH secretion, inhibits action of GnRH on the pituitary and antagonizes the action of gonadotropins on the ovaries.
- Ovaries are inactive, ovulation is inhibited and estrogen and progesterone output falls to low levels.
- So the chance of a nursing female of becoming pregnant is very low and is a birth control mechanism.

31. What is P50?

Refer answer short answer 12.

32. What are the types of hypoxia?

Refer answer short note 12.

33. Mention common refractory errors of the eye.

- **Myopia—shortsightedness:** Eyeball may be elongated and therefore parallel rays of light from a distant object are brought to focus in front of the retina. It may be genetic or acquired. It can be corrected by using biconcave lenses.
- **Hypermetropia—farsightedness:** Here the parallel rays of light from a distant object are brought to focus behind the retina. It occurs due to decrease in anteroposterior diameter of the eye. It can be corrected by using biconvex lenses.
- **Astigmatism:** The problem here is the corneal surface is not spherical. One meridian of the cornea is different from the other. So the parallel rays of light are not able to converge to a point of focus as there is unequal refraction from the different meridians. So a blurred image is seen. It can be corrected using cylindrical lenses.
- **Presbyopia:** It is commonly seen in aged people above the age of 40 years. The near point has receded beyond the normal reading distance due to loss of plasticity of lens. The loss of plasticity results in loss of accommodation property of the lens. It is corrected using convex lens for near work and plain glasses for far work and it is given as the bifocal lenses.

34. SA node as pacemaker.

- SA node is the pacemaker of the heart and it is said to be the pacemaker as it discharges electrical impulses at a rapid rate than the other regions and this depolarization spreads through the conducting system to other regions before they depolarize on their own.

- It is located at the junction of SVC with the right atrium.
- SA node contains cells which are round with gap junctions. They are 'P' cells or the pacemaker cells.
- They are supplied by sympathetic and parasympathetic nerves.
- They fire at a rate of 100/min.

35. PR interval.
- It is between beginning of P wave to beginning of Q wave.
- The normal duration is 0.12–0.2 sec (Average 0.18 sec).
- This denotes atrial depolarization and conduction to AV node.
- Prolonged PR interval signifies AV conduction block.

36. Reflex arc.
- Reflex is defined as the involuntary response to a threshold stimulus obtained by stimulating a sensory receptor.
- The simplest reflex arc has a single synapse.
- **Components of a reflex arc:** Receptor → afferent nerve → Integrating center → Efferent nerve → Effectors (*refer* **Fig. 59**).

37. Functions of cerebrospinal fluid.
- CSF offers mechanical protection by acting as a shock absorber.
- CSF offers the optimum chemical environment for accurate neuronal signaling.
- CSF acts as a circulating medium for exchange of nutrients and waste products between the blood and nervous tissue.
- Continuous formation and drainage removes metabolic wastes.
- Acts as lymph

- Provides nutrition
- Reduces the weight of brain

38. What is righting reflex?
- Righting reflexes help to maintain the normal standing position and keep the animal's head upright.
- These reflexes are integrated in the nuclei of midbrain.

39. Name the nuclei responsible for hunger and satiety in human being.
- Feeding center (hunger)—lateral nucleus
- Satiety center—ventromedial nucleus

40. What is referred pain?
Refer answer to short answer 17.

41. Extracellular fluid volume and blood volume in an adult male weighing 70 kg.
- ECF volume in a 70 kg adult (20% of the body weight)—14 L
- Blood volume is calculated = 100/100-hematocrit. Plasma volume is 3.5 L and Hct is 38.
- So total blood volume = 3500 × 100/100-38 = 5645 mL.

42. Calcium transporters on the membrane of sarcoplasmic reticulum.
Calcium transporters on SR membrane are Ryanodine receptors, IP3 receptor and Ca^{2+}-Mg^{2+} ATPase.

43. Mechanism of edema in congestive cardiac failure.
In congestive heart failure, there is increase in venous pressure which results in increased capillary pressure. This leads to increased filtration pressure and thereby increased interstitial fluid and edema.

44. State a manifestation of hypocalcemic tetany. Give one cause leading to this condition.
Carpopedal spasm is a feature of tetany—the hand takes a peculiar posture-flexion at metacarpophalangeal joints, extension at interphalangeal joints and opposition of

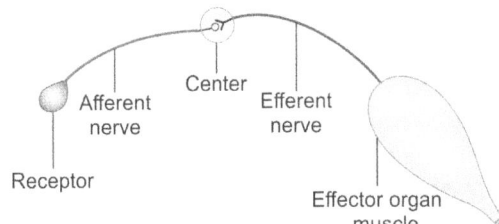

Fig. 59: Reflex arc.

thumb. Spasm of feet is rare and if it happens there is plantar flexion of toes and the toes are drawn up.
It is seen in hypoparathyroidism.

45. List the vitamin K-dependent coagulation factors.

- In the liver, the following clotting factors synthesis depends upon vitamin K:
- Factor II or prothrombin
- Factors VII, IX and X
- Protein C

46. Rh status of mother, father and child for occurrence of Rh incompatibility.

For Rh incompatibility to occur the Rh status are:
- Mother is Rh negative
- Father is Rh positive
- Fetus is Rh positive

47. Role of tropomyosin in muscle contraction.

- Tropomyosin is a regulatory protein.
- It is double stranded and is placed in the groove in the actin filament.
- It covers the myosin binding sites of actin.
- On release of Ca^{2+} from SR, Ca^{2+} binds to troponin C.
- After the binding of troponin C and Ca^{2+}, tropomyosin is lifted from the myosin binding sites and the myosin binding sites of actin are exposed and the myosin heads bind to actin.
- This brings about cross-bridge cycling and muscle contraction.

48. Type of acetylcholine receptor on skeletal muscle and its function.

- The type of acetylcholine receptor on the muscle fiber is nicotinic acetylcholine receptor.
- It is a non-specific cation channel by itself.
- When two molecules of acetylcholine binds to the receptor, the channel opens and allows entry of Na^+, as it is the major cation in the ECF.
- Na^+ influx results in development of depolarizing end-plate potential (EPP) in the motor end plate.
- EPP excites the neighboring muscle membrane which in turn generates Action potential.

49. Hormones secreted by hypothalamus.

They are:
- Growth hormone releasing hormone (GHRH)
- Growth hormone inhibiting hormone (GHIH) or somatostatin
- Prolactin inhibiting factor (PIF) or Dopamine
- Thyrotropin releasing hormone (TRH)
- Corticotropin releasing hormone (CRH)
- Gonadotropin releasing hormone (GnRH)

50. Hormonal defect in (a) Addison's disease (b) Conn's syndrome.

- Addison's disease—decreased synthesis of mineralocorticoids and glucocorticoids
- Conn's syndrome—primary hyperaldosteronism—increased synthesis of aldosterone

51. List the calcium transporters on the sarcoplasmic reticular membrane in the ventricular Muscle.

The calcium transporters on the SR membrane of ventricular muscles are—ryanodine receptors and IP3 receptors on the SR membrane to release Ca^{2+} and Ca^{2+}- Mg^{2+} ATPase to pump back calcium into the SR.

52. State Starling's law of the heart.

Frank-Starling's law states that, within physiological limits the force of contraction is directly proportional to the initial length of the muscle.

53. What is the effect of 2,3 diphosphoglycerate on the oxygen-hemoglobin dissociation curve? Does it help in loading or unloading of oxygen?

- 2,3 DPG is a product of glycolysis via Embden-Meyerhof pathway got from 3-phosphoglyceraldehyde.
- It is a highly charged anion that binds to deoxyhemoglobin
- $HbO_2 + 2,3\ DPG \leftrightarrow Hb - 2,3\ DPG + O_2$. So in presence of 2,3 DPG the affinity

hemoglobin to O_2 decreases and it releases O_2. So the oxy-Hb dissociation curve shifts to the right.
- It helps in unloading of O_2.

54. What are the types of hypoxia?

Refer answer to short note 12.

55. Region of the cochlea which vibrates most for the highest sound frequency in the audible range.

The basilar membrane at the base of the cochlea vibrates the most for the highest sound frequency in the audible range.

56. Visual field defect when the optic chiasma is cut in the center.

In the crossing of optic chiasma, the nasal retinal fibers from both the eyes are damaged and the field defect here is **bitemporal hemianopia**.

57. State the refractive error in astigmatism. How is it corrected?

Refer answer to short answer 33.

58. What is 'Blind spot'?

The optic nerve leaves the eye and the retinal blood vessels enter the eye at a point 3 mm medial to and slightly above the posterior pole of the eye.

It is called as the optic disk and is viewed through the ophthalmoscope.

There are no receptors of vision (Rods and Cones) in this area, so called as the 'blind spot'.

59. Receptors for vestibular sensation.

- The vestibular apparatus in the inner ear consists of—3 semicircular canals and 2 sac, such as structures—utricle and saccule.
- The receptors for vestibular sensation are the hair cells and they are located in the cristae in the ampulla of semicircular canals and the macula or otolithic organ of the utricle and saccule.
- The receptors in the canals and the utricle and saccule are the **hair cells** located in unique structures.
- The hairs of the hair cells are embedded in thick gelatinous substance called the **cupula**.

60. Name of tracts made up by second order neurons in the pathway for (a) fine touch, (b) pain.

- **Fine touch:** Dorsal column pathway
- **Pain:** Lateral spinothalamic tract

Answers to 2014 Question Paper

ANSWER ALL QUESTIONS

I. Essay Questions   **(15 Marks each)**

1. Describe the physiological roles of the different types of granulocytes circulating in blood.
2. Define glomerular filtration rate (GFR). What are its determinants? Discuss the phenomenon of autoregulation of GFR. Describe the best test for estimation of GFR. What is the routinely used clinical test to assess renal function?
3. Define the terms cardiac output and total peripheral resistance and discuss their determinants.
4. What are the neural mechanisms involved in spontaneous breathing? Discuss chemical regulation of respiration. Distinguish between the two types of respiratory failure.
5. What is the composition of gastric juice? Describe the mechanism of HCl secretion. Give a detailed account on the regulation of gastric secretion.
6. Define blood pressure. Discuss in brief the various factors which influence the pressure. Add a note on hypertension.
7. Define anemia. Classify them. List the important investigations to confirm the various types of anemia.
8. Define cardiac cycle. Describe the sequence of events during cardiac cycle in detail with suitable diagrams.

II. Short Notes   **(2.5 Marks each)**

1. cAMP signaling pathway, with an example.
2. Colloid oncotic pressure and its importance.
3. Excitation-contraction coupling in skeletal muscle.
4. Types of polycythemia and complications due to this condition.
5. Findings of 'tests of hemostasis' in hemophilia.
6. Functions of macrophages.
7. Physiological role of corticosteroids.
8. Function of any one hormone of posterior pituitary.
9. Composition of bile and the physiological role (if any) of the components.
10. Pathophysiology of peptic ulcer.
11. Describe the 3 bipolar limb leads of ECG. What is the significance of (a) PR interval (b) ST segment in an ECG?
12. Discuss the changes in ventricular volume during different phases of the cardiac cycle with a diagram.
13. Discuss any two pulmonary function tests which can detect obstructive lung disease.
14. Trace the pathway for perception of fine touch.
15. Operant conditioning.
16. Clinical features of cerebellar lesions.
17. Define muscle tone and discuss the phenomenon responsible for it. What conditions lead to alterations of tone?
18. Endogenous opioid peptides.
19. Refractory errors of the eye.
20. Discuss the phenomena by which sound waves in air induce action potentials in the cochlear nerve.
21. Hypersecretion of growth hormone.
22. Tissue macrophage system.
23. Neural regulation of respiration.
24. Functions and tests of cerebellum.

25. Transport across cell membrane.
26. Ovarian and endometrial changes of menstrual cycle.
27. Brown-Séquard syndrome.
28. Oxygen dissociation curve.

III. Short Answers   (1 Mark Each)

1. Membrane transporters involved in clearance of calcium from cytoplasm.
2. Concentrations of sodium and potassium in intra- and extracellular fluids.
3. Phenomena involved in the act of swallowing.
4. Role of ATP in relaxation of muscle.
5. Draw a schematic diagram of the sarcomere and label its components.
6. Opsonins.
7. Cells which express major histocompatibility complex II.
8. Significance of glycosylated hemoglobin.
9. Name 4 enzymes in pancreatic secretion.
10. Hormonal imbalance causing (a) acromegaly (b) cretinism.
11. List the types of shock.
12. Define preload and state its effect on cardiac function.
13. Baroreceptor reflex.
14. What is myocardial infarction? State one ECG change in this condition.
15. Role of myelin sheath in conduction of nerve impulse.
16. Conditions where plantar response is 'extensor'.
17. Finding in Weber's test in conduction deafness of the left side.
18. Muscle actions responsible for (a) normal expiration (b) forced expiration.
19. Oxygen carrying capacity of blood.
20. Hypoxic vasoconstriction—where does it occur and what are its complications?
21. Permissive action of hormone.
22. Role of vitamin D in calcium homeostasis.
23. Contraception in males.
24. Corpus luteum.
25. Vitamin-K dependent clotting factors.
26. Atonic bladder.
27. Functions of skin.
28. Secondary active transport.
29. Motor unit.
30. Refractory period.
31. Heart sounds.
32. Waves of ECG in Lead II.
33. Different types of hypoxia.
34. Aphasia.
35. Stages of sleep.
36. Optic pathway.
37. Functions of ascending reticular activating system.
38. Components of vestibular apparatus.
39. Features of Parkinson's disease.
40. Functions of middle ear.
41. Functions of plasma proteins.
42. Nonexcretory functions of kidney.
43. Myasthenia gravis.
44. Stages of spermatogenesis.
45. Cystometrogram and its significance.
46. Hormones regulating calcium homeostasis.
47. Enterohepatic circulation.
48. Enzymes involved in digestion of fat.
49. Structure of platelets.
50. Functions of saliva.
51. Dead space.
52. Hering Breuer reflex.
53. Korotkoff sounds.
54. Draw a diagram of the pathway of crude touch and label it.
55. Functions of CSF.
56. Fluent aphasia.
57. Receptor potential.
58. Motor homunculus.
59. Attenuation reflex.
60. Taste pathway.

I. ESSAY QUESTIONS

1. **Describe the physiological roles of the different types of granulocytes circulating in blood.**

Granulocytes in blood are:
❐ Neutrophils
❐ Eosinophils
❐ Basophils (*refer* **Fig. 1**)

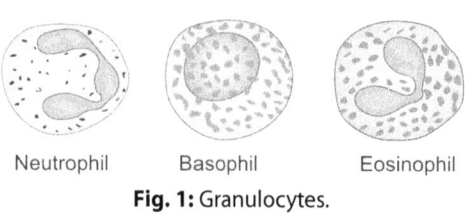

Fig. 1: Granulocytes.

Physiological Roles of Neutrophils

- Neutrophils are the first line of defense
- It does the defense mechanism by phagocytosis.

Phagocytosis

- Neutrophils are the first ones to reach the site of infection followed by macrophages.
- They come out of the blood vessels by a process called **emigration**.
- Adhesion molecules like *selectins* and *integrins* help in emigration.
- Phagocytes are attracted to sites of infection or inflammation by **chemotaxis**.
- Substances inducing chemotaxis are called **chemotaxins.**
- On reaching the pathogens or tissue debris, phagocytes adhere to them—**adherence**.
- Then they put out processes—Pseudopods and ingest the particles—**ingestion**.
- The ingested particle is enclosed in a vesicle—**phagosome** (*refer* Fig. 2).
- Phagosome attaches to lysosomes in the neutrophil to form— **phagolysosome**.
- The lysosomes put out hydrolytic enzymes like *lysozymes*.
- The phagocytes have oxidative enzymes in them which form lethal oxidative metabolites like—O_2^-, H_2O_2 and **hypochlorites**.
- **Antimicrobials: Defensins** in phagocytes kill the microorganisms.
- By all these killing mechanisms the microbes are killed and degraded or form **residual bodies**.

Other Functions

- Neutrophils release many chemical mediators like leukotrienes, thromboxane A2 which mediate inflammatory reaction.
- It mediates febrile response by releasing endogenous pyrogens.

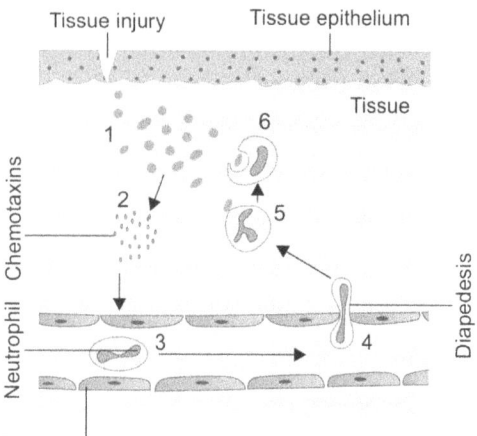

Fig. 2: Phagocytosis—Neutrophils marginate towards the wall of capillary followed by diapedesis, chemotaxis and engulfing the microbes: (1) Entry of microorganisms; (2) Chemotaxis; (3) Margination; (4) Diapedesis; (5) Fusion of microbe with lysosome; (6) Formation of phagolysosome.

Eosinophils

Structure of Eosinophils

- Size is same as that of neutrophils (10–14 µm)
- Bilobed nucleus and lobes are connected by thick chromatin strand—gives a spectacle-shaped appearance.
- Cytoplasm has coarse, orange pink granules.
- **Granules contain:** Eosinophil peroxidase, eosinophilic cationic protein, major basic protein, histaminase, catalase, etc.
- Mostly present in tissues.

Physiological Roles

- Leave the capillaries and enter tissue spaces where allergic reactions occur.
- Releases an enzyme, histaminase that combats the effects of histamine released by basophils.
- They inhibit mast cell degranulation
- They are weakly phagocytic and phagocytose Ag-Ab complexes
- Eosinophils also release substances (Major basic protein) which kill the parasitic worms.
- So eosinophil counts increase in allergy and worm infestation.

Basophils

- They are similar to mast cells.
- They are mildly phagocytic
- They enter tissues at sites of infection or tissue damage and release histamine, heparin and serotonin.
- These chemicals are responsible for the inflammatory reactions.
- They also release eosinophilic chemotactic factor which attracts eosinophils to combat the inflammatory reactions by removing Ag-Ab complexes.
- Mast cells and basophils release the inflammatory mediators and are responsible for allergic reactions.
- Basophils release heparin which is an anti-coagulant and thereby removes minute clots and prevents clotting of blood.

---

2. Define glomerular filtration rate (GFR). What are its determinants? Discuss the phenomenon of auto-regulation of GFR. Describe the best test for estimation of GFR. What is the routinely used clinical test to assess renal function?

- **Glomerular filtration rate is defined as the volume of plasma filtered by all the nephrons of both the kidneys per unit of time.**
- Normal value is 125 mL/min or 180 L/day.

The determinants of GFR are:

- **Filtration co-efficient (Kf):** It is the product of permeability of the glomerular membrane and its surface area. As the Kf increases GFR increases and as Kf decreases GFR decreases.
- **Glomerular capillary hydrostatic pressure (P_{GC}):** It is dependent on arterial blood pressure, renal blood flow and afferent and efferent arteriolar resistance. P_{GC} is directly proportional to GFR.
- **Capillary oncotic pressure (π_{GC}):** GFR is inversely proportional to π_{GC}.
- **Hydrostatic pressure in Bowman's space:** It opposes filtration and GFR is inversely related to GFR.
- **Sympathetic stimulation:** Stimulation leads to vasoconstriction and decreased RBF and GFR.

Autoregulation of GFR

- The autoregulatory mechanism of GFR is similar to autoregulation of renal blood flow.
- Autoregulation of GFR maintains a constant rate of filtration in spite of change in arterial pressure within the range of 80–180 mm Hg (MAP).
- There are two autoregulatory mechanisms of GFR—Myogenic mechanism and tubuloglomerular feedback.

Myogenic Mechanism

- As the renal blood pressure increases, the afferent arteriole is stretched and the stretch induces reflex contraction smooth muscles lining the wall of the afferent arteriole.
- This result in vasoconstriction of afferent arteriole and thereby decreases renal blood flow and thereby decreases GFR.

Tubuloglomerular (TG) Feedback

- TG feedback is an autoregulatory mechanism in the kidneys to regulate the renal blood flow (RBF) and thereby the GFR.
- This feedback mechanism is dependant on the NaCl content in the tubular fluid.
- The NaCl content in the tubular fluid is sensed by the macula densa cells and signals are sent to the afferent arterioles to regulate the RBF and GFR.
- Increased renal arterial pressure increases glomerular capillary pressure and thereby increases filtration.
- The increased GFR leads to increased NaCl content in the tubular fluid.
- This is sensed by the macula densa cells and they send signals to cause vasoconstriction of the afferent arterioles and thereby decrease RBF and GFR and NaCl content is brought back to normal.
- If NaCl content is less, it is sensed by the macula densa cells and signals are sent to the afferent arterioles resulting in

```
↑Renal arteriolar pressure ←----• (-)
         ↓                        |
↑Glomerular capillary pressure    |
         ↓                        |
       ↑GFR                       |
         ↓                        |
Increased NaCl delivery to tubule |
         ↓                        |
  Sensed by macula densa          |
         ↓                        |
Signals sent to afferent arteriole|
         ↓                        |
Afferent arteriole vasoconstriction----'
```

Fig. 3: Tubuloglomerular feedback.

vasodilation followed by increased RBF and GFR (*refer* **Fig. 3**).
- The mediating chemicals may be Thromboxane A2 or Adenosine for vasoconstriction and NO for vasodilation and they are released by the macula densa cells.

The Best Test to Estimate GFR
- It is done by assessing renal clearance of Inulin.
- Renal clearance is defined as the volume of plasma that is cleared of substance in a minute by excretion of the substance in urine.

It is Calculated by using the Formula

C = UV/P
- C = Clearance of the substance
- U = Urinary concentration of the substance
- V = Rate of urine flow
- P = Plasma concentration of substance in plasma
  - Inulin is used to measure GFR as it is freely filtered and neither reabsorbed or secreted by the tubules.
  - It is biologically inert and nontoxic and is neither metabolized nor stored.

Methodology
- A loading dose of Inulin is administered intravenously followed by a continuous infusion to keep the plasma level a constant.
- After the inulin has equilibrated in the body fluids, an accurately timed urine sample of urinary specimen is collected and half way through plasma sample is obtained.
- Then with the plasma and urinary concentrations the clearance is calculated by using the above formula.

$$U_{IN} = 35 \text{ mg/mL}$$
$$V = 0.9 \text{ mL/min}$$
$$P_{IN} = 0.25 \text{ mg/mL}$$
$$C_{IN} = U_{IN} V/P_{IN}$$
$$= 35 \times 0.9/0.25$$
$$= 126 \text{ mL/min}$$

Routinely used Clinical Test used to Assess Renal Function
- A fall in GFR is the first and only clinical sign of kidney disease.
- So measurement of GFR is used to assess kidney diseases.
- Since measurement of GFR by inulin clearance is cumbersome in clinical setting, plasma creatinine is measured and its level is inversely proportional to GFR.
- But the fall in GFR should be substantial for the rise in plasma creatinine

---

3. Define the terms cardiac output and total peripheral resistance and discuss their determinants.

Cardiac output is defined as the amount of blood ejected by each ventricle per minute.
Cardiac output = Stroke volume × Heart rate
Normal value = 5–6 L/min.

Determinants of Cardiac Output
- CO = Stroke volume (SV) × Heart rate (HR)
- So factors affecting either of them will alter CO.

Factors Affecting SV
- Preload
- After load
- Contractility

Factors Affecting HR

HR is affected by nerves supplying heart (Sympathetic and parasympathetic nerves) and cardiac centers

Preload

- The initial muscle length is the **preload** (the extent to which the muscle is stretched before contraction).
- Preload is decided by the **end-diastolic volume (EDV)**.
- EDV is decided by the **venous return (VR)**.
- **Preload affecting stroke volume is based on the Frank-Starling's law:** It states that within physiological limits, the force of contraction is directly proportional to the initial length of the muscle.

Causes for Application of Frank-Starling's Law

- Increase in EDV →↑stretch of muscle fiber → Interaction of thick and thin filament increases →↑ force of contraction.
- Stretch of muscle fibers → Opens stretch sensitive Ca^{2+} channels on sarcolemma →↑ Ca^{2+} influx →↑ force of contraction.
- ↑Ca^{2+} influx →↑ Ca^{2+} release from SR (CICR) →↑ force of contraction.
- ↑stretch of muscle fiber →↑ Affinity of troponin for Ca^{2+}

EDV is dependent on:

- **Venous return, which is dependent on:**
  - *Skeletal muscle pump:* Contraction of limb muscles press on the veins and increases forward movement of blood in the veins
  - *Thoracic pump:* Increase in respiration depresses the diaphragm and decreases intrathoracic pressure and thereby, it acts like a suction force to increase VR
  - *Abdominal pump:* During respiration compression of abdominal muscles press on the veins and favors venous emptying
  - *Cardiac pump:* Vis A Tergo (Force from behind), Vis A Fronte (Force from front)
  - *Total blood volume:* As the blood volume increases VR increases and vice versa
  - *Capacity of venous system:* Sympathetic stimulation to the veins causes venoconstriction and thereby increases venous emptying
  - *Body position:* On standing, there is venous pooling due to gravity and it may decrease the VR.
- **Atrial pump activity:** Contributes 20% ventricular filling and stimulated by sympathetic stimulation.
- **Ventricular compliance:** Affected by damage to myocardium as in MI, pericardial effusion and cardiac tamponade.

This type of regulation of stroke volume in relation to change in initial length of muscle fiber is said to be **heterometric regulation**.

Contractility

Contractility is increase in force of contraction and thereby increase in stroke volume without increase in initial muscle length.

- Ventricles are able to do more work per stroke at a given EDV.
- Factors which affect contractility—inotropic agents.
- There are positive and negative inotropic agents.

Contractility is increased by:

- **Autonomic activity** (Sympathetics are positively inotropic)
- **Muscle mass:** Increase in myocardial mass increases contractility as after regular exercise
- Concentration of hormones and chemicals
- **Heart rate:** Force frequency relationship

Factors increasing contractility, positive inotropic agents:

- Sympathetic stimulation
- Circulating catecholamines
- Force frequency relationship
- Digitalis
- Glucagon
- Insulin
- Thyroxine
- Chemicals like xanthine, theophylline

Factors decreasing contractility, negative inotropic agents:

- Loss of myocardium as in myocardial infarction
- Hypoxia
- Hypercapnia
- Acidosis
- Acetylcholine

Regulation of stroke volume by affecting contractility of myocardium is **homometric regulation**. Here the force of contraction is affected without much change in muscle length.

Afterload

- It is the force against which the heart muscle shortens
- Cardiac output is inversely proportional to afterload
- **Cardiac output α 1/afterload (anrep effect)**
- It is decided by peripheral resistance
- **Peripheral resistance is decided by:**
  - Vessel diameter
  - Viscosity of blood
- **This is also included in homometric regulation.**

Determinants of Peripheral Resistance

- **Total peripheral resistance is defined** as the resistance offered to the blood flow in the blood vessels.
- There is a resistance to blood flow in the peripheral circulatory system and it is said to be the peripheral resistance.
- Arterioles are the site of major resistance to blood flow in the vascular system. Therefore, they are called as the 'resistance vessels'.
- The walls of the arterioles are having more of smooth muscles than elastic tissue and these muscles are supplied by noradrenergic fibers and they are in partial contraction at rest—Vasomotor tone.
- The constriction and relaxation of the arterioles in any organ is responsible for the tissue perfusion.
- The resistance is decided by the vasoconstriction or dilatation. There are other factors also which decide the total peripheral resistance (TPR).
- Important factors responsible for TPR are—radius of the vessel and viscosity of blood.

Radius of the Vessel

- Radius of the vessel is decided by the sympathetic nerves.
- Decrease in radius increases TPR and increase will decrease TPR.
- Even a decrease in resistance by half will increase the TPR 16 times.
- When the radius is doubled the resistance is reduced by 6% of its previous value

Viscosity of Blood

- Viscosity of blood also affects TPR.
- But the most commonly occurring change in TPR is due to change in the radius of blood vessel.
- Viscosity of blood is decided by the cellular components of blood, especially RBCs and composition of plasma and resistance of cells to deformation. Temperature also affects viscosity.
  - *Hematocrit:* Viscosity of blood is mostly dependent on the hematocrit. In large vessels increase in hematocrit largely increases viscosity. In smaller vessels, the effect of viscosity on TPR is less due to difference in nature of blood flow. So the net effect of viscosity of blood on TPR is less in vivo than in vitro, unless there is severe polycythemia. In anemia, TPR is decreased as viscosity is decreased.
  - *Composition of plasma:* Viscosity is increased in diseases where there is marked increase in plasma proteins as in multiple myeloma.
  - *Effect of deformed cells:* There is rise viscosity in hereditary spherocytosis
  - *Effect of temperature:* Increase in body temperature decreases viscosity and decrease in body temperature increases viscosity.

4. What are the neural mechanisms involved in spontaneous breathing? Discuss chemical regulation of respiration. Distinguish between the two types of respiratory failure.

Neural Regulation of Respiration

- Breathing is an automatic process occurring throughout life without conscious effort.
- Respiration is a process which is highly regulated.

- Spontaneous respiration is due to rhythmic discharge of neurons from respiratory centers supplying the inspiratory muscles.
- This is under cortical (voluntary) and medullary and pontine control (Automatic).
- These centers in turn are regulated by alterations in the PCO_2, PO_2 and pH of arterial blood and other nonchemical influences.

Cortical Control or Voluntary Control of Respiration

Impulses from cerebral cortex
↓
Corticospinal tract
↓
Motor neurons supplying the inspiratory muscles

- Impulses also reach the innervation of expiratory muscles.
- There is a reciprocal inhibition between the motor neurons supplying the I and E neurons.
- There is an exception for this at the start of expiration were the "I" neurons are active.
- The inspiratory muscles are active for some time during expiration to brake the elastic recoil of lungs and make expiration smooth.

Automatic Control of Respiration

Impulses from brainstem respiratory centers in pons and medulla → supplies neurons in intermediolateral horn cells of cervical and thoracic segments → supplies inspiratory muscles.

Medullary Respiratory Centers

- **Dorsal respiratory group of neurons (DRG):** Has 'I' neurons
- **Ventral respiratory group of neurons (VRG):** Has 'I' and E' neurons (*refer* **Fig. 4**)
- **Central pattern generator (CPG):** Pre-Bötzinger complex (*refer* **Fig. 5**)

Dorsal Respiratory Group of Neurons

- Located near nucleus tractus solitarius (NTS)
- Contains only inspiratory neurons
- They project to cell bodies of phrenic nerves in spinal cord.

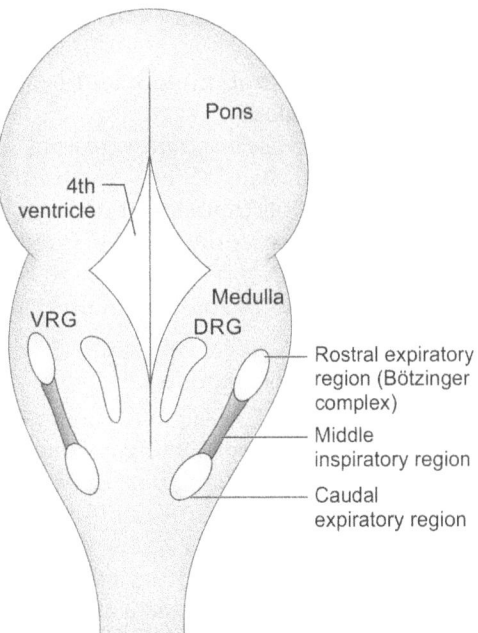

Fig. 4: Respiratory centers in medulla.
[DRG: dorsal respiratory group of neurons (has only inspiratory neurons); VRG: ventral respiratory group of neurons (has both inspiratory and expiratory neurons)]

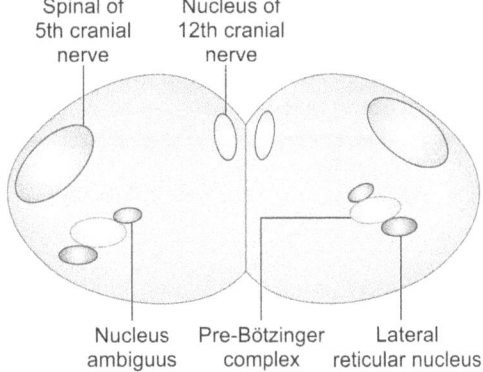

Fig. 5: Location of pacemaker (Pre-Bötzinger complex) for rhythm generation in medulla.

- Its activity is weaker to start with and gradually increases in a ramp fashion for 2 seconds and abruptly stops for 3 seconds.
- The ramp signal helps in steady increase in lung volume during inspiration
- Receives input from peripheral chemoreceptors through 9th and 10th cranial nerves.

Ventral Respiratory Group of Neurons

- Located in ventrolateral medulla in region of nucleus ambiguus (NA)

- Contains both inspiratory and expiratory group of neurons
- 3 regions—Rostral, middle and caudal inspiratory regions
- Middle region has inspiratory neurons
- Rostral and caudal has expiratory neurons—supply expiratory muscles.
- They are active only during forceful respiration.
- I and E neurons reciprocally inhibit each other

Pacemaker Cells for Respiration
- Located close to DRG and VRG neurons
- Present in the pre-Bötzinger complex between nucleus ambiguus and lateral reticular nucleus.
- They are pacemaker cells and are responsible for generating respiratory rhythm → Rhythmically activate phrenic nerves.
- It receives input from higher centers

Pontine Centers

There are two centers:
1. **Pneumotaxic center:**
   - Located in nucleus parabrachialis and Kölliker-Fuse nucleus in the upper part of pons (*refer* **Fig. 6**)
   - Active during both inspiration and expiration.
   - On stimulation, it shortens the duration of inspiration. When its activity is less, the duration of inspiration is longer.
   - Its major function is to limit inspiration, by inhibiting apneustic center
   - It coordinates switching between inspiration and expiration.
2. **Apneustic center:**
   - Present in lower part of pons (*refer* **Fig. 6**).
   - On stimulation → Leads to prolonged inspiratory spasms—APNEUSIS
   - It sends inputs to DRG to cause a prolonged inspiration
   - It is constantly stimulating DRG.
   - But its actions are kept in check by inputs from pneumotaxic center and vagal afferents from airways.

Mechanism of Breathing
- The neurons in DRG discharge steadily and spontaneously in a ramp like fashion for 2–3 seconds.
- Muscles of inspiration contract steadily resulting in expansion of the lung and chest wall resulting in inspiration.
- As the inspiration happens, the stretch receptors in lungs and airways are stimulated and impulses from here travel through vagus nerve to stop the firing of DRG neurons.
- Impulses from pneumotaxic center through inhibition of apneustic center stops the firing of DRG (*refer* **Fig. 7**).
- Inspiratory muscles relax and the lung and chest wall recoils and induces expiration.
- At the end of expiration, the next cycle starts.

Factors Influencing Respiratory Centers
- **Afferents from higher centers:** Cerebral cortex, limbic system, hypothalamus
- **Afferents from peripheral receptors:** Baroreceptors, chemoreceptors, J receptors, pain receptors, proprioceptors, pulmonary stretch receptors and thermoreceptors.

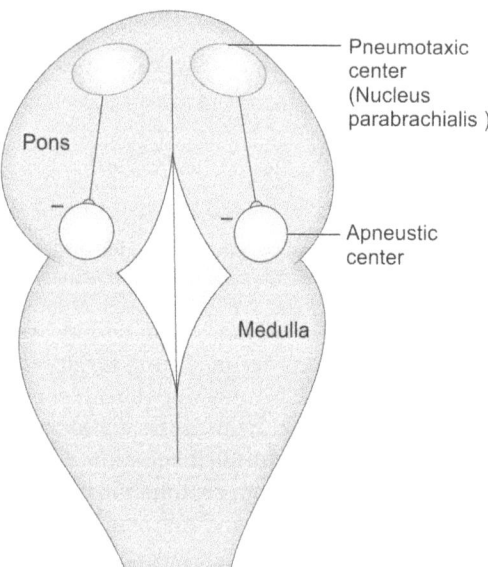

Fig. 6: Respiratory centers in pons, pneumotaxic and apneustic centers.

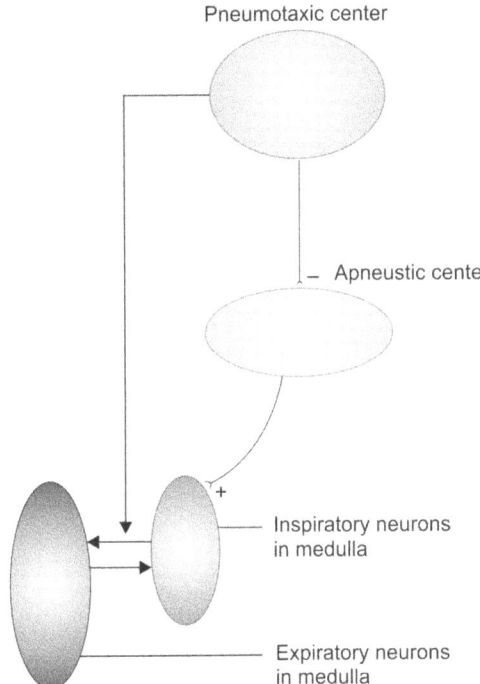

Fig. 7: Interaction of medullary and pontine centers in regulation of respiration.

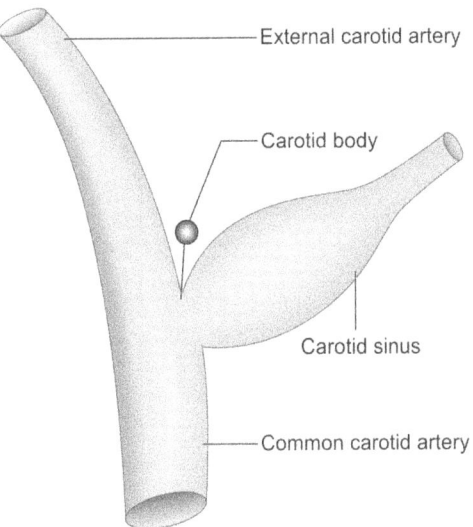

Fig. 8: Location peripheral chemoreceptors at bifurcation of common carotid artery; the carotid body. Carotid sinus is the dilatation in internal carotid artery; the baroreceptor.

- **Reflexes:** Hering-Breuer reflex, sneezing reflex, swallowing reflex, cough reflex, speech

Chemical Regulation of Respiration

- Chemical regulation of respiration is also through the modulation of activities of neural centers through chemoreceptors.
- There are 2 sets of chemoreceptors responding to changes in arterial PO_2, PCO_2 and pH
- They are peripheral and central chemorecptors.

Peripheral Chemoreceptors

- Carotid and aortic bodies (*refer* **Fig. 8**).
- They have high blood flow (2000 mL/ 100 g/min) and high metabolic rate.
- Their metabolic needs are met by dissolved O_2.
- So they are highly sensitive to ↓PO_2, ↑PCO_2 and ↓pH.
- These receptors are not stimulated in anemia or carbon monoxide poisoning.
- They are stimulated in ↓PO_2, vascular stasis, cyanide poisoning

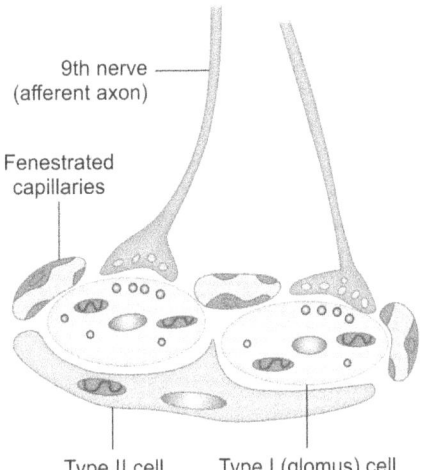

Fig. 9: Cells in carotid body—Type I (glomus cells) and Type II (supporting cells). Glomus cells are supplied by 9th cranial nerve and are close to fenestrated capillaries.

- They have 2 types of cells—glomus and sustentacular cells.

Sensitivity of Peripheral Chemoreceptors (PCR)

- Glomus cells are the sensors (*refer* **Fig. 9**)
- Hypoxia is the major stimulus. Neurotransmitter is Dopamine
- PCRs also responds to ↑PCO_2 and ↓pH

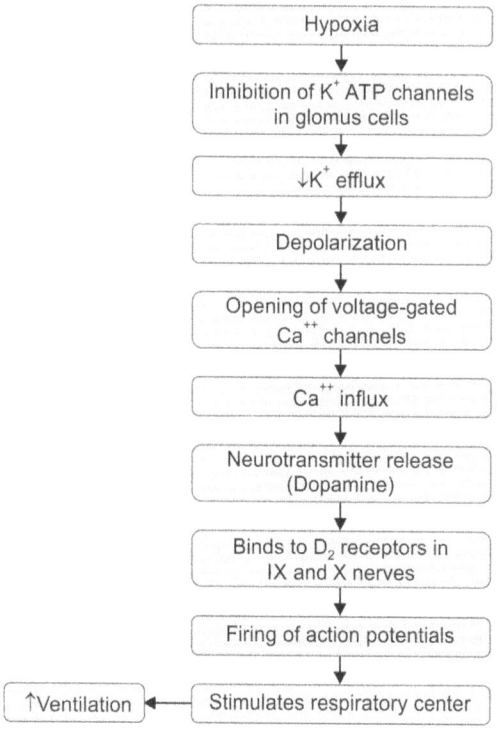

Fig. 10: Effect of hypoxia on peripheral chemoreceptors.

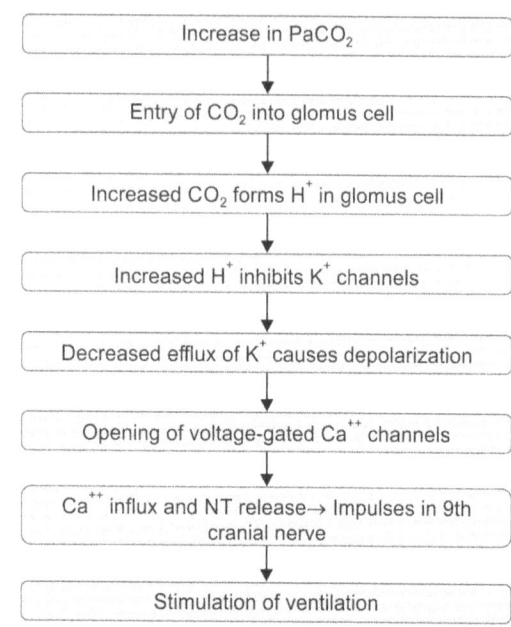

Fig. 11: Effect of hypercapnia on peripheral chemoreceptors.

- When PO_2 <100 mm Hg, there is firing rate of the nerves supplying them (9th and 10th cranial nerves)
- Response is maximum when PO_2 falls <60 mm Hg
- Effect of hypoxia is less when PO_2<60 mm Hg because:
  - Hypoxia → Hyperventilation → CO_2 blow out → ↓$PaCO_2$ → ↓ventilation
  - Deoxy-Hb has more affinity for H+ → ↓arterial [H+] → ↓ventilation

Mechanism of Hypoxia Stimulating PCR
Hypoxia inhibits K+ channels by:
- O_2 sensor in the glomus cell is a heme containing protein and is associated with O_2. In hypoxia the lack of O_2 inhibits the K+ channels (*refer* Fig. 10).
- In hypoxia there is increase in cAMP in glomus cells which inhibits cAMP sensitive K+ channels.

Effect of CO_2 on PCR
Refer Fig. 11.

Integrated Effects of Arterial—PCO_2, PO_2 and pH on Ventilation, by Stimulating PCR
- At low P_{ACO_2} level with hypoxia, ventilation is not stimulated till PO_2 <60 mm Hg.
- High P_{ACO_2} levels (as in ↑metabolic rate/breathing CO_2 mixtures) →↑ventilation. But if CO_2 content in breathed air is >7% → CNS depression → CO_2 narcosis
- Hypercapnia with hypoxia, shifts the CO_2 curve to left and slope is increased.
- Acidosis by itself (as in diabetic ketoacidosis) can stimulate ventilation by stimulating PCR. (Even in absence of hypoxia or hypercapnia)

Central Chemoreceptors (CCR)
- Located in the medulla and is different from the other respiratory neurons.
- There are also other such CCR in and around the brainstem nuclei—Nucleus tractus solitarius, nucleus ambiguus (*refer* Fig. 12).
- They respond maximally to changes in [H+] in brain CSF and ISF which is in turn decided by P_{ACO_2} and HCO_3^- of CSF.

↑Arterial PCO_2
↓
↑Brain ECF CO_2 level

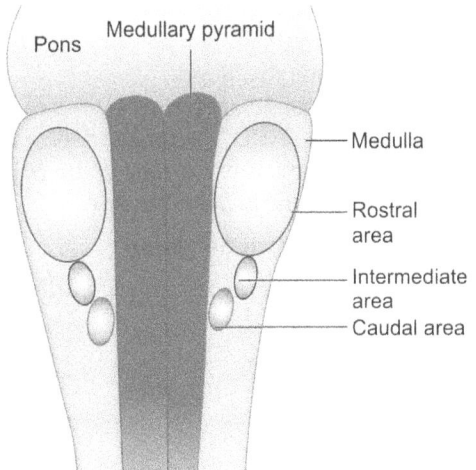

Fig. 12: Location of central chemoreceptors in ventral medulla. There are rostral, intermediate and caudal centers.

$$CO_2 + H_2O \rightarrow H_2CO_3 \rightarrow H^+ + HCO_3^-$$
↓
Increase in brain ECF H⁺ level
↓
Stimulation of CCR
↓
Stimulation of medullary inspiratory center
↓
Firing of neurons supplying diaphragm and external intercostal muscles
↓
Increase in ventilation

Two Types of Respiratory Failure

Respiratory failure is due to inadequate gas exchange. There are two types of failures—Type 1 and Type 2 failure.
1. **Type 1 failure:** Here only the PO_2 level in the arterial blood is low and PCO_2 level is either normal or low. It may be due to mismatch in ventilation/perfusion ratio and the defect here is poor oxygenation of blood.
2. **Type 2 failure:** Here PO_2 level is below 60 mm Hg and also hypercapnea is present, PCO_2 is > 50 mm Hg. Seen in conditions of increased airway resistance like bronchial asthma, decreased breathing effects as in brainstem lesion, skeletal deformity like kyphosis and a decrease in diffusion area as in chronic bronchitis.

5. What is the composition of gastric juice? Describe the mechanism of HCl secretion. Give a detailed account on the regulation of gastric secretion.

Composition of Gastric Juice

- 2–2.5 L/day
- pH 1–2
- Water—99.45%
- Solids—0.55%
- Electrolytes—Na^+, K^+, Mg^{2+}, Cl^-, HCO_3^-, HPO_4^-, SO_4^-
- Enzymes—pepsin, lipase, gelatinase
- Mucus—insoluble and soluble
- Intrinsic factor

Mechanism of HCL Secretion

- In stomach, hydrochloric acid is secreted by the parietal cells which are present in the main gastric glands in body of the stomach.
- Pure secretion from the parietal cell has a pH of 0.82 and is isotonic (150 mEq of H^+ and 150 mEq of Cl^+).
- Parietal cell is polarized with an apical side facing the lumen and a basolateral side facing the interstitium.
- There are many tubulovesicular structures in the parietal cell which are studded with H^+-K^+ ATPase which pump H^+ into the lumen in exchange for K^+.
- These cells are highly metabolizing and they put out lot of CO_2. The cell is also rich in the enzyme carbonic anhydrase.

HCl secretion from the parietal cells happens in 2 steps:
1. Secretion of H^+ into the lumen
2. Secretion of Cl^- into the lumen.

The steps involved in HCl secretion are:
1. CO_2 in the cell is hydrated in the presence of Carbonic anhydrase, $CO_2 + H_2O \rightarrow H_2CO_3$
2. $H_2CO_3 \rightarrow H^+ + HCO_3^-$
3. The H^+ is pumped into the lumen by the H^+-K^+ATPase pump on the apical side. For one H^+ pumped out of cell one K^+ is taken into the cell which later diffuses back into the lumen (*refer* **Fig. 13**).

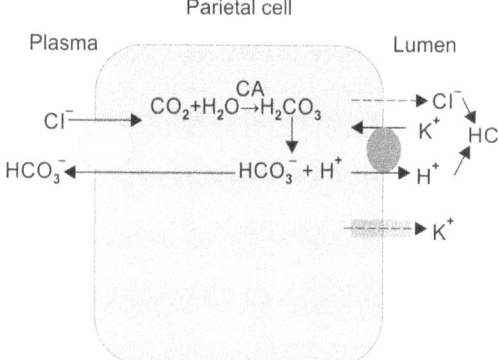

Fig. 13: Mechanism of HCl secretion.
(CA: Carbonic anhydrase)

4. HCO_3^- is extruded in the basolateral side through an anion exchanger in exchange for one Cl^-.
5. The Cl^- which enters the cell will diffuse across the apical membrane into the lumen.
6. So for every H^+ secreted, one Cl^- is also secreted into the lumen and one HCO_3^- is absorbed into the blood.

So when gastric secretion is increased after a meal, the HCO_3^- getting added to the blood is increased, thereby raising the pH of blood—*Postprandial alkaline tide*.

Regulation of Gastric Secretion

Neural, humoral and reflex regulation of secretion.

Factors that Stimulate
- Vagus nerve
- Gastrin
- Histamine

Factors that Inhibit
- Low pH in the stomach
- Somatostatin
- Prostaglandin E2 (*refer* **Fig. 14**)

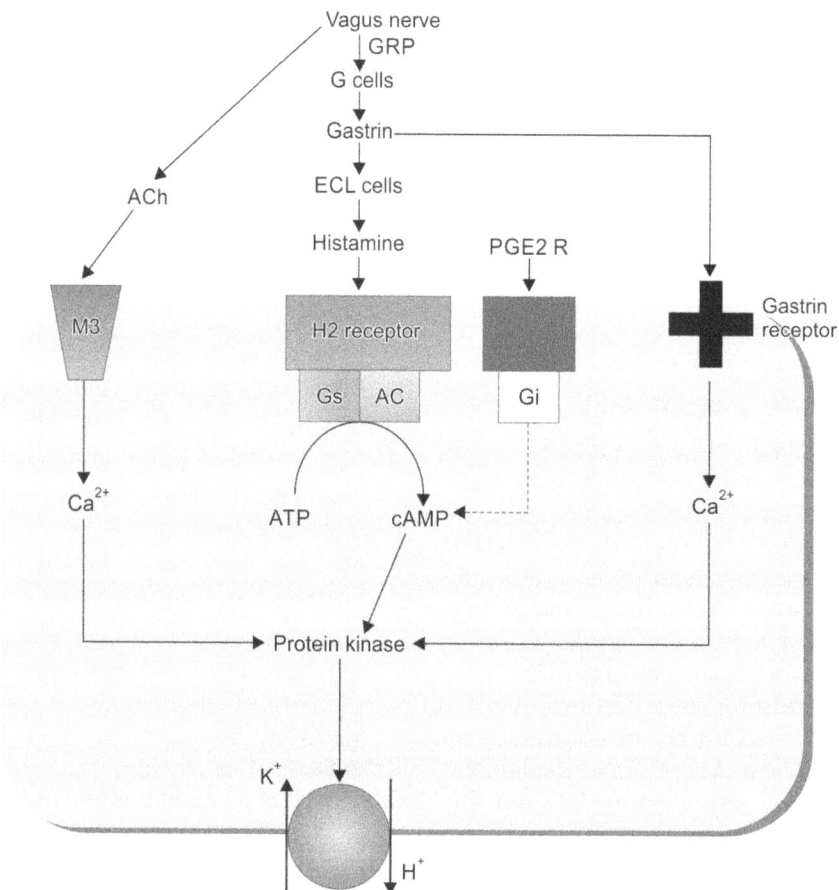

Fig. 14: Parietal cell with the regulating factors for HCl secretion.
(PGE2R: Prostaglandin E2 receptor; M3: Muscarinic receptor)

Regulation is discussed in terms of:
- Cephalic phase
- Gastric phase
- Intestinal phase

Cephalic Phase
- Nearly 500 mL/hr (45% of total secretion)
- Initiated by thought, sight, smell, taste of food through stimulation of vagus nerve.
- Emotions also affect secretion (*refer* Fig. 15)

Gastric Phase
- About 50% of total secretion. Food in stomach induces secretion by:
  - Distension of body of stomach (through reflexes—Vagal reflex)
  - Distension of antrum (through gastrin secretion)
  - By products of partial digestion of protein (through gastrin secretion)

Intestinal Phase
- It begins when chyme enters the intestine.
- Intestinal influence is inhibitory by:
  - *Enterogastric reflex:* By distension, presence of acid and products of digestion—inhibits secretion.

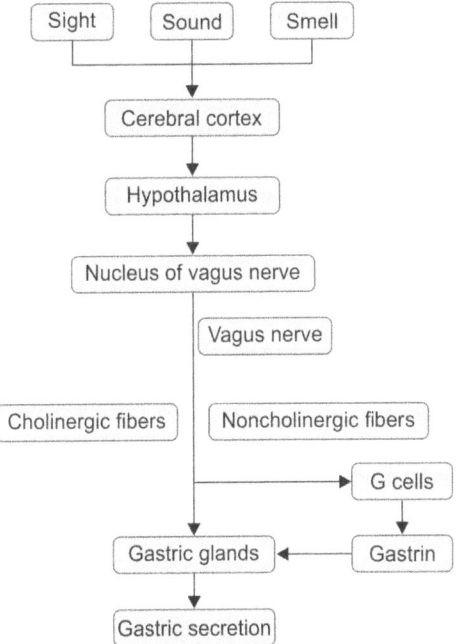

Fig. 15: Cephalic phase of regulation of HCl secretion. This phase of gastric secretion is regulated through vagus nerve.

- *Hormonal mechanism:* CCK, secretin, GIP, neurotensin, etc., enterogastrone.

---

6. Define blood pressure (BP). Discuss in brief the various factors which influence the pressure. Add a note on hypertension.

- BP is defined as the lateral pressure exerted by the moving column of blood on the vessel wall. Normal value = 120/80 mm Hg.

Components of BP
- Systolic BP
- Diastolic BP
- Pulse pressure
- Mean arterial pressure

Factors Influencing BP
- Blood pressure = Cardiac output × Peripheral resistance.
- Cardiac output = Stroke volume × Heart rate

Stroke Volume

It is decided by:
- **End-diastolic volume (preload):** Preload is directly proportional to stroke volume and cardiac output. It is based on Frank-Staling's law.
  Factors affecting preload are—blood volume, skeletal muscle pump, thoracic pump as in respiration, ventricular compliance and atrial contraction
- **Contractility:** Force of contraction of the myocardium without increase in initial length of the muscle fiber. It is said to be the inotropic property of the heart. Sympathetic stimulation, catecholamines, glucagon and digitalis are positively inotropic. Hypoxia, hypercapnia, acidosis are negatively inotropic.
- **Afterload:** It is the peripheral resistance against which the heart contracts. It is determined by peripheral resistance. Afterload is inversely related to stroke volume and cardiac output
  - **Heart rate (HR)**
  - **It is regulated by:**
    - Parasympathetic nerves—decrease HR
    - Sympathetic nerves—increase HR

Peripheral Resistance
- **Diameter of blood vessels:** Vasomotor tone—regulated by sympathetic nerve supply (Increases the tone). Vasoconstriction increases the PR and thereby the blood pressure is increased.
- **Viscosity of blood:**
  - Plasma proteins
  - Number of RBCs

Hypertension
- It is defined as the sustained elevation of systemic arterial pressure.
- Blood pressure is determined by cardiac output and peripheral resistance.
- Systolic BP is determined by cardiac output and therefore affected by stroke volume and heart rate. These determinants are subjected to daily activities. Therefore elevation in systolic BP is not usually considered as hypertension.
- Diastolic BP is determined by peripheral resistance. PR is in turn decided by caliber of blood vessel and viscosity of blood. Sustained elevation of diastolic BP results in hypertension. It is usually associated with elevation of systolic BP also.
- 120/80 mm Hg is normal BP
- 120–139/80–89 mm Hg—prehypertension
- Above 140/90 mm Hg—hypertension

Types of hypertension (HT):
1. Primary or essential hypertension
2. Secondary hypertension

Primary or Essential Hypertension
- In over 90% of the individuals with hypertension, the cause is unknown. This is said to be primary HT. It could be due to sympathetic hyperactivity, increased sodium intake, increase in blood volume, etc.
- It can be in the benign form or it can progress to malignant HT.

Benign Form
- There could be moderate or great increase in BP up to 210/110 mm Hg. But there is also fluctuation of systolic BP. So, it is called as labile HT.
- In late stages, systolic BP is increased and fixed and does not come back to normal.
- Antihypertensives are prescribed.
- It causes cardiac hypertrophy, arteriosclerosis of the vessels and increased incidence of myocardial infarction. There are renal changes, such as albuminuria, hematuria, etc.

Malignant Hypertension
- BP is very much increased even up to 260/150 mm Hg.
- There are arteriolar lesions
- Patients show symptoms of papilledema, cerebral symptoms and renal failure.
- If patient is not treated, usually death occurs within 6 months to 2 years.

Secondary Hypertension
Blood pressure is increased due to some other underlying disease.

It can be due to:
- **Renal diseases**, such as glomerulonephritis, pyelonephritis, renal tumors, polycystic kidney disease, etc.
- **Goldblatt hypertension:** Due to renal artery stenosis. They are of two types:
  1. *One kidney one clip Goldblatt hypertension:* One kidney is removed and the renal artery of the other kidney is stenosed. Here rise in BP is independent of renin levels.
  2. *Two kidney one clip Goldblatt hypertension:* Two kidneys are present and constriction of the renal artery of one kidney. The rise in BP is dependent on increased Renin levels.
- **Cardiovascular diseases**, such as atherosclerosis
- **Endocrinal diseases:**
  - Pheochromocytoma
  - Cushing's syndrome
  - Primary hyperaldosteronism or Conn's syndrome
  - Acromegaly
  - Glucocorticoid-remediable hyperaldosteronism
  - Myxedema
- Neurogenic hypertension: These are done experimentally to demonstrate the role of baroreceptors in regulating blood pressure.

- Bilateral clamping of the carotid arteries proximal to carotid sinuses results in increase in BP.
- Similar changes are seen when the carotid sinus nerves (IXth cranial nerve) on each side are cut.
- The rise is not too high as the aortic sinuses are still functioning.
- If the vagus nerve from the aortic sinus is also cut it results in rapid rise in BP even upto 300/200 mmHg.
- Similar results are seen when the NTS in medulla is bilaterally damaged. This can even be fatal.
- These forms of hypertension are said to be neurogenic hypertension.
- **Hypertension in pregnancy:** Due to pressor peptides secreted from placenta hypertension is present with pre-eclampsia or eclampsia.
- **Congenital diseases**, such as Liddle's syndrome where there is excessive retention of salt and water.
- **Coarctation of aorta:** Congenital narrowing of the aorta especially the thoracic aorta results in severe hypertension in upper half of the body.
- **Chronic treatment with oral contraceptive pills:**
  - OC pills contain estrogen and progesterone.
  - Estrogen increases production of angiotensinogen resulting in elevated angiotensin II levels.
  - Normally this would decrease renin secretion and that brings Ang II levels to normal.
  - But in consumption of OC pills this feedback is incomplete resulting in hypertension—pill hypertension.

Effects of Hypertension

On the Heart

- The consistent increase in peripheral resistance leads to increase in afterload which increases the work of the myocardium resulting in left ventricular hypertrophy.
- Myocardial oxygen requirement increases due to increased ventricular muscle mass.
- So even minimal narrowing of coronary vessels results in ischemia.
- Gradually the ability to compensate for the high peripheral resistance is exceeded and the heart fails.

On the Blood Vessels

- There is increased incidence of atherosclerosis.
- High BP also leads to stiffness of vessels and their compliance is lost.
- They are prone for cerebral thrombosis and cerebral hemorrhage.

Kidneys

- Atherosclerosis of renal vessels affects renal functions, such as filtration and tubular functions.
- Renal failure is an important complication in HT.

---

7. Define anemia. Classify them. List the important investigations to confirm the various types of anemia.

- **Anemia is defined as the decrease in red cell count or hemoglobin content in blood.**
- Anemia is classified based on the cause of anemia and based on the structure of red cells.

Morphological Classification or Wintrobe's Classification

Based on the size and the presence of hemoglobin content inside the cell it is classified as:

1. **Normocytic normochromic anemia:** The RBC size (MCV) and the hemoglobin content (MCH and MCHC) is normal. It is seen in hemorrhagic anemia, hemolysis and aplastic anemia.
2. **Microcytic hypochromic anemia:** The cell volume and the hemoglobin content are decreased. MCV, MCH and MCHC are below normal. It is seen in iron deficiency anemia.
3. **Macrocytic anemia:** MCV is above normal range. There is macrocytosis and the hemoglobin concentration is normal. This type is normally seen in vitamin B_{12} and folic acid deficiency.

Etiological Classification or Wintrobe's Classification

Anemia is usually due to either decreased production from the bone marrow or increased destruction.

Classification of Anemia

1. **Decreased red cell production:**
   - Decreased production due to stem cell failure—Aplastic anemia
   - *Dietary deficiencies:*
     - Iron deficiency anemia
     - Megaloblastic anemia—due to deficiency of folic acid and vitamin B_{12} deficiency.
     - Pernicious anemia—anemia due to vitamin B_{12} deficiency due to deficiency of intrinsic factor.
     - Protein deficiency
2. **Increased destruction of red cells:** Hemolytic anemias—congenital and acquired.
   Congenital:
   - *Membrane defects:* Hereditary spherocytosis and hereditary elliptocytosis
   - *Hemoglobin defects:*
     - Hemoglobinopathies (defects in hemoglobin): Sickle cell anemia (HbS, in the beta chain in the 6th position glutamic acid is replaced by Valine), abnormal hemoglobin like HbC, HB E, Hb D
     - Thalassemias (Deficiencies of hemoglobin—deficiency of a or b chain)—major and minor.
   - *Enzyme defects:* Deficiency of Glucose-6-Phosphate dehydrogenase and pyruvate kinase.

   Acquired:
   - Due to antigen-antibody reactions—Erythroblastosis fetalis, incompatible blood transfusions, etc.
   - Infections—malaria
   - Drug induced—quinine, aspirin, etc.
   - Snake venom
   - Hypersplenism—excessive destruction of RBCs
   - Burns
3. **Blood loss anemia:**
   - *Acute hemorrhage:* Trauma, surgery, etc.
   - *Chronic blood loss:* Menorrhagia, worm infestation
4. **Anemia due to chronic renal failure:** Due to decreased production of erythropoietin
5. Anemia associated with chronic diseases

Investigations to Detect the Types of Anemia

Iron-deficiency Anemia

- ❏ **Blood picture and red cell indices:**
  - Hb concentration↓
  - RBCs in peripheral smear are microcytic hypochromic
  - Red cell indices, such as MCV, MCH, MCHC are reduced
- ❏ **Bone marrow findings:**
  - Erythroid hyperplasia
  - Marrow is iron—deficient
- ❏ **Biochemical findings:**
  - Serum iron decreases <50 µg% (normal 60–160 µg%)
  - Serum ferritin low
  - TIBC is increased

Megaloblastic Anemia

- ❏ **Blood changes:**
  - RBCs are macrocytic normochromic.
  - RBC count decreases < 1 million/cumm
  - Hb decreases <12 g/dL
  - MCV increases 95–160 fl (Normal 78–94 fl)
  - MCH increases to 50 pg
  - MCHC normal as both MCV and MCH has increased
  - Peripheral smear there are nucleated RBCs.
  - Reticulocyte count increases >5%
  - WBC and platelet counts decrease.
- ❏ **Biochemical findings:**
  - Plasma concentration of vitamin B_{12} decreases in pernicious anemia.
  - Serum folate level decreases in anemia due to folic acid deficiency.

---

8. Define cardiac cycle. Describe the sequence of events during cardiac cycle in detail with suitable diagrams.

Definition

- ❏ Cardiac cycle is defined as the cycle of mechanical and electrical events taking

place from beginning of one beat to the beginning of next beat.
- It is given as the changes in volume, pressure and flow in different cardiac chambers, the electrical activities occurring (through ECG) and coinciding heart sounds (using PCG) in various phases of cardiac cycle.
- Duration of a cardiac cycle is 0.8 s when heart rate is 75/min.

Phases of Cardiac Cycle and their Duration
1. Atrial systole—0.1 s
2. Atrial diastole—0.7 s
3. Ventricular systole—0.3 s
4. Ventricular diastole—0.5 s
- Atrial diastole merges with ventricular systole.
- So, the phases described here are atrial systole, ventricular systole and diastole.
- **Ventricular systole: 2 phases—0.3 s**
  - Isovolumetric contraction phase-0.05 s
  - Phase of ejection 0.25 s
    - Phase of rapid ejection—0.1 s
    - Phase of reduced ejection—0.15 s
- **Ventricular diastole: 0.5 s**
  - Protodiastole—0.04 s
  - Isovolumetric relaxation phase—0.06 s
  - Rapid ventricular filling—0.11 s
  - Diastasis—0.19 s
- **Atrial systole: 0.1 s**

Atrial Systole
- Duration is 0.1 sec
- This follows the phase of diastasis
- Begins from peak of "P" wave in ECG to peak of "QRS" complex
- Atria contracts and increases intra-atrial pressure. Blood is pumped into ventricles.
- Final filling of ventricle takes place here (Last 25-30%).
- Already the ventricles are in diastole and 75% of filling is complete.
- 4th heart sound is recorded in phonocardiogram.

Ventricular Systole

Isovolumic Contraction Phase
- Starts at peak of 'QRS' complex. Duration is 0.05 sec.

- Rise in ventricular pressure closes the AV valves and semilunar valves have not yet opened.
- 1st heart sound (S1) is heard, due to closure of AV valves.
- Ventricular pressure rises (>80 mm Hg) steeply and ventricular volume remains same.
- There is bulging of AV valves into the atria due to ventricular contraction. This creates 'C' wave in JVP curve.
- Phase ends with opening of semilunar valves and ejection of blood.

Ventricular Ejection
- **Rapid ejection phase: (0.1s)**
  - Semilunar valves open and blood is rapidly ejected (2/3rd of stroke volume) into aorta/pulmonary artery.
  - Steep fall in ventricular volume and steep increase in aortic flow
  - Ventricular pressure increases to a peak (120 mm Hg in the left and 25 mm Hg in the right)
  - Aortic pressure also increases.
  - Corresponds to ST segment in ECG
- **Reduced ejection phase: (0.15 s)**
  - Duration is 0.15 sec
  - Ventricular and aortic pressure decreases but aortic pressure is greater.
  - Aortic blood flow decreases. Only 1/3rd of stroke volume is ejected here.
  - Ventricular volume further decreases.
  - Momentum keeps blood flowing into aorta.
  - 'T' wave appears in ECG

Ventricular Diastole—0.5 s
1. Protodiastole—0.04 s
2. Isovolumetric relaxation—0.06 s
3. Phase of rapid ventricular filling—0.11s
4. Phase of reduced filling or diastasis—0.19s
5. Phase of second rapid filling—0.1 s

1. **Protodiastole:**
   - Duration is 0.04 sec
   - As the reduced filling phase ends, the ventricles start relaxing.
   - Intraventricular pressure drops.
   - This phase ends when aortic valve closes.

2. **Isovolumetric relaxation phase:**
   - Duration is 0.06 sec
   - This phase is between closure of semilunar valves and opening of AV valves.
   - Second heart sound (S2) appears due to closure of semilunar valves.
   - Closure of semilunar valves creates '**dicrotic notch**' in aortic pressure curve
   - Ventricular volume remains the same and pressure drops steeply as the ventricles relax (2–3 mm Hg) (*refer* **Fig. 16**).
   - When intraventricular pressure drops below atrial pressure, AV valves open.
3. **Rapid ventricular filling:**
   - Duration is 0.11 sec
   - As the AV valves open there is rapid inrush of blood into ventricles.
   - This is because the atria are filled with venous return and pressure is high here.
   - This vibration of ventricular wall creates the 3rd (S3) heart sound.
   - Major filling takes place here.
4. **Diastasis:**
   - Duration 0.19 sec.
   - This is a slow filling phase.
   - Ventricular volume rises slowly.
   - Ventricular and atrial pressures reduce and remain same (Little >0 mm Hg).
   - Nearly 75% of filling has occurred.

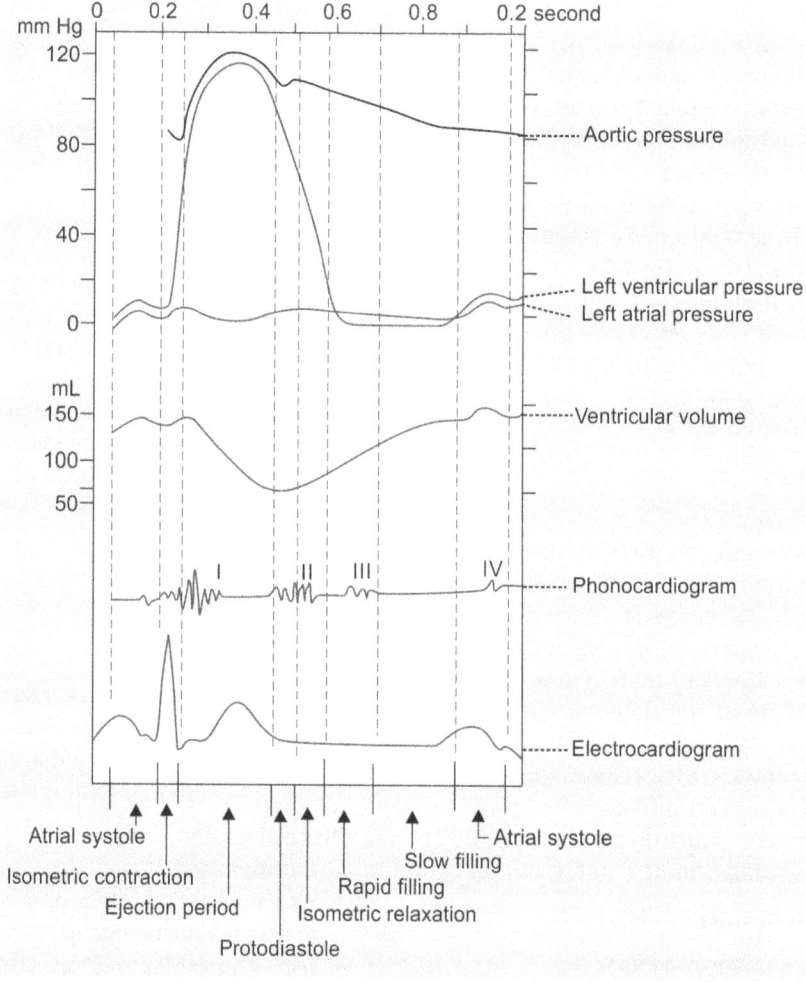

Fig. 16: Cardiac cycle with pressure volume changes in aorta, left ventricle, left atrium, ECG and phonocardiogram.

5. **Last rapid filling:**
   - Duration 0.1 sec.
   - Atria contracts and pumps the last 25% of blood into ventricles.
   - At rest, this volume is not essential.
   - But in tachycardia (as in exercise) when the duration of diastole decreases this volume assumes importance.

II. SHORT NOTES

1. cAMP signaling pathway, with an example

- cAMP is an important second messenger for peptide hormones.
- Many chemicals, such as norepinephrine, ACTH, ADH, angiotensin II, calcitonin, CRH, FSH, LH, etc., act via cAMP.
- It is said to be the cAMP-Adenylyl cyclase pathway.

The following is the signaling pathway:
- Peptide hormone binds to the membrane bound receptor
- The receptor is bound to G-protein.
- On binding of hormone to receptor, GDP is released from G-protein and replaced by GTP and G-protein is activated.
- Activated G-protein in turn stimulates or inhibits the membrane bound enzyme adenylyl cyclase.
- Adenylyl cyclase catalyzes the conversion of cytoplasmic ATP to cAMP. When the G-protein is stimulatory (Gs) the cAMP levels increase and when the G-protein is inhibitory (Gi) The cAMP is decreased (*refer* **Fig. 17**).
- cAMP in turn activates a cascade of enzyme system like protein kinase A.
- Protein kinase A catalyzes the phosphorylation of proteins, changing their confirmation and functions.
- cAMP is inactivated to 5'AMP by the enzyme phosphodiesterase and activity is terminated.

For example, the activation of phosphoryl kinase enzyme in the liver by epinephrine via cAMP and protein kinase A is given below:

Epinephrine
↓
β2 receptor
↓
Gs
↓
Adenylyl cyclase

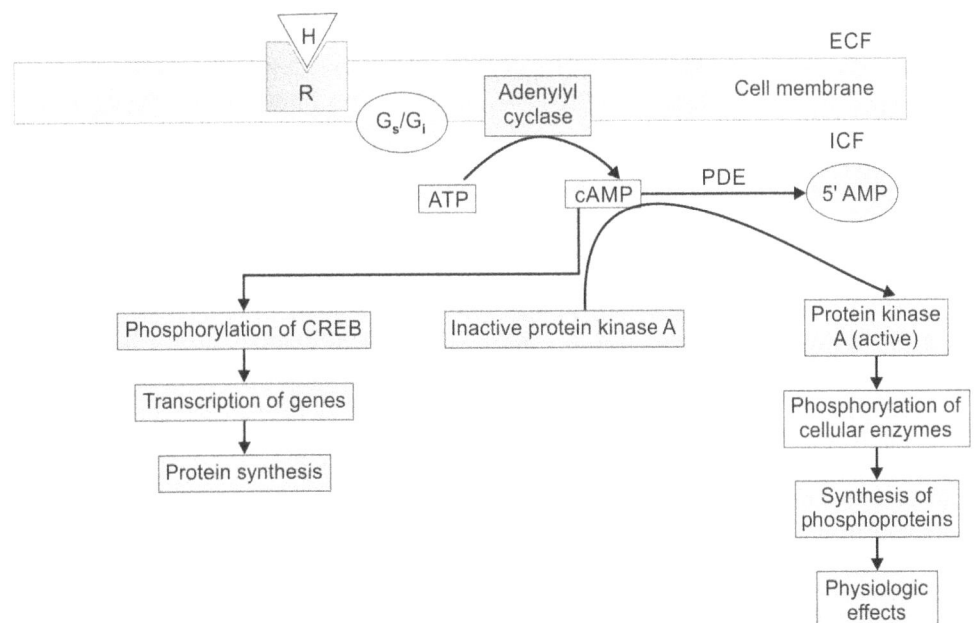

Fig. 17: Activation Gs-adenylyl cyclase-cAMP pathway signaling pathway.

↓
ATP → cAMP
↓
Protein kinase A activated
↓
Inactive phosphorylase
b kinase +ATP → Activated phosphorylase b kinase
↓
Phosphorylase b +ATP → Phosphorylase A
↓
Glycogen → Glucose-1-phosphate

2. Colloid oncotic pressure and its importance.

- Colloidal oncotic pressure is the osmotic pressure generated by larger molecules, especially proteins in plasma.
- The oncotic pressure exerted by plasma proteins is 26–28 mm Hg.
- It is the important force involved in fluid movement across the capillaries.
- Among the plasma proteins, albumin is the major protein to exert the oncotic pressure.
- The pores in between the endothelial cells are smaller in size and therefore do not allow the movement of proteins and other colloids across them.
- The colloids have a high molecular weight and are present in large amounts.
- Therefore, the capillary membrane is like an impermeable membrane to colloids and they exert an osmotic pressure of an average of 25 mm Hg.
- The rate of filtration of fluid across the capillary wall at any time is dependent upon the balance of Starling's forces.
- One of the Starling's forces is the plasma oncotic pressure and other forces are—Capillary hydrostatic pressure, interstitial hydrostatic pressure and osmotic pressure in the interstitium.
- So the hydrostatic pressure gradient (Hydrostatic pressure in capillary—hydrostatic pressure in interstitium) and the osmotic pressure gradients (Colloidal oncotic pressure in capillary—colloidal osmotic pressure in interstitium) decide filtration across capillaries.
- In the arteriolar end of the capillaries, the hydrostatic pressure is 36 mm Hg and the interstitial hydrostatic pressure varies in different tissues, it is subatmospheric in subcutaneous tissues, positive in liver and 6 mm Hg in the brain.
- The oncotic pressure in capillary is 25 mm Hg and in the interstitium it is negligible.
  - So fluid movement = $K[(Pc + \pi i) - (Pi + \pi c)]$
  - K = Filtration co-efficient
  - Pc = Hydrostatic pressure in capillary (37 mm Hg in arteriolar end and 17 mm Hg in venous end))
  - Pi = Hydrostatic pressure in interstitium (1 mm Hg)
  - πc = Colloidal oncotic pressure in plasma (25 mm Hg)
  - πi = Colloidal osmotic pressure in interstitium (0 mm Hg)
  - Pc and πi favors filtration and Pi and πc opposes filtration.
- In the arteriolar end of capillaries the hydrostatic pressure in capillaries exceeds the oncotic pressure and therefore filtration of fluid happens here.
- Along with the fluid filtered, nutrients also enter the tissues.
- As fluid moves out of the capillaries, in the venous end, the hydrostatic pressure in capillaries drops to 17 mm Hg and the colloid oncotic pressure is 25 mm Hg and this favors reabsorption in the venous end of capillaries along with the metabolic wastes.
- In the glomerulus, throughout length of the capillary, the hydrostatic pressure exceeds the oncotic pressure and therefore fluid moves out of the capillaries throughout the length of the capillary.

Applied Aspects
In hypoproteinemia due to malnutrition, liver diseases (synthesis of protein is less) and in nephrosis (albumin is lost in urine), the plasma colloidal oncotic pressure decreases resulting in edema.

3. Excitation contraction coupling in skeletal muscle.

The process by which the muscle membrane is excited and followed by muscle contraction is given as excitation-contraction coupling.

The steps are given below:

- The action potential generated following the end-plate potential (EPP) moves through the T-tubule and activates the voltage-gated dihydropyridine receptors (DHPRs) which are present in the T tubule membrane.
- The activated DHPRs open the Ca^{2+} channels named as the Ryanodine receptors which are located in the terminal cisterns of the sarcoplasmic reticulum (SR).
- This releases Ca^{2+} from the SR into the cytoplasm and the Ca^{2+} concentration in cytosol rises by 2000 times that of the resting state.
- The Ca^{2+} now gets attached to the troponin C subunit.
- Troponin C-Ca^{2+} complex now induce a conformational change in the tropomyosin and the tropomyosin is lifted up, exposing the myosin binding sites on actin molecules.
- So the myosin heads bind to the actin molecules and cross-bridge cycling starts resulting in muscle contraction.

4. Types of polycythemia and complications due to this condition

Polycythemia is increase in the RBC count above the normal value. It can be physiological or pathological.

Physiological Polycythemia

- **Age:** At birth, the count is high (6–7 million cells/cumm) and after birth it starts decreasing due to destruction of RBCs.
- **High altitude:** Hypoxia in high altitude stimulates production of erythropoietin which in turn stimulates RBC production.
- Excessive exercise

Pathological Polycythemia—2 Types

1. **Primary polycythemia or polycythemia vera:** It is said to be a member of myeloproliferative syndrome and is due to the cancerous condition of the bone marrow. The counts increase more than 10 million cells/cumm. A high WBC count may also be seen. In this condition, erythropoietin levels may be very low.
2. **Secondary polycythemia:** It happens due to hypoxic conditions in the body as in lung (Emphysema, COPD) and cardiovascular diseases (Cyanotic heart diseases). The hypoxia stimulates synthesis of erythropoietin and thereby increased production of RBCs.

Complications of Polycythemia

Increase in RBC count, increases the viscosity of blood and thereby increases the peripheral resistance leading to hypertension and left heart failure.

5. Findings of 'tests of hemostasis' in hemophilia.

Hemophilia is a bleeding disorder due to the absence of clotting factor VIII. It is a genetic disorder and is X-linked recessive disease. The males are always affected and the females are careers.

The laboratory tests in hemophilia:

- **Bleeding time** is normal as the platelet count and the capillary integrity is normal
- **Capillary fragility test** is normal
- **Platelet count** is also normal
- **Coagulation time:** It is the time taken for the blood to clot in a capillary tube by formation of fibrin thread. It is prolonged in hemophilia.
- **Prothrombin time:** It is done by Quick's one stage method. Here the anticoagulated plasma of the patient is mixed with commercially available tissue thromboplastin and calcium chloride solution and is incubated at 37°C. The time at which a gel is formed is taken to be the PT. Normally it is around 11–16 seconds. Only extrinsic pathway is assessed by this method and therefore it is normal in hemophilia.
- **Partial thromboplastin time (PTT):** Here to the anticoagulated plasma, Kaolin (surface agent), calcium chloride and cephalin are added and incubated at 37°C. The time taken to form the gel is the PTT. It gives an idea about the intrinsic pathway.

Normal PTT is 40 seconds. It is prolonged in hemophilia.
- **Thromboplastin generation test:** This test assesses the intrinsic pathway of coagulation and the normal value is 12 seconds. It is prolonged in hemophilia.

6. Functions of macrophages.

The macrophages have the following functions:
1. **Phagocytosis:** As a phagocyte, it is very powerful and it emigrates into the tissues following the bacterial invasion. But this happens 24 hours after the neutrophil action and therefore it is said to be the **second line of defense**. It engulfs the bacteria and digests it; the process of digestion of bacteria is similar to that of the neutrophils—by producing free radicals—H_2O_2 and lowering the pH. It can also engulf other substances like the cell debris, dead RBCs, foreign bodies, etc.
2. **Secretory function:** Monocytes and macrophages secrete many chemicals like interleukins, IL-1, TNF-α, binding proteins like transferrin, lysozyme, proteases, acid hydrolase, etc.
   - IL-1 has many important functions—it acts as a WBC growth factor in red bone marrow, it is an endogenous pyrogen, etc.
   - TNF α—it induces shock in septicemia due to gram-negative bacterial infections, destroys invading bacteria, etc.
   - Transferrin is an iron-binding protein in plasma to carry iron and also makes it unavailable for bacteria and thereby prevents its multiplication.
3. **Role in lymphocyte-mediated immunity:** Macrophages act as antigen presenting cells in immune reactions. It engulfs the microorganism and digests it and attaches the antigenic component to the MHC II molecule in the macrophage. The antigen-MHCII complex now moves towards the membrane of the macrophage and is inserted there. This macrophage moves towards the lymph nodes and the antigen is presented to the lymphocytes. The lymphocytes with the receptor for the antigen binds to the APC and is activated for further differentiation and division.
4. Monocyte-macrophage secretory products also play a **key role in healing and repair**.

7. Physiological role of corticosteroids.

Metabolic actions of glucocorticoids are:
1. **Effects on carbohydrate metabolism:**
   - Increases gluconeogenesis in liver → increased glycogen stores.
   - Antagonizes the action of insulin on muscle and adipose tissue—prevents glucose uptake.
   - This spares glucose for the brain.
   - Increases glucose output from liver.
   - Results in hyperglycemia
2. **Effects on protein metabolism:**
   - It is proteolytic in action
   - Breaks down proteins into AA and inhibits protein synthesis.
   - Amino acids are used for gluconeogenesis
   - Therefore, increased cortisol levels drain the protein stores in the body
3. **Effects on lipid metabolism:**
   - Cortisol is permissive for the lipolytic action of catecholamines.
   - But high cortisol levels increase total body fat by 2 mechanisms:
     a. Cortisol stimulates appetite → obesity due to increased caloric consumption.
     b. High cortisol →↑ blood glucose →↑ insulin secretion → lipogenesis.
- Pattern of fat distribution—**centripetal**—concentrated in trunk, but wasting is seen in arms and legs.

Permissive Action

Cortisol amplifies effects of certain processes of other hormones where it does not act directly.

Examples:
A. It does not induce glycogenolysis itself but augments glycogenolysis by glucagon.
B. It also augments vaso-responsiveness of blood vessels to catecholamines.

Actions on Bones

Increases bone resorption by:

Cortisol decreases renal and GIT absorption of calcium
↓
Lowers serum calcium levels
↓
Parathyroid hormone secretion stimulated
↓
Mobilizes calcium from bone by resorption and demineralization

- Also inhibits action of osteoblasts and suppresses collagen formation. Hence high cortisol levels results in **osteoporosis**

Actions on CVS

- Cortisol is permissive for the vasopressor effects of catecholamine and Ang ll.
- Hence it is necessary for maintenance of normal BP.
- Stimulates erythropoietin synthesis and so increases RBC production.

Actions on Connective Tissue

Cortisol inhibits fibroblast proliferation and collagen formation
↓
So excess cortisol levels
↓
Thinning of skin and walls of capillaries
↓
Easy damage to skin and easy bruising of capillaries
↓
Intracutaneous hemorrhage

Action on Kidneys

- Cortisol inhibits ADH secretion and action, so in absence of cortisol a water load leads to water intoxication.
- Cortisol also has a weak mineralocorticoid action → ↑Na⁺ and H₂O reabsorption.
- **Increases GFR:**
  - By increasing cardiac output
  - By direct action on kidneys

Action on Muscles

- Cortisol has complex action on muscles.
- Excess cortisol results in muscle weakness due to:
  - Proteolysis
  - Hypokalemia

Actions on GIT

- Cortisol has a trophic action on GIT.
- It also increases appetite → weight gain in hypercortisolism.
- Increased acid secretion → acidity, gastritis

Action on CNS

- Glucocorticoids alters mood and behavior
- REM sleep ↓, but slow wave sleep ↑
- In excess—insomnia, elevated or depressed mood, ↓ memory.
- Frank psychosis occurs with excess or reduced cortisol levels.
- Dampens the acuity to olfactory, gustatory, auditory and visual stimuli.

Action in Fetus

- Facilitates maturity of CNS, retina, skin, GIT and lungs.
- During the last week of pregnancy, the synthesis of surfactant is stimulated by cortisol.
- So if premature delivery suspected weekly doses of cortisol given to mother till delivery.

Action on Inflammation and Immune System

- Cortisol is frequently used clinically for its anti-inflammatory property
- It inhibits synthesis of mediators of inflammation.
- Inhibits migration of leukocytes to site of injury.
- Decreases the number of circulating eosinophils.
- Inhibits fibroblast proliferation at inflammatory site which is a defense mechanism in the body to prevent spreading of infection.
- Excess cortisol inhibits normal defense mechanisms of body against infection

Effect on Immune Response

- Cortisol inhibits immune response in the body.
- At high doses it decreases the number of T lymphocytes (helper T-cells) and their migration to antigenic site.
- B lymphocytes and antibody production are not affected directly.

- Because of these effects, glucocorticoids are used for immunosuppression after organ transplantation.

Effect on Stress

- Protects the body against stress
- During stress there is increased secretion of CRH from hypothalamus.
- This increases the secretion of ACTH from anterior pituitary
- Therefore, glucocorticoid secretion increases
- Cortisol facilitates lipolysis by catecholamine and increases release of free fatty acids which supplies the energy needed to cope up with stress.
- It is also permissive for the vasoconstriction induced by catecholamines which is needed for maintaining BP during stress.

8. Function of any one hormone of posterior pituitary.

- Oxytocin is an oligopeptide with 9 amino acids and is secreted from the Posterior pituitary.
- It is synthesized from magnocellular neurons of paraventricular nucleus of hypothalamus and is secreted into circulation from posterior pituitary.

Functions of oxytocin in:

- It stimulates milk ejection reflex
- It induces parturition reflex
- It also acts on nonpregnant uterus to facilitate sperm transport
- In males, it is secreted during ejaculation and causes contraction of smooth muscles of vas deferens to propel the sperm towards urethra.

9. Composition of bile and the physiological role (if any) of the components.

Composition of Bile

Bile is formed from hepatocytes in liver. Some substances are added to bile from (e.g., bile pigments).

The composition of bile is:

- It contains water and solids
- Water—97.5%
- Solids—2.5%
- Solids includes organic and inorganic substances
- Organic substances—bile salts, bile pigments, cholesterol, fats, fatty acids, lecithin, mucin
- Inorganic substances – Na^+, K^+, Cl^-, HCO_3^- and Ca^{++}.

Functions of Bile Salts

- **Digestion and absorption of fats:** Bile salts have detergent action and emulsifies fats into smaller molecules on which the pancreatic lipase acts and aids in digestion of fats.
- **Absorption of fats:** The bile salts along with lecithin forms micelles because of their amphipathic nature. The lipids are kept in the core of the micelles and are made soluble in water in intestinal lumen and are carried to the enterocytes. They micelle move to the brush border of the enterocytes and the lipids diffuse out of the micelle and is absorbed into the brush border.
- **Choleretic action:** Bile salts are present in the bile and they stimulate further secretion of bile from the liver.
- Bile salts on entering the intestine are converted into bile acids and are added to the bile acid pool of the body.
- Bile salts also help in *absorption of fat-soluble vitamins.*
- Bile salts along with lecithin solubilize cholesterol and *prevent formation of gallstones.*
- Bile salts are synthesized from cholesterol and when its excretion is increased more *cholesterol is lost from the circulation.*
- HCO_3^- in bile decreases the acidity of gastric secretion and protects the intestinal mucosa.
- Bilirubin, a break down product of hemoglobin gives color to feces and is excreted in stools.

10. Pathophysiology of peptic ulcer.

There are two types of ulcers:
1. **Duodenal ulcer**
2. **Gastric ulcer**

Ulcer is due to disruption of the mucosal barrier or excess secretion of gastric juice.

Acid or pepsin in gastric juice digests the mucosa leading to ulcer.

Mucosal barrier is formed by:
- **Mucus** secreted by the neck cells and surface mucosal cells in the mucosal lining. It also contains mucin, phospholipid, HCO_3^- and water.
- **Prostaglandins** secreted by epithelial cells have antisecretory activity (HCl) and increases HCO_3^- and mucus.
- **Epithelium of mucosa:** Low permeability, rapid turnover and HCO_3^-, mucus secretions from there.
- **Bicarbonate secretion** from gastric mucosal cells increases the pH.

Factors which Impair Mucosal Defense
- Defective mucus secretion
- **Drugs, such as NSAIDs, cortisol, etc.:** They inhibit secretion of mucus and bicarbonate
- Alcohol
- Type of Food
- **Smoking:** ↓ mucus and pancreatic secretions. Causes reflux of duodenal contents.
- Stress
- Reflux of gastric contents
- Delayed gastric emptying
- **H. pylori infection:** Causes local inflammation in antral mucosa and disrupts the barrier

Factors which Increase Secretion
- **Genetic factors:** Increased parietal cell mass, increased postprandial gastrin response
- **Psychosomatic factors:** Anxiety increases secretion
- **Food:** Alcohol, tea, coffee, spicy food
- Rapid gastric emptying
- **Zollinger-Ellison syndrome:** It is a gastrin secreting tumor of pancreas

---

11. Describe the 3 bipolar limb leads of ECG. What is the significance of (a) PR interval (b) ST segment in an ECG?

- In bipolar leads both the electrodes are active and one electrode is connected to the negative terminal and the other electrode is connected to the positive terminal of the electrocardiogram.
- The placements of three bipolar limb leads are based on the Einthoven's triangle.
- It is an equilateral triangle with each side of the triangle as the axis of each lead and heart as source of current in the center.
- The 3 corners of the triangle are formed by the two shoulders and the pubic region. Since the body fluid acts as a good conducting media the leads can be placed in the two arms and left foot.
- The two electrodes have to be placed in the corners of the triangle
- Bipolar limb leads—Lead I, II and III

Lead I: The two active electrodes are placed in the right and left arms. Left arm is connected to positive terminal and right arm is connected to negative terminal.

Lead II: It is between the right arm and left foot. Right arm is connected to negative terminal and left arm to positive terminal (*refer* **Fig. 18**)

Lead III: It is between left arm and left foot. Left foot is connected to positive terminal and left arm is connected to negative terminal.

As the electrical activity of the heart moves toward the positive lead an upward deflection is recorded in that lead.

PR Interval
- It is between the onset of P wave to the onset of QRS complex.
- The normal duration is 0.12–0.2 seconds
- It is the time taken for impulse conduction from SA node to the AV node.
- Prolonged PR interval signifies AV conduction block

ST Segment
- It is an isoelectric line between the end of QRS complex and beginning of T wave (*refer* **Fig. 19**).
- Normal duration is 0.04–0.08 seconds
- It is in relation to ventricular repolarization.
- ST segment is clinically segment as it is 'the indicator' of myocardial infarction.

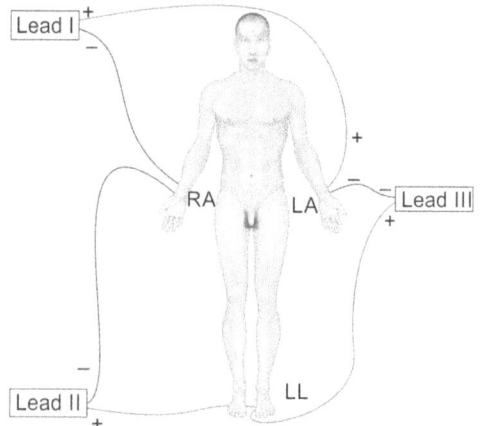

Fig. 18: Placement of bipolar limb leads.

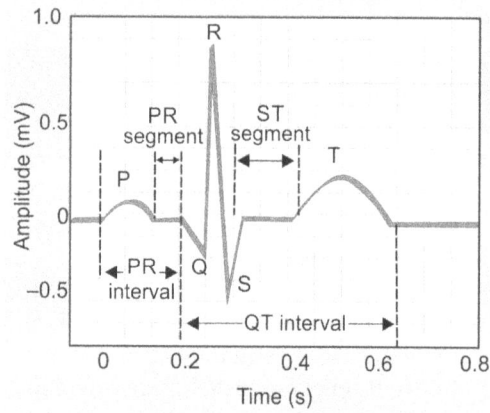

Fig. 19: Waves, segments and intervals in a normal ECG recorded in lead II.

12. Discuss the changes in ventricular volume during different phases of the cardiac cycle with a diagram.

Volume Changes in the Ventricles During Various Phases of Cardiac Cycle

Ventricular Systole

Isovolumetric contraction phase: There is no change in the volume of the ventricle in this phase.

Ventricular ejection phase:
- During this phase, blood is ejected out of both the ventricles—stroke volume. It is about 80 mL.
- The end-diastolic volume is about 130 mL and therefore after ejection 50 mL remains in the ventricle—end-systolic volume.
- Ejection fraction is the ratio of EDV ejected per systole.

Ventricular Diastole
- **Protodiastole** is the phase just before closure of semilunar valves. There is continuous drop in ventricular pressure and no blood flowing into the ventricles. So volume does not change.
- **Isovolumetric relaxation phase:** As the name implies no change in ventricular volume as the AV valves and semilunar valves are closed and therefore no blood flows in or flows out (*refer* **Fig. 16**).
- **First rapid filling phase and diastasis:** This phase starts with opening of AV valves. The ventricular pressure is very low, almost zero and there is pressure gradient allowing rapid inrush of blood into the ventricles. Almost 75% of the ventricular filling happens in this phase (105 mL of EDV).
- **Atrial systole or second rapid filling phase:**
  - The last 25% of ventricular filling happens due to atrial contraction or systole.
  - The EDV of 130 mL is reached in both the ventricles.

13. Discuss any two pulmonary function tests which can detect obstructive lung disease.

- The major problem in obstructive lung disease is during expiration. The major feature is decrease in expiratory flow rate.
- The most important tests done to detect the obstructive airway diseases are—maximum mid-expiratory flow rate (MMEFR) and FEV_1/FVC ratio.

MMEFR
- It is the flow rate in the middle 50% of FVC.
- It is given as forced expiratory flow rate at 25–75% of the lung volume ($FEF_{25-75\%}$)
- Normally it is around 300 L/min
- This parameter indicates the patency of the smaller airways and therefore is affected in chronic obstructive lung disorders like bronchial asthma.

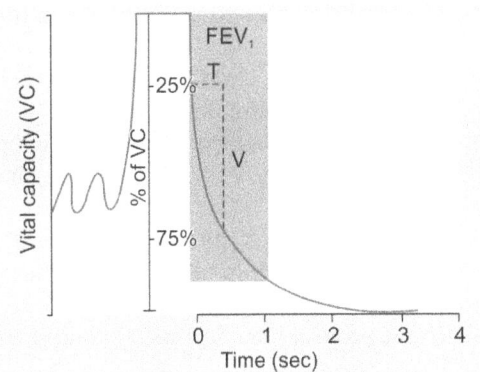

Fig. 20: Timed vital capacity in normal individuals. FEV1 is around 80% of FVC. The same recording can be used to calculate forced expiratory flow rate between 25 and 75% of expiratory flow with T as time and V as volume in the curve.

Timed Vital Capacity

- Timed vital capacity (TVC) or Forced vital capacity (FVC) is the maximum volume of air which has been breathed out as maximally, forcefully and rapidly as possible following a maximum inspiration. As it includes the words rapidly, time factor is included here. So, it is a dynamic lung volume and is divided into the following components:
- **FEV_1**: It is the volume of FVC forcefully breathed out in the first second of expiration and the normal value is 80% of FVC (refer **Fig. 20**).
- **FEV_2**: It is the volume of FVC forcefully breathed out in the first two seconds of expiration. Normal value is 95% of FVC.
- **FEV_3**: It is the volume of FVC forcefully breathed out in the first 3 seconds of exhalation. Normal value is 98–100% of FVC.
- In obstructive lung disorders, the vital capacity is normal but the FEV_1 is decreased.
- FEV_1 less than 72% is a definite indicator of obstructive lung disorder.

---

14. Trace the pathway for perception of fine touch.

- The posterior or dorsal column consists of the tracts of Goll and Burdach and they carry the fine touch sensation.

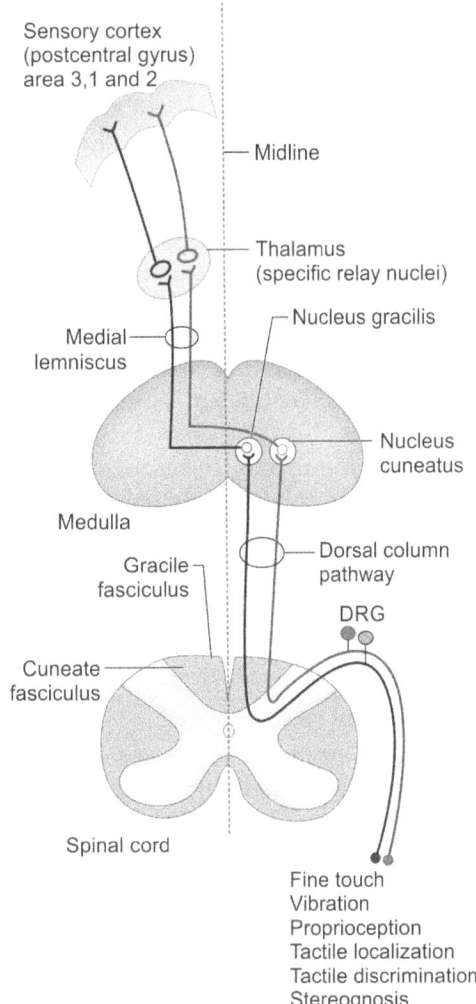

Fig. 21: Pathway of Dorsal column tract

- They ascend up in two fasciculi—fasciculus gracilus and fasciculus cuneatus
- They are made up of large myelinated fibers which carry sensations, such as touch, pressure, vibration, stereognosis, tactile localization, tactile discrimination and proprioception.
- Gracile fasciculus lies medially and carries these sensations from the hind limb and trunk, the cuneate fasciculus lies laterally and carries impulses from the upper half of the body and upper limbs.
- It is also called as the lemniscal system (refer **Fig. 21**)
- First order neurons have their cell bodies in the dorsal root ganglia.

- The peripheral axons of these neurons are nerve fibers from the receptors.
- The central axons from the dorsal root ganglia enter the spinal cord and ascend up in the dorsal column as the dorsal column tract.
- Gracile and cuneate fasciculi reach medulla and synapse with ipsilateral nucleus gracilis and nucleus cuneatus respectively.
- From these nuclei, the second order neurons arise and cross to the opposite side and ascend up as the medial lemniscus.
- Medial lemniscus terminates on the Ventroposterolateral nucleus (VPLN) of the opposite side thalamus.
- Third order neuron arises from the thalamus and terminates in the somatosensory area 1 (Broadmann's area 3, 1, 2) in post-central gyrus.

15. Operant conditioning.

- It is a reflex response to a stimulus, that previously elicited little or no response, acquired by repeatedly pairing the stimulus with another stimulus which normally produces a response.
- The stimulus that normally produces a response is the unconditioned stimulus (UCS) and the stimulus which elicits a response after pairing with UCS is the conditioned stimulus (CS)
- There are two types of conditioned reflexes—classical conditioning and operant conditioning.

Operant Conditioning

- It is a form of conditioning in which the animal is taught to do a task in order to obtain a reward or to avoid a punishment.
- UCS is the pleasant or unpleasant event and CS is light or an event which alerts the animal to do the task.
- For example, the animal kept in a skinner box where there is a lever and when the animal presses the lever it can escape an electric shock to its feet.
- The animal learns to avoid pressing the lever.
- This is called as conditioned avoidance reflex or negative reinforcement.
- Similarly in another experiment when the animal presses the lever it is provided with food pellet.
- Initially, it presses the lever accidentally and then it continues to do learning that it receives the food pellet.
- This is positive reinforcement of learning

16. Clinical features of cerebellar lesions.

- Patients with cerebellar lesion do not show much abnormalities when they are at rest.
- The symptoms are well established when they move.
- There is **no paralysis or sensory defects.**
- The effect of lesion is manifested on the same side of lesion
- But there is marked incoordination of movements—**Ataxia**.
- This is due to errors in rate, range, force and direction of movement.
- There is hypotonia.

Ataxia is expressed as:
- Instability during walking which is expressed as **drunken gait or wide-based gait**.
- There are also defects in skilled movements like **scanning of speech**.
- **Past pointing or dysmetria:** Attempting to touch an object with one finger results in overshooting to one side or the other. This is followed by correction of the overshoot which results in overshooting to the other side.
- Therefore, the finger oscillates back and forth resulting in **intention tremors**.
- It is called so as it is seen when the person attempts to do an action.
- The person with cerebellar lesion is unable to brake a movement or stop a movement. For example, in a normal person flexion of the forearm against resistance is kept in check when the resistance is suddenly released. But in a person with cerebellar lesion the patient is unable to brake the

movement and the forearm flies backward in an arc—**rebound phenomenon**.
- They also show the feature of **adiadochokinesia**—Inability to do rapid alternating opposite movements, such as repeated supination and pronation of the hands.
- They show **decomposition of movement**: The movements are dissected into individual components and carried out in each joint at a time.
- Defects in flocculonodular lobe (Vestibulocerebellum) results in **vertigo, nystagmus and motion sickness**.

17. Define muscle tone and discuss the phenomenon responsible for it. What conditions lead to alterations of tone?

- Muscle tone is the partially contracted state of the muscle at rest. It is the resistance offered by the muscle to stretching.
- All muscles exhibit a tone but it is more pronounced in the antigravity muscles. Therefore, it helps in maintaining body posture and equilibrium.
- It is due to stretch reflex which is integrated at the level of the spinal cord.
- There is a continuous asynchronous, low frequency discharge from the motor neurons in the anterior horn.
- The alpha motor neurons discharge continuously because of impulses coming from the muscle spindles present within the muscles.
- The muscle spindle is in turn stimulated by either stretching of the muscles or the gamma motor neurons discharge.

Stretch Reflex
- It is a monosynaptic reflex integrated at the level of spinal cord and helps in regulating the length of the muscle. The components of the reflex arc are:
- Stimulus—stretch of the muscle
- Receptor—muscle spindle
- Afferent nerve—Ia and II sensory fibers
- Center—spinal cord
- Efferent nerve—alpha motor nerve fiber
- Effector—extrafusal muscle fiber
- Response—contraction of extrafusal fibers (*refer* **Fig. 22**).
- Muscle tone is altered in UMN and LMN lesions.
- In UMN lesions, the inhibitory control of higher centers over the stretch reflex is removed and therefore there is hypertonia in the muscles.
- In LMN lesion, the final common pathway to the muscles is affected which results in hypotonia in the muscles.
- In cerebellar lesion there is hypotonia.

18. Endogenous opioid peptides.

- Presence of opioid receptors in the body has led to the search for endogenous opioids.
- There are precursors identified, which form opioid peptides.

The first one to be recognized is enkephalins:
- Met-enkephalin and Leu-enkephalin.
- They are found in the nerve endings of GIT and in brain. They are also present in substantia gelatinosa of spinal cord where gating of pain happens.

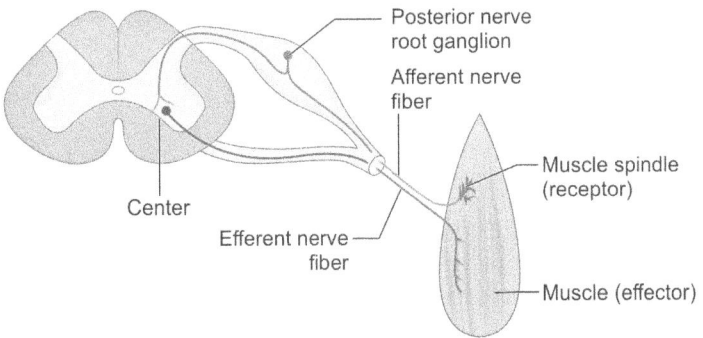

Fig. 22: Stretch reflex pathway.

- It is also present in the brainstem.
- They bind to the δ and μ opioid receptors

β-endorphin
- It is an opioid peptide and is a part of proopiomelanocortin produced from the anterior and intermediate lobe of pituitary gland.
- It has 31 amino acid residues.
- It is present in the brain and the blood coming from the pituitary gland.

The next precursor is prodynorphin:
- It contains **Dynorphins** and α and β **Neoendorphins.**
- Dynorphins are present in the duodenum, posterior pituitary and hypothalamus.
- **Neoendorphins** are also present in the hypothalamus.
- Endorphins bind only to μ receptors whereas other opioids bind to various receptors.

Effect of Stimulation of the Following Opioid Receptors

- **μ receptor:** They get activated on binding to opioids and results in activation of second messengers. This leads to K^+ conductance and thereby hyperpolarizes the neurons.
  Effects of stimulation: Analgesia, respiratory depression, constipation, euphoria, sedation, increased secretion of growth hormone and prolactin and miosis.
- **κ receptor:** It is bound by dynorphins. Activation of these receptors results in closure of Ca^{2+} channels.
  Effect of stimulation: Analgesia, diuresis, sedation, miosis and dysphoria.
- **δ receptor:** Bound by all the above types of opioids. Activation of these receptors results in closure of Ca^{2+} channels.

Effect of stimulation: Analgesia

---
19. Refractory errors of the eye.

- **Myopia—short-sightedness:** Eyeball may be elongated and therefore parallel rays of light from a distant object are brought to focus in front of the retina. It may be genetic or acquired. It can be corrected by using biconcave lenses. The lens diverges the light rays before they strike the cornea and then they are converged by the lens in the eye, so that the object is focused on the retina. It is the most common error of refraction (*refer* **Fig. 23**).
- **Hypermetropia—far-sightedness:** Here the parallel rays of light from a distant object are brought to focus behind the retina. It occurs due to decrease in anteroposterior diameter of the eye. It can be corrected by using biconvex lenses so that they converge the light rays before they fall on the cornea and therefore the light rays fall on the retina (*refer* **Fig. 23**).

Astigmatism

The problem here is the corneal surface is not spherical. One meridian of the cornea is different from the other. So, the parallel rays of light are not able to converge to a point of focus as there is unequal refraction from the different meridians. So, a blurred image is seen. It can be corrected using cylindrical lenses.

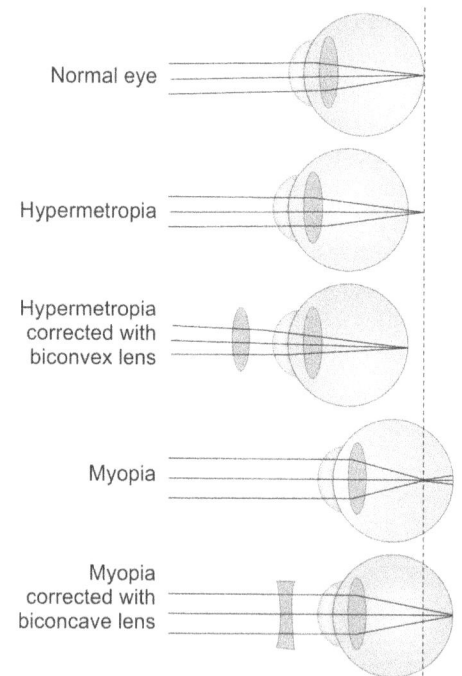

Fig. 23: Refractory errors with corrections. Hypermetropia is corrected with convex lens and myopia is corrected with concave lens.

Presbyopia

It is commonly seen in aged people above the age of 40 years.

The near point has receded beyond the normal reading distance due to loss of plasticity of lens. The loss of plasticity results in loss of accommodation property of the lens. It is corrected using convex lens for near work and plain glasses for far work and it is given as the bifocal lenses.

---

20. Discuss the phenomena by which sound waves in air induce action potentials in the cochlear nerve.

Conduction of Sound Waves

Sound waves travel in the air medium and enter the external ear, travel through the middle ear and reach the inner ear.

Conduction in External Ear

- External ear consists of the pinna and the external auditory meatus.
- Pinna collects the sound waves and passes it to the external auditory meatus. It helps in identifying the source of sound.
- The external auditory meatus funnels the sound towards the tympanic membrane at a high pressure.
- When the sound waves strike the tympanic membrane, it vibrates according to the frequency of the sound and stops promptly when the sound disappears. It is critically dampened.

Conduction in Middle Ear

- Middle ear has the 3 ossicles—malleus, incus and stapes.
- The manubrium of malleus is attached to the umbo of tympanic membrane.
- Head of malleus articulates with body of incus
- Long process of incus articulates with head of stapes.
- The footplate of stapes is attached to oval window (*refer* **Fig. 24**).
- As the sound waves hit the tympanic membrane, it vibrates and the vibration is transmitted to the ossicles and they vibrate as a single unit.
- The sound waves have been travelling in the air media and when they reach the inner ear it is transmitted to a fluid medium. This results in loss of sound energy by 30 db.
- This is prevented by the **impedance matching** mechanism in the middle ear.
- Impendence matching is done by the differences in surface area of the tympanic

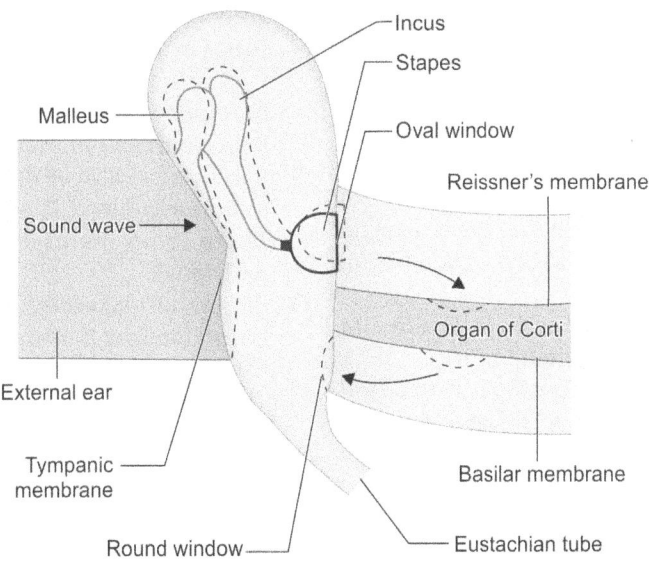

Fig. 24: Conduction of sound waves in the external, middle ear and internal ear. Dashed lines indicate the movement of structures following transmission of sound waves in the ear.

membrane and the membrane covering the oval window.
- Tympanic membrane surface area is much greater than the surface is of membrane covering the oval window. This helps in concentrating sound in a smaller area and thus amplifying it.
- Lever action of the ossicles also amplifies the sound. There is an overall increase in sound pressure by 28 folds.

Conduction in the Inner Ear
- The movement of the stapes vibrates the membrane covering the oval window.
- This creates a spreading wave in the perilymph in scala vestibuli of the cochlea.
- The wave is transmitted directly to perilymph in scala tympani.
- As the wave moves up the cochlea it reaches a maximum height and then drops off.
- The point in cochlea where it reaches a maximum height is dependent on the frequency of the sound detected.
- High pitched waves reach a maximum near the base of cochlea and the low frequency waves reach a maximum near the apex.
- The waves in the scala vestibuli cause the basilar membrane to vibrate.
- The movement of the basilar membrane makes the organ of Corti to move up and down.
- The tops of hair cells in organ of Corti are held rigid by the reticular lamina and the hairs of outer hair cells are embedded in the tectorial membrane.
- When the stapes moves due to sound transmission both membranes move in the same direction but they are hinged on different axes and this causes bending of the hairs.
- The hairs of inner hair cells are not attached to tectorial membrane.
- But it can be moved or bent by the fluid moving between the tectorial membrane and the hair cells.

Transduction of Sound Energy
- The hairs in the hair cells are arranged with taller hair in one end and smaller hairs in descending order.
- The largest hair is the kinocilium and the smaller ones are the stereocilia.
- When the smaller hairs bend towards the larger hairs there is depolarization of the hair cells and when the movement is in the opposite direction there is hyperpolarization of the cells.
- When the movement of basilar membrane moves the organ of Corti upwards and this causes lateral bending of stereocilia which results in depolarization.
- This is due to opening of K^+ channels in the hair cells due to the pull provided by the tip link protein.
- K^+ in the endolymph of scala media, the compartment in which the organ of Corti is placed, enters through the channel and depolarizes the hair cells.
- This result in release of the neurotransmitter, glutamate which stimulates the nerve fibers in the bases of hair cells and these nerves together form the cochlear branch of vestibulocochlear nerve.
- Now the electrical impulse travels through the VIII cranial nerve to the higher centers.

21. Hypersecretion of growth hormone.

Acromegaly
- It is a clinical condition due to excess secretion of growth hormone (GH) in adults (After the fusion of the epiphyseal plates in the long bones).
- It is usually due to a tumor of growth hormone producing cells (somatotrophs) in the anterior pituitary gland.
- Rarely, it can also be due to hypothalamic tumors secreting GH releasing hormone.
- There is no increase in height of the individual.
- But because of excess levels of GH, there is thickening of bones and proliferation of soft tissues like connective tissue and skin.
- This leads to coarse disfigured appearance. "Acro" means extremity and "megaly" is large.

Clinical Features of Acromegaly
- The tumor in the anterior pituitary compresses the optic chiasma resulting in visual disturbances.

- Enlargement of sella turcica and headache.
- Enlarging tumor may destroy other pituitary cells and decrease in levels of other hormones secreted from anterior pituitary may happen.

Clinical features due to excess GH levels:
- **Acromegalic face:** Jaw and cheek bones become more prominent, lips are thickened, nose is broad and thick, enlarged brows and coarse skin.
- **Prognathism:** Protrusion of the lower jaw due to elongation and thickening of mandible.
- Enlarged spade like hands, broad fingers and large feet.
- Body hair is increased
- **Kyphosis:** Since the vertebral bones continue to grow, the person has kyphosis.
- They develop osteoarthritis
- **Organomegaly:** Internal organs like heart, liver, spleen and kidneys are enlarged.
- High levels of GH decreases insulin sensitivity in the tissues and the patient has hyperglycemia and are prone to develop diabetes mellitus.

Gigantism

It is due to hypersecretion of GH in children before the closure of epiphysis.

Symptoms
- Abnormal height (7-8 ft tall)
- Enlarged hands and feet
- Gynecomastia
- Loss of libido
- Hyperglycemia which may result in diabetes mellitus
- They also have symptoms similar to acromegaly due to the compression of tumor on neighboring neural structure.

22. Tissue macrophage system.

- Monocytes are formed in the bone marrow. They circulate in blood for 10-20 hours.
- They are the largest blood cells, 12-20 μm in size (2-2.5 times the size of RBCs).
- Nucleus occupies almost 50% of the cell volume and the rest is the cytoplasm. The granules in cytoplasm do not take the regular staining and therefore not visible—so is an agranulocyte
- Monocytes after circulation, enter various tissues through the capillary membrane and swell up to become the macrophage.
- They live for months to years as a tissue **macrophage.**
- They exist as either fixed macrophages or mobile macrophage.
- The monocytes, macrophages and specialized endothelial cells in bone marrow, spleen and lymph nodes are grouped as **reticuloendothelial system**.
- They are destroyed once their phagocytic action is over.
- Tissue macrophages are named according to the sites where they are present.

Following are the tissue macrophages:

1. **Pulmonary alveolar macrophage (PAM):** The PAMs are present in the walls of the alveolus. It is one of the routes of entry of microbes from the environment. Macrophages phagocytose the microorganisms and if possible digests them and release them into the lymph.

2. **Kupffer cells in the liver sinusoids:** The other route of entry for microorganisms is through GIT. Bacteria absorbed from ingested food enters the portal circulation and reaches the liver and are phagocytosed and destroyed by Kupffer cells lining the sinusoids.

3. **Macrophages in the spleen and bone marrow:** Trabeculae of red pulp and sinuses of the spleen are lined by macrophages and they are very narrow passages and when blood squeezes through this path, unwanted debris and older cells like senile RBCs are phagocytosed and removed by the macrophages.

   In the bone marrow also there are macrophages to take care of microorganisms that enter through other routes of entry into the body.

4. **Tissue macrophages in skin and subcutaneous tissues (Histiocytes):**

Normally skin forms a protective barrier to prevent entry of microorganisms, but in case of break-age of the protective skin barrier infections may enter and they are taken care by the skin macrophages.
5. **Macrophages in lymph nodes:** There are macrophages in lymph nodes also.
6. **Osteoclasts:** Osteoclasts also belong to the family of monocytes and when they come in contact with stromal cells of bone marrow, they get converted to osteoclasts and they erode the bone and help in its remodeling.
7. **Microglia:** Microglia is a type of neuroglial cell and it belongs to the monocyte family and they have the property of scavenging foreign particles in the nervous system.

Functions of Monocyte-macrophage System

☐ Active phagocytosis, they are the second line of defense.
☐ They enter tissues to become macrophages. They are given different names in various tissues—Kupffer cells in liver, PAM in lungs, etc.
☐ They also take part in immune response (As APCs)
☐ They synthesize many substances like IL-1, TNF-α, lysozyme, proteases, etc.
☐ They also help in healing and repair of tissue.

---

23. Neural regulation of respiration.

Refer answer to Essay 4

---

24. Functions and tests of cerebellum.

Functions of Cerebellum

1. **Control of posture and equilibrium:**
   - Vestibulocerebellum or the flocculonodular lobe controls posture and equilibrium.
   - It receives inputs from vestibular apparatus directly and also through vestibular nuclei about position of head and body.
   - It sends efferents to vestibular nuclei from which the vestibulospinal tract arises to regulate posture.
   - Vestibulocerebellum is also concerned with regulating vestibulo-ocular reflex.

2. **Control of muscle tone and stretch reflex:**
   - Spinocerebellum influences the muscle tone through its output via fastigial nucleus which in turn controls the vestibulospinal and reticulospinal tract (arising from pontine reticular formation).
   - The major influence of cerebellum on tone is facilitatory.
   - Vestibulospinal tract is facilitatory to α motor neurons and reticulospinal tract is facilitatory to γ motor neurons.
   - Since control of cerebellum is on both α and γ motor neurons it has an important role in α-γ linkage.

3. **Control of voluntary movements:**
   - Paravermal portion of spinocerebellum controls skilled voluntary movements.
   - It does not initiate movements but it coordinates voluntary movements.
   - Coordination of movements is by regulating the time, rate, range, force and direction of movements.
   - All three functional divisions of the cerebellum work together as "comparator of servomechanism".

Comparator servomechanism:
   - Impulses for voluntary movements are planned and programmed in the premotor cortex and it is sequenced in primary motor area and the command to skeletal muscles is sent through the corticospinal tract.
   - A copy of the plan or intended movement is also sent to the spinocerebellum.
   - Cerebellum also gets feedback from the proprioceptors about the actual movement performed by the muscles and joints.
   - It also receives other sensory inputs from eye, ear and vestibular apparatus.
   - Now the cerebellum compares the intended movement and the executed movement along with other sensory inputs mentioned above.

- It thereby modifies appropriately the ongoing movement.
- If any corrections have to be done in programming of movements the error signals are sent to the motor cortex.

4. **Control of body movements of one side:**
   - Motor cortex of one side is connected to opposite cerebellum through a closed feedback loop; Cerebral-cerebellar-cerebral circuit, the cortico-ponto-dentato-thalamo-cortical pathway.
   - So each cerebellar hemisphere controls the opposite cerebral cortex.
   - But the corticospinal tract descending down from the motor cortex decussates in medulla and controls the opposite side of the body.
   - Since there is double decussation, it is that cerebellum controls same side of the body.

5. **Planning and programming of movements:** Cerebrocerebellum has extensive connections with motor cortex and therefore is involved in planning and programming of movements.

6. **Learning of skills:**
   - Cerebellum always tends to make changes in ongoing movements and therefore it improves by learning.
   - Another evidence is that there are increased activities in the climbing fibers when a new skill is learnt.
   - So cerebellum has a great role in learning skills.

7. **Eyeball movement:** Pyramis of cerebellum is concerned with eyeball movement.

Tests of Cerebellum

- **Finger-nose test:** The patient is asked to extend the hand and to bring the tip of his index finger and touch the tip of nose. He is asked to repeat it alternately with both the hands rapidly.
- **Adiadochokinesis:** Rapid and alternate pronation and supination of the forearm
- **Finger-to-finger test:** The patient is asked to bring his arms to the sides and then asked to bring the tips of index fingers together in front as an arc and to touch the tips.
- **Drawing a circle in air** with finger tip
- **Buttoning** and unbuttoning the shirt
- **Heel-knee test:** The subject is asked to place the heel of one leg on the knee of another leg and to move the heel along the medial side of the tibia.
- **Walking in straight line**

25. Transport across cell membrane.

The cell membrane, being a semipermeable one, does not allow all substances to pass through it.

It is easier for lipids and lipid-soluble substances to pass through the bilipid layer.

Water and water-soluble substances need channels/carriers to be transported across the membrane.

Substances on either side of the membrane differ in their concentrations also, therefore they either move along the gradients or against the gradients.

So transport across the cell membrane is classified as:
- Active transport
- Passive transport
- Vesicle-mediated transport

Passive Transport

Here the movement of substances is along the concentration or electrical gradient and there is no energy expenditure.

Types:
1. Simple diffusion
2. Facilitated diffusion
3. Osmosis
4. Filtration
5. Bulk flow
6. Solvent drag

Simple Diffusion

- **Lipid soluble** substances diffuse by dissolving in the membrane and diffuse to either side of membrane—O_2, N_2, steroids, etc.
- **Water-soluble** substances move through water filled channel proteins.
- No energy expenditure.
- Moves substances along concentration gradient

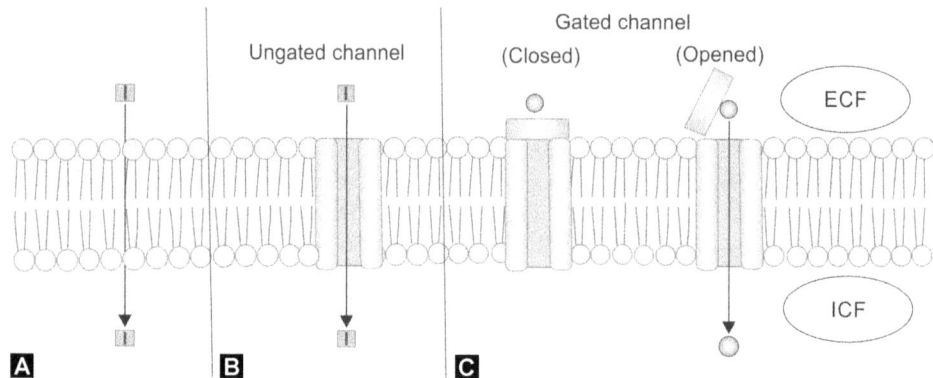

Figs. 25A to C: (A) Simple diffusion through lipid membrane; (B) Simple diffusion through nongated channels; (C) Diffusion through gated channels.

Diffusion Through Channels
- Channels are water-filled pores.
- This allows water-soluble substances to move across the membrane.
- The channels have selective permeability.
- They may be gated or nongated (*refer* **Figs. 25A to C**)
- Gates could be either change in—voltage, binding ligands or stretch (Mechanical).

Factors Affecting Net Diffusion
1. **Cell membrane permeability:**
   - *Thickness of membrane:* Inversely proportional
   - *Lipid solubility:* Directly proportional
   - Distribution of protein channels in membrane
   - *Temperature:* Directly proportional
   - *Size of molecule:* Inversely proportional
   - *Area of membrane:* Directly proportional
2. **Concentration gradient—directly proportional**
3. **Electrical gradient**
4. **Pressure gradient—directly proportional**

Facilitated Diffusion
- Large water-soluble substances (e.g., glucose) are carried by a protein which changes configuration on binding (*refer* **Fig. 26**).
- This change in configuration shifts the molecule in or out.
- Highly selective and specific
- **Types:**
  - Uniport
  - Symport
  - Antiport

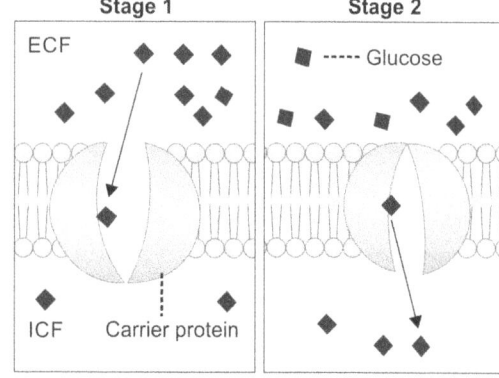

Fig. 26: Facilitated diffusion. A uniport transporting glucose molecules.

- **Characteristics:**
  - Specificity
  - Saturation
  - Competition

Osmosis
Diffusion of water or other solvent molecules through a semipermeable membrane (i.e., membrane impermeable to solute and not to solvent) from a solution containing lower concentration of solutes to the solution containing higher concentration of solutes—**Osmosis**.

Filtration and Bulk Flow
Filtration or movement of water and solutes through the capillary wall are examples of filtration.

If filtration involves movement of greater volume of water it is called bulk flow.

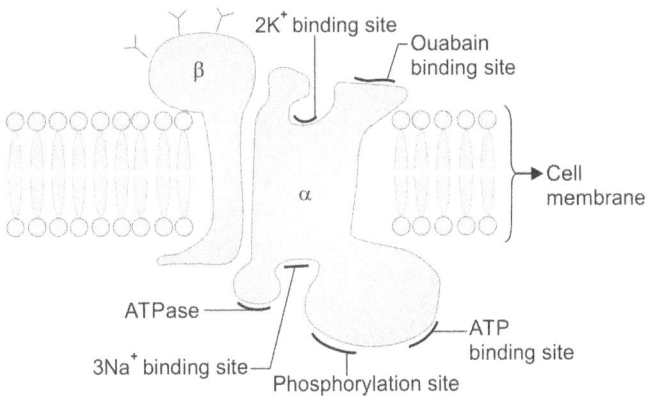

Fig. 27: Sodium-potassium pump; primary active transporter.

Solvent Drag

During bulk flow if solvents are carried along—solvent drag.

Active Transport

- It is also carrier mediated
- Moves substances uphill against concentration gradient.
- So associated with energy expenditure. Energy is derived from ATP, either directly or indirectly
- **Types:**
  - Primary active transport
  - Secondary active transport

Primary Active Transport

Here substances are moved uphill across the cell membrane with the help of pumps. It involves energy expenditure which is directly derived from break down of ATP.

Example:

- Na^+- K^+ Pump (*refer* **Fig. 27**)
- H^+-K^+ Pump
- Ca^{++} ATPase

Secondary Active Transport

In the secondary active transport, the substances are moved against the concentration gradient with the help of energy derived indirectly from the ATP. Na^+- K^+ pump, when it pumps out Na^+ from the cell, creates a concentration gradient for Na^+ into the cell. This gradient for Na^+ is utilized for movement of other ions across the cell membrane. So, the transporters of secondary active transport move Na^+ in exchange (Sodium counter-transporter) or along (Sodium cotransporter) with another molecule (both organic and inorganic substances).

Example:

- Na^+—Glucose symport
- Na^+—Amino acid symport
- Na^+—H^+ exchanger
- Na^+—Ca^{++} exchanger (*refer* **Fig. 28**)

Vesicle-mediated Transport

- Large polar molecules—like protein hormones in endocrine glands are transported across the cell as membrane wrapped vesicles.
- **Types:**
  - Endocytosis
  - Exocytosis

Endocytosis

It is the process by which substances are internalized within the cell. There are 3 types:

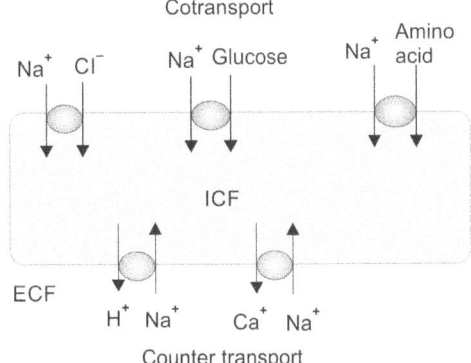

Fig. 28: Secondary active transporters; Na^+—Glucose symporter, Na^+ Amino acid symport, Na^+-H^+ exchanger, Na^+- Ca^{2+} exchanger.

1. Phagocytosis
2. Pinocytosis
3. Receptor-mediated endocytosis

1. **Phagocytosis:** Engulfing of solid substances (Cell eating) as that of microorganisms by the neutrophils
2. **Pinocytosis:** Engulfing the liquid components (Cell drinking)
3. **Receptor-mediated endocytosis:** Here the substances to be internalized get attached to a receptor protein present on the cell membrane and the whole complex is engulfed.

Exocytosis

It is the process by which substance are extruded from the cell. It is the reversal of endocytosis. The substances to be extruded are in the vesicle which moves towards the cell membrane and gets attached to the membrane and is later pinched out of the cell.

26. Ovarian and endometrial changes of menstrual cycle.

Ovarian Changes During the Menstrual Cycle

There are 3 phases of ovarian changes during the cycle.

They are:
1. Follicular phase
2. Ovulatory phase
3. Luteal phase

Follicular Phase
- In the female fetus, at the time of birth there are many primordial follicles. Inside each follicle there is an immature ovum.
- At the start of each menstrual cycle 6–12 primordial follicles start to grow in size and mature.
- This is due to the increase of FSH and LH release from the anterior pituitary gland. FSH levels are more than LH levels.
- After 5–7 days, one follicle continues to grow and mature (Dominant follicle), while the other follicles start to degenerate and undergoes atretic changes.
- The follicle, which will mature and become dominant, will be based on the ability of it to secrete estrogen.

Changes happening in the maturing follicle are:
- Ovum inside the follicle grows in size and the surrounding granulosa cells multiply in number—**Primary follicle**
- Outer to the granulosa cell layer, spindle-shaped cells in the interstitium of the ovary develop into theca cells. They get differentiated to theca interna and theca externa cells—**Preantral follicle**.
- The granulosa and the theca cells start secreting estrogen. Granulosa cells secrete a follicular fluid which gets accumulated as the antrum—**Early antral follicle**
- Till this phase, growth of the follicle is due to high levels of FSH. The FSH and estrogen together increase the LH receptors on the granulosa cells.
- As estrogen levels in the follicle increase, follicular growth is increased at a greater rate. The antrum increases in size and ovum also enlarges. The ovum is pushed to one pole surrounded by granulosa cells—**Mature graffian follicle**.
- Mature follicle reaches the size of 1 to 1.5 cm.
- The cycle reaches the 14th day.

Ovulatory Phase
- In a female with a 28 days cycle, ovulation occurs on the 14th day.
- Just before ovulation, outer wall of the follicle swells and a small protrusion, the stigma is seen.
- After a few minutes a fluid starts oozing out followed by the release of ovum along with the corona radiata around it.

Hormonal changes:
- Two days before ovulation, estrogen levels increase and there is a positive feedback regulation of estrogen on LH secretion.
- LH levels reach 6–10 times the normal value and peaks 10–12 hours before ovulation.
- High LH levels are essential for the final growth, maturation and ovulation.
- LH acts on the granulosa cells to increase progesterone secretion.

This causes:
- Theca externa cells to release proteolytic enzymes from lysosomes, which will

dissolve the follicular capsule and degeneration of stigma.
- Blood vessels grow rapidly into the follicle and prostaglandins are secreted into the follicle.
- Both these events cause the follicle to swell and break the stigma and release the ovum.

Luteal Phase
- As soon as the follicle is ruptured and ovum released, the follicle is filled with blood—**corpus hemorrhagicum.**
- The granulosa and theca cells are laden with fat droplets and are luteinized, the cells are now in yellow color—**corpus luteum**.
- LH induces luteinization of the follicle and favors its hormonal function.
- The corpus luteum starts producing estrogen and progesterone, progesterone levels are more than estrogen levels.
- Corpus luteum continues to grow for the next 7-8 days.
- High estrogen and progesterone levels negatively inhibit the LH and FSH secretion from anterior pituitary.
- Also, inhibin released from corpus luteum inhibits FSH secretion.
- If ovum is not fertilized, as the FSH and LH levels decrease, by 26th day of the cycle, the corpus luteum completely involutes and becomes a scar tissue—**corpus albicans**.
- As corpus luteum regresses, estrogen and progesterone levels decrease suddenly and the inhibition on FSH and LH is removed. FSH and LH levels start rising and a new set of follicles start developing and the next cycle starts.
- If the ovum is fertilized, corpus luteum continues to secrete progesterone under the influence of hCG till the placenta takes over the secretion of progesterone.

Changes in the Uterine Endometrium

The uterine changes are given in 3 phases:
1. Proliferative phase
2. Secretory phase
3. Menstrual phase

Proliferative Phase
This phase correlates with follicular phase of ovarian cycle. Estrogen secreted from the follicle stimulates growth of uterine endometrium and therefore it thickens. Glands in the endometrium and the blood vessels grow. This phase is from day 5 till the day of ovulation.

Secretory Phase
This phase is from day of ovulation to 25th day. It correlates with the luteal phase of the ovarian cycle. Progesterone levels are high and they make the endometrium secretory by acting on the glands. Maximum action is 5-7 days after ovulation. The secretion is rich in glycogen and can nourish the fertilized ovum. Secretory endometrium is favorable for implantation of fertilized ovum.

If fertilization does not happen the corpus luteum starts to regress and the progesterone and estrogen levels drop. Withdrawal of hormonal support of the endometrium and release of prostaglandins result in vasoconstriction of the spiral arteries, uterine ischemia happens and endometrial necrosis and shedding of endometrium happens

Menstrual Phase
It starts with the menstrual bleeding with the shedding of outer 2/3rd of endometrium, unfertilized ovum and continues for 5 days.

27. Brown-Sequard syndrome.

Hemisection of spinal cord is called Brown-Sequard syndrome. It involves lesion of one lateral half of spinal cord.

Following injury to the spinal cord there are these following stages:
1. Stage of spinal shock
2. Stage of reflex activity
3. Stage of reflex failure

Immediately after the lesion, there is complete loss of function below the level of lesion. This happens because of sudden removal of impulses from higher centers.

The symptoms of Brown-Sequard are seen in the second stage. Symptoms are explained as the features above the level of lesion, at the level and below the level of lesion, on the same side and opposite side of lesion.

	Sensory		Motor	
	Same side	Opposite side	Same side	Opposite side
Above the level of lesion	Small area of hyperesthesia	Normal	Normal	Normal
At the level of lesion	Complete loss of sensation (anesthesia)	Not affected	Lower motor neuron type of paralysis	Not affected
Below the level of lesion	Damage to dorsal column fibers: Loss of fine touch, tactile localization, two-point discrimination, vibration sense, stereognosis and position sense	Damage to lateral and anterior spinothalamic tract: Loss of pain, temperature and crude touch sensations. All other sensations are intact	Upper motor neuron type of paralysis as the inhibition from higher centers is removed. Temporary loss of vasomotor tone	Not usually affected

28. Oxygen dissociation curve.

- This curve compares the partial pressure of O_2 and % saturation of Hb with O_2.
- It is sigmoid in shape.
- The shape is sigmoid because of the change in configuration of hemoglobin from T to R state and therefore there is gradual increase in affinity for O_2 and then it gets saturated.
- It has a steep and plateau phase (refer Fig. 29).
- About 90% saturation of Hb takes place at a PO_2 of 60 mm Hg.
- P_{50} is the partial pressure at which 50% of the hemoglobin is saturated with oxygen.
- P_{50} is inversely related to the affinity of hemoglobin for oxygen.
- The **steep phase** denotes the unloading zone where even a minimum drop in PO_2 results in unloading of large amounts of oxygen to the tissues.
- The **plateau phase** denotes the loading zone, where O_2 is taken up by hemoglobin in the lungs and once all the four sites in Hb are loaded with O_2 there is no further uptake and thereby a plateau phase is reached.
- The curve gets shifted to right are left in conditions of decreased or increase in affinity of hemoglobin for O_2 respectively.

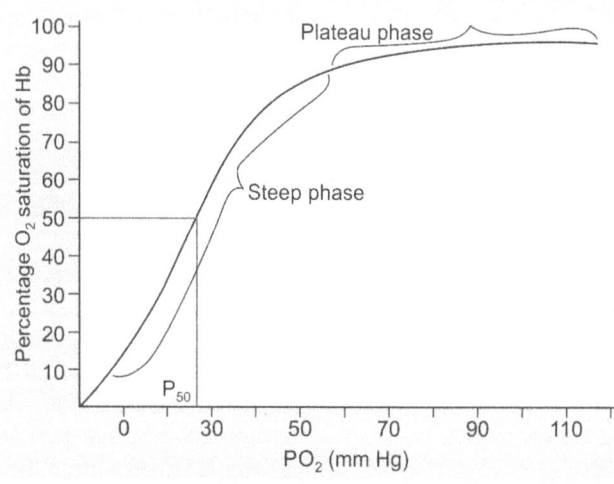

Fig. 29: Oxygen-hemoglobin dissociation curve. P_{50} is the partial pressure of O_2 at which 50% of hemoglobin is saturated with O_2. It is around 27 mm Hg. There are two phases—steep phase and plateau phase.

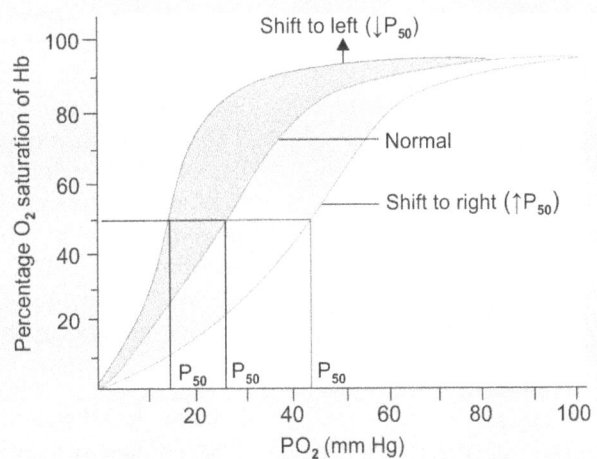

Fig. 30: Right and left shift of O_2-Hb dissociation curve. P_{50}, PO_2 at which hemoglobin is 50% saturated is 27 mm Hg. Right shift denotes decrease in hemoglobin affinity for O_2 and left shift increased affinity for O_2.

Conditions where O_2-Hb dissociation curve is shifted to right:
- Hypoxia
- ↑PCO_2
- ↑temperature
- ↑2,3-DPG levels in RBC
- ↑H^+ concentration (Acidosis)

Conditions where O_2-Hb dissociation curve is shifted to left:
- High PO_2
- Low PCO_2
- Low body temperature
- Presence of fetal hemoglobin
- Alkalosis
- Low 2,3-DPG levels in RBC (refer **Fig. 30**)
- Carbon monoxide poisoning

III. SHORT ANSWERS

1. Membrane transporters involved in clearance of calcium from cytoplasm.

- Ca^{2+} transporters to clear Ca^{2+} from cytoplasm of a cell is by the following transporters in the cell membrane— Ca^{2+}-H^+ ATPase and Na^+-Ca^{2+} exchanger.
- Ca^{2+} ATPase is the transporter on the sarcoplasmic reticulum membrane in skeletal muscles to pump back Ca^{2+} into SR resulting in muscle relaxation.

2. Concentrations of sodium and potassium in intra- and extracellular fluids.

	Intracellular concentration (mmol/L of H_2O)	Extracellular concentration (mmol/L of H_2O)
Na^+	15	150
K^+	150	5.5

3. Phenomena involved in the act of swallowing.

Deglutition is a reflex response integrated in the medulla in nucleus tractus solitarius and nucleus ambiguus.

There are 3 phases:
1. Oral or voluntary phase
2. Pharyngeal or involuntary phase
3. Esophageal phase

Oral Phase

The tongue forms a bolus of food and pushes it to the oropharynx by pushing up and against the hard palate.

Pharyngeal Phase

- It starts when food enters the pharynx.
- Soft palate elevated and closes nasopharynx
- Larynx rises, vocal cords approximate and epiglottis closes laryngeal opening

- Deglutition apnea follows.
- Palatopharyngeal folds approximate for selective material to move out.
- Cricopharyngeus relaxes and bolus enters upper esophagus.

Esophageal Phase

- There are 2 sphincters in the esophagus—UES and LES.
- UES is formed by cricopharyngeus muscle. It opens reflexly after the beginning of swallow.
- Food on reaching esophagus is pushed into the stomach by peristalsis—primary and secondary peristalsis.
- Primary peristalsis is initiated by swallowing, coordinated by vagus nerve.
- Secondary peristalsis is initiated by food in the esophagus and it sweeps the food, coordinated by intrinsic nerves.

4. Role of ATP in relaxation of muscle.

- After the cross-bridge cycling of the energized head of myosin, the head stays attached to actin molecule.
- For the head to get detached another molecule of ATP has to get attached to the myosin head so that the head is removed from the attachment site.
- The final relaxation happens after the cytoplasmic Ca^{2+} is decreased by pumping the Ca^{2+} into the sarcoplasmic reticulum.
- This is done by the primary active transporter Ca^{2+} - ATPase.
- A single molecule of ATP is broken to provide energy for the pumping of Ca^{2+} into SR.

5. Draw a schematic diagram of the sarcomere and label its components.

See **Fig. 31**.

6. Opsonins.

- Opsonins are chemical substances which coat the microorganisms and make it tastier for phagocytosis by the neutrophils or macrophages.
- Complementary protein C3b and the immunoglobulin IgG are opsonins.

Sarcomere at rest

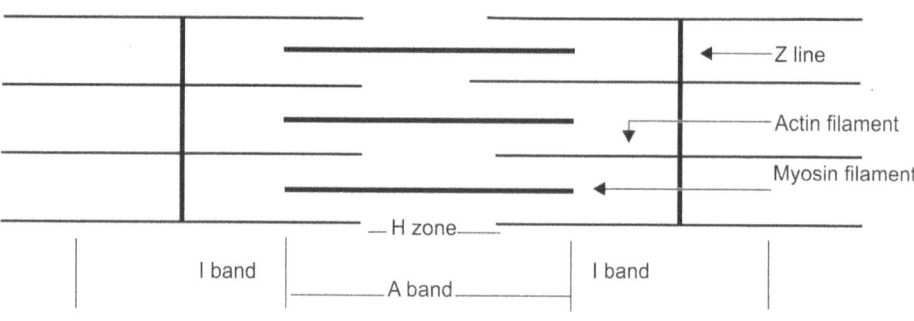

Sarcomere during contraction

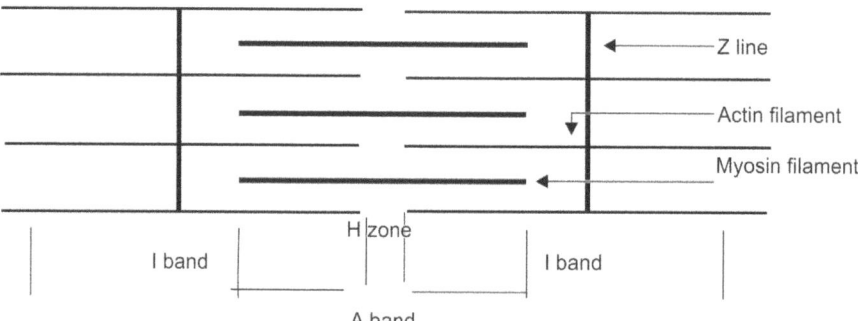

Fig. 31: Structure of sarcomere.

7. Cells which express major histocompatibility complex II.

MHC II proteins are present in the antigen presenting cells like macrophages, dendritic cells and B cells and activated T cells.

8. Significance of glycosylated hemoglobin.

- There are small amounts of hemoglobin A derivatives closely associated with hemoglobin A that represent glycated hemoglobin.
- One of these is hemoglobin A_{1c} (HbA_{1c}). It has a glucose attached to the terminal valine in each β chain and is of special interest because its quantity increases in poorly controlled diabetes mellitus.
- It gives an idea about the average blood glucose levels for the past 3 months.

9. Name 4 enzymes in pancreatic secretion.

- Trypsin, chymotrypsin, carboxypeptidase—proteolytic enzymes
- Pancreatic amylase—enzyme for digesting carbohydrates

10. Hormonal imbalance causing (a) acromegaly (b) cretinism.

- **Acromegaly:** Hypersecretion of growth hormone in adults after the fusion of epiphysis
- **Cretinism:** Hypothyroidism in children

11. List the types of shock.

Types of Shock
- Hypovolemic shock
- Distributive shock
- Cardiogenic shock
- Obstructive shock

12. Define preload and state its effect on cardiac function.

- Preload is the tension developed in the muscle before the muscle starts contracting. In cardiac muscle, the initial muscle length is the **preload** (the extent to which the muscle is stretched before contraction).
- Preload is decided by the **end-diastolic volume (EDV)**.
- EDV is decided by the **venous return**.
- According to Frank-Starling's law "**Within physiological limits, the force of contraction is directly proportional to the initial length of the muscle**".
- Therefore preload is directly proportional to stroke volume and to cardiac output.

13. Baroreceptor reflex.

Baroreceptors
- There are two types of baroreceptors (BRs). High pressure and low-pressure baroreceptors.
- High pressure BRs are present in the carotid and aortic sinuses (*refer* **Fig. 32**).
- Low pressure BRs are present in the great veins, right and left atria.
- High pressure BRs are there to monitor and correct the day-to-day change in BP as in change of posture from supine to standing position.
- They regulate BP maximally when the MAP is between 70–110 mm Hg and stops firing when MAP falls <40 or rises above 150 mm Hg.

The Reflex
- Most important reflex to regulate BP
- Also called as sinoaortic reflex
- Receptor—carotid and aortic sinuses
- Stimulus—stretch of baroreceptors (as in increased BP)
- Afferents—IXth (supplies carotid sinus) and Xth cranial nerves (aortic sinus)

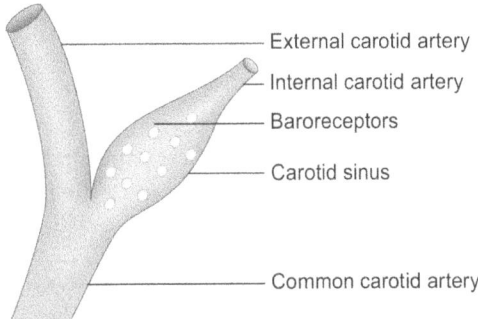

Fig. 32: Baroreceptor—carotid sinus.

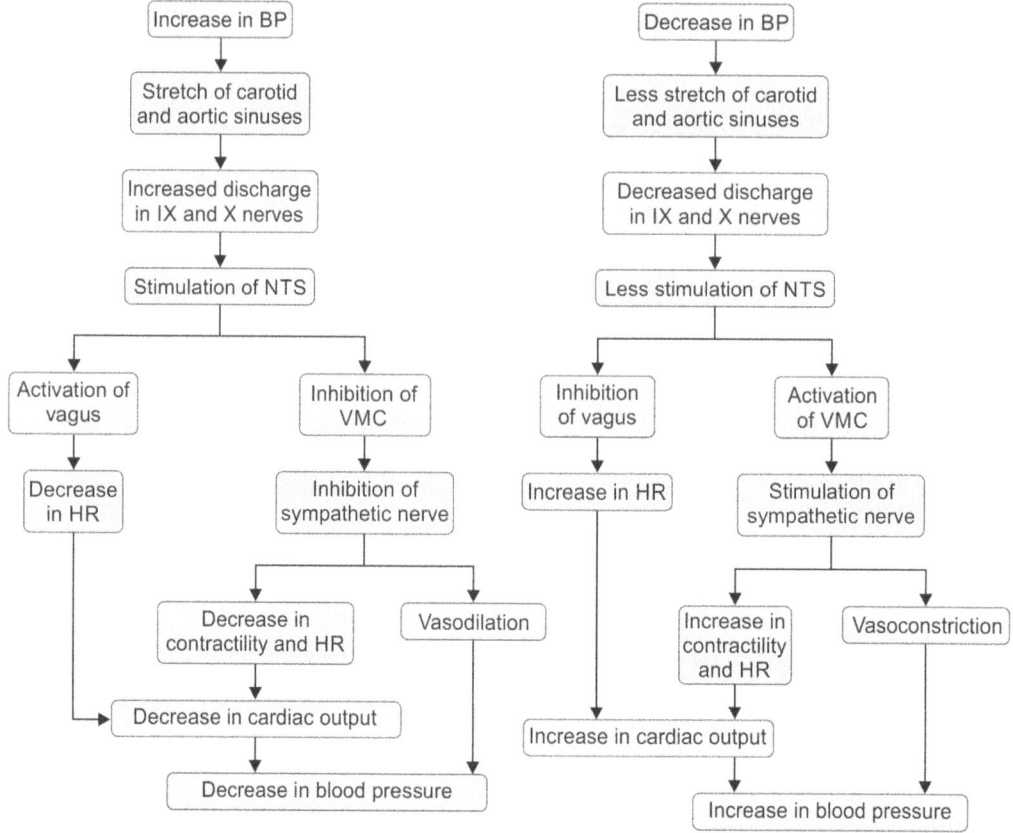

Fig. 33: Regulation of BP by baroreceptors.

- Efferents—sympathetic nerves and vagus nerve
- Effector—heart and blood vessels
- Response—decrease in BP (*refer* Fig. 33).

14. What is myocardial infarction? State one ECG change in this condition.

- Myocardial infarction (MI) is myocardial cell death due to ischemia. It happens when the ischemia is prolonged and the obstruction of coronary vessels is more than 75%.

ECG Change in MI

- The most significant ECG change in MI is elevation of the ST segment in the leads overlying the infarct.

15. Role of myelin sheath in conduction of nerve impulse.

- Myelin sheath is present outside axolemma
- In peripheral nervous system, it is formed by Schwann cells.
- In CNS by oligodendrocytes
- Initially axons near the Schwann cells invaginate into its membrane.
- This forms Mesaxon. This winds around many times with lipids in between—Myelin sheath.
- Outside this a thin layer of Schwann cell cytoplasm—Neurilemma is present.
- Along the axon, Schwann cells surround for 1 mm.
- In between two wrappings of Schwann cells is the nodes of Ranvier
- The myelin sheath acts as an insulator and prevents transmission of impulse across it
- But in the nodes of Ranvier the voltage-gated sodium channels are concentrated more in number (2000–12000 per square micrometer of the membrane)

- Conduction of action potentials happens in the form of circular currents (current sinks).
- In unmyelinated neurons these current sinks happen in the neighboring parts of the membrane and therefore the conduction of impulse is slower.
- In the myelinated neurons since the myelin sheath acts as an insulator and the nodes of Ranvier are concentrated with voltage-gated sodium channels are concentrated the impulses jumps from one node to the other node. This type of conduction is said to be **saltatory conduction**.
- It is a faster conduction and myelinated nerves conduct impulses 50 times faster than the unmyelinated nerve fibers.
- The other factors which affect the conduction of impulses are the thickness or the diameter of the nerve and the temperature.
- As the diameter increases, the resistance to flow of axoplasmic current is less and therefore impulse transmission is faster in large diameter nerves.
- Temperature is directly proportional to conduction velocity.

16. Conditions where plantar response is 'extensor'.

Normal response to plantar reflex is plantar flexion of big toe and flexion and adduction of other toes.

Babinski's Sign

- It is an extensor plantar response. There is dorsiflexion of big toe and abduction and dorsiflexion of other toes.
- It is seen infants in physiological conditions and in upper motor neuron lesion, especially corticospinal tract lesion in pathological conditions.

17. Finding in Weber's test in conduction deafness of the left side.

- Weber's test is a tuning fork test.
- Here the base of the vibrating tuning fork is placed on the vertex or in the forehead.
- In normal conditions the subject hears equally in both the ears through bone conduction.
- In conduction deafness, on placing the tuning fork sounds are heard better in the deaf ear due to the absence of masking sounds.

18. Muscle actions responsible for (a) normal expiration (b) forced expiration.

- Muscles involved in normal expiration—normal expiration happens by passive recoil of the lungs. There is no muscle action during normal expiration.
- Muscles involved in forced expiration—anterior abdominal wall muscles and the internal intercostal muscles.

19. Oxygen carrying capacity of blood.

- Oxygen is carried in blood in two forms—dissolved form and as oxyhemoglobin.
- The maximum amount of oxygen that can be carried by hemoglobin is called as the oxygen carrying capacity of blood
- **O_2 transported as oxyhemoglobin**—1.34 mL of O_2 is carried by each gram of hemoglobin. In an average adult, 15 g of hemoglobin is present in each deciliter of blood.
- Therefore 1.34 × 15 = 20.1 mL of blood is carried in 100 mL of arterial blood. So 20.1 mL/100 mL of O_2 is the O_2 carrying capacity of blood.

20. Hypoxic vasoconstriction—where does it occur and what are its complications?

- Hypoxic vasoconstriction is seen in the pulmonary arteries.
- In systemic arteries hypoxia induces vasodilatation and thereby increases blood flow to remove the hypoxic stimulus.
- Hypoxic vasoconstriction diverts the blood flow from under ventilated airways towards normal alveoli. Hypoxia directly causes contraction of vascular smooth muscles.

21. Permissive action of hormone.

Cortisol amplifies effects of certain processes of other hormones where it does not act directly.

Example:
- It does not induce glycogenolysis by itself but augments glycogenolysis by glucagon.
- It also augments vaso-responsiveness of blood vessels to catecholamines.
- Lipolytic actions of catecholamine is possible only in the presence of cortisol
- Thyroid hormone is essential for inducing the growth promoting effects of growth hormone.

22. Role of vitamin D in calcium homeostasis.

- Vitamin D has a potent effect in increasing the blood calcium levels. Vitamin D by itself does not increase blood calcium levels.
- It gets converted to 1,25-dihydroxycholecalciferol in the skin, liver and kidneys.
- 1,25-Dihydroxycholecalciferol or calcitriol is the active form of vitamin D.

Actions of Calcitriol
- It acts in the intestines to increase absorption of calcium from ingested food. It acts by inducing the calcium binding protein on the intestinal cells and thereby transports calcium from intestinal lumen to the cell cytoplasm. It also increases activity of Ca^{2+} stimulated ATPase in the brush border of cell membrane.
- It decreases Ca^{2+} excretion through the kidneys by stimulating reabsorption of Ca^{2+} from the renal tubules.
- It also plays an important role in both bone resorption and deposition of calcium.

23. Contraception in males.

Temporary Methods
- Natural method
- Barrier method
- Pills

Natural Method or Coitus Interruptus
Withdrawal of penis before ejaculation prevents deposition of semen in the vagina. This method needs practice and timing is very important. The disadvantages are that the precoital secretions may contain sperms and it can lead to pregnancy.

Barrier Method
Condoms are the widely used barrier method in males. It is made of fine latex sheet. It prevents deposition of semen in the vagina and prevents fertilization of ovum. It can be used to prevent transmission of sexually transmitted diseases.

Pills
- Drugs are used to inhibit spermatogenesis.
- Gossypol and testosterone are used.
- **Gossypol:** It is derived from cottonseed oil. It decreases sperm count.
- **Testosterone:** High testosterone levels inhibit sperm production.

Permanent Methods

Vasectomy: A small portion of vas deferens is removed after clamping. Both the open ends are ligated and sutured.

24. Corpus luteum.

- On the 14th day of the menstrual cycle after the release of ovum from the graafian follicle the inside of the follicle is filled with blood—***Corpus hemorrhagicum***
- The granulosa and the thecal cells of the follicle proliferate and the clotted blood is replaced with yellowish lipid rich luteal cells forming the ***corpus luteum***. Following this starts the luteal phase of menstrual cycle. The luteal cells start secreting estrogen and progesterone.
- If pregnancy occurs, the corpus luteum persists and continues to produce progesterone which is essential for the survival of the fetus. Its function is maintained by hCG secreted from trophoblasts.
- If fertilization has not occurred the corpus luteum regresses and degenerates 4 days before the next menstrual cycle. Gradually it is replaced by a scar tissue—***Corpus albicans***.

Functions of Corpus Luteum
- Corpus luteum secretes estrogen and progesterone during the luteal phase of menstrual cycle.

- The progesterone secreted from the corpus luteum prepares the endometrium for the implantation of the fertilized ovum.
- On fertilization of the ovum, the corpus luteum continues to secrete progesterone till the placenta takes over the function of secreting progesterone.

25. Vitamin K dependent clotting factors.

- Vitamin K is a cofactor for the enzyme which catalyzes conversion of glutamic acid residues to—γ carboxyglutamic acid residues in the liver.
- Six clotting factors, synthesized in the liver, require the conversion of glutamic acid to γ carboxyglutamic acid.
- They are factors—II, VII, IX and X, and protein C and S.

26. Atonic bladder.

- Atonic bladder is due to deafferentation of the bladder.
- Destruction of the afferent nerves to bladder results in inhibition of impulses from the bladder due to stretching of the bladder while it is getting filled.
- Loss of afferent impulses results in absence of micturition reflex.
- All bladder reflexes are lost in spite of intact efferent control to bladder.
- Instead of emptying of bladder it gets filled to its capacity and there is overflow dribbling of urine.
- It happens in tabes dorsalis and crush injury to spinal cord.

27. Functions of skin.

- It forms a **protective covering** for the body and prevents entry of microorganisms and other toxic substances from the environment.
- Helps in **body temperature regulation:** Evaporation of sweat from skin and the loss of water by insensible perspiration help in temperature regulation.
- It is the **largest sensory organ** in the body as it has many receptors in the skin and hair follicle.
- **Synthesis of 1,25-dihydroxycholecalciferol** By the action of sunlight on the skin 7-dehydrocholesterol is formed from vitamin D. It is the precursor for 1,25-dihydroxycholecalciferol.
- **Protects the body from U-V radiations** due to the presence of melanin pigment.
- It is a form of **innate immunity** and thereby provides resistance against infections.

28. Secondary active transport.

- In secondary active transport, substances are moved against the concentration gradient with the help of energy derived indirectly from ATP. Na$^+$- K$^+$ pump, when it pumps out 3 Na$^+$ from the cell, creates a concentration gradient for Na$^+$ influx into the cell.
- This inward gradient of Na$^+$ is utilized for movement of other ions across the cell membrane.
- So the transporters of secondary active transport moves Na$^+$ in exchange (Sodium counter-transporter) or along (Sodium cotransporter) with another molecule (both organic and inorganic substances).

Ex.
- Na$^+$- Glucose symport (*refer* **Fig. 34**)
- Na$^+$- Amino acid symport
- Na$^+$- H$^+$ exchanger
- Na$^+$- Ca^{++} exchanger

29. Motor unit.

- Motor unit is a single motor neuron with all its branches and all the muscle fibers supplied by it.
- The size of the motor unit is decided by the muscle fibers supplied by it (*refer* **Fig. 35**).
- The ones which supply the intrinsic muscles of the hand supply only less than

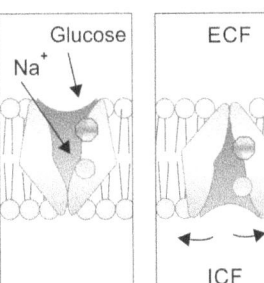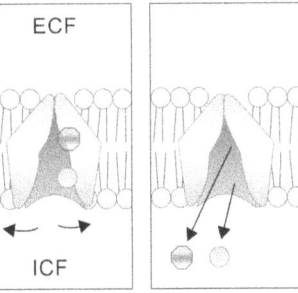

Fig. 34: Na$^+$—Glucose symport, a secondary active transporter.

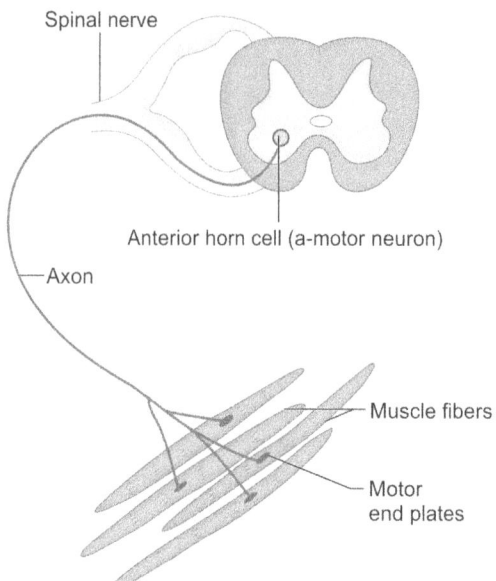

Fig. 35: Motor unit.

10 fibers and produce less tension but the ones which supply back muscles are large motor units and have hundreds of fibers.
❐ All the muscle fibers in a single motor unit are of the same type, i.e., either oxidative type or glycolytic type.
❐ Based on this, the motor units may be classified as either oxidative or slow and glycolytic or fast motor units.

30. Refractory period.

❐ Following the development of action potential in a part of the membrane, the same area does not respond to a second stimulus.
❐ Refractory period is defined as the length of time during which the membrane does not respond to a second stimulus. They are of two types—absolute and relative refractory periods.
 • **Absolute refractory period:** It is the time period in action potential during which no stimulus, no matter how strong and how ever long given, does not excite the membrane. In nerve action potential it corresponds to the period from the time the firing level is reached until the repolarization is 1/3rd completed.
 • **Relative refractory period:** During relative refractory period stronger than normal stimuli can cause excitation. It falls between the end of relative refractory period to the start of after-depolarzation.

31. Heart sounds.

Refer **Fig. 36**.

Heart sounds	Events responsible	Duration	Frequency	Others
First sound (S_1)	Due to vibrations set by sudden closure of AV valves at the onset of ventricular systole	0.15 sec	25–45 Hz In PCG recorded as 9–13 waves	Soft and long, heard as "LUBB"
Second sound (S_2)	Associated with closure of aortic and pulmonary valves after the end of ventricular systole	0.12 sec	50 Hz In PCG recorded as 4–6 waves	Normally S2 can be split due to early closure of aortic valve, heard as "Dup"
Third sound (S_3)	Is heard at 1/3rd of diastole due to rapid filling of ventricle due to vibrations set by inrush of blood		0.1 sec In PCG recorded as 1–4 waves	Normally audible only in children and young adults
Fourth sound (S_4)	Heard just before (S_1) Occurs during atrial contraction Due to ventricular filling		20 cyc/sec In PCG recorded as 1–2 waves	Rarely heard in normal adults Heard in vent hypertrophy and CCF

Fig. 36: Heart sounds; their causes and characteristics.

Heart Sounds can be Recorded by Phonocardiogram

Significance of Heart Sounds

- **1st sound:** Increased in exercise, hyperkinetic states like anemia and decreased in shock, MI, pericardial effusion.
- **2nd sound:** Loud in hypertension, low in aortic and pulmonary stenosis. Splitting is common.
- **3rd sound:** Increased in MR. Important sign of heart failure.
- **4th sound:** Always seen in abnormal conditions. Seen in left ventricular hypertrophy.

32. Waves of ECG in Lead II.

Normal ECG in Lead II

- Lead II is a bipolar limb lead between right arm (negative electrode) and left arm (positive electrode).
- The ECG tracing in Lead II shows both negative and positive deflections equally and therefore used as a standard recording.
- There are intervals and segments in the ECG

ECG Waves

- There are positive and negative waves are deflections in the ECG tracing.
- There are 4 waveforms—P wave, QRS complex, T wave and U wave (*refer* **Fig. 37**).

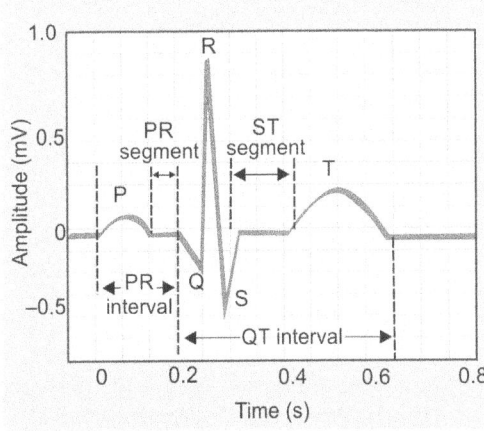

Fig. 37: Normal ECG in Lead II with waves, segments and intervals.

1. **P wave:** This is the first positive wave in ECG and is due to atrial depolarization. Duration is 0.1 second
2. **QRS complex:** Consists of a negative Q wave, positive R wave and negative S wave. This complex is due to ventricular depolarization. Normal duration is 0.08 seconds.
3. **T wave** is a positive deflection following QRS complex and is due to ventricular repolarization. Normal duration is 0.27 seconds
4. **U wave** is also positive deflection and is normally not seen. It is seen in slow depolarization of the papillary muscle. Duration is 0.08 seconds.

33. Different types of hypoxia.

- **Hypoxia is defined as deficiency of O_2 at tissue level.**
- **Types:**
  1. Hypoxic hypoxia
  2. Anemic hypoxia
  3. Stagnant hypoxia
  4. Histotoxic hypoxia

34. Aphasia.

Fluent Aphasia or Wernicke's Aphasia

- Lesion in the sensory speech area—Wernicke's area (Area 22). It can happen due to blockage of vessels supplying the area or injury.
- Also called as fluent aphasia.
- Here the person is able to hear spoken words or identifying written words
- But cannot comprehend spoken or written words.
- Motor speech is intact. So speech is not disturbed. Person speaks excessively.
- Impairment of written words as they are not able to comprehend written words also.

Nonfluent Aphasia or Broca's Aphasia

- In lesion of Broca's area there is normal comprehension of speech but there is poverty of speech.
- This type of aphasia is called as nonfluent aphasia.

- Broca's area is the motor speech area (Area 44) and is located in the foot of the primary motor cortex (Area 4).

Global Aphasia

- Lesion in both the Wernicke's area and Broca's area results in Global aphasia.
- All aspects of speech are impaired.
- The patient is not able to comprehend or repeat words.

Anomic Aphasia

- It is a type of difficulty in speech due to lesion in the angular gyrus (Area 39).
- The person has no difficulty in speech or understanding of auditory information.
- But there is trouble in understanding written language and pictures because the visual information is not processed and transmitted to Wernicke's area.
- It is also called as word blindness.

35. Stages of sleep.

- Sleep is said to be a state of altered consciousness or partial unconsciousness from which a person can be aroused.
- Sleep has two components—non-rapid eye movement (NREM) and Rapid eye movement (REM) sleep
- NREM sleep has four stages, each with different EEG activities.

Stage 1

- Stage of transition between wakefulness and sleep.
- Lasts for 1–7 minutes.
- Person is relaxed with eyes closed and fleeting thoughts.
- Alpha waves which were present will diminish.
- People when awakened at this stage will say that they were not sleeping.

Stage 2

- Stage of light sleep.
- It is little more difficult to wake the person.
- Fragments of dreams maybe experienced.
- Eyes may role from side to side.
- EEG shows sleep spindles—bursts of sharply pointed waves occurring at a frequency of 12–14 Hz and lasts 1–2 seconds.

Stage 3

- It is a period of moderately deep sleep.
- Body temperature and BP decrease.
- It is difficult to wake the person
- EEG shows mixture of sleep spindles and large, low frequency waves.
- This stage occurs 20 minutes after falling asleep.

Stage 4 or Slow Wave Sleep

- Deepest level of sleep.
- Brain metabolism drops significantly.
- Body temperature slightly falls.
- Muscle tone is decreased only slightly.
- Reflexes are intact.
- EEG shows slow, large amplitude Delta waves.

A person during sleep will go from stage 1–4 in about 1 hour. Then has the REM sleep.

REM Sleep

- In a period of sleep of 7–8 hours, REM and NREM sleep alternate.
- REM sleep occurs 3–5 times during the sleep alternating with NREM sleep.
- Initial episode of REM sleep will be lasting for 10–20 minutes. Then with each episode it prolongs and the final episode is for 50 minutes.
- In adults REM sleep totals for about 90–120 minutes. With age period of REM sleep decreases.
- 50% of an infant's sleep is REM sleep. 35% for 2-year-old infant, 25% for adults.
- REM sleep is thought to be important for maturation of brain in infants.
- This has been identified by the high percentage of REM sleep in infants.
- Bruxism, erection of penis, twitching of facial muscles.

36. Optic pathway.

- The visual pathway starts in the retina.
- Retina has ten layers. Rods and cones are in the innermost close to choroid.
- The light passes through all the layers and fall on rods and cones.

- The layer close to vitreous chamber is made of ganglion cells. The axons of these cells form the optic nerve.
- The optic nerve leaves the eye through the optic disc, the blind spot.
- The fibers from temporal part of retina receive impulses from nasal field of vision and travels in the lateral half of the nerve and the fibers from nasal part of retina receive impulses from temporal field of vision and travels in medial half of the nerve.
- The optic nerves cross in the optic chiasma. The medial fibers alone cross over and join the uncrossed fibers of the opposite optic nerve.
- On each side medial crossed fibers and lateral uncrossed fibers join to form the optic tract.
- The optic tract reaches the lateral geniculate body of the thalamus and relays there.
- The next order of fibers which originate in the LGB is termed the geniculocalcarine fibers and they reach the primary visual area in the occipital cortex (area 17).
- From here impulses reach the visual association areas (Area 18 and 19).

37. Functions of ascending reticular activating system.

- RAS plays a role in sleep-wakefulness. It also induces alertness.
- It plays a role in development of EEG waves, learning and memory.
- Controls muscle tone—mainly through the descending RF.
- Since many visceral areas are located here it regulates visceral functions

38. Components of vestibular apparatus.

- It is the sensory organ which detects the sensation of equilibrium.
- It is made of membranous tubes and chambers in the petrous part of temporal bone.
- It consists of 3 semicircular canals and 2 sac like structures—utricle and saccule and the membranous labyrinth within (*refer* **Fig. 38**)

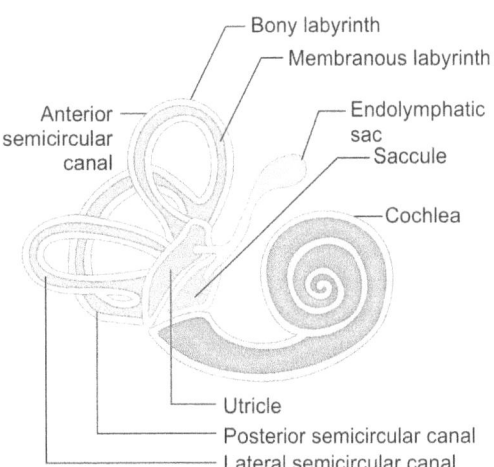

Fig. 38: Components of inner ear. It contains the vestibular apparatus—saccule, utricle and three semicircular canals. Inner ear also contains cochlea, the organ of hearing.

- Semicircular canals detect angular acceleration and thereby help in regulation of body posture and visual fixation.
- Utricle and saccule detect linear acceleration and position of head in relation to gravity.

39. Features of Parkinson's disease.

- Also called as paralysis agitans
- Due to destruction of nigrostriatal dopaminergic neurons (fibers to putamen is mostly affected) of basal ganglia.

Characterized by:
- **Hyperkinetic features:**
  - *Rigidity:* Lead pipe or cogwheel
  - *Tremors:* Resting tremors, 6-8 Hz frequency
- **Hypokinesia:**
  - Weakness of movements and lack of initiation of movements—akinesia
  - Bradykinesia
- **Lack of automated movements**
- **Mask like face without expression**
- **Festinant or short shuffling gait**

40. Functions of middle ear.

- **Tympanic reflex:** It is a protective reflex. When a loud sound is transmitted through the ossicles in middle ear a reflex is initiated with a latent period of

40–80 msec. Contraction of stapedius and tensor tympani pulls the tympanic membrane medially and membrane covering oval window laterally. This makes the ossicular system rigid and there is reduction in transmission of sounds. This reduces the intensity of sound by 30–40 decibels. It is also called as **attenuation reflex**.

Functions of this reflex:
- This reflex protects the cochlea from damaging loud sounds.
- It filters the low frequency sounds
- It prevents hearing one's own speech

☐ **Transmission of sound waves from external ear to internal ear**
☐ **Impedance matching:**
- As the sound waves travel from rarer (air in external and middle ear) to denser medium (Fluid in the inner ear) they are dampened (by 30 db).
- This loss in sound energy is prevented in the middle ear by impedance matching which is:
  - By area differences
  - By lever action
  - By buckling factor
    - *Area difference:* Area of tympanic membrane is greater than foot plate of stapes and therefore there is convergence of sound and pressure is increased by 17 times.
    - *Lever action of the ossicles* increases pressure by 1.32 times
    - *Buckling factor:* Tympanic membrane is conical in shape and the handle of malleus is attached to the umbo. As the tympanic membrane moves in and out, the buckling of membrane moves the handle of malleus less and this increases the force and decreases the velocity.

41. Functions of plasma proteins.

Plasma proteins are categorized as albumin (55%), globulin (38%) and fibrinogen (7%). They are classified based on their electrophoretic pattern.

Albumin
☐ Their levels are 4.8 g/dL.
☐ Molecular weight is the least and is 69000.
☐ They are synthesized in the liver.
☐ They regulate plasma colloidal oncotic pressure.
☐ It helps in transport of bilirubin, hormones, ions, fatty acids, metals, etc.
☐ It also helps in regulating acid-base balance.

Globulin
☐ Normal level is 2–3 g/dL.
☐ Their molecular weight is 90000–156000.
☐ There are—α, β and γ globulins with subtypes for each one.
☐ There are different forms of globulins—glycoprotein, lipoprotein, transferrin, haptoglobins, ceruloplasmin and immunoglobulins.
☐ They act as transport proteins as in transferrin transports iron, ceruloplasmin copper, lipoproteins lipids, etc.
☐ The immunoglobulins provide immunity.
☐ The normal albumin:Globulin ratio is 1.5–2.5:1 ratio.

Fibrinogen
☐ Normal value is 0.3 g/dL.
☐ Their molecular weight is 500,000.
☐ It has the highest molecular weight.
☐ It helps in coagulation of blood and provides viscosity of blood.
☐ There are other plasma proteins like prealbumin, prothrombin, etc.
☐ There are nearly 100s of plasma proteins.
☐ All the above proteins are amphoteric in nature since they have both the NH_2 and COOH groups, they act as buffers for both acids and bases.

42. Nonexcretory functions of kidney.

☐ **Endocrine functions of kidneys:** Kidneys help in synthesis of 1,25-dihydroxycholecalciferol, erythropoietin, renin, prostaglandins and thromboxane A2.
☐ **Regulation of acid-base balance:** Kidneys excretes H^+, titrable acid, NH_4 and

reabsorbs HCO_3^- and thereby regulates plasma pH.
- **Regulation of ECF volume:** Kidneys are capable of excretion and reabsorption of water as per the requirements of the body. Hormones, such as ADH, aldosterone and ANP act on the kidneys to regulate ECF volume.
- **Regulation of blood pressure:** Kidneys play a major role in long-term regulation of blood pressure. Renin-angiotensin-aldosterone mechanism acts through the kidneys to regulate BP.
- **Regulation of ECF osmolality:** Kidneys reabsorbs Na, Cl and water and thereby regulates EFC osmolality.
- Kidneys also help in **gluconeogenesis** in conditions of starvation.

43. Myasthenia gravis.

- It is disease of the neuromuscular junction.
- It is an autoimmune disorder and auto-antibodies are produced against the nicotinic acetylcholine receptors in the motor end plate.
- Women are affected more.

The antibodies act by:
- Competes with acetylcholine to bind to acetylcholine receptor
- Induces endocytosis of acetylcholine receptors
- Damages the postsynaptic membrane

Symptoms:
- It is characterized by weakness and fatigability of skeletal muscles and it gets worsened after repeated usage. Patient is better in the morning and weakness develops in the evening and improves after sleep.
- Extraocular muscles are involved in the early stages resulting in ptosis and diplopia
- Proximal limb muscles are affected early
- Later on respiratory muscles are involved and their paralysis results in death.

Treatment:
- Acetylcholinesterase inhibitors—prevents breakdown of acetylcholine and thereby increase ACh levels in NMJ.
- Antibodies can be removed by plasmapheresis and thymectomy
- Immunosuppressants can also be used.

44. Stages of spermatogenesis.

- Spermatogenesis involves both mitotic and meiotic divisions and spermiogenesis.

Mitotic Division

- The primitive germ cell, spermatogonia, in the basal lamina of the seminiferous tubule undergoes mitotic divisions to form primary spermatocytes.
- Each spermatogonium divides 5 times to produce 32 spermatogonia.
- 32 spermatogonia (44+X+Y) reach the adluminal side of the tubule and undergo mitosis to become 64 primary spermatocytes (44+X+Y).
- Primary spermatocytes are large cells with diploid number of chromosomes (2n)

Meiotic Divisions

- The primary spermatocytes with diploid number of chromosomes undergo the first meiotic division to form the secondary spermatocyte which is haploid in nature.
- The second meiotic division results in formation of spermatids (22+X or Y).
- A total of 512 spermatids are derived from single spermatogonia.

Spermiogenesis

- The spermatids do not undergo further divisions but structural changes take place as the spermatids mature into sperm—spermiogenesis.
- This process happens in the deep folds of Sertoli cells.

The changes taking place are:
- The amount of cytoplasm is reduced in spermatids
- The nucleus elongates to become the head of sperm
- The acrosomal cap is formed
- The tail and middle piece are formed.

Spermiation

- After the maturation, the sperms stay attached to the Sertoli cells.
- The release of sperms into the tubule is called spermiation.

45. Cystometrogram and its significance.

- Smooth muscles which make up the urinary bladder show the property of plasticity, a property when a muscle is stretched, the tension initially developed is not maintained. So there is no length-tension relationship in the bladder wall muscle.
- A study is done to assess the relation between the intravesicular pressure and intravesicular volume. The bladder is catheterized and fully emptied. Then volumes of fluid in increments of 50 mL are filled into the bladder through the catheter. This test is said to be the *Cystometry*.
- A graph is plotted relating the intravesicular volume and intravesicular pressure, this is the cystometrogram.
- There are 3 components in this graph – Ia, Ib and II.
  - **Ia:** There is an initial rise in the pressure of 10 cm of H_2O when the bladder is filled with the first 100 mL of fluid.
  - **Ib:** Further increments of fluid up to 300–400 mL produces not much rise in the pressure and a flat segment is seen in the cystometrogram. This segment is said to follow the Law of Laplace which states that the distending pressure (P) in a spherical viscus is equal to twice wall tension (T) divided by the radius (r). $P = 2T/r$. As the bladder gets filled, the wall tension increases, so does the radius of the bladder and therefore the pressure increase is less till the organ is full.
  - **II:** As the volume in the bladder reaches 400 mL there is a sharp rise in the pressure resulting in initiation of the micturition reflex (*refer* **Fig. 39**).
- Beyond 600 mL, the urge to empty the bladder is unbearable.

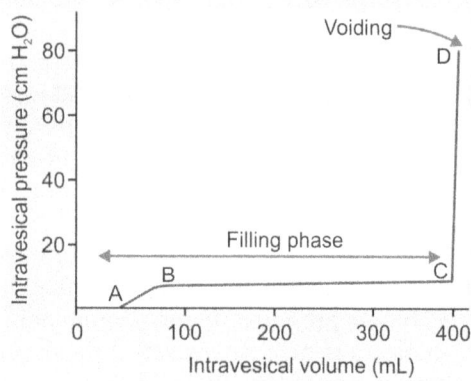

Fig. 39: Cystometrogram, Phase 1a (Mild increase in pressure when 100 mL of water is infused into bladder), Phase 1b (Not much rise in pressure from 100–400 mL intravesical volume) and Phase II (Steep rise in pressure when intravesicular volume reaches 400 mL and stimulates micturition reflex).

46. Hormones regulating calcium homeostasis.

- Parathormone
- 1,25-Dihydroxycholecalciferol or calcitriol
- Calcitonin

Parathormone and calcitriol increase serum calcium levels and calcitonin decreases calcium levels.

Calcium homeostasis is done by these hormones.

47. Enterohepatic circulation.

- Bile acids and salts present in the bile on entering the intestine are absorbed from the terminal part of the ileum and re-enter the portal vein to be secreted back into the bile from hepatocytes.
- This process repeats many times— enterohepatic circulation.
- The conjugated bile salts are absorbed and recirculated in the above manner.
- Also, bile salts are unconjugated and some of it is also absorbed.
- Colonic bacteria act on free bile acids and are converted to secondary bile acids and a part of it is also absorbed back into the portal vein.
- About 95% of secreted bile salts are absorbed by the enterohepatic circulation and only 200–500 mg/day are excreted.

Significance of Enterohepatic Circulation

- Only the amount of bile salts which are excreted, are synthesized and replaced daily, to maintain the pool of bile salts in the body which are essential for digestion and absorption of fats.
- The total amount of bile salts is 2–4 g.
- This amount is circulated daily many times to digest and absorb fats in the diet taken.

48. Enzymes involved in digestion of fat.

- There are fat-digesting enzymes in the mouth, stomach and pancreatic juice.
- **Lingual lipase** is secreted by the Ebner's gland on the dorsal surface of tongue.
- Lingual lipase starts its action while in the stomach and digests 30% of triglycerides. **Gastric lipase** is of little importance in digestion of fats except in conditions of pancreatic insufficiency.
- Most of the digestion of fats begin in the duodenum by the action of **pancreatic lipase.**
- It acts on the fats emulsified by bile salts.
- Action of lipase is potentiated by the action of **colipase**, an enzyme which is also present in the pancreatic juice.
- The other lipase present in pancreatic juice is **bile salt-activated lipase, cholesteryl ester hydrolase and phospholipase A2.**

49. Structure of platelets.

- Platelets are in a diameter of 2-4 μm. They are colorless, disc shaped and do not have nucleus.
  - **The membrane** of platelets is made of lipids, cholesterol, carbohydrates, proteins and glycoproteins. There are many receptors present in the cell membrane for collagen and fibrinogen
  - Below the cell membrane microtubules made of tubulin is present and helps in regulating the shape of the platelets.

Cytoplasm

- Organelles like endoplasmic reticulum, Golgi apparatus and mitochondria are present in the cytoplasm.
- It also contains contractile proteins like actin, myosin and thrombosthenin and are responsible for contraction of platelets which causes clot retraction.
- Cytoplasm contains two types of granules— Dense granules and Alpha granules (*refer* **Fig. 40**).

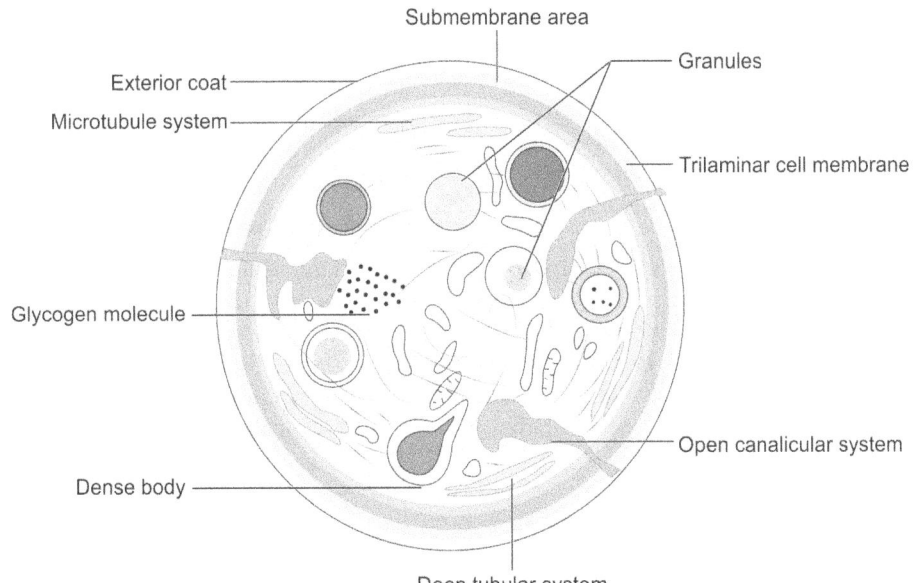

Fig. 40: Structure of platelets.

- Alpha granules contain—Von Willebrand factor, platelet-derived growth factor (PDGF), platelet activating factor (PAF), fibronectin, plasminogen, platelet fibrinogen, thrombospondin, etc.
- Dense granules—nonprotein substances, such as serotonin, ADP, calcium, ATP and pyrophosphate.

50. Functions of saliva.

- Ptyalin (α-amylase) in saliva splits starches. Action of amylase is maximum at a pH of 6.8. Digestion continues in stomach for some time till the pH becomes less than 4.
- **Protective function:** Saliva cleans the mouth after a meal and prevents growth of harmful bacteria.
- Saliva contains lysozyme, IgA and lactoferrin for protection. Lysozymes are bactericidal and lactoferrin is bacteriostatic in action.
- Saliva facilitates speech.
- It helps in taste of food.
- Mucus in saliva helps in lubrication of food, mastication and swallowing
- It buffers the gastric juice in stomach.
- Proline rich proteins in the saliva protect the enamel of tooth.
- Saliva dilutes hot and irritant foods and protects buccal mucosa. It also dilutes regurgitated bile and HCl
- In animals, it helps in temperature regulation.
- Helps in excretion of heavy metals, alcohol, morphine, thiocyanate, etc.

51. Dead space.

- Dead space is the space in the airways in which the volume of air present does not take part in gaseous exchange.
- There are 3 types of dead spaces—anatomical dead space, alveolar dead space and physiological or total dead space.
  - **Anatomical dead space** is the conducting zone of the respiratory pathway in which the gaseous exchange does not take place and the volume of air is said to be the dead space air.
  - **Alveolar dead space** is the alveoli which do not have blood supply and the volume of air in these alveoli do not take part in gas exchange and is considered to be wasted ventilation.
  - **Physiological dead space** is the sum of the above two dead spaces.
- Since in normal conditions, there are no alveolar dead spaces, physiological dead space is equal to anatomical dead space.
- In a normal adult, of the 500 mL of tidal volume inhaled, 150 mL remains in the anatomical dead space, which is also the physiological dead space.

52. Hering–Breuer reflex.

There are two types of Hering-Breuer reflexes:

Hering-Breuer Inflation Reflex

- Hering and Breuer found that, over inflation of the lungs during inspiration, results in decreased output through the phrenic nerves to the diaphragm and thereby stimulates expiration.
- This reflex is a protective reflex to prevent over inflation of the lungs.
- The receptors are slowly adapting nerve endings of the myelinated vagus nerves in the airways of the lungs.
- This reflex is stimulated by steady increase in lung volume resulting in immediate and prolonged expiration.
- It is more useful in infants than adults and it regulates the tidal volume in infants.

Hering-Breuer Deflation Reflex

- This reflex is activated during expiration and stops expiration and stimulates inspiration.
- It decreases the duration of expiration.
- It is seen in conditions like pneumothorax and atelectasis.
- It helps in opening of collapsed alveoli
- The receptors are slowly adapting stretch receptors in airways and lung parenchyma and the impulses are carried by vagus nerve.
- The efferent is also vagus nerve.

53. Korotkoff sounds.

- These sounds are heard during recording of arterial BP by auscultatory method.
- This is based on the principle that streamline flow in an artery is silent and turbulent flow creates sounds.
- While recording blood pressure by auscultatory method by using a sphygmomanometer, Riva-Rocci cuff is tied in the upper arm overlying the brachial artery.
- The cuff is inflated well above the systolic pressure in the artery.
- At this point, on auscultation over the artery no sounds are heard as the artery is completely occluded by the inflated cuff.
- Now the cuff pressure is gradually released and auscultation is done over the brachial artery.
- At the point at which the cuff pressure is just below the systolic pressure, there is a spurt of blood, flowing through the vessel only during systole.
- Since the vessel is still constricted the flow is intermittent and turbulent it creates an intermittent tapping sound.
- These sounds are called as Korotkoff's sounds.
- As the cuff pressure is lowered further, the sounds become louder, dull, muffled and then disappear as the artery is full open and thereby the flow becomes streamline again.

Korotkoff sounds are described in 5 phases:
- **Phase 1:** It starts appearing with a tapping sound. It denotes systolic BP. This phase lasts for 10-12 mm Hg fall in BP
- **Phase 2:** Sounds become murmur-like and is for 14-15 mm Hg fall in mercury column.
- **Phase 3:** Sounds become clear, knocking or banging in quality. It is heard for 14-15 mm Hg fall in mercury column
- **Phase 4:** Sounds again become muffled in quality. It is dull and faint. It lasts for 4-5 mm Hg fall in mercury column.
- **Phase 5:** No sounds are heard here. It is taken to be the diastolic BP.

54. Draw a diagram of the pathway of crude touch and label it.

- Anterior or ventral spinothalamic tract carries crude touch.
- It is an ascending tract.
- It is a part of the anterolateral system.
- It carries the sensation of crude touch.
- The first order neurons are present in the dorsal root ganglion. They are of pseudo-unipolar type of neurons.
- The central axons of these neurons terminate on second order neurons located in the laminae III, IV and V.
- Second order neurons fibers from these laminae cross to the opposite side and occupy the anterior white column.
- It ascends in the anterior white column of spinal cord and enters medulla.
- It joins with lateral spinothalamic tract and ascends up as spinal lemniscus (*refer* **Fig. 41**).
- The second order neurons terminate in the ventroposterolateral nucleus (VPLN) in thalamus.
- From the VPLN of thalamus, the third order neurons ascend up to terminate in the opposite somatosensory area I (Area 3, 1,2) and somatosensory area II.

55. Functions of CSF.

- CSF offers mechanical protection by acting as a shock absorber.
- CSF offers the optimum chemical environment for accurate neuronal signaling.
- CSF acts as a circulating medium for exchange of nutrients and waste products between the blood and nervous tissue.
- Continuous formation and drainage removes metabolic wastes from brain.
- Acts as lymph
- Provides nutrition
- Reduces the weight of brain

56. Fluent aphasia.

- Lesion in the sensory speech area—Wernicke's area (area 22).
- It can happen due to blockage of vessels supplying the area or due to injury.

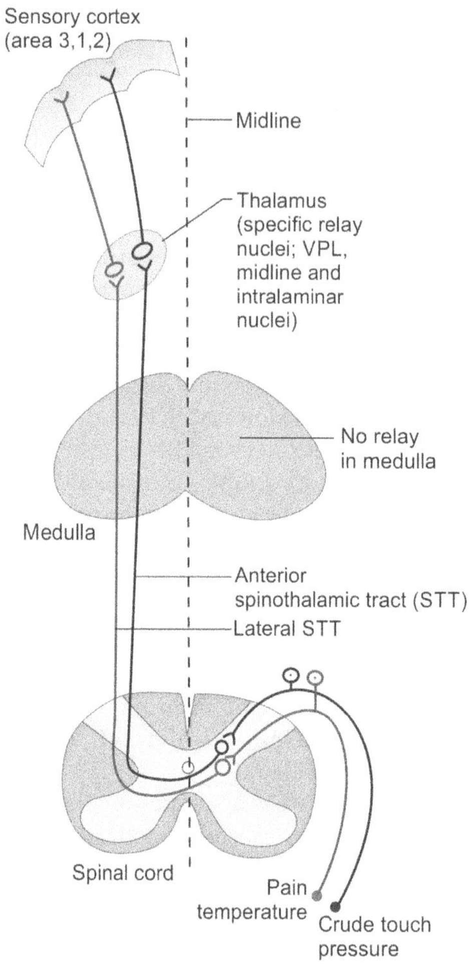

Sensory cortex (area 3,1,2)
Midline
Thalamus (specific relay nuclei; VPL, midline and intralaminar nuclei)
No relay in medulla
Medulla
Anterior spinothalamic tract (STT)
Lateral STT
Spinal cord
Pain temperature
Crude touch pressure

Fig. 41: Anterior and lateral spinothalamic tracts.

- Here the person is able to hear spoken words or identify written words
- But cannot comprehend spoken or written words.
- Motor speech is intact. So, speech is not disturbed. Person speaks excessively.
- There is impairment of reply to written words as they are not able to comprehend written words also.

57. Receptor potential.

- Receptor potential is a graded potential.
- The experimental study to identify the receptor potential was done with the Pacinian corpuscle.
- It is a receptor for touch and vibration.
- It is quiet larger and therefore can be isolated and studied.
- Each capsule has concentric lamellae of connective tissue surrounding the unmyelinated ending of the sensory nerve fiber.
- Myelin sheath for the terminal starts within the corpuscle.
- The first node of Ranvier is also located inside the corpuscle and the second node is located at the point where the nerve leaves the corpuscle.
- On placing recording electrodes, over the nerve leaving the corpuscle and when graded pressure is applied, a non-propagated depolarizing potential is recorded.
- It is said to be the generator potential or the receptor potential.
- As the pressure is increased the amplitude of the potential increases and as the potential reaches 10 mV an action potential is fired.
- It has been experimentally identified that the generator potential is generated in the unmyelinated nerve terminal of the sensory nerves.
- The receptor has converted the mechanical energy to electrical energy.
- The generator potential depolarizes the sensory nerve at the first node of Ranvier and generates the action potential there.

58. Motor homunculus.

- Parts of the whole body are represented in the primary motor area (area 4) and this is said to be the motor homunculus.
- Face is represented bilaterally whereas, other body parts have unilateral representation.
- The whole body is represented upside down with the feet above and the face and hands in the lower part of area 4.
- The area of representation for each part of the body is based on the level of skilled activities performed.
- So the fingers and hand have larger area of representation than the trunk and lower limbs.
- The area of representation for lips and tongue are also larger since they are involved in speech.

59. Attenuation reflex.

It is a protective reflex. When a loud sound is transmitted through the ossicles in middle ear a reflex is initiated with a latent period of 40-80 msec. Contraction of stapedius and tensor tympani pulls the tympanic membrane medially and membrane covering oval window laterally. This makes the ossicular system rigid and there is reduction in transmission of sounds. This reduces the intensity of sound by 30-40 decibels. It is also called as **tympanic reflex**.

Functions of this reflex:
- This reflex protects the cochlea from damaging loud sounds.
- It filters the low frequency sounds
- It prevents hearing one's own speech

60. Taste pathway.

The taste receptors are present in the taste buds which are located on the tongue in the papillae.
- There are 10,000 taste buds.
- Taste buds are located in—fungiform, foliate and vallate papillae.
- Cells in taste buds—Type 1 and 2—supporting cells.
- Type 3 cells—receptor epithelial cells have microvilli projecting into taste pore.
- They are receptors are replaced constantly in 10 days.
- Each bud is innervated by 50 nerves at bases of receptor cells.
- Each nerve innervates 5 taste buds.
- The sensory fibers from the taste buds travel through 3 nerves—Chorda tympani branch of facial nerve (from anterior 2/3rd of the tongue), glossopharyngeal nerve (from posterior 1/3rd of the tongue) and vagus nerve from epiglottis, pharynx and palate (*refer* **Fig. 42**).
- They all reach the medulla and terminate on the same side nucleus tractus solitarius of the same side.

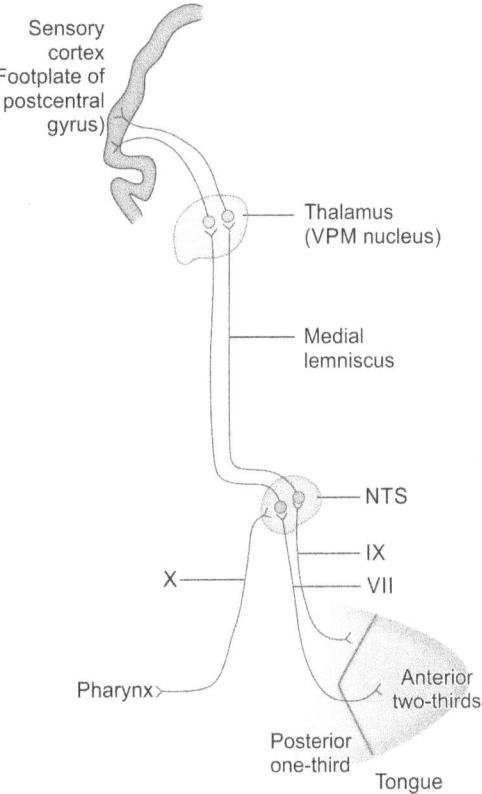

Fig. 42: Taste pathway. Sensation of taste is carried through VIIth cranial nerve from anterior 2/3rd of tongue, by glossopharyngeal nerve (IX) from anterior 1/3rd of tongue, from pharynx, epiglottis by vagus nerve (X) to nucleus tractus solitarius (NTS).

- From here the second order neurons travel along with medial lemniscus to reach ventral posteromedial nucleus of ipsilateral thalamus.
- Some fibers from medulla go to the vomiting center, hypothalamus, limbic system and salivary nucleus.
- The 3rd order neurons arise from the thalamus and they reach the foot of post-central gyrus on the same side (area 43).
- From there impulses are also transmitted to the insula and lateral orbitofrontal cortex.

Answers to 2015 Question Paper

ANSWER ALL QUESTIONS

I. Elaborate on (10 Marks each)
1. Describe the synthesis, storage, release, functions, and regulation of secretion of thyroid hormone. Add a note on hypothyroidism.
2. Define cardiac output. Explain the factors regulating cardiac output. Add a note on ejection fraction.
3. Describe the mechanism of coagulation of blood.
4. Describe in detail the pyramidal tract. List out the differences between UMN and LMN lesions.
5. Discuss in detail the gastric secretions with experimental evidences. Add a note on peptic ulcer.
6. Explain the chemical regulation of respiration. Add a note on oxygen toxicity.

II. Write notes on (5 Marks each)
1. Give an account on micturition.
2. Classify the blood groups and indications and complications of blood transfusion.
3. Auditory pathway with suitable diagram.
4. Adjustment in respiratory physiology at high altitudes.
5. Cushings syndrome.
6. Succus entericus.
7. Functions of hypothalamus.
8. Baroreceptor reflex.
9. Factors necessary for erythropoiesis.
10. Explain the actions of glucocorticoids.
11. Effects of lesions in optic pathway.
12. Determinants of blood pressure.

III. Short answers (3 Marks each)
1. Fetoplacental unit.
2. Importance of dietary fibers.
3. Neuromuscular transmission
4. ESR-clinical significance.
5. Movements of small intestine.
6. Diabetes insipidus.
7. Red cell indices.
8. Extracellular edema.
9. Functions of Sertoli cells.
10. Tests for ovulation.
11. Accommodation reflex.
12. Conducting system of the heart.
13. Artificial respiration.
14. Conditioned reflexes.
15. Surfactant.
16. Central analgesic system.
17. VO_2 max.
18. Functions of CSF.
19. Decompression sickness.
20. Babinski's sign and its clinical significance.
21. Resting membrane potential.
22. Define all or none law. How is this law applicable in the skeletal and cardiac muscle?
23. Name the muscle proteins. What is the role of troponin C in muscle contraction?
24. Inulin clearance.
25. Countercurrent exchanger mechanism in kidney.
26. Somatomedin.
27. Action of thyroxine on CVS.
28. Positive feedback mechanism.
29. How does temperature influence spermatogenesis?

30. Effects of estrogen on the uterine endometrium.
31. Dark adaptation.
32. Periodic breathing.
33. Pacemaker potential.
34. Cardiac reserve.
35. Referred pain theories.
36. Features of shock.
37. Peak expiratory flow rate.
38. Oxygen debt.
39. Mass reflex.
40. Impedance matching.
41. Dwarfism.
42. Functions of lymphocytes.
43. Proximal tubular events.
44. Acromegaly.
45. Hormones produced by placenta.
46. Stages of deglutition.
47. Renin angiotensin system.
48. Oral contraceptives.
49. Chronaxie and rheobase.
50. Significance of glycosylated hemoglobin.
51. Phasic changes in coronary blood flow.
52. AV nodal delay.
53. Properties of reflex.
54. Splanchnic circulation.
55. Functions of middle ear.
56. Nitrogen narcosis.
57. Effects of positive 'g'.
58. Papez circuit.
59. Heart sounds.
60. Differentiate REM and NREM sleep.

I. ELABORATE ON

1. Describe the synthesis, storage, release, functions, and regulation of secretion of thyroid hormone. Add a note on hypothyroidism.

Hormones synthesized from thyroid gland are:

- From follicular cells—thyroxine (T4) and triiodothyronine (T3)
- From parafollicular cells—calcitonin.

Synthesis of Thyroid Hormone

- Synthesis takes place in the follicular cells and the hormone is stored in follicular

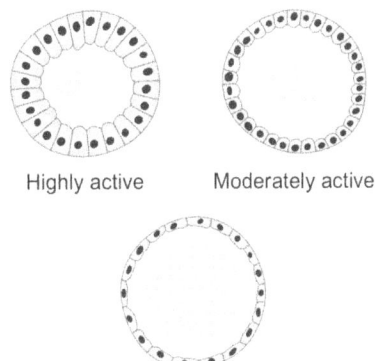

Fig. 1: Thyroid follicle—active follicle, moderately active follicle, and inactive follicle with colloid content. Inactive follicle is lined by flattened epithelial cells and the colloid content is more. In an active follicle, the cells are columnar and colloid content is less.

lumen as colloid. Size and shape of follicles vary based on the activity of the gland (refer **Fig. 1**).

- Thyroid hormones are Iodothyronines, formed by coupling of iodinated tyrosine molecules by ether linkages.

Following are the steps in synthesis of thyroid hormones:

1. Iodide trapping
2. Thyroglobulin synthesis
3. Oxidation of iodide
4. Organification
5. Coupling
6. Storage
7. Release

Iodide Trapping

- Iodide is transported from the blood in thyroid capillaries to the follicular cell through **sodium-iodide symporter (NIS)**.
- NIS transports I-against electrochemical gradient.
- TSH stimulates I-trapping and concentration in the gland.
- Iodide immediately moves towards the apical membrane of the follicular cell.

Thyroglobulin Synthesis

- As iodide is being trapped, thyroglobulin is also synthesized in the endoplasmic

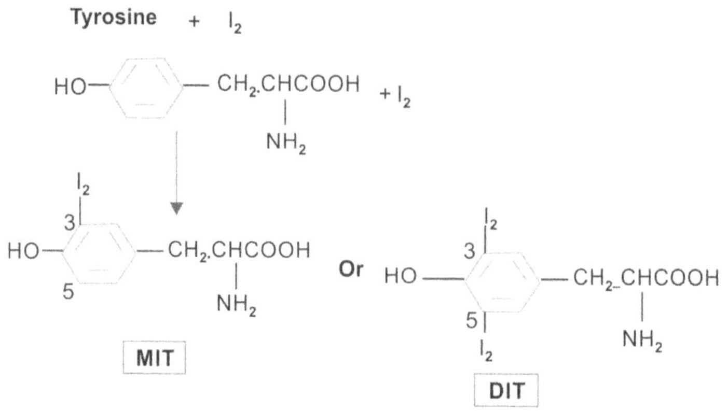

Fig. 2: Organification reaction—I_2 molecule is bound to tyrosine molecules. If it is bound in one position (3) then MIT (Monoiodotyrosine) is formed. If I_2 is bound in two positions (3 and 5) it is DIT (Diiodotyrosine).

reticulum of follicular cells and transferred to colloid.

- TG is a glycoprotein. Has 131 tyrosine amino acids.

Oxidation of Iodide

- Iodide on reaching the colloid—apical membrane interface is oxidized to iodine.
- This reaction is catalyzed by thyroid peroxidase enzyme (TPO) present in the colloid-membrane interface.
- $2I^- + H_2O_2 \rightarrow I_2 + 2\,HO^-$

Organification

- The tyrosine molecules of thyroglobulin get iodinated in the colloid to form iodotyrosines.
- This is **organification** and is catalyzed by TPO (*refer* **Fig. 2**).
- It forms either monoiodotyrosine (MIT) or diiodotyrosine (DIT) depending on the number of iodine attached to tyrosines.

Coupling Reaction

Two DIT molecules couple to form tetraiodotyrosine (T_4) or thyroxine.

Or

One molecule of MIT and DIT couple to form triiodothyronine (T_3)

Or

One molecule of DIT and MIT couple to form Reverse T_3 (RT_3), an inactive component formed in the follicular cells.

This is coupling reaction and is catalyzed by TPO (*refer* **Fig. 3**).

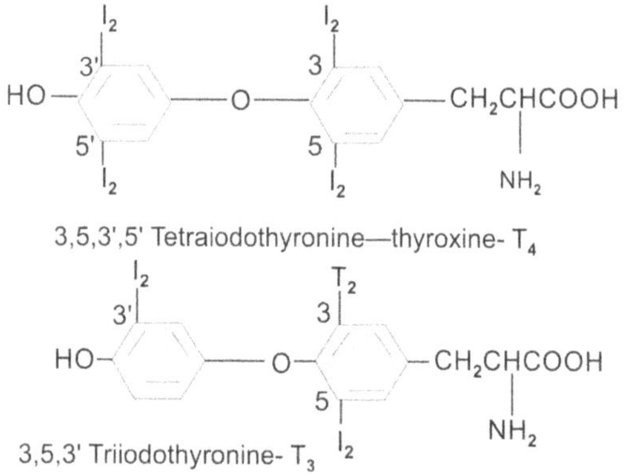

Fig. 3: Coupling reaction. Two MITs couple to form T_4 (Thyroxine) and one MIT and one DIT binds T_3 (Triiodothyronine) is formed.

Storage

- TG after iodination is stored in the colloid until release.
- In each molecule of thyroglobulin (TGB): MIT-7, DIT-6, T_4- 2, T_3- 0.2 molecules are present.
- The gland is capable of storing secretions needed for 100 days.

Release of the Hormone

- On stimulation by thyroid stimulating hormone (TSH), colloid droplets (with TG and T3 and T4) are endocytosed through megalin into the cell.
- The droplet gets attached to a lysosome and forms a phagosome.
- Proteolytic enzymes of the phagosome break the peptide bonds between thyroid hormone (TH) and TG (*refer* **Fig. 4**).

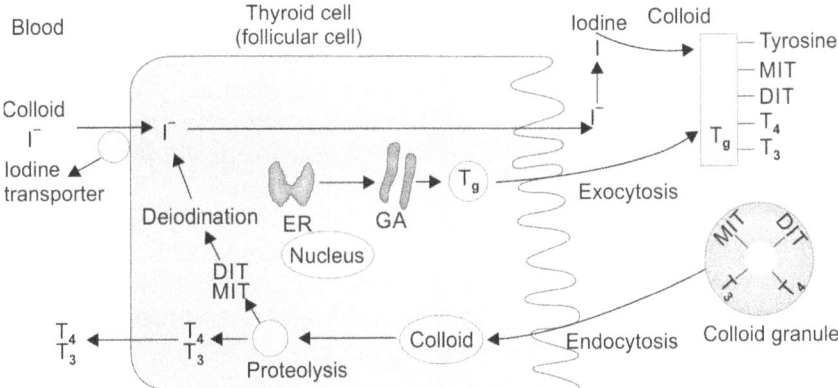

Fig. 4: Synthesis of thyroid hormone in follicular cell.
(DIT: diiodotyrosine; MIT: monoiodotyrosine; ER: endoplasmic reticulum; GA: Golgi apparatus; Tg: thyroglobulin; T4: thyroxine; T3: triiodothyronine)

- This releases T_3, T_4, MIT and DIT.
- Released thyroid hormones enter into the capillaries by diffusion.
- MIT and DIT are deiodinated by the enzyme, **thyroid deiodinases**, which are selective for iodotyrosines and not for iodothyronines.
- Small amounts of TG are also released.

Functions of Thyroid Hormone

The actions of thyroid hormone are grouped as:
- Metabolic actions
- Developmental effects
- Effects on various systems

Metabolic Actions
- Calorigenesis
- Regulation of intermediary metabolism (of carbohydrate, lipid, and protein metabolism).
- Vitamin metabolism.

Calorigenesis:
- It increases heat production
- The major role of thyroid hormone is to increase O_2 consumption and BMR. In hyperthyroidism, BMR and O_2 consumption increases 50–100% and in hypothyroidism it decreases by 30–40%.

Effects on protein metabolism:
- Thyroid hormone stimulates protein synthesis and degradation.
- TH increases cellular uptake of amino acids and formation of proteins.
- In hypothyroidism, small doses of TH helps in protein anabolism.
- High levels of TH increase protein catabolism

Effects on carbohydrate metabolism:
- Thyroid hormone acts on all aspects of carbohydrate metabolism.
- Increases glucose uptake from GIT.
- Increases insulin resistance and degradation.
- Glycogen synthesis and degradation is also affected.
- Increases gluconeogenesis.

Effects on lipid metabolism:
- Thyroid hormones affect all aspects of lipid metabolism—lipogenesis, fat mobilization and lipolysis.
- TH increases cholesterol synthesis and also its clearance by increasing LDL synthesis.
- So in hypothyroidism serum, cholesterol levels increase and in hyperthyroidism, it is decreased.

Effects on vitamin metabolism:
- Thyroid hormones are needed for the conversion of β carotene to vitamin A
- In hypothyroidism carotene accumulate in blood and give yellow discoloration—**carotenemia**.

Effects on Growth, Development, and Maturation

Thyroid hormone has an important action on growth and maturation. This effect has been evidenced in metamorphosis of tadpoles. Thyroid hormone levels increase sharply just before the major step of metamorphosis.

In hypothyroid humans, puberty is delayed or absent. The bone maturation is also delayed.

Effects on Other Systems

- **Effects on skeletal system:** Thyroid hormone stimulates linear growth of bone and maturation of epiphyseal center GH secretion and actions are potentiated by TH. Adequate thyroid hormones are needed for normal growth.
- **Effects on respiratory system:** The respiratory rate, minute ventilation and response to hypercapnia, and hypoxia are increased. O_2 carrying capacity is increased by increase in red cell mass.
- **Effects on cardiovascular system:** The main action on CVS is to increase blood supply to tissues to deliver more O_2.

In hyperthyroidism:
- Heart rate and stroke volume ↑→↑ cardiac output
- Systolic BP ↑ and diastolic BP ↓→ widened pulse pressure.
- Diastolic BP is decreased due to decreased peripheral resistance.

In hypothyroidism:
- Heart rate and stroke volume decrease.
- Peripheral resistance is usually increased.
- The cutaneous vasoconstriction is responsible for the cold skin in hypothyroids.

- **Effect on nervous system:**
  - Thyroid hormones are important for the growth and development of the brain in fetal and neonatal period. So TH deficiency in this period leads to irreversible brain damage and mental retardation.
  - The parts in CNS mostly affected are cerebral cortex, basal ganglia, and cochlea.
  - Many actions of excessive TH resemble increased sympathetic activity like: Tachycardia, tremor, increase in metabolism.

Hypothyroidism

Hypothyroidism due to thyroid gland dysfunction is primary hypothyroidism.
- Hypothyroidism may also occur due to disease in the pituitary gland or in hypothalamus.
- Symptoms of hypothyroidism vary in children and adults.
- In children hypothyroidism due to iodine deficiency—**cretinism**.

Symptoms
- **In newborns:** Respiratory distress syndrome, poor feeding, hoarse cry, umbilical hernia, retarded bone age, no visible symptoms detected, so early thyroid screening and TH replacement is essential to prevent mental retardation.
- **In children:** Mental retardation, stunted growth, potbelly, enlarged and protruding tongue, delayed or absent sexual maturity, deaf mutism with rigidity, precocious puberty can also occur.
- **In adults: Hypothyroidism in adults is Myxedema—**
  ↓BMR, hypothermia and cold intolerance, skin is dry and cold.

  CNS symptoms:
  - They are dull and lethargic, speech and mentation slow, reflex time is prolonged
  - Depression, excess sleep, Frank psychosis (Myxedema madness)

  CVS symptoms:
  - Bradycardia, ↓ myocardial contractility, cardiac output ↓, hypertension
  - S. Cholesterol TGL levels ↑ - Atherosclerosis

  Skin:
  - Nonpitting edema (Myxedema)
  - Hoarseness of voice, thick skin, thick facial features, enlarged tongue, hair is brittle, thin, coarse and lacks luster

  GIT symptoms:
  - ↓Appetite and food intake, constipation, BMR and caloric use ↓→ weight gain

- Amenorrhea is present, conception is difficult, still births and abortion common.

2. Define cardiac output. Explain the factors regulating cardiac output. Add a note on ejection fraction.

- Cardiac output (CO) is defined as the amount of blood ejected by each ventricle per minute.
  - CO = Stroke volume (SV) × Heart rate (HR)
  - NV = 70 mL/beat × 70/min = 4900 mL/min

Determinants of Cardiac Output

- CO = Stroke volume (SV) × Heart rate (HR)
- So, factors affecting either of them will alter CO.
  Factors affecting SV:
  - Preload
  - After load
  - Contractility
- **Factors affecting HR:** HR is affected by nerves supplying heart (symp and parasympathetic nerves) and cardiac centers (*refer* **Fig. 5**).

Preload

- The initial muscle length is the **preload** (the extent to which the muscle is stretched before contraction).
- Preload is decided by the **end diastolic volume (EDV)**.
- EDV is decided by the **venous return (VR)**.
- **Preload affecting stroke volume is based on the Frank-Starling's law:**
  It states that within physiological limits, the force of contraction is directly proportional to the initial length of the muscle (*refer* **Fig. 5**).

Causes for application of Frank-Starling's law:

- Increase in EDV →↑ stretch of muscle fiber → Interaction of thick and thin filament increases →↑ force of contraction.
- Stretch of muscle fibers → Opens stretch sensitive Ca^{2+} channels on sarcolemma →↑ Ca^{2+} influx →↑ force of contraction.
- ↑Ca^{2+} influx →↑ Ca^{2+} release from SR (CICR) →↑ force of contraction.
- ↑Stretch of muscle fiber →↑ affinity of troponin for Ca^{2+}

EDV is dependent on:

- **Venous return, which is dependent on:**
  - *Skeletal muscle pump:* Contraction of limb muscles press on the veins and

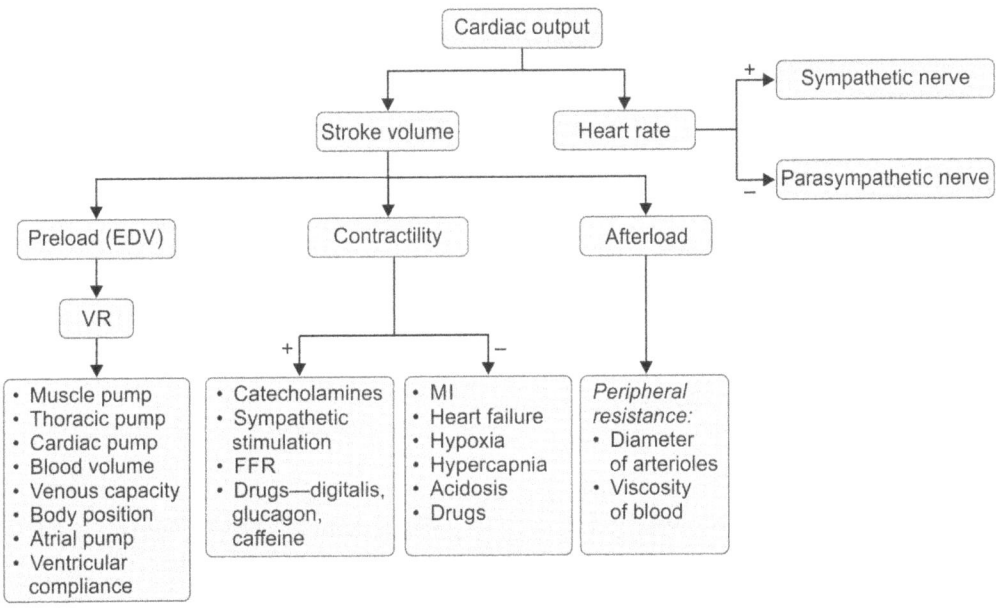

Fig. 5: Regulation of cardiac output.
(FFR: force-frequency relation; MI: myocardial infarction)

increases forward movement of blood in the veins
- *Thoracic pump:* Increase in respiration depresses the diaphragm and decreases intrathoracic pressure and thereby it acts like a suction force to increase VR
- *Abdominal pump:* During respiration compression of abdominal muscles press on the veins and favors venous emptying
- *Cardiac pump:* Vis A Tergo (Force from behind), Vis A Fronte (Force from front)
- *Total blood volume:* As the blood volume increases VR increases and vice versa
- *Capacity of venous system:* Sympathetic stimulation to the veins causes venoconstriction and thereby increases venous emptying
- *Body position:* On standing, there is venous pooling due to gravity and it may decrease the VR.
☐ **Atrial pump activity:** Contributes 20% ventricular filling and stimulated by sympathetic stimulation.
☐ **Ventricular compliance:** Affected by damage to myocardium as in MI, pericardial effusion, cardiac tamponade.

This type of regulation of stroke volume in relation to change in initial length of muscle fiber is said to be **heterometric regulation.**

Contractility

Contractility is increase in force of contraction and thereby increase in stroke volume without increase in initial muscle length.
☐ Ventricles are able to do more work per stroke at a given EDV.
☐ Factors which affect contractility—**inotropic agents.**
☐ There are positive and negative inotropic agents.

Contractility is increased by:
☐ Autonomic activity (Sympathetics are positively inotropic)
☐ *Muscle mass:* Increase in myocardial mass increases contractility as after regular exercise

☐ Concentration of hormones and chemicals
☐ *Heart rate:* Force frequency relationship

Factors increasing contractility, positive inotropic agents:
☐ Sympathetic stimulation
☐ Circulating catecholamines
☐ Force frequency relationship
☐ Digitalis
☐ Glucagon
☐ Insulin
☐ Thyroxine
☐ Chemicals, such as xanthine, theophylline

Factors decreasing contractility, negative inotropic agents:
☐ Loss of myocardium as in myocardial infarction
☐ Hypoxia
☐ Hypercapnia
☐ Acidosis
☐ Acetylcholine

Regulation of stroke volume by affecting contractility of myocardium is **homometric regulation.** Here the force of contraction is affected without much change in muscle length.

Afterload
☐ It is the force against which the heart muscle shortens
☐ Cardiac output is inversely proportional to after load
☐ **Cardiac output α 1/after load (anrep effect)**
☐ It is decided by peripheral resistance
☐ **Peripheral resistance is decided by:**
- Vessel diameter
- Viscosity of blood
☐ This is also included in **homometric regulation.**

Regulation of Heart Rate
☐ Heart rate is also a factor affecting CO.
☐ HR is in turn regulated by autonomic nerves.
☐ Sympathetics →↑Heart rate
☐ Parasympathetics →↓ HR
☐ Normally ↑HR →↑ CO
☐ But in severe tachycardia →↓ duration of diastole →↓ Ventricular filling →↓ CO

Ejection Fraction

- It is the percentage of end diastolic volume which is ejected per beat.
- Stroke volume is given as the percentage of EDV
- EF = SV/EDV × 100
- Normal value is about 65%
- It is a good indicator of left ventricular functioning.

3. Describe the mechanism of coagulation of blood.

- Blood while flowing in the vessels is fluid in nature, but when the vessel wall is injured or the blood is removed from the body and collected in a test tube it becomes a jelly like mass—The Clot.
- Clotting or coagulation of blood involves a series of cascade of events in which many clotting factors (Proteins in the plasma) are activated in a serial manner. There are many such clotting factors.

They are:

- **Factor I:** Fibrinogen
- **Factor II:** Prothrombin
- **Factor III:** Thromboplastin
- **Factor IV:** Calcium
- **Factor V:** Labile factor or proaccelerin
- **Factor VI:** Nonexistent
- **Factor VII:** Stable factor or proconvertin
- **Factor VIII:** Antihemophilic factor
- **Factor IX:** Christmas factor or plasma thromboplastic component (PTC) or antihemophilic factor B
- **Factor X:** Stuart-Prower factor
- **Factor XI:** Plasma thromboplastin antecedent (PTA) or antihemophilic factor C.
- **Factor XII:** Hageman factor or glass factor or contact factor
- **Factor XIII:** Laki-Lorand factor or fibrin stabilizing factor
- **HMWK:** High molecular weight kininogen or Fitzgerald factor
- Pre-Ka (Prekallikrein or Fletcher factor)
- **Kallikrein:** Ka
- **PL:** Platelet phospholipid

The coagulation process involves three major steps:
1. Formation of prothrombin activator
2. Conversion of prothrombin to thrombin
3. Conversion of fibrinogen to fibrin

Formation of Prothrombin Activator is by 2 Mechanisms

1. Extrinsic pathway
2. Intrinsic pathway

Intrinsic Pathway

This pathway is activated when there is injury to vessel wall and exposure of collagen or blood itself.

Steps involved are:

- Injury to vessel wall exposes collagen activates factor XII to XIIa
- Factor XIIa activates factor XI to XIa
- Factor XIa activates factor IX to IXa
- Factor IXa in the presence of VIII, Ca^{2+} and platelet phospholipids (PPL) activates factor X to Xa.
- The activated factor Xa, platelet phospholipids, factor Va and Ca^{2+} forms the **prothrombin activator** (*refer* **Fig. 6**).

Extrinsic Pathway

The extrinsic pathway is triggered when the injury involves damage to the blood vessels and the surrounding tissues. The damaged tissue releases tissue thromboplastin, a protein-phospholipid mixture which activates factor VII. This triggers the extrinsic pathway.

- Inactive factor VII is activated to active factor VIIa
- VIIa in the presence of Ca^{++}, platelet phospholipid (PL) and tissue thromboplastin, activates factors IX and X.
- Active factor Xa, Va, Ca^{++} and PL, forms the prothrombin activator.
- Prothrombin activator converts prothrombin to thrombin.
- Thrombin catalyzes the conversion of fibrinogen to fibrin

Conversion of Prothrombin to Thrombin

Prothrombin activator in the presence of Ca^{2+} converts prothrombin to thrombin.

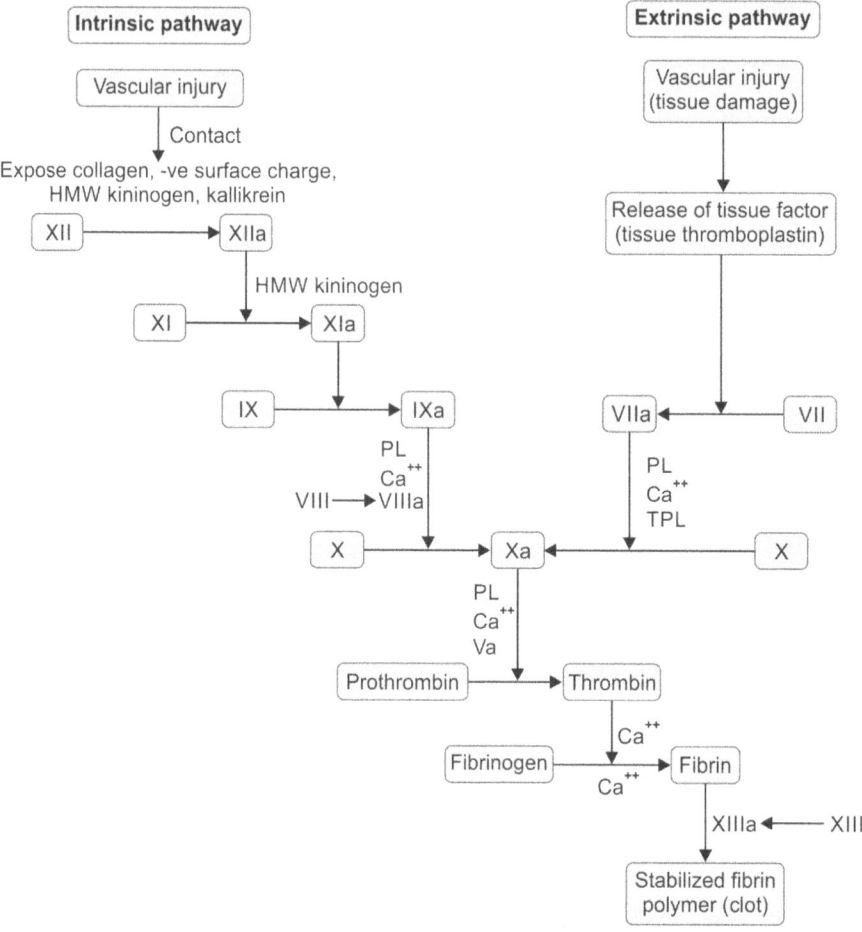

Fig. 6: Mechanism of clotting.
(TPL: tissue phospholipid; PL: platelet phospholipid)

This happens at the surface of platelets. Thrombin is a proteolytic enzyme.

Conversion of Fibrinogen to Fibrin

- Thrombin, a proteolytic enzyme removes two pairs of polypeptide chains from each fibrinogen molecule and converts it to fibrin monomer.
- The fibrin monomers now polymerize to form long fibrin threads. The fibrin is initially a loose mesh of interlacing strands. This meshwork traps the blood cells.
- It is later converted to a dense tight aggregate by formation of covalent cross-linkages. This is catalyzed by factor XIII and Ca^{2+}. The stabilized fibrin mesh with the trapped blood cells forms the CLOT.

---

4. Describe in detail the pyramidal tract. List out the differences between upper motor neuron (UMN) and lower motor neuron (LMN) lesions.

Pyramidal Tract

Origin of CST

Corticospinal tract (CST) arises from the following areas in the cerebral cortex:
- 30% fibers arise from the primary motor are (area 4).
- 30% fibers arise from premotor area (area 6).
- 40% fibers arise from somatosensory area 1 (area 3, 1, 2).

Course of CST

- The fibers, after originating from the above areas pass through the corona radiata and then pass through the posterior limb of internal capsule.
- In corona radiata they are spread out and appear fan-like.
- On entering the internal capsule (IC), they are arranged in a very compact manner (*refer* **Fig. 7**).

Internal Capsule (IC)

In IC, CST is present in the anterior 2/3rd of the posterior limb of the capsule. The body is represented here from anterior to posterior aspect.

Midbrain

CST passes through pes pedunculi and occupies the middle 3/5th of it. Here the representation of body is, head in the medial aspect and legs laterally and trunk in the middle.

Pons

In pons, the fibers are dispersed as they pass through the pontine nuclei and pontocerebellar fibers.

Medulla oblongata

- The split fibers reunite here to form a single bundle which appears as a bulge in the anterior aspect and which is said to be the **pyramid**. Therefore, it gets the name—**pyramidal tract**.
- In medulla, 75% of the fibers cross over to the opposite side and forms the lateral corticospinal tract (LCST). 25% of the fibers descend down on the ipsilateral side as the anterior corticospinal tract (ACST).

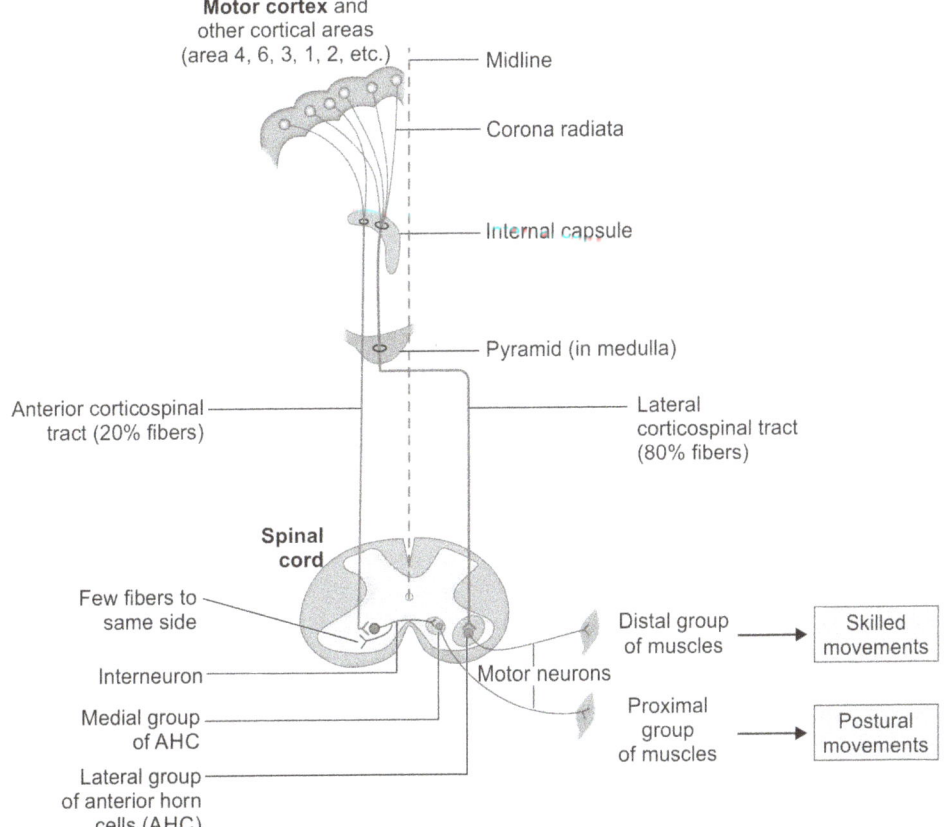

Fig. 7: Origin, course and termination of pyramidal tract. Lateral corticospinal tract supplies distal limb muscles and anterior corticospinal tract supplies proximal limb and trunk muscles.

Spinal cord

- The crossed and uncrossed fibers descend down in spinal cord (SC) as the ACST and LCST. The LCST fibers end on the internuncial neurons in SC, which in turn synapse with anterior horn cells (α motor neurons) and they supply the distal limb muscles are responsible for the fine voluntary movements.
- Uncrossed ACST fibers reach the respective spinal segment and they cross over at the segment to opposite side and end on internuncial neurons which in turn synapse on the anterior horn cells. ACST fibers supply the proximal limb muscles and trunk muscles and are responsible for regulation of posture and tone.
- There are many inputs which converge on the spinal motor neurons. These suprasegmental inputs come from other spinal segments, brain stem and cerebral cortex. These neurons which converge on the anterior horn cells of spinal cord are the **upper motor neurons**. It includes the pyramidal and extrapyramidal tracts.
- Anterior horn cells and their fibers which supply the muscles form the **lower motor neurons**. So, they are called as the **"final common pathway"**.

Functions of Pyramidal Tract

- LCST supplies the distal limb muscles and therefore they control voluntary fine movements, such as writing, stitching, etc.
- VCST supplies axial and proximal limb muscles and they control posture and gross movements, such as balancing, climbing, etc.
- LCST facilitates superficial reflexes and in its lesion, superficial reflexes are lost.
- CST facilitates muscle tone.
- CST also communicates with other areas controlling motor activities, such as basal ganglia, cerebellum, and brain stem.
- Some fibers from the cortex also terminate on cranial nerve nuclei (corticobulbar fibers) and therefore supplies facial muscles.

Differences between UMN and LMN lesions:

Sl. No.	Upper motor neuron lesion	Lower motor neuron lesion
1.	Damage to motor tracts above anterior horn cell	Damage to the anterior horn cells and below
2.	Muscles affected in groups	Individual muscles affected
3.	Spastic type of paralysis	Flaccid type of paralysis
4.	Deep reflexes are exaggerated	Deep reflexes are lost
5.	There is no muscle atrophy	Paralyzed muscles are atrophied
6.	Babinski's sign is positive	Plantar reflex is normal
7.	Muscle tone is increased (Hypertonia)	Muscle tone is decreased (Hypotonia)
8.	Common site of lesion is at the Internal capsule	Injury to peripheral nerves, Poliomyelitis
9.	No involuntary movements	Fasiculations are present
10.	Nerve conduction study is normal	Nerve conduction velocity is decreased

5. Discuss in detail the gastric secretions with experimental evidences. Add a note on peptic ulcer.

Composition of Gastric Juice

- 2–2.5 L/day
- pH—1–2
- Water—99.45%
- Solids—0.55%
- Electrolytes—Na^+, K^+, Mg^{2+}, Cl^-, HCO_3^-, HPO_4^-, SO_4^-
- Enzymes—pepsin, lipase, gelatinase
- Mucus—insoluble and soluble
- Intrinsic factor

Mechanism of HCl Secretion

- In stomach, hydrochloric acid is secreted by the parietal cells which are present in the main gastric glands in body of the stomach.

- Pure secretion from the parietal cell has a pH of 0.82 and is isotonic (150 mEq of H^+ and 150 mEq of Cl^+).
- Parietal cell is polarized with an apical side facing the lumen and a basolateral side facing the interstitium.
- There are many tubulovesicular structures in the parietal cell which are studded with H^+-K^+ ATPase which pump H^+ into the lumen in exchange for K^+.
- These cells are highly metabolizing and they put out lot of CO_2. The cell is also rich in the enzyme carbonic anhydrase.

HCl secretion from the parietal cells happens in 2 steps:
1. Secretion of H^+ into the lumen
2. Secretion of Cl^- into the lumen.

The steps involved in HCl secretion are:
1. CO_2 in the cell is hydrated in the presence of Carbonic anhydrase, $CO_2 + H_2O \rightarrow H_2CO_3$
2. $H_2CO_3 \rightarrow H^+ + HCO_3^-$
3. The H^+ is pumped into the lumen by the H^+-K^+ ATPase pump on the apical side. For one H^+ pumped out of cell one K^+ is taken into the cell which later diffuses back into the lumen
4. HCO_3^- is extruded in the basolateral side through an anion exchanger in exchange for one Cl^- (*refer* **Fig. 8**).
5. The Cl^- which enters the cell will diffuse across the apical membrane into the lumen.
6. So for every H^+ secreted, one Cl^- is also secreted into the lumen and one HCO_3^- is absorbed into the blood.

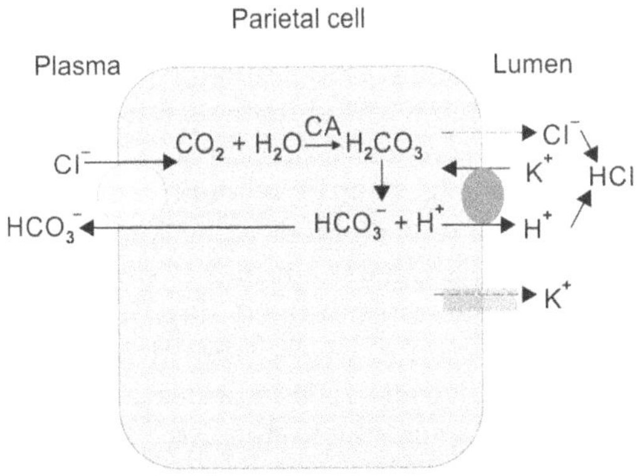

Fig. 8: Mechanism of HCl secretion. (CA: Carbonic anhydrase).

So when gastric secretion is increased after a meal, the HCO_3^- getting added to the blood is increased, thereby raising the pH of blood—*Postprandial alkaline tide.*

Regulation of Gastric Secretion

Neural, humoral and reflex regulation of secretion

Factors that Stimulate
1. Vagus N
2. Gastrin
3. Histamine

Factors that Inhibit
1. Low pH in the stomach
2. Somatostatin
3. Prostaglandin E2 (*refer* **Fig. 9**)

Regulation is discussed in terms of:
1. Cephalic phase
2. Gastric phase
3. Intestinal phase

Cephalic Phase
- Nearly 500 mL/hr (45% of total secretion)
- Initiated by thought, sight, smell, taste of food through vagus nerve.
- Emotions also affect secretion (*refer* **Fig. 10**)

Gastric Phase

About 50% of total secretion. Food in stomach induces secretion by:
- Distension of body of stomach (through reflexes—vagal reflex)
- Distension of antrum (through gastrin secretion)
- By products of partial digestion of protein (through gastrin secretion)

Intestinal Phase
- It begins when chyme enters the intestine.
- Intestinal influence is inhibitory by:
  - **Enterogastric reflex:** By distension, presence of acid and products of digestion—inhibits secretion.
  - **Hormonal mechanism:** CCK, Secretin, GIP, Neurotensin, etc.,—**Enterogastrone**.

Experimental Evidences

Phasic regulation of gastric secretion is studied by many experimental procedures conducted in animals.

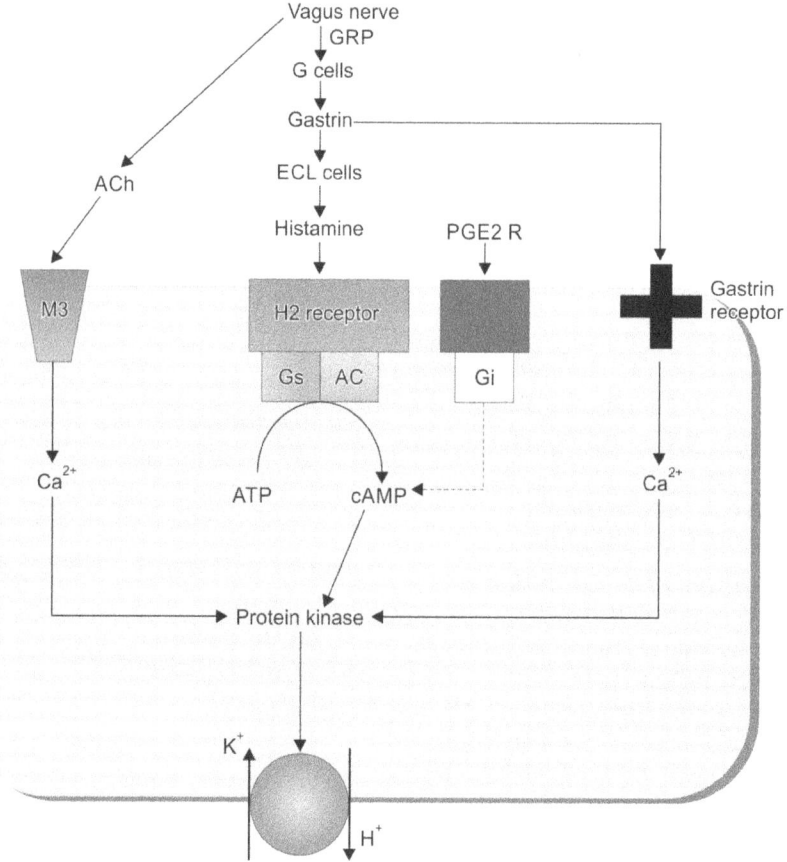

Fig. 9: Parietal cell with the regulating factors for HCl secretion.
(PGE2 R: prostaglandin E2 receptor; M3: muscarinic receptor)

1. **Experimental evidence for cephalic phase of gastric secretion:**
   - It is demonstrated by sham feeding experiment in dogs.
   - The esophagus of the dog is divided in the middle and both the cut ends are brought and fixed to the abdominal surface.
   - Now the dog is made to swallow food, but the food comes out of the cut end.
   - The gastric secretion in this phase is due to the cephalic phase as this is due to the smell, sight, and taste of food.
   - The secretion from the stomach is collected from the stomach through a tube connected to the lower cut end of esophagus.
2. **Experiment to demonstrate that vagus stimulates gastric secretion by Pavlov's pouch:**
   - Under anesthesia, a pouch of the stomach is created with intact nerve and blood supply and is separated from the stomach. The mucosa is incised and muscle layer is kept intact. The main section of stomach is restored by applying sutures.
   - An outlet is made from the pouch and is sutured with abdominal wall to drain the secretions from stomach.
   - The vagus nerve is identified in the neck and divided. After some days, the peripheral cut end is stimulated in the anesthetized dog. There is secretion of gastric juice rich in HCl and pepsin which indicates that vagus is secretomotor to stomach.
3. **Heidenhain's pouch to demonstrate gastrin-mediated regulation of gastric seceretion:**

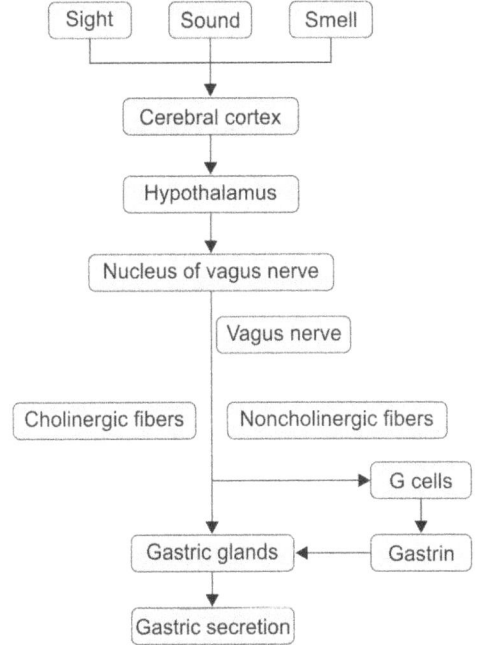

Fig. 10: Cephalic phase of regulation of Hcl secretion. This phase of gastric secretion is regulated through Vagus nerve.

- Heidenhain's pouch is a modified Pavlov's pouch in which the denervated antral part of stomach is seperated with intact blood supply.
- When this pouch is distended, there is gastric secretion. Since it is denervated, there is a blood-borne mechanism which mediates the secretion, which could be due to gastrin.
- It is confirmed by injecting gastrin and following which there is similar gastric secretion from the Heidenham's pouch.

Pathophysiology of Peptic Ulcer

There are two types of ulcers:
1. **Duodenal ulcer**
2. **Gastric ulcer**

Ulcer is due to disruption of the mucosal barrier or excess secretion of gastric juice.

Acid or pepsin in gastric juice digests the mucosa leading to ulcer.

Mucosal barrier is formed by:

- **Mucus** secreted by the neck cells and surface mucosal cells in the mucosal lining. It also contains mucin, phospholipid, HCO_3^- and water.
- **Prostaglandins** secreted by epithelial cells have antisecretory activity (Hcl) and increases HCO_3^- and mucus.
- **Epithelium of mucosa:** Low permeability, Rapid turnover and HCO_3^-, mucus secretions from there.
- **Bicarbonate secretion** from gastric mucosal cells increases the pH.

Factors which Impair Mucosal Defense

1. Defective mucus secretion
2. **Drugs, such as NSAIDs, cortisol, etc.:** They inhibit secretion of mucus and bicarbonate
3. Alcohol
4. Type of food
5. **Smoking:** ↓mucus and pancreatic secretions. Causes reflux of duodenal contents.
6. Stress
7. Reflux of gastric contents
8. Delayed gastric emptying
9. **H. Pylori infection:** Causes local inflammation in antral mucosa and disrupts the barrier

Factors which Increase Secretion

- **Genetic factors:** Increased parietal cell mass, Increased postprandial gastrin response
- **Psychosomatic factors:** Anxiety increases secretion
- **Food:** Alcohol, tea, coffee, spicy food
- Rapid gastric emptying
- **Zollinger-Ellison syndrome:** It is a gastrin secreting tumor of pancreas.

---

6. Explain the chemical regulation of respiration. Add a note on oxygen toxicity.

- Chemical regulation of respiration is also through the modulation of activities of neural centers through chemoreceptors.
- There are 2 sets of chemoreceptors responding to changes in arterial PO_2, PCO_2, and pH
- They are **peripheral and central chemorecptors.**

Peripheral Chemoreceptors

- Carotid and aortic bodies (*refer* **Fig. 11**).
- They have high blood flow (2000 mL/100 g/min) and high metabolic rate.

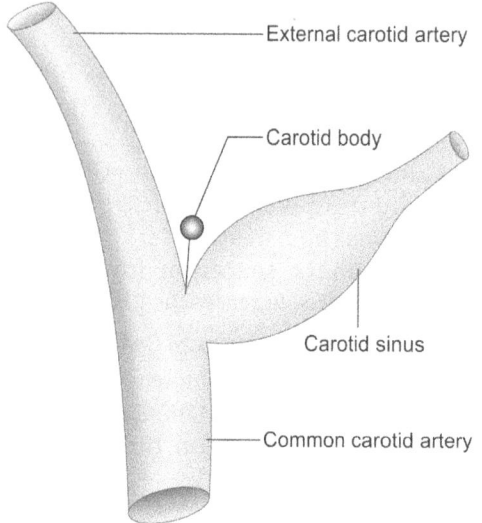

Fig. 11: Location peripheral chemoreceptors at bifurcation of common carotid artery; the carotid body. Carotid sinus is the dilatation in internal carotid artery; the baroreceptor.

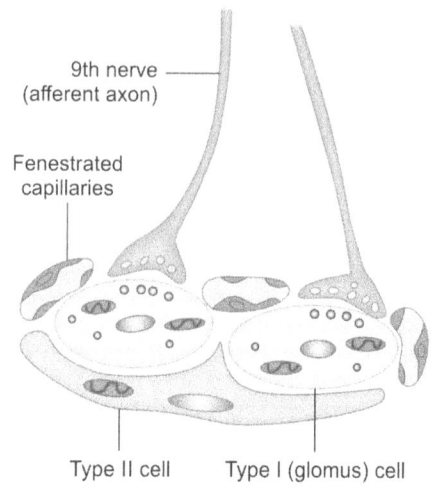

Fig. 12: Cells in carotid body—Type I (glomus cells) and Type II (supporting cells). Glomus cells are supplied by 9th cranial nerve and are close to fenestrated capillaries.

- Their metabolic needs are met by dissolved O_2.
- So they are highly sensitive to ↓PO_2, ↑PCO_2 and ↓pH.
- These receptors are not stimulated in anemia or carbon monoxide poisoning.
- They are stimulated in ↓PO_2, vascular stasis, cyanide poisoning
- They have 2 types of cells—glomus and sustentacular cells.

Sensitivity of Peripheral Chemoreceptors (PCR)

- Glomus cells are the sensors (*refer* **Fig. 12**).
- Hypoxia is the major stimulus. Neurotransmitter is Dopamine
- PCRs also responds to ↑PCO_2 and ↓pH
- When PO_2 <100 mm Hg there is ↑firing rate of the nerves supplying them (9th and 10th cranial nerves)
- Response is maximum when PO_2 falls <60 mm Hg
- Effect of hypoxia is less when PO_2<60 mm Hg because:
  - Hypoxia → Hyperventilation → CO_2 blow out →↓$PaCO_2$ →↓ventilation (*refer* **Fig. 13**)
  - Deoxy-Hb has more affinity for H+ →↓arterial [H+] →↓ventilation

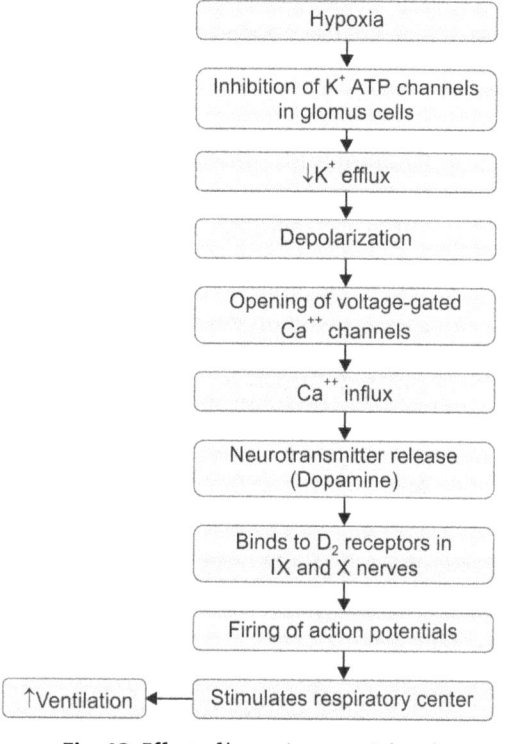

Fig. 13: Effect of hypoxia on peripheral chemoreceptors.

Mechanism of Hypoxia Stimulating PCR
Hypoxia inhibits K+ channels by:
1. O_2 sensor in the glomus cell is a heme containing protein and is associated with

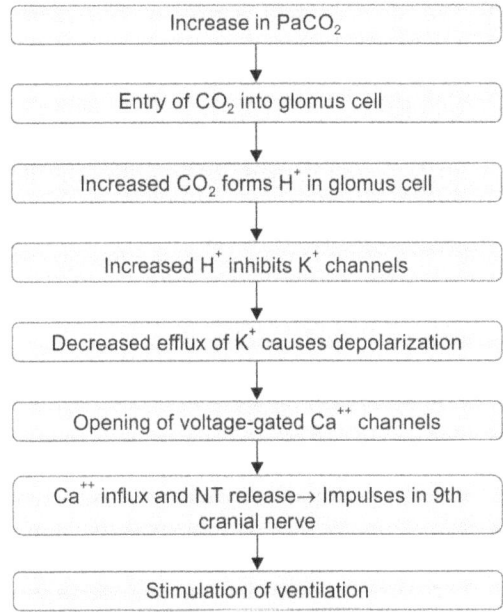

Fig. 14: Effect of hypercapnia on peripheral chemoreceptors.

O_2. In hypoxia the lack of O_2 inhibits the K^+ channels (*refer* **Fig. 13**).
2. In hypoxia, there is increase in cAMP in glomus cells which inhibits cAMP sensitive K^+ channels.

Effects of CO_2 on PCR
Refer **Fig. 14**.

Integrated Effects of Arterial—PCO_2, PO_2, and pH on Ventilation, by Stimulating PCR
- At low $PaCO_2$ level with hypoxia, ventilation is not stimulated till PO_2 <60 mm Hg.
- High $PaCO_2$ levels (as in ↑metabolic rate/breathing CO_2 mixtures)→↑ ventilation. But if CO_2 content in breathed air is >7% → CNS depression → CO_2 Narcosis
- Hypercapnia with hypoxia, shifts the CO_2 curve to left and slope is increased.
- Acidosis by itself (as in Diabetic ketoacidosis) can stimulate ventilation by stimulating PCR (even in absence of hypoxia or hypercapnia).

Central Chemoreceptors (CCR)
- Located in the medulla and is different from the other respiratory neurons.
- There are also other such CCR in and around the brain stem nuclei—nucleus tractus solitarius, Nucleus ambiguous (*refer* **Fig. 15**).
- They respond maximally to changes in [H^+] in brain CSF and ISF which is in turn decided by $PaCO_2$ and HCO_3^- of CSF.

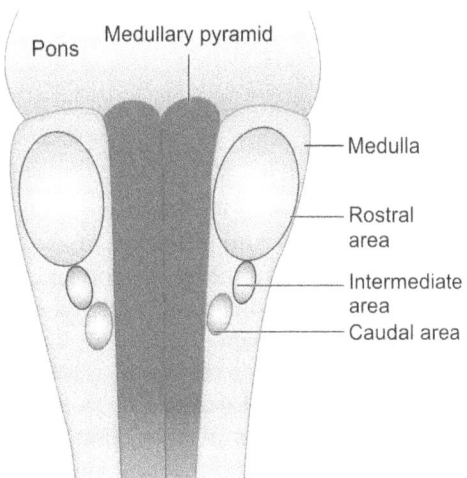

Fig. 15: Location of central chemoreceptors in ventral medulla. There are rostral, intermediate, and caudal centers.

↑Arterial PCO_2
↓
↑Brain ECF CO_2 level
↓
$CO_2 + H_2O \rightarrow H_2CO_3 \rightarrow H^+ + HCO_3^-$
↓
Increase in brain ECF H^+ level
↓
Stimulation of CCR
↓
Stimulation of medullary inspiratory center
↓
Firing of neurons supplying diaphragm and external intercostal muscles
↓
Increase in ventilation

O_2 Toxicity
- O_2 toxicity may appear when 100% O_2 is given at a pressure of 4 atm.
  - It is due to formation of Free radicals (like O_2^-, H_2O_2).
  - They oxidize PUFA and destroy the cellular enzymes.

- **Symptoms:**
  - Nausea
  - Irritability
  - Dizziness, tinnitus
  - Disorientation
  - Muscle twitching
  - Convulsions and in severe cases coma
  - Congestion and irritation of airways →tracheobronchial secretions →↓ Surfactant → Pulmonary edema
  - Blurring of vision
  - In newborns it results in retrolental fibroplasia (formation of opaque vascular tissue in eyes) that in turn results in premature retinopathy.
  - When given for longer periods results in bronchopulmonary dysplasia and branchial cyst in newborns when they are treated with 100% O_2 for respiratory distress syndrome.

II. WRITE NOTES ON

1. Give an account on micturition

Nerve supply of urinary bladder

- Urinary bladder is a triangular-shaped sac like structure. The bladder extends down as the urethra.
- The bladder wall is made of detrusor, a smooth muscle and there are two sphincters—internal and external urethral sphincters.
- Internal sphincter is at the neck of the bladder and is made of smooth muscle. It is supplied by sympathetic and parasympathetic nerves.
- External sphincter is made of skeletal muscle and is supplied by somatic motor nerve (pudendal nerve).
- The bladder wall is also supplied by sympathetic and parasympathetic nerves.
- Parasympathetic nerves (pelvic nerve) have both afferents and efferents to bladder wall and internal sphincter. They arise from S2–S4 segments of spinal cord. When they are stimulated, they cause contraction of bladder wall and relaxation of internal sphincter and therefore emptying of bladder (refer **Fig. 16**).
- The sympathetic nerves (hypogastric nerve) also have afferents and efferents and they arise from L1–L3 segments of spinal cord. They also supply the bladder wall and internal sphincter. When stimulated, they cause relaxation of bladder wall and contraction of internal sphincter and therefore filling of bladder.

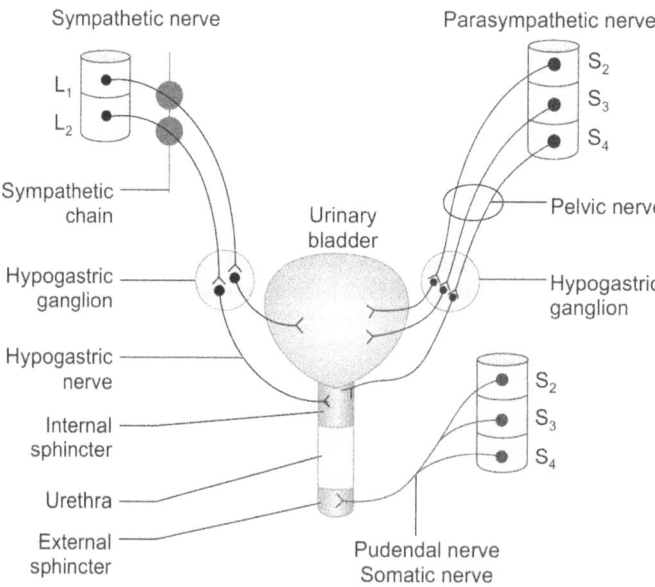

Fig. 16: Nerve supply of urinary bladder

- Somatic nerve (pudendal nerve) to external sphincter arises from S2–S4 segments of spinal cord and have control from higher centers. It is under voluntary control.
- Once urine enters the renal pelvis, it flows through the ureters and enters the bladder, where urine is stored.

Micturition Reflex

- **Micturition is the process of emptying the urinary bladder.**
- **Two processes are involved:**
  1. The bladder fills progressively until the tension in its wall rises above a threshold level, and then
  2. A nervous reflex called the micturition reflex occurs that empties the bladder (*refer* **Fig. 17**).

  The micturition reflex is an automatic spinal cord reflex; however, it can be inhibited or facilitated by centers in the brainstem and cerebral cortex.

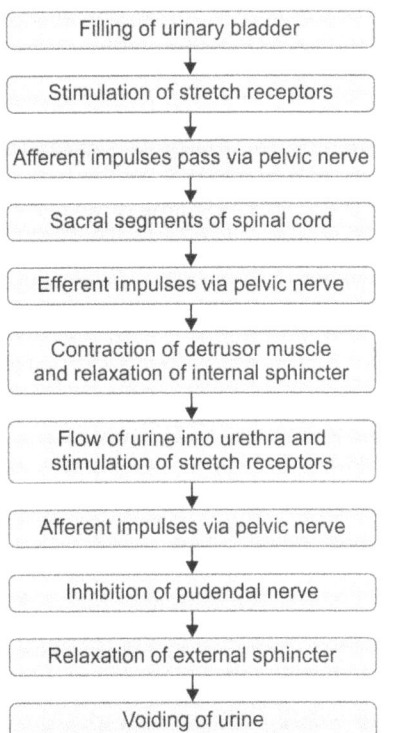

Fig. 17: Micturition reflex.

The reflex pathway:
- **Initiation:** Reflex initiated by stimulation of stretch receptors in bladder wall.
- **Stimulus:** Filling of bladder up to 300–400 mL
- **Afferents:** Through pelvic nerves (PS) to reach S2–S4 segments in spinal cord.
- **Efferents:** PS motor fibers from S2–S4 end in the detrusor muscle (excitatory) and internal sphincter (inhibitory).
- **Response:** Causes contraction of bladder wall and relaxation of internal sphincter. Once it becomes powerful another reflex through pudendal nerve relaxes the ES → voiding.

2. Classify the blood groups and indications and complications of blood transfusion.

Classification of Blood Groups

- The blood groups are divided based on the presence of antigens or agglutinogens on the membranes of RBCs.
- An individual with a particular antigen will not possess the corresponding antibody or agglutinin in his plasma.
- This forms the basis of blood grouping.
- There are more than 30 blood group systems based on the presence of nearly 400 antigens.
- The blood group systems are: ABO system, Rh system, MNS, Lutheran, P, Kell, Kidd, Duffy, Lewis, etc.
- Most of the antigens are cold antigens and therefore they do not react in body temperature.
- The ABO and Rh systems are the major blood group systems as they react in body temperature and when they react with their corresponding agglutinins they produce major reactions.

Indications of Blood Transfusion

- Acute blood loss
- Chronic anemia
- Bone marrow failure
- Preparation for surgery or during surgery
- Burns—only plasma is given

- Clotting diseases—fresh frozen plasma given

Complications of Blood Transfusion

Due to Mismatched Transfusion

Happens immediately → Agglutination of RBCs → Hemolysis—acute hemolytic transfusion reactions. Usually happens in ABO incompatibility

Complications are:
- Shivering and fever
- Hemoglobinemia and hemoglobinuria
- Jaundice
- Acute renal failure
- Clumped RBCs block vessels of vital organs

Due to Faulty Techniques of Giving Blood
- Thrombophlebitis
- Air embolism

Febrile Reactions

Due to pyrogens in the blood

Allergic Reactions

Itching, erythema, nausea, vomiting, and anaphylaxis

Transmission of Diseases

Hepatitis, malaria, AIDS, syphilis, etc.

Due to storage of blood: Increased K^+ content of plasma → on infusion leads to arrhythmias and cardiac arrest

3. Auditory pathway with suitable diagram.

The action potentials generated in the cochlear division of VIII cranial nerve travels in the following pathway.

Organ of Corti
↓
Bipolar cells of spiral ganglion
↓
Cochlear nuclei (Dorsal and ventral) in brain stem
↓
Superior olivary nuclei of both sides
↓
Lateral lemniscus (both sides)
↓
Inferior colliculus (both sides)
↓
Medial geniculate body in thalamus (both sides)
↓
Primary auditory cortex (Area 41) (both sides) (*refer* **Fig. 18**)
↓
Auditory association areas (Areas 42, 22) (both sides)

4. Adjustment in respiratory physiology at high altitudes.

Physiological Changes at High Altitude

- Effects of high altitude is due to low barometric pressure → ↓ P_{IO2}
- Hypoxic symptoms appear at 10,000 ft and are severe at 15,000 to 18,000 ft.
- There are various compensatory mechanisms by which the O_2 supply to tissue is increased. They are:
  - First and foremost—**hyperventilation**
  - In high altitude, there is no drive for ventilation till PO_2 is <60 mm Hg (at 14,000 ft) and on reaching <60 mm Hg, there is hyperventilation, because:
  - **1st stage:**
  - Hypoxia acts on peripheral chemoreceptors (PCR) → stimulation of ventilation → CO_2 blow out → ↓PCO_2 → arterial pH → ↓ ventilation.
  - **2nd stage:**
  - Ventilation slowly decreases and then increases and becomes stable after 8–10 hours, due to: pH of CSF is more alkaline in the acute phase. But later ventilation increases by ↓pH, by movement of HCO_3^- out of CSF
  - There is renal compensation for the alkaline nature because the kidneys excrete more HCO_3^- into the urine → ↓pH

Acclimatization to High Altitude

- When a person ascends to high altitudes and stays there for some time he gets adapted.
- It starts by 12 hours and takes several days.
- The maximum height up to which acclimatization possible is 18,000 ft.

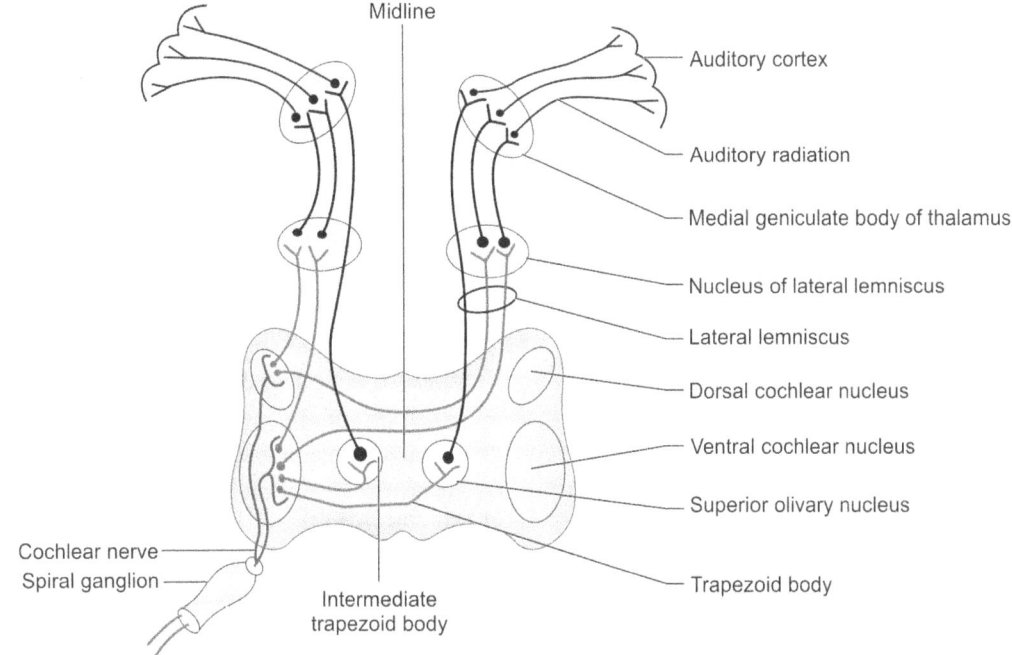

Fig. 18: Auditory pathway from right cochlea. There is bilateral route through brainstem and bilateral cortical representation.

Changes during Acclimatization to High Altitude

Respiratory Changes

- **Initial changes:**

  Hyperventilation by hypoxia stimulating PCR

  ↓

  CO_2 washout

  ↓

  Renal compensation and HCO_3^- excretion out of CSF

  ↓

  Stimulates central chemoreceptors and ventilation

  ↓

  After 4 days ventilation slowly increases and is dependent on altitude

Hematological Changes

- Hypoxia stimulates erythropoietin production by kidneys →↑RBC production (starts after 3 days) →↑O_2 delivery to tissues.
- There is also increase in 2,3-DPG levels in RBC →↑O_2 delivery to tissues.

CVS Changes

- There is ↑in HR, cardiac output (CO) and BP due to activation of sympathoadrenal activity →↑CO and ↑HR →↑blood flow.
- Vasodilatation due to hypoxia →↑ blood flow

Changes in Tissues

- ↑in number of capillaries
- ↑in number of mitochondria in cells
- ↑in activity of oxidative enzymes like cytochrome oxidase
- ↑in myoglobin content
- Angiogenesis

5. Cushings syndrome.

It is due to **hypersecretion of glucocorticoids**:

Causes

- Pharmacological use of exogenous glucocorticoids—ACTH levels are low here.
- ACTH secreting pituitary tumor—Cushing's disease—ACTH levels are high, skin pigmentation present (Because of MSH like activity of ACTH).

- Primary hypercortisolism due to adrenal tumor—ACTH levels are low.

Symptoms

- Obesity with characteristic centripetal distribution of fat, sparing the limbs.
- Face is rounded and cheeks red due to polycythemia.
- Loss of bone mass → osteoporosis → vertebral fractures and necrosis of hip.
- Loss of connective tissue integrity → fragile capillaries, easy bruisability and purple striae in abdomen.
- Increased protein catabolism → atrophy and weakness of skeletal muscles.
- Poor wound healing and response to infection due to loss of protein.
- Disturbances in glucose metabolism—blood glucose levels are high resulting in glucose intolerance, insulin resistance, hyperglycemia or even diabetes mellitus.
- Mineralocorticoid activity of glucocorticoids leads to Na^+ and H_2O retention → Hypertension.
- Excess androgen secretion in women → hirsutism, male pattern baldness, clitoral enlargement.

Diagnosis

- Elevated plasma cortisol or urinary free cortisol levels.
- Loss of diurnal pattern of secretion of cortisol.
- Loss of suppressive effect of exogenous dexamethasone.

6. Succus entericus.

- Secretions of small intestine is called as succus entericus
- It is isotonic in nature
- Daily secretion rate is 1000-2000 mL/day

Composition

- **Mucus:**
  - Secreted by Brunner's glands in duodenum and goblet cells in mucosa of small and large intestines.
  - Stimulated by cholinergic stimulus and chemicals and physical irritation.
  - Protective against HCl and chyme from damaging the mucosa.
- **Enzymes:**
  - They are brush border enzymes and not secreted into the lumen.
  - The brush border enzymes are—peptidases (proteolytic enzymes), disaccharidases (carbohydrate digesting enzymes), intestinal lipases, and enterokinase
- Water and electrolytes

Regulation of Secretion

- Vagal stimulation increases secretion
- Local distension and irritation of mucosa increases secretion.
- Hormones like VIP also increase the secretion.

Functions of Succus Entericus

- Proper mixing of chyme to favor its digestion and absorption.
- Brush border enzymes digest nutrients.
- Mucus in the secretion protects mucosa and also traps bacteria.
- Mucus also contains Ig A for providing mucosal immunity.
- Brunner's gland secretions protect duodenum from damage due to stomach acid.

7. Functions of hypothalamus.

- Regulation of food intake
- Regulation of body temperature
- Regulation of thirst
- Regulation of anterior pituitary hormones
- Regulation of posterior pituitary hormones
- Regulation of sleep wake cycle
- Control of autonomic nervous system
- Control of reproduction
- Control of emotions
- Control of circadian rhythm
- Role in stress
- Role in visceral and somatic function
- Role in reward and punishment

Regulation of Food Intake

There are two groups of neurons involved in food intake:

1. Ventromedial N (Satiety center)
2. Lateral N (Feeding center)

Feeding center stimulates appetite and increases food intake and satiety center inhibits feeding center and brings satiety.

Regulation of Food Intake

These are the hypothesis regulating food-intake:

- **Glucostatic hypothesis:** Activity of satiety center is regulated by glucose utilization of the neurons. When the glucose utilization is low their activity is less and vice versa. When satiety center activity is less the feeding center's activity is unchecked and the person feels hungry. When utilization is high, the glucostat activity is unchecked and there is inhibition of feeding center and the person feels sated. Hypoglycemia is an appetite stimulant and the decrease in plasma glucose decreases the utilization of glucose by the cells.
- **Lipostatic hypothesis:** This hypothesis is based on the fact that the adipose tissues send humoral signals like Leptin, a hormone secreted by adipose tissue. When fat depots are more, the leptin levels increase and it decreases food intake and increases energy output.
- **Gut-peptide theory:** After food intake, there are hormones released from the GIT which act on the hypothalamus and thereby inhibits food intake
- **Thermostatic theory:** Food intake is increased in cold weather and decreased in warm weather.

Hormones and NT Regulating Food Intake

- **Hormones increasing food intake:**
  - Neuropeptide Y
  - Orexins
  - Ghrelin
  - MCH
  - AGRP (Agouti-related peptide)
  - Galanin
  - GHRH
- **Hormones decreasing food intake:**
  - Estrogen
  - Dopamine
  - α MSH
  - Cocaine- and amphetamine-regulated transcript (CART)
  - Corticotrophin releasing hormone (CRH)
  - Gut hormones
  - Cholecystokinin
  - Leptin

Temperature Regulation

- Humans need to maintain body temperature at 37°C.
- Preoptic region of anterior hypothalamus has a role in regulation of body temperature in warmth. When body temperature goes above set point it stimulates heat dissipating mechanisms like vasodilation and sweating.
- Posterior hypothalamus acts in cool temperature and involved in heat conserving mechanisms like vasoconstriction, pilo-erection and sympathetic stimulation.

Regulation of Thirst

- Thirst center is located in the hypothalamus.
- It is located in the lateral hypothalamus.
- It is stimulated by osmoreceptors in increase in tonicity of body fluids.
- A decrease in ECF volume also stimulates thirst center.

Regulation of ECF Volume

Achieved by regulation of ADH, Aldosterone and thirst mechanism.

Regulation of Endocrine Functions

- Hypothalamus controls anterior pituitary and through anterior pituitary it regulates secretion of other endocrine glands.
- It secretes posterior pituitary hormones.
- Hypothalamus is considered to be the master of endocrine orchestra.
- It is a part of the brain and therefore is the link between neural and endocrine systems.

Control of Reproduction

- Hypothalamus releases GnRH which regulates the release of FSH and LH from anterior pituitary gland.
- They in turn control reproductive function in males and females.

- They regulate spermatogenesis, development of accessory sex organs in males and menstrual cycle and secondary sexual characteristics in females.
- Also the sexual behavior are influenced by hypothalamus (preoptic and anterior hypothalamus)

Regulation of Sleep Wake Cycle

- Hypothalamus regulates sleep wake cycle.
- There are two sleep centers:
  1. Diencephalic sleep zone
  2. Basal forebrain sleep zone
- Stimulation of these areas at the frequency of 8 Hz induces slow wave sleep

Control of ANS

- Hypothalamus controls and integrates the activities of ANS.
- Through ANS it is a major regulator of visceral activities.
- Stimulation of posterior hypothalamus results in increase in HR, BP, pupillary dilatation, piloerection (sympathetic system stimulated).
- Stimulation of anterior hypothalamus results in decreased HR, increased HCl secretion, urination, etc. (Parasympathetic system stimulated).

Regulation of Emotional and Behavioral Patterns

- With the limbic system, it participates in the expressions of emotions.
- The circuit given below is responsible for emotions (refer Fig. 19).

Regulation of Circadian Rhythm

- The suprachiasmatic nucleus establishes patterns of awakening and sleep that occur on a circadian (daily) schedule.
- This is mediated through Retinohypothalamic tract.
- **Examples**
  - Cortisol secretion
  - Body temperature
  - ACTH secretion
  - Melatonin secretion
  - Sleep-wakefulness

Regulation of Reward and Punishment Areas

- Hypothalamus along with LS and cortex integrate and bring about smooth responses for reward and punishment.
- VM nucleus is associated with reward and posterior and lateral N of hypothalamus with punishment.

8. Baroreceptor reflex.

Baroreceptors

- There are two types of baroreceptors (BRs). High-pressure and low-pressure baroreceptors.
- High-pressure BRs are present in the carotid and aortic sinuses (refer Fig. 20).
- Low-pressure BRs are present in the great veins, right, and left atria.
- High-pressure BRs are there to monitor and correct the day-to-day change in BP as in change of posture from supine to standing position.

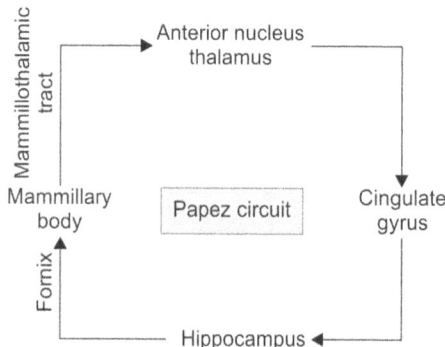

Fig. 19: Papez circuit.

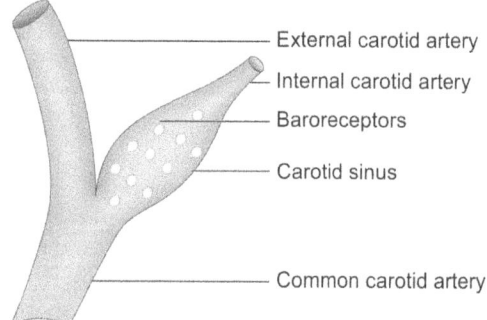

Fig. 20: Baroreceptor—carotid sinus.

- They regulate BP maximally when the MAP is between 70–110 mm Hg and stops firing when MAP falls <40 or rises above 150 mm Hg.

The Reflex

- Most important reflex to regulate BP
- Also called as sino-aortic reflex
- **Receptor:** Carotid and aortic sinuses
- **Stimulus:** Stretch of baroreceptors (as in increased BP)
- **Afferents:** IXth (Supplies carotid sinus) and Xth cranial nerves (Aortic sinus)
- **Efferents:** Sympathetic nerves and vagus nerve
- **Effector:** Heart and blood vessels
- **Response:** Decrease in BP (*refer* **Fig. 21**).

9. Factors necessary for erythropoiesis.

Regulation of Erythropoiesis

There are general and special factors regulating erythropoiesis.

General Factor—Hypoxia

- Major function of RBC is to carry oxygen to the tissues.
- So when there is decrease in tissue oxygen levels, it induces production of RBCs.
- Hypoxia stimulates the interstitial cells of the kidneys to synthesize the hormone **erythropoietin**.
- It acts on bone marrow to stimulate the erythropoietin sensitive stem cells to become proerythroblasts and thereby stimulates formation of RBCs.

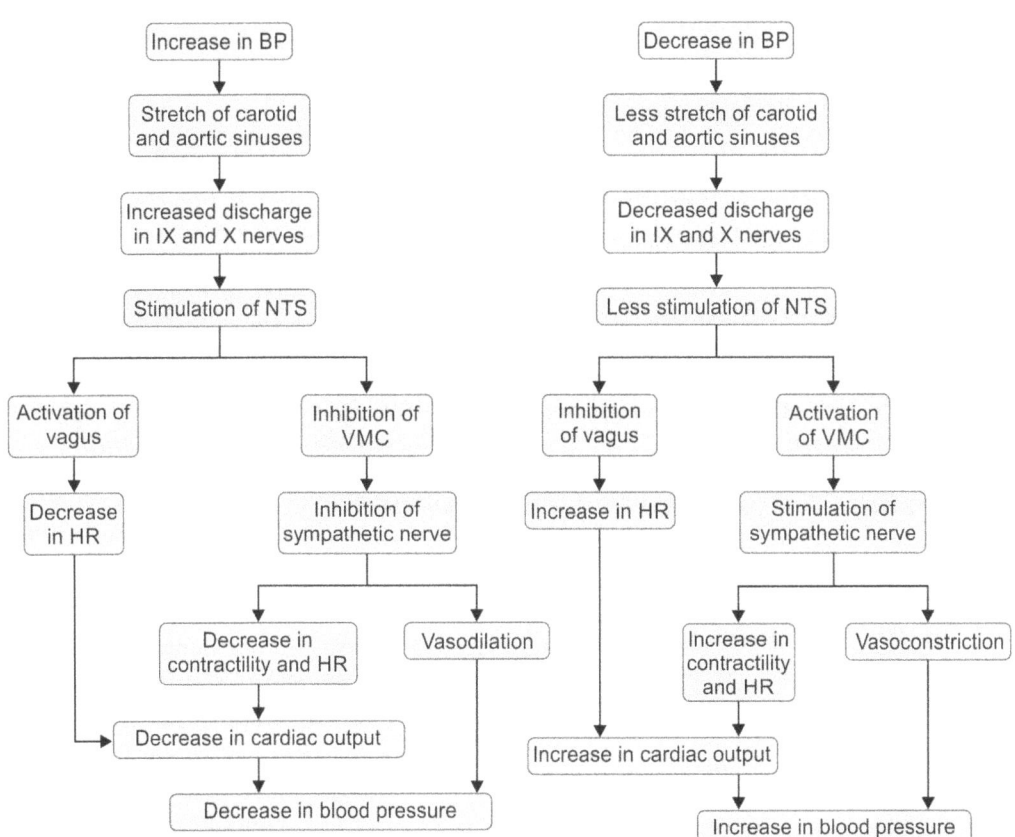

Fig. 21: Regulation of BP by baroreceptors.

- It also increases the release of reticulocytes from the bone marrow.

Factors Increasing Erythropoietin Production
- Hypoxia
- Catecholamines
- Thyroxine
- Testosterone

Special Maturation Factors

Dietary factors:
- Proteins help in globin formation
- Iron helps in heme formation
- Copper, cobalt and nickel also helps in heme formation
- Calcium helps in absorption of iron from GIT
- Vitamin C also helps in iron absorption
- Vitamin B12 and folic acid helps in synthesis of nucleic acids and final maturation of RBC
- Intrinsic factor synthesized in the stomach by the parietal cells help in absorption of vitamin B12.

---

10. Explain the actions of glucocorticoids.

Metabolic actions of glucocorticoids are:
- **Effects on carbohydrate metabolism:**
  - Increases gluconeogenesis in liver → increased glycogen stores.
  - Antagonizes the action of insulin on muscle and adipose tissue—prevents glucose uptake.
  - This spares glucose for the brain.
  - Increases glucose output from liver.
  - Results in hyperglycemia
- **Effects on protein metabolism:**
  - It is proteolytic in action
  - Breaks down proteins into AA and inhibits protein synthesis.
  - Amino acids are used for gluconeogenesis
  - Therefore, increased cortisol levels drain the protein stores in the body
- **Effects on lipid metabolism:**
  - Cortisol is permissive for the lipolytic action of catecholamines.
  - But high cortisol levels increase total body fat by two mechanisms:
    1. Cortisol stimulates appetite → obesity due to increased caloric consumption.
    2. High cortisol →↑ blood glucose →↑ insulin secretion → lipogenesis.
- Pattern of fat distribution—**centripetal**—concentrated in trunk, but wasting is seen in arms and legs.

Permissive Action

Cortisol amplifies effects of certain processes of other hormones where it does not act directly.

Examples
- It does not induce glycogenolysis itself but augments glycogenolysis by glucagon.
- It also augments vaso responsiveness of blood vessels to catecholamines.

Actions on Bones

Increases bone resorption by:
Cortisol decreases renal and GIT absorption of calcium
↓
Lowers serum calcium levels
↓
Parathyroid hormone secretion stimulated
↓
Mobilizes calcium from bone by resorption and demineralization
- Also inhibits action of osteoblasts and suppresses collagen formation. Hence, high cortisol levels results in **osteoporosis**

Actions on CVS
- Cortisol is permissive for the vasopressor effects of catecholamine and Ang ll.
- Hence, it is necessary for maintenance of normal BP.
- Stimulates erythropoietin synthesis and so increases RBC production.

Actions on Connective Tissue

Cortisol inhibits fibroblast proliferation and collagen formation:

So excess cortisol levels
↓
Thinning of skin and walls of capillaries
↓
Easy damage to skin and easy bruising of capillaries
↓
Intracutaneous hemorrhage

Action on Kidneys
- Cortisol inhibits ADH secretion and action, so in absence of cortisol a water load leads to water intoxication.
- Cortisol also has a weak mineralocorticoid action →↑Na⁺ and H_2O reabsorption.
- **Increases GFR:**
  - By increasing cardiac output
  - By direct action on kidneys

Action on Muscles
- Cortisol has complex action on muscles.
- Excess cortisol results in muscle weakness due to:
  - Proteolysis
  - Hypokalemia

Actions on GIT
- Cortisol has a trophic action on GIT.
- It also increases appetite → weight gain in hypercortisolism.
- Increased acid secretion → acidity, gastritis

Action on CNS
- Glucocorticoids alters mood and behavior
- REM sleep ↓, but slow wave sleep ↑
- In excess—insomnia, elevated or depressed mood, ↓ memory.
- Frank psychosis occurs with excess or reduced cortisol levels.
- Dampens the acuity to olfactory, gustatory, auditory, and visual stimuli.

Action in Fetus
- Facilitates maturity of CNS, retina, skin, GIT, and lungs.
- During the last week of pregnancy the synthesis of surfactant is stimulated by cortisol.
- So if premature delivery suspected weekly doses of cortisol given to the mother till delivery.

Action on Inflammation and Immune System
- Cortisol is frequently used clinically for its anti-inflammatory property
- It inhibits synthesis of mediators of inflammation.
- Inhibits migration of leucocytes to site of injury.
- Decreases the number of circulating eosinophils.
- Inhibits fibroblast proliferation at inflammatory site which is a defense mechanism in the body to prevent spreading of infection.
- Excess cortisol inhibits normal defense mechanisms of body against infection

Effect on Immune Response
- Cortisol inhibits immune response in the body.
- At high doses, it decreases the number of T lymphocytes (helper t-cells) and their migration to antigenic site.
- B lymphocytes and antibody production are not affected directly.
- Because of these effects, glucocorticoids are used for immunosuppression after organ transplantation.

Effect on Stress
- Protects the body against stress
- During stress there is increased secretion of CRH from hypothalamus.
- This increases the secretion of ACTH from anterior pituitary
- Therefore glucocorticoid secretion increases
- Cortisol facilitates lipolysis by catecholamine and increases release of free fatty acids which supplies the energy needed to cope up with stress.
- It is also permissive for the vasoconstriction induced by catecholamines, which is needed for maintaining BP during stress.

11. Effects of lesions in optic pathway.

Injury in the visual pathway leads to visual field defects. The type of lesion depends on the site of lesion (*refer* **Figs. 22A to D**).
- Complete loss of vision—**anopia**
- Loss of vision in one half of the visual field—**hemianopia**
  - **Lesion in optic nerve:** There is complete loss of vision (anopia) on the same side visual field.
  - **Lesion in optic chiasma (crossed fibers):** Bitemporal hemianopia
  - **Lesion in optic chiasma (uncrossed fibers):** Damage happens due to

carotid artery aneurysm—leads to binasal hemianopia.
- **Lesion in optic tract:** Lesion in one side will cause homonymous hemianopia of the opposite side, like lesion in left optic tract will cause right homonymous hemianopia.
- **Lesion in geniculocalcarine tract:** Homonymous hemianopia
- **Optic radiation (medial fibers):** Homonymous lower quadrantinopia
- **Optic radiation (lateral fibers):** Homonymous upper quadrantinopia.
- **Lesion in visual cortex:** Homonymous hemianopia with macular sparing. Macula is spared because it has a larger area of representation in the visual cortex.

---

12. Determinants of blood pressure.

❏ BP is defined as the **lateral pressure exerted by the moving column of blood** on the vessel wall. Normal value = **120/80 mm Hg.**

Components of BP

❏ Systolic BP
❏ Diastolic BP
❏ Pulse pressure
❏ Mean arterial pressure

Determinants of BP

❏ Blood pressure is determined by **cardiac output** and **peripheral resistance**.
❏ Cardiac output is determined by **stroke volume** and **heart rate**.
❏ Stroke volume is determined by cardiac contractility and **end diastolic volume (EDV)**
❏ EDV is determined by **venous return**. Venous return is determined by **skeletal muscle pump, cardiac pump, blood**

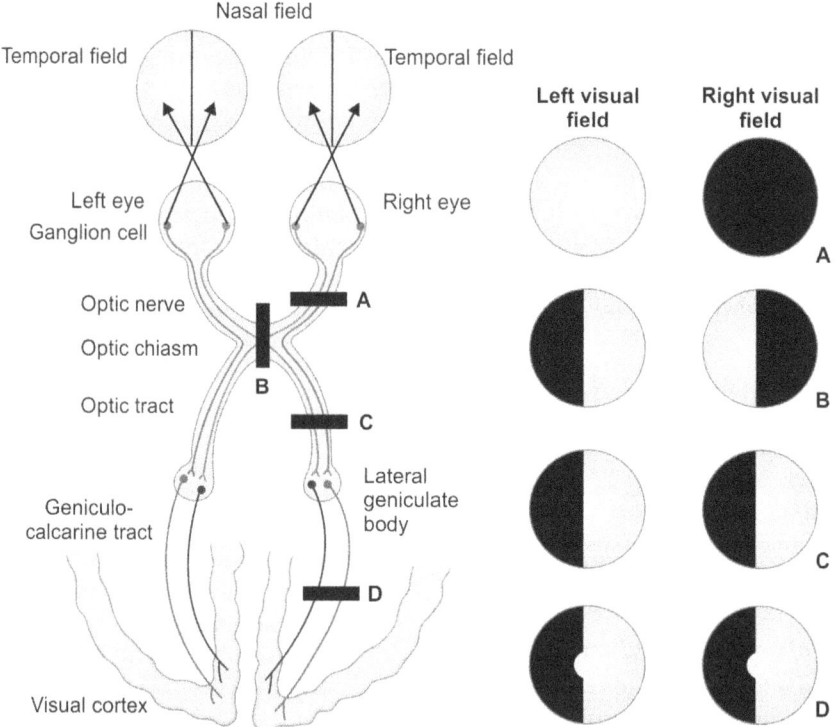

Figs. 22A to D: Visual pathway and lesions: (A) Lesion in right optic nerve causes right anopia; (B) Lesion of nasal fibers of optic chiasm causes bitemporal heteronymous hemianopia; (C) Lesion of right optic tract, causes left homonymous hemianopia; (D) Lesion in geniculocalcarine tract causes left homonymous hemianopia with macular sparing.

volume, **respiratory pump, sympathetic stimulation.**
- **Contractility** is determined by **sympathetic stimulation, hypoxia, acidosis,** etc.
- **Heart rate** is modulated by **sympathetic and parasympathetic nerves.**
- **Peripheral resistance** is determined by afterload, which in turn is determined by **caliber of arterioles and viscosity of blood.**
- **Systolic BP** is determined by **cardiac output** and **diastolic BP** is determined by **peripheral resistance.**

III. SHORT ANSWERS

1. Fetoplacental unit.

- Placenta produces steroidal hormones; estrogen and progesterone with the interaction of the fetal adrenals.
- Placenta forms pregnenolone and progesterone from cholesterol.
- Some of this pregnenolone enters the fetal circulation and along with the pregnenolone from fetal liver, forms the substrate for the formation of dehydroepiandrosterone (DHEA) and 16-OH DHEAS in fetal adrenals (*refer* **Fig. 23**).

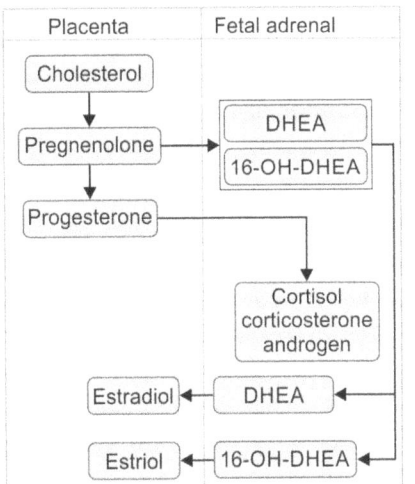

Fig. 23: Fetoplacental unit. Placenta and fetal adrenals, together synthesize progesterone and estrogen.
(DHEA: dehydroepiandrosterone; 16-OH DHEA: 16-hydroxy dehydroepiandrosterone)

- DHEAS and 16-OH DHEAS are transported back to the placenta where DHEAS forms estradiol and 16 OHDHEAS forms estriol.
- Estriol is the major estrogen, and since its formation requires fetal adrenals, urinary excretion of estriol by mother is a good indicator of well-being of fetus.

2. Importance of dietary fibers.

- Dietary fibers include cellulose, hemicellulose, lignin, etc.
- These substances when ingested are not digested due to lack of microorganisms for digesting them.
- So they pass out without getting digested.

Functions of dietary fibers are:

- The undigested fibers when they are present in the colon, they tend to hold water and increase the bulk of feces and therefore can be **used for treating constipation.**
- It **decreases the rate of absorption** of nutrients form intestines and thereby prevents sudden increase in blood glucose levels after food intake. Due to slow absorption of carbohydrates, insulin demand is also decreased. So, it can be used as a **supplementary treatment in diabetes mellitus.**
- It **decreases blood cholesterol levels** by excreting bile salts. Bile salts get trapped in the fiber and is excreted. The rate of formation of bile salts are increased and cholesterol is used for it. So, it is used for **controlling hypercholesterolemia,** obesity, etc.
- It **prevents colon cancer** by diluting the carcinogens and minimizing their contact with the colon.

3. Neuromuscular transmission

It is the junction between the motor neuron and the muscle fiber it supplies.

Structure of NMJ

- The NMJ is formed by the axon terminal of the motor neuron.
- On approaching the muscle fiber, the axon it loses its myelin sheath and divides into

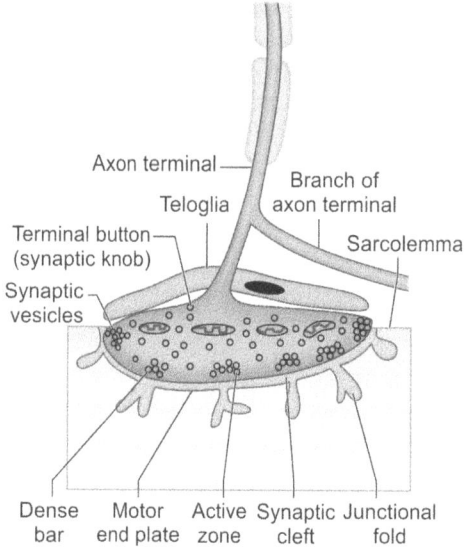

Fig. 24: Neuromuscular junction.

many branches and the nerve terminals bulge to form the terminal buttons which approaches the muscle fiber at its center.
- NMJ has a presynaptic membrane, synaptic cleft and postsynaptic membrane (*refer* Fig. 24).

Presynaptic Terminal
- It is the membrane of the terminal button of the axon.
- It has many ACh vesicles and mitochondria within the membrane.
- The membrane is studded with many voltage-gated Ca^{2+} channels.

Synaptic Cleft
- It is a space of 50–100 nm width between the presynaptic and postsynaptic membranes.
- It has ECF in it and acetylcholinesterase enzyme is present in it.

Postsynaptic Membrane
- It is the muscle membrane in contact with the nerve terminal and it is thrown into many folds—junctional folds and is thickened and deepened—synaptic trough.
- The muscle membrane here is called as the **motor end plate**.
- It contains the nicotinic acetylcholine receptors.

Impulse Transmission in NMJ

Stimulation of nerve fiber
↓
AP generated in nerve fiber
↓
Conduction of AP in nerve fiber
↓
Impulse reaches nerve terminal
↓
Voltage-gated Ca^{2+} channels in nerve terminal open
↓
Ca^{2+} influx into presynaptic membrane
↓
Exocytosis of ACh vesicles and ACh is released into synaptic cleft
↓
ACh moves across the cleft and binds to Nicotinic ACh receptors in muscle membrane
↓
The receptor is a nonspecific cation channel which opens on binding with ACh
↓
Influx of Na^+ ions into postsynaptic membrane
↓
Local depolarization of muscle membrane—**end plate potential**
↓
Generation of action potential in the neighboring muscle membrane by the EPP

4. ESR-clinical significance.

It is the rate at which the RBCs settle down/sediment when the blood is anticoagulated and allowed to stand in a long narrow tube for some time. It is expressed as millimeter/hour.

Factors which affect ESR
- **Number of RBCs:** Increase in number of RBCs decreases ESR and decrease in number raises the ESR.
- Increase in size of RBCs increase ESR.
- **Rouleaux formation:** Increased rouleaux forming tendency increases ESR.

Fibrinogen and globulin in plasma as in inflammation will increase rouleaux and increase in ESR.

Clinical Significance

- Normal value of ESR is 3–7 mm/h in males and 5–9 mm/h in females by Westergren method.
- It is elevated in chronic inflammatory conditions.
- It is of no diagnostic value but it gives an idea about the progress of the patient under treatment and therefore is of prognostic value.

---

5. Movements of small intestine.

- **Five types of movements in the normal state:**
  1. Peristalsis—propulsive movement
  2. Mixing movements—segmentation contraction and tonic contraction
  3. Migrating motor complexes (MMC)
  4. Movements of Villi
  5. Contractions of muscularis mucosa
- **Abnormal movements:** Peristaltic rushes.

MMC

- Migrating motility complexes are motility present in the interdigestive period.
- These are bursts of electrical and mechanical activities in GIT
- It starts in the esophagus and spreads through the stomach and ileum to the ileocaecal valve
- Occurs once in 90 minutes and lasts for 10–20 min.
- It clears the GIT for the next meal.
- Occurs in 3 phases—Phases I, II and III
- **Phase I:** No spike potential, no contractions
- **Phase II:** Irregular spike potentials and contractions
- **Phase III:** Regular spike potentials and contractions

Mixing Movements

Segmentation Contractions

- These are ring like contractions present in short segments of the intestine of 1–2 cm.
- They are present in regular intervals.
- Their frequency matches the slow wave frequency.
- Slow waves are waves generated in the pacemaker cells located in the wall of duodenum and it spreads through the muscular wall of the intestines.
- Strength of the contraction depends on the spike waves superimposed on the slow waves.
- These ring-like contractions appear in one segment and the nearby segment relaxes, this is followed by another set of contractions in the segments between the previous contractions.
- These contractions appear sausage shaped and they cut into the bolus and move it to and fro and increase their exposure to the absorptive surface of the mucosa (*refer* **Fig. 25**).
- Therefore, these contractions help in mixing the bolus with digestive juices and in digestion and absorption of food.

Tonic Contractions

- These are prolonged contractions of one segment of intestine and the segment appears to be isolated from the rest of the ileum.
- Segmentation and tonic contractions delay the passage of chyme and thereby

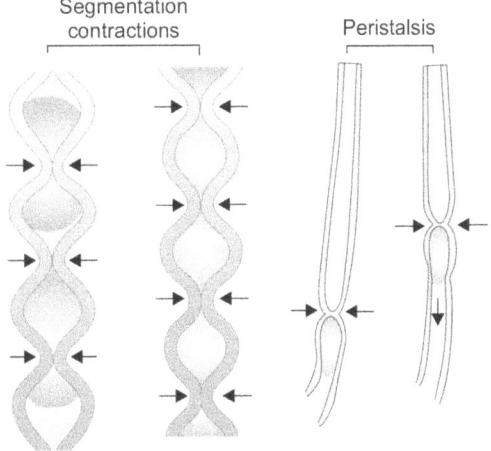

Fig. 25: Segmentation contractions and peristalsis

allow contact of chyme with enterocytes and favor absorption.

Peristalsis

- This is a type of propulsive movement which helps to move the chyme forward. It is a reflex initiated by the stretch of the intestinal wall following the entry of food.
- Stretch of the intestinal wall initiates a ring of constriction behind the bolus and a relaxation in front of the bolus.
- The ring of contraction behind pushes the bolus to the relaxed segment in front of the bolus.
- Next ring of contraction now appears in the previous relaxed segment and the bolus is pushed further.
- These waves always propel the contents from the oral to caudal direction and never in the opposite direction—law of the gut.
- These waves appear even in the absence of nerve supply but they can be modified by the autonomic nerves, parasympathetic nerves increase the activity and sympathetic nerves decrease the activity.
- The propelling speed varies from 2–25 cm/s.
- Sometimes the peristaltic waves can be very fast and they empty the contents faster—peristaltic rushes, seen in acute diarrhea.
- Antiperistalsis happens in vomiting.

Contractions of Muscularis Mucosa

- Irregular in nature.
- Occurs at a frequency of 3/min.
- It helps in mixing the contents and in absorption.

Contraction of Villi

- The type of contraction seen as elongation and shortening of the villi.
- It helps in emptying of central lacteals of the villi and increases the absorptive surface area.
- It is stimulated by the hormone Villikinin.

Functions of Movements of Small Intestine

- Mixing the chyme with the digestive juices and helps in digestion
- Propelling the chyme forward
- Presenting the chyme to absorptive surface and helps for absorption

6. Diabetes insipidus.

- Lack of ADH action—diabetes insipidus (DI):
  - **Central or neurogenic DI:** ADH is not synthesized and secreted from posterior pituitary. It can be treated with DDVAP (Desmopressin), clofibrate, chlorpropamide
  - **Nephrogenic DI:** The synthesis of ADH is normal. But the receptors for ADH in the kidneys do not respond to ADH due to genetic mutations. It is treated with diuretics like Hydrochlorothiazide
- Features of DI:
  - Polyuria—urine output is 3–20 L/day
  - Polydipsia—increase in thirst sensation
  - Osmolality of urine is very low (<300 mosm/L)
  - Dehydration happens if water intake is decreased

7. Red cell indices

Mean Corpuscular Volume (MCV)

It refers to the average volume of a single RBC. It is calculated by dividing PCV by the red cell count.

$$MCV = PCV \times 10/RBC \text{ count}/\mu L$$
$$= 45 \times 10/5 = 90 \ \mu m^3$$

Normal value of MCV is 78–94 μm^3
Decrease in MCV = Microcytosis
Increase in MCV = Macrocytosis

Mean Corpuscular Hemoglobin (MCH):

MCH is average weight of hemoglobin contained in each RBC. It is calculated by dividing the amount of Hb in 1 L of blood by RBC count in 1 L of blood.

$$MCH = Hb \text{ g in L/RBC in L}$$
$$= Hb \text{ g\%} \times 10/RBC \text{ in } \mu L \times 10^{12}$$
$$= 15 \times 10/5 \times 10^{12} = 30 \times 10^{-12} \text{ g}$$
$$= 30 \text{ pg}$$

Normal value of MHC is 27–30 pg.

Mean Corpuscular Hemoglobin Concentration (MCHC)

It is the amount of hemoglobin expressed as a percentage of RBC volume.

$$MCHC = Hb\ g\%/PCV \times 100\ mL \times 100$$
$$= 15/45 \times 100 = 33.3\%$$

Normal value = 30–38%

In iron deficiency anemia, the RBCs are hypochromic and MCHC is less

Color Index (CI)

It is the ratio of Hb to RBC.

CI = Percentage of normal Hb/Percentage of normal RBC count
= 100/100 = 1

Normal value of CI = 0.85 to 1.15

8. Extracellular edema.

It is the accumulation of abnormally large volumes of fluid in the interstitium.

Causes for Edema

- **Increased filtration pressure:**
  - Arteriolar dilation
  - Venous constriction
  - Increased venous pressure—heart failure, venous obstruction, effect of gravity, increased ECF volume
- **Decreased osmotic gradient across vessel wall:**
  - Decreased plasma protein level
  - Accumulation of osmotically active substances, such as the metabolites in interstitium
- **Increased capillary permeability:** By chemicals like histamine, kinins, and substance P
- **Lymphatic obstruction:**
  - **Lymph** is the fluid present in the lymphatic ducts.
  - Normally across the capillaries, fluid efflux (in arteriolar end) is more than the fluid influx (in venous end).
  - The extra fluid which stays back in the interstitium cannot afford to be lost from circulation.
  - This volume is returned back to the circulation through the lymphatic ducts which empties through the thoracic duct into the internal jugular vein.
- The normal lymph flow is 2–4 L/day.
- If there is obstruction for the drainage of this fluid, it remains in the interstitium and results in edema.
- But the fluid is rich in proteins and long-term retention leads to inflammation and fibrosis.
- This leads to nonpitting edema.
- Example for this type of edema is filariasis, where the parasites block the lymphatics and this result in accumulation of fluid especially in legs and scrotum—elephantiasis.

9. Functions of Sertoli cells.

- They play a major role in the maturation of spermatozoa. Spermatids mature into spermatozoa in the deep folds of cytoplasm in the Sertoli cells.
- They provide nutrition to the developing spermatozoa and help in spermiation
- They take part in the formation of Blood-testis barrier which selectively allows certain substances to enter seminiferous tubule.
- They phagocytose damaged germ cells.
- They secrete seminal fluid
- **Sertoli cells produce substances like:**
  - *Mullerian inhibiting substance (MIS):* Causes regression of Mullerian duct and promotes development of structures from the Wolffian duct.
  - *Inhibin:* Inhibits FSH secretion
  - *Activin*
  - *Androgen binding protein (ABP):* This helps to maintain a high concentration of androgens in the seminiferous tubule which is essential for spermatogenesis
  - Estrogen is produced from androgen in the presence of Aromatase which is present in the Sertoli cells.

10. Tests for ovulation.

- **Rise of basal body temperature:** There is a rise in 0.5°C in basal body temperature after ovulation. The rise is due to the thermogenic effect of progesterone which

is secreted by corpus luteum. It is recorded first thing in the morning, orally, before getting up from bed, before eating or drinking anything.
- **Mittelschmerz:** After ovulation, bleeding into the ruptured follicle happens, some amount of blood is also split into the abdominal cavity close to the ovary and results in fleeting abdominal pain.
- **Spinnbarkeit:** During proliferative phase, under the influence of estrogen, cervical mucus is very thin and at the time of ovulation it is the thinnest and a drop of mucus between the thumb and index finger can be stretched to 10 cm, this is Spinnbarkeit.
- Sometimes following ovulation **mild spotting** can also be present
- **Fern test:** At the time of ovulation, under the effect of estrogen, the cervical mucous is thin and when spread on a slide and viewed under the microscope gives a fern shape. In the luteal phase when progesterone is present this fern pattern is absent.
- **Demonstration of LH peak:** LH surge is seen just before ovulation and therefore regular estimation of LH levels can give us an idea about ovulation.
- **Laparoscopic examination**
- **Ultrasound scanning of pelvis**

11. Accommodation reflex.

- When the eye is focusing on a close object the curvature of the lens increases to get a clear image on retina—accommodation of lens.
- This occurs due to contraction of ciliary muscles
- Results in increase of curvature of lens—adds 12 diopters to the power of the lens, power of lens increases (>70 D)
- **Near point:** 10 cm in young adult.
- **Presbyopia:** Near point increases (83 cm).

Other changes of accommodation are:

- Constriction of pupil
- Convergence of eyeball

Accommodation Reflex Pathway

Impulses from retina for near vision
↓
Optic nerve
↓
Optic chiasma
↓
Optic tract
↓
Lateral geniculate body
↓
Visual cortex (area 17)
↓
Frontal eye field
↓
Edinger-Westphal nuclei of both sides (parasympathetic fibers)
↓
Efferents go through the oculomotor nerves → medial rectus → convergence of eyeball
↓
Ciliary ganglion
↓
Supplies the sphincter pupillae and the ciliary muscles
↓
Constriction of pupil and anterior curvature of lens increases
↓
Accommodation of eye

12. Conducting system of the heart.

- These impulses originated in the SA node are conducted down through the specialized conducting system as mentioned above.
- The impulses from SA node are transmitted to the AV node through three internodal bundles which are socialized tissues for conduction of impulses from SA node to AV node in a faster way.
- The atrial tissues also conduct impulses but they are slower.

The three bundles are:

1. Anterior internodal tract of Bachman
2. Middle internodal tract of Wenckebach
3. Posterior internodal tract of Thorel

4. Through these bundles the impulses reach the AV node.

Interatrial Tract of Bachman
- This bundle starts in the SA node and ends in the left atrium.
- The left atrium is also depolarized simultaneously

AV Node
- It is located beneath the endocardium on the right side of lower part of atrial septum near the tricuspid valve.
- The conduction velocity through the AVN is very slow because the fibers are smaller with less number of gap junctions.
- There is a delay of 0.1 s
- The delay provides time for atrial contraction and final ventricular filling.
- It also prevents transmission of all impulses from atria to ventricles in supraventricular tachycardia.
- It is supplied by sympathetic and PS nerves which alter the conduction rate

Atrioventricular Bundle of His
- This bundle starts in the AV bundle and descends down the fibrous skeleton and divides into right and left branches and they supply the right and left ventricles.
- The bundles divide into many small branches, the Purkinje fibers.

Purkinje Fibers

They are present in the endocardium and reaches all parts of ventricles.

Ventricles
- The spread of depolarization in the ventricular muscles are from the AVN to the His bundle → Purkinje fibers → Ventricles.
- The conduction velocity of the AP through ventricular muscles are 0.3–0.4 msec.
- This results in depolarization of both ventricles at the same time and leads to contraction of both ventricles at the same time (*refer* **Fig. 26**).
- In ventricle, the spread of depolarization is from endocardium to epicardium.

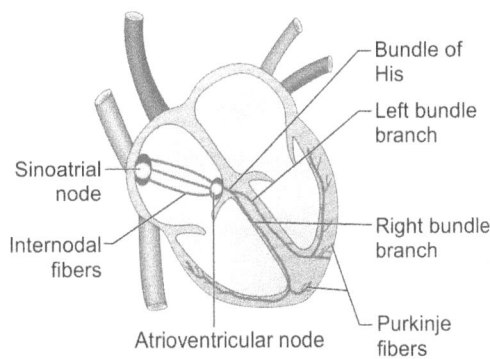

Fig. 26: Conducting system of the heart.

13. Artificial respiration.

When there is respiratory deficiency or respiratory arrest artificial respiration is given.

Conditions

Drowning, gas poisoning, electric shock, anesthesia, accidents, etc.

Methods

Instrumental and manual methods.

Instrumental Methods
- Used when there is a need for prolonged support.
- **Three types:**
  1. Positive pressure method
  2. Negative pressure method
  3. Boyle's apparatus

Positive Pressure Method:
- Used in operation theatres
- Here air or O_2 mixture is used to inflate the lungs at positive pressures either continuously or intermittently.
- It impairs venous return.

Negative Pressure Method:
- Achieved by alternate compression and relaxing the chest wall.
- **They are:**
  - *Drinker's method* (Iron lung chamber)
  - *Bragg-Paul method*: Use of hollow elastic rubber bag.
  - Others

Drinker's Method (Iron Lung Method)
- The instrument contains an airtight iron chamber with a bellow on one side of the instrument.
- When the bellow moves in and out it creates a rise and fall of pressure inside the chamber.
- The person is placed inside the chamber with the head and neck outside the chamber.
- When the pressure rises inside the chamber expiration happens for the patient and when the pressure falls in the chamber there is inspiration.

Bragg-Paul Method
- Here an elastic rubber bag is tied around the chest of the patient.
- The bag is connected to a pump which can inflate and deflate the bag.
- When the bag is inflated it compresses the chest and air is expired.
- When the pressure is released, the chest enlarges passively and air is drawn in.

Boyel's Apparatus

This apparatus is used in the hospitals for artificial ventilation. It is an automatic instrument in which rate and depth of ventilation and composition of inspired can be altered.

Manual Methods

Holger–Neilson Method
- The subject is made to lie prone and the head is turned to one side **(Fig. 27A)**.
- The shoulder is abducted and flexed at the elbow and the hands are placed under the cheek.
- The operator is in kneeling position at the head of the patient and he places his hands spread on the back of the subject and bends forward to press on his back **(Fig. 27B)**.
- The pressure on the back of the subject and compresses on the chest and expels the air out **(Fig. 27C)**.
- Then he holds the arm above the elbow of the subject and pulls the arm forward **(Fig. 27D)**.
- This enlarges the chest and results in inspiration. It is repeated 12/min. This is an exhaustive method for the examiner.

Eve's Rocking Method
- Here the subject is made to lie prone on board which is rocketed on a pivot so that it can move up and down like a see-saw.
- When the board is tilted head down the abdominal organs push on the diaphragm resulting decrease in thoracic volume and expiration happens.
- When the board is tilted in the opposite direction the inspiration happens.

Mouth-to-Mouth Respiration
- It can be direct or indirect method. In direct method, the operator places his mouth directly on the subject's mouth and in indirect method it is done with a small tube.

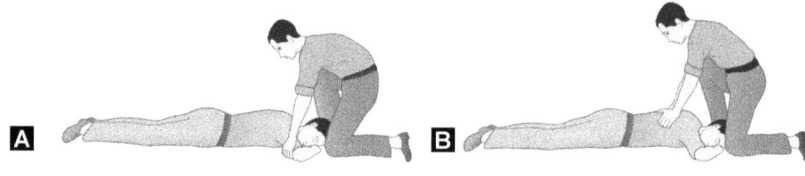

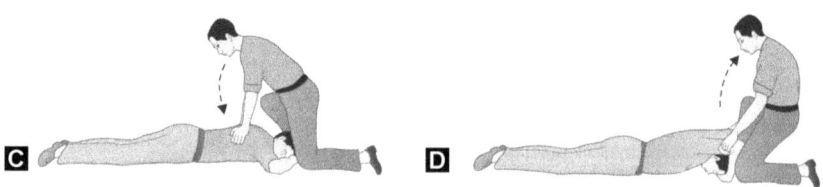

Figs. 27A to D: Holger-Nielsen method of artificial respiration

- The subject is made to lie supine; the airway is kept clean from vomitus, foreign body, etc.
- The subject's head is extended, the operator sits on the side of the subject holds the lower jaw with his left hand and opens the mouth and with his right hand clips the nostrils.
- The operator then inhales deeply and places his mouth on the subject's mouth or the tube placed in the subject's mouth and blows into the subject's mouth smoothly, volume twice that of the tidal volume.
- This inflates the lungs of the subject and then the examiner removes his mouth from the subject's mouth and the lungs recoil resulting in expiration.
- It is repeated 12 times a minute.
- *Advantages*: Can be applied immediately, can achieve large tidal volumes, CO_2 stimulates respiration, simple technique.
- *Disadvantages*: Infection may spread, volunteer may get exhausted.

14. Conditioned reflexes.

- It is a reflex response to a stimulus, that previously elicited little or no response, acquired by repeatedly pairing the stimulus with another stimulus which normally produces a response.
- The stimulus that normally produces a response is the unconditioned stimulus (UCS) and the stimulus which elicits a response after pairing with UCS is the conditioned stimulus (CS)
- There are two types of conditioned reflexes—classical conditioning and operant conditioning.

15. Surfactant

- It is a protein-lipid complex secreted by the Type II alveolar epithelial cells lining the alveoli.
- Surfactant is a mixture of dipalmitoyl phosphatidylcholine (DPPC), other lipids and proteins—SP-A, SP-B, SP-C and SP-D (*refer* **Fig. 28**).
- It acts as a detergent to reduce the surface tension of the fluid lining the alveoli and prevent its collapse during expiration.
- The phospholipids have hydrophobic tails and a hydrophilic head. They arrange themselves with the tails facing the alveolar lumen and intersperse between water molecules.

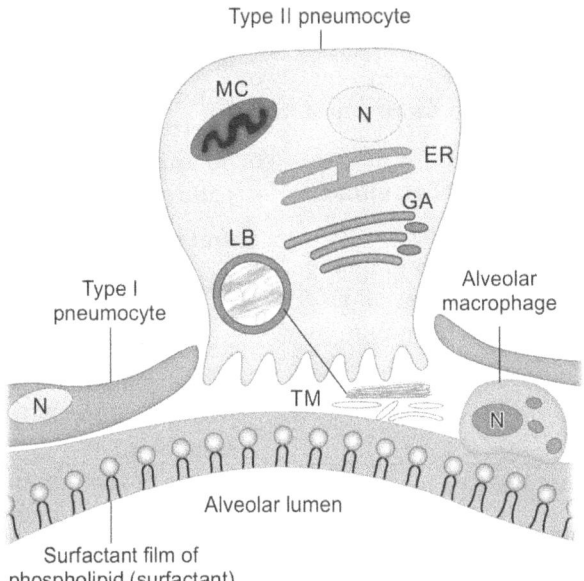

Fig. 28: Arrangement of surfactant molecules in alveolar lumen.
(N: nucleus; MC: mitochondria; ER: endoplasmic reticulum; GA: Golgi apparatus; LB: lamellar body; TM: tubular myelins)

- So, during inspiration as the alveoli enlarge the surfactant molecules move apart and surface tension of water increases and during expiration, they come closer and the surface tension is lowered.
- Surfactant is important at birth. After birth, the infant tries to breathe and makes inspiratory movements and the lungs expand after which the lung tends to recoil and the presence of surfactant prevents the collapse of the alveoli.
- Surfactant deficiency results in alveolar collapse, which results in infant respiratory distress syndrome (IRDS)
- Maturation of surfactant in the lungs is enhanced by glucocorticoids. During term, the fetal and maternal cortisol increases and favors maturation of surfactant.

Other Functions of Surfactant
- Stabilizes the lung alveoli
- It also decreases the effect of surface tension, which if not countered will increase the pulmonary capillary hydrostatic pressure and thereby fluid accumulation in the alveolus. So, surfactant prevents pulmonary edema.
- As it prevents alveolar collapse, it decreases the work of breathing
- They help in immunity

Regulation of Secretion of Surfactant

It is regulated by hormones—glucocorticoids, insulin and thyroxine promote secretion of surfactant.

Factors which affect Surfactant Secretion
- High O_2 content affects surfactant secretion as in O_2 therapy in patients undergoing cardiac surgery using pump oxygenator
- Occlusion of pulmonary bronchus or pulmonary artery
- Long-term inhalation of 100% O_2
- Cigarette smoking

---

16. Central analgesic system.

Analgesic System in the Brain
- **Pain modulation takes place in two places:**
  1. At the peripheral nerve endings
  2. At the spinal cord level

Peripheral Nerve Endings

Endorphins and enkephalins combine with nociceptors and decrease the response to stimuli.

At the Spinal Cord
- **Peripheral mechanism: By gate control theory**—large Aβ fibers (when stimulated by touching or rubbing the painful area) ↓ nociception in C fibers.
- **Central pain suppressing mechanism:** Opioids secreted from areas in brain stem inhibit pain transmission in the spinal cord.

Gate control mechanism:
- Pain sensation is carried by Aδ and unmyelinated C fibers and they ascend up as spinothalamic tract.
- Touch and pressure sensations are carried by large myelinated Aβ fibers and they ascend up as dorsal column tract in spinal cord.
- Dorsal column fibers in the spinal cord give a branch to inhibitory interneurons which secrete enkephalins and which in turn end on the second order neurons in pain pathway.
- So, when there is pain in an area, touching or pressing that region stimulates the large Aβ fibers which in turn inhibit pain pathway and thereby there is decreased pain perception.
- So the large Aβ fibers gate the pain pathway.

Central pain suppressing mechanism:
- Pain pathway, as it ascends up gives branches to periaqueductal grey (PAG) in midbrain.
- There is a pain suppressing descending pathway from PAG to medulla and to spinal cord.
- Axons of the neurons in PAG terminate on serotonergic neurons in raphe magnus nuclei in medulla.
- They secrete enkephalin here.
- Axons of serotonergic neurons in raphe magnus nuclei descend and terminate on

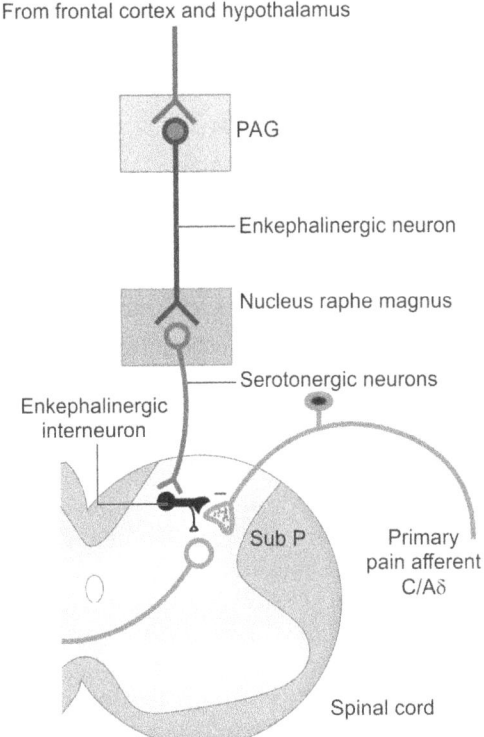

Fig. 29: Endogenous pain inhibition by spinal cord and brainstem structures. PAG—periaqueductal gray. It has enkephalinergic neurons which end on serotonergic neurons of raphe magnus nucleus in medulla. They send out axons which end on enkephalinergic neurons in spinal cord and decreases pain.

the inhibitory interneurons in spinal cord (*refer* **Fig. 29**).
- They secrete serotonin and stimulate internuncial neurons which in turn inhibit second order neurons in the pain pathway by secreting enkephalin.

17. VO$_2$ max.

- Normal O$_2$ uptake at rest is 250 mL/min. It can increase to 3 L/min during exercise.
- So, it is given as the maximum amount of O$_2$ consumed by an individual during exercise or VO$_{2max}$.
- VO$_{2max}$ is the product of maximal cardiac output and maximal O$_2$ extraction by the tissues.
- VO$_{2max}$ improves with training. In a sedentary individual it is around 3 L/min and in athletes it is up to 5 L/min.

18. Functions of CSF.

- CSF offers mechanical protection by acting as a shock absorber.
- CSF offers the optimum chemical environment for accurate neuronal signaling.
- CSF acts as a circulating medium for exchange of nutrients and waste products between the blood and nervous tissue.
- Continuous formation and drainage removes metabolic wastes from brain.
- Acts as lymph
- Provides nutrition
- Reduces the weight of brain

19. Decompression sickness.

- Also called as "Dysbarism, The bends, Caissons disease, Divers palsy".
- This happens when a person breathing compressed air ascends up rapidly.
- At high pressures, N$_2$ dissolves in body fluids and stays dissolved.
- When the person ascends up to sea level gradually N$_2$ is converted to air gradually and is blown out.
- But when he ascends up rapidly the dissolved N$_2$ does not have enough time to be converted to air and to be blown out and therefore it stays in the tissues as N$_2$ bubbles.
- N$_2$ dissolved in tissues forms bubbles while escaping from tissues due to rapid ascent.
- Gas bubbles block the blood vessels and stay in tissues to create symptoms.

Symptoms are:
- Pain in joints and muscles of legs or arms.
- Sensation of numbness
- The chokes—shortness of breath, pulmonary edema, etc.
- Paralysis of muscles
- Coronary ischemia
- Neurological symptoms

Treatment: Recompression in pressurized chamber followed by slow decompression

20. Babinski's sign and its clinical significance.

- It is an abnormal plantar reflex.
- On eliciting a plantar reflex, the normal response is adduction and plantar flexion of all the toes.
- In Babinski's sign, there is dorsiflexion of big toe and fanning out of all the other toes.
- It is a normal response in infants below 2 years of age as the myelination of pyramidal tract is not complete till this age.
- In adults if this response is seen it is due to lesion of pyramidal tract.

21. Resting membrane potential.

There is a potential difference across the membrane of all cells and the inside of the cell is more negative than the outside of the cell. This is said to be the membrane potential. The membrane potential at rest in a cell is said to be the resting membrane potential (RMP).

The RMP in excitable cells like the nerve and muscle cells are important as the change in the potential makes the cell to become more excited or inhibited.

RMP is due to unequal distribution of ions on either side of the membrane and various forces acting on the membrane. They are:
- Unequal distribution of ions across the cell membrane (*refer* **Fig. 30**)
- Differences in the permeability of the membrane to various ions.
- Na^+ - K^+ pump or Na^+ - K^+ ATPase

The RMP of Various Cells

- RMP of the nerve is –70 mV
- RMP of skeletal membrane is –90 mV
- RMP of cardiac muscle is –90 mV
- RMP of smooth muscles is variable

Selective Permeability of the Membrane to Ions

The membrane allows certain molecules to move freely across and restrict movements of certain ions. It is highly permeable to K^+ and chloride at rest and only moderately permeable to Na^+. It is totally impermeable to intracellular proteins and phosphates which are anions. The high permeability for K^+ allows it to move out of the cells and the anions are impermeable and they line up along the interior of the membrane to create the negative membrane potential.

There are gated channels for other ions in the membrane which allows movements of ions in various situations.

Concentration of Ions in ICF and ECF

- **Cations:** Na^+ are high in the ECF (140 mEq/L) and K^+ are high in the ICF (150 mEq/L).
- **Anions:** Cl^- and HCO^- are high in ECF and in ICF proteins and PO^- are high.

Na^+-K^+ Pump

This pump, by creating a gradient for Na^+ helps to maintain the RMP. It also contributes minimally for genesis of RMP as the pump extrudes 3 Na^+ ions out of the cell and 2 K^+ ions into the cell. So a loss of a single positive ion creates a net negativity inside the membrane.

Factors Responsible for Genesis of RMP

- *Permeability of membrane to K^+*: Membrane is highly permeable to K^+ at rest and K^+ gradient is outward and the outward movement creates negativity inside the cell.
- *Permeability of membrane to Na^+*: At rest there is always an inward gradient for Na^+ and the membrane is less permeable to Na^+ than K^+ and therefore the Na^+ influx will not balance K^+ efflux and so inside the cell the potential is negative.

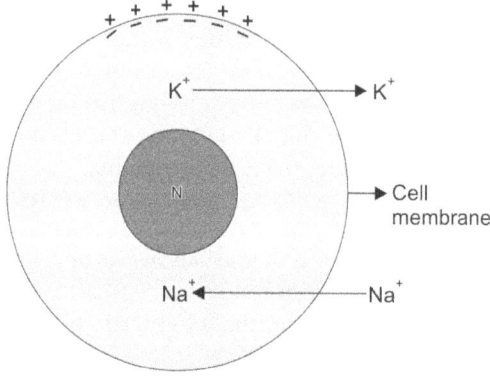

Fig. 30: Genesis of RMP. At rest, an electrical potential difference exists across the membrane of a cell with the inside being negative than the outside of a cell. This is because the cell membrane is more permeable to K^+ at rest than to Na^+. So, K^+ efflux is more than Na^+ influx. This is responsible for the RMP.

- *Permeability of membrane to anions*: The membrane is totally impermeable to anions and therefore they remain inside the cell to create negativity along the inner aspect of the membrane.
- Na^+-K^+ *Pump*: They offer minimum role in genesis of RMP but they help to maintain RMP.

22. Define all or none law. How is this law applicable in the skeletal and cardiac muscle?

- Only a stimulus of threshold intensity can excite the tissues.
- If the stimulus is of subthreshold intensity, it does not induce an action potential.
- If a suprathreshold stimulus is given, action potentials are produced of the same amplitude as that of the threshold stimulus response.
- In skeletal and cardiac muscles when the action potentials are generated, it produces maximum response.
- In skeletal muscle fiber, when a threshold stimulus is given, it induces an action potential followed by contraction of the individual muscle fiber and results in force generation by the single fiber.
- But in a cardiac muscle, since there are gap junctions in between ventricular myocytes and atrial myocytes, when a threshold stimulus is given whole of the atria and ventricles get excited at the same time and each of them contract as individual syncitia. This is needed for the efficient pumping of blood by the myocardium.

23. Name the muscle proteins. What is the role of troponin C in muscle contraction?

There are three types of proteins in the muscles—structural proteins, contractile proteins and regulatory proteins.

Structural Proteins

- **Actinin:** Binds actin to Z lines
- **Titin:** Connects Z line to M line, provides scaffolding to sarcomere
- **Desmin:** Binds Z lines to plasma membrane

Contractile Proteins

- **Actin and myosin:** Myosin heads bind to attaching sites on actin and bring about cross-bridge cycling and thereby contraction.

Regulatory Proteins

- **Troponin:** There are three subunits— Troponin I, T, and C. Troponin I inhibits the interaction of myosin with actin, troponin T binds other troponins to tropomyosin and Troponin C binds to calcium ions. Binding of Ca^{2+} to troponin C results in movement of tropomyosin away from the Myosin binding sites of actin, exposing the binding sites which results in cross-bridge cycling and it results in muscle contraction (*refer* **Fig. 31**).
- **Tropomyosin:** Covers the myosin binding site of actin. On binding of troponin C to Ca^{2+} tropomyosin is lifted and exposes the myosin binding sites on actin molecules (*refer* **Fig. 32**).

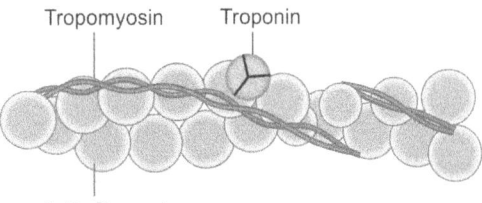

Fig. 31: Muscle proteins in thin filament. It consists of actin, tropomyosin, and troponin. Troponin is made of three subunits – I, T, and C.

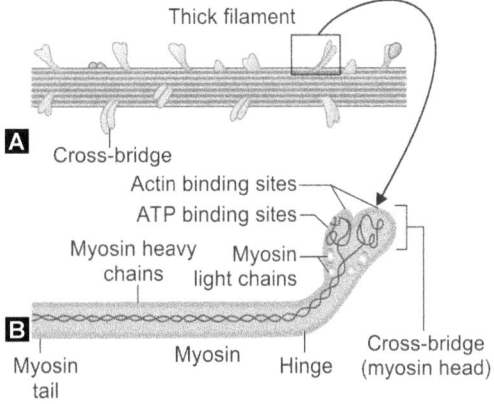

Fig. 32: (A) Arrangement of myosin molecule in thick filament; (B) Structure of myosin molecule.

24. Inulin clearance.

- Clearance is defined as the quantity of plasma cleared of a particular substance per unit time.
- Clearance of various substances are used to assess the functions of the kidneys.
- Clearance of a substance, which is excreted from the body by only filtration and is neither reabsorbed or secreted or metabolized, is used to measure GFR.
- It should be also nontoxic
- Inulin is a polymer of fructose and meets the above criteria.

Methodology

- A loading dose of inulin is administered intravenously followed by a continuous infusion to maintain its plasma arterial levels.
- After equilibration of inulin in plasma, a timed sample of urine and a sample of plasma are collected half way through.
- Plasma and urine concentrations of inulin are calculated.
- Clearance of inulin is calculated by the formula:

$$C_{IN} = U_{IN} \cdot V/P_{IN}$$

U_{IN} = Urinary concentration of inulin
V = Volume of urine excreted
P_{IN} = Plasma concentration of inulin

25. Counter-current exchanger mechanism in kidney.

- Counter-current mechanism in general is a mechanism in which fluids flow in opposite directions in closely placed structures.
- In kidneys, the counter-current mechanism is used to generate and maintain a hyperosmolar gradient from the outer to inner region of the medulla, the highest osmolality is at the tip of the renal papillae.
- Hyperosmolar medullary interstitium is essential for the process of concentration of urine.
- Only in the presence of this hyperosmolar interstitium ADH can reabsorb water from the collecting ducts.
- The counter-current system in the kidneys has two components—the counter-current multiplier and the counter-current exchanger.
- The descending and ascending loops of Henle act as the counter-current multiplier. Flow of fluid in descending loop is towards the deeper parts of medulla and is highly permeable to water and in the ascending limb the flow of fluid is towards the cortex and it is totally impermeable to water and permeable to solutes. This selective permeability of the loops of Henle helps in generating a hyperosmolar gradient in the medulla (*refer* **Fig. 33**).
- Vasa recta acts as the counter-current exchanger. The flow of blood in the ascending and descending limbs of the vasa recta helps in maintaining the hyperosmolar environment created by the counter-current multiplier.
- The ascending and descending limbs of vasa recta are also selectively permeable to water and solutes.

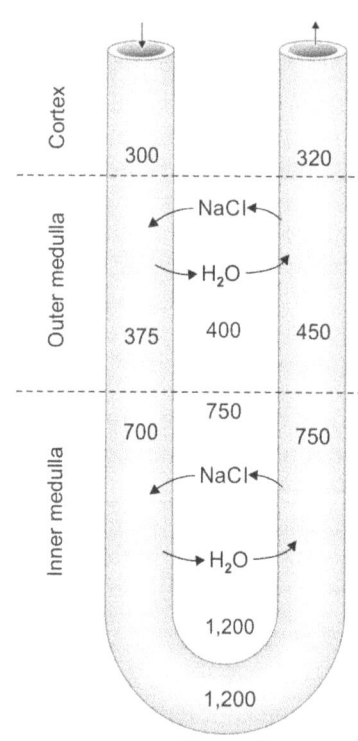

Fig. 33: Vasa recta (counter-current exchanger).

- Solutes come out of the ascending limb and enters descending limb and water enters the ascending limb and moves out into the general circulation. Solutes get circulated in the deeper parts of the medulla and thereby the vasa recta prevent the dilution of solutes in the medullary interstitium.
- This is the mechanism by which the counter-current exchanger is able to maintain the hyperosmolar medullary gradient generated by the counter-current multiplier.

26. Somatomedin.

- Somatomedins are polypeptide growth factors secreted by the liver and other tissues.
- They resemble insulin, except for the c peptide, they are called as insulin like growth factors (IGF).
- There are two types; somatomedin C (IGF-1) and insulin like growth factor II (IGF-II).

IGF-I

- The secretion of IGF, I is independent of GH in fetal period and is dependent on GH after birth.
- It is low during childhood, reaches a peak in puberty and declines thereafter.
- Receptors of IGF-I are similar to insulin receptor.
- They induce skeletal and cartilage growth and protein metabolism.
- They stimulate collagen formation.

IGF-II

- Its secretion is independent of GH levels and is always constant.
- Receptors of IGF-II are mannose 6-phosphate receptors
- IGF-II plays a major role in fetal growth.

27. Action of thyroxine on CVS.

Thyroxine increases metabolic rate and therefore, main action of CVS is to increase blood supply to tissues to deliver more O_2.

In Hyperthyroidism

- Heart rate and stroke volume ↑→↑ Cardiac output
- Systolic BP ↑ and diastolic BP ↓ → Widened pulse pressure.
- Diastolic BP is decreased due to decreased peripheral resistance. Decrease in PR is due to vasodilatation which in turn is due to increased heat production due to increase in metabolism.

In Hypothyroidism

- Heart rate and stroke volume decrease.
- Peripheral resistance is usually increased.
- The cutaneous vasoconstriction is responsible for the cold skin in hypothyroids.

28. Positive feedback mechanism.

- Most of the control systems in the body are negative feedback regulations.
- There are negative and positive feedback mechanisms.

Positive Feedback Mechanism

- In positive feedback regulation the output of the control system is enhanced or amplified so that controlled variable continues to move in the direction of the initial change.
- For example: Parturition reflex (*refer* Fig. 34)
- Positive feedback occurs in only certain instances whereas the negative feedback regulation is the most common one happening in the body.

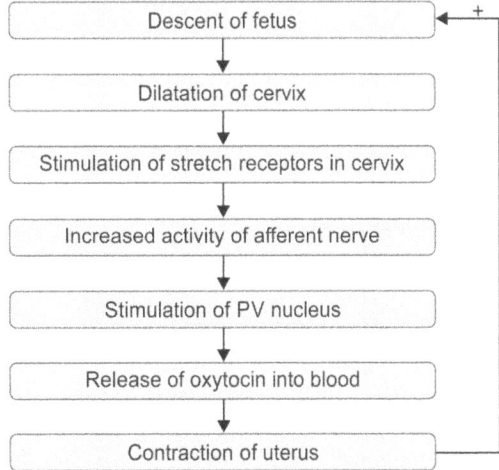

Fig. 34: Parturition reflex (positive feedback regulation).

29. How does temperature influence spermatogenesis?

Body temperature: Spermatogenesis takes place in a temperature less than the inner body temperature. The testes are kept at a temperature of 32°C. If the testis is exposed to higher temperatures the tubular walls degenerate, inhibits spermatogenesis and sterility results.

30. Effects of estrogen on the uterine endometrium.

Proliferative Phase

- This phase correlates with follicular phase of ovarian cycle.
- Estrogen secreted from the follicle stimulates growth of the uterine endometrium and therefore it proliferates.
- The glands in the endometrium and the blood vessels also grow. This phase is from day 5 till the day of ovulation.

Secretory Phase

- This phase is from day of ovulation to 25th day.
- It correlates with the luteal phase in the ovarian cycle.
- Progesterone levels are high and they make the estrogen primed endometrium to become secretory by acting on the glands.
- Maximum action is 5–7 days after ovulation.
- The secretion is rich in glycogen and can nourish the fertilized ovum.
- The secretory endometrium is favorable for implantation of fertilized ovum.

Menstrual Phase

- If fertilization does not happen, corpus luteum starts to regress and progesterone and estrogen levels drop.
- Withdrawal of hormonal support of the endometrium and release of prostaglandins result in vasoconstriction of the spiral arteries → uterine ischemia happens and endometrial necrosis and shedding of endometrium happens.
- It starts with menstrual bleeding with the shedding of outer 2/3rd of endometrium, unfertilized ovum and continues for 5 days.

31. Dark adaptation.

- When a person moves from a brightly illuminated place to a dark environment, he is not able to see anything. But gradually the eyes get accommodated to the darkness and his vision improves. This is said to be **dark adaptation**. Complete adaptation happens in 20 minutes.
- The changes happening in the eye in darkness are—dilatation of pupil, shifting of cone vision to rod vision and regeneration of rhodopsin in darkness.
- The changes happening are discussed under neural adaptation and chemical adaptation.

Neural Adaptation

- The dark adaptation happens in two phases.
- The first phase is due to cone adaptation and it happens in the first 5–10 minutes.
- This increases the retinal sensitivity to light 100 times.
- In the second phase of adaptation, the rod sensitivity to light increases and the retinal sensitivity increases by 1000–10,000 times.
- Once rod adaptation has happened even a single photon of light is visible to the eye.

Chemical Adaptation

- When a person stays in bright light, the rod pigment rhodopsin is bleached and is converted to all-transretinal and opsin.
- Therefore, rods are insensitive to light and do not respond to light.
- The rod sensitivity can increase only when the rhodopsin is resynthesized and this takes several minutes to happen.
- That is why the dark adaptation by rods takes 20 minutes (*refer* **Fig. 35**).
- The rods are present in the retina 15–20 degrees away from the fovea. That is the reason there is dilatation of the pupil to expose the retina rich in rods to light.

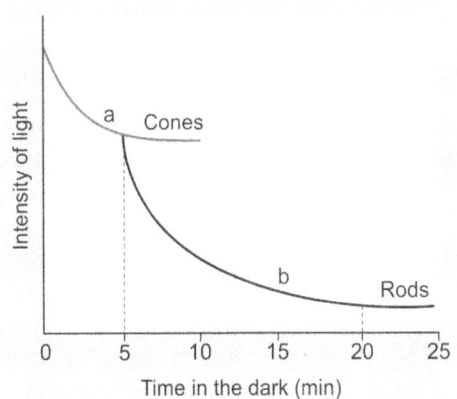

Fig. 35: Dark adaptation curve. There are two curves, curve a shows cone adaptation and curve b shows rod adaptation

- The time taken for dark adaptation depends on the degree of brightness of light to which the eye is exposed and for how long it is being exposed.
- Brighter the light and longer the duration later it takes for dark adaptation.

32. Periodic breathing.

Periodic breathing means respiratory activity alternating with apnea.

Cheyne–Stokes Respiration

- It is an abnormal respiratory pattern with waxing and waning of respiration separated by periods of apnea.
- Duration of each cycle is 1 minute
- Arterial PO_2 and PCO_2 levels fluctuate in different phases of respiration.
- Seen in conditions like drug over-dosage, brain diseases, congestive cardiac failure, uremia and hypoxia due to other causes.
- It is also seen in physiological conditions like—sleep and during voluntary hyperventilation, also in persons with increased sensitivity to CO_2.
- There is usually disruption of neural pathways that inhibit respiration.

Cheyne–Stokes Respiration in Voluntary Hyperventilation

Following hyperventilation there is apnea→ accumulation of CO_2→ stimulation of respiratory center→ gradual increase in respiration → as PCO_2 decreases → CO_2 is blown out → apnea

Cheyne-Stokes Respiration in CCF

- In patients with heart failure the circulation time of blood is longer (as the pumping of heart is inefficient).
- So, it takes a longer time for the changes in blood PCO_2 to reach the respiratory centers.
- As these patients hyperventilate the PCO_2 levels are lowered and since the circulation time is prolonged it takes time for this lowered PCO_2 levels to be detected (*refer* **Fig. 36**).
- By the time the PCO_2 levels are further lowered in pulmonary capillaries and when this blood reaches the brain, the low PCO_2 inhibits respiratory center producing apnea.
- Therefore, the respiratory control system oscillates because the negative feedback loop between brain and lungs is lengthened.

Biot's Breathing

- Has one or more large tidal volumes separated by apnea (*refer* **Fig. 37**).
- It is seen in irregular intervals
- It is seen only in pathological conditions
- Present in diseases ↑ intracranial tension— tumors, meningitis, pontine hemorrhage, central medullary lesions.

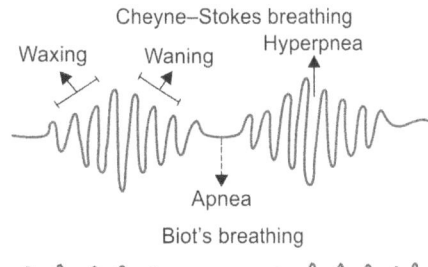

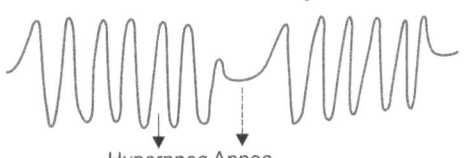

Fig. 36: Periodic breathing; Cheyne-stokes breathing and Biot's breathing.

33. Pacemaker potential.

- In the mammalian heart, sino-atrial node is the pace maker. It is said to be the pace maker as it generates impulses by itself without neural input at a faster rate.
- Other tissues of the heart—AV node, atria and ventricle are also capable of generating impulses but SA node generates impulses at a faster rate and therefore said to be the pacemaker of the heart.

Pacemaker Potential

- The ventricular and atrial muscle cells have a resting membrane potential of –90 mV. On stimulation, the membrane depolarizes and produces an action potential.
- The pacemaker cells are smaller and rounded (P cells) and they do not have a stable resting membrane potential and RMP is around –55 to –60 mV.
- From –60 mV, there is a slow depolarization slope which reaches the firing level of –40 mV and there is a rapid depolarization followed by rapid repolarization back to –60 mV and again there is a slow depolarization slope rising to firing level.
- This slope which takes the membrane to firing level is the **pacemaker potential or prepotential**.

Ionic Events Responsible for Pacemaker Potential

- At –60 mV the K^+ channels start closing down thereby preventing K^+ efflux. This is responsible for the first part of prepotential (the slope).
- Next part is due to opening up of **'f'** type Na^+ channels (The Na^+ current in this channel is said to be funny current as the channel opens in hyperpolarization)
- Last part of depolarization of the prepotential is due to opening of T-type (Transient) Ca^{2+} channels allowing Ca^{2+} influx (*refer* **Fig. 37**).
- Now as the firing level is reached (–40 mV), the long lasting Ca^{2+} channels (L-type) open and produces a rapid depolarization and the action potential.
- Then the K^+ channels open and the K^+ efflux bring about rapid repolarization and membrane potential reaches –60 mV. Then the next prepotential starts.
- So in the pacemaker cells, it is a Ca^{2+} dependent depolarization rather than Na^+

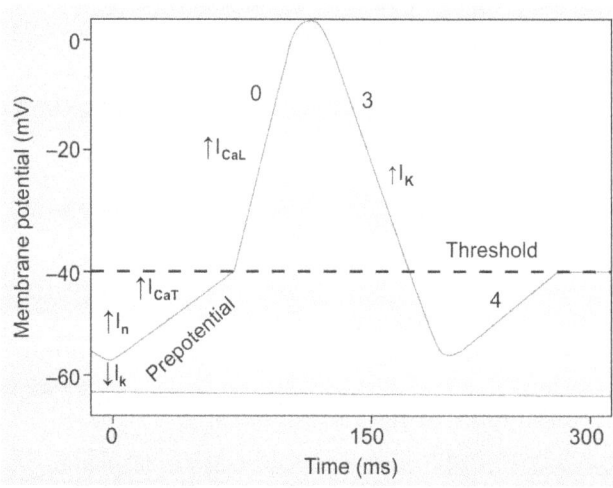

Fig. 37: Pacemaker potential. Slope of pacemaker potential (Phase 4), the prepotential is due to three events; first part of depolarization is due to closure of K^+ channels, 2nd part is due to Na^+ influx through sodium channel and last part of depolarization is due to Ca^{2+} influx through T-type Ca^{2+} channels. Rapid depolarization (Phase 0) is due to opening of L-type Ca^{2+} channels and repolarization (Phase 3) due to opening of K^+ channels.

dependent depolarization as in ventricular muscles.
- The pacemaker cells are supplied by sympathetic and parasympathetic nerves.
- On stimulation by sympathetic nerves the prepotential slope becomes steeper and the rate of spontaneous discharge increases thereby increasing the heart rate.
- On stimulation by the parasympathetic nerves, the slope of the prepotential decreases and spontaneous firing also decreases thereby heart rate decreases.

34. Cardiac reserve.
- It is the amount of blood that can be pumped out of each ventricle in excess of the normal cardiac output.
- Normal value is 15–25 L/min

35. Referred pain theories.
Irritation of a vicus or viscera usually produces pain which is not usually felt in the location of the viscus but in a somatic structure that is in a distance from the viscus. This is **referred pain**.

For example:
- Cardiac pain is usually referred to the inner aspect of the left arm or to the neck.
- When there is an irritation of central region of diaphragm there is pain in the tip of the shoulder.
- Pain in the testicle due to distension of ureter as in ureteric calculus.

Theories of Referred Pain

The pain in viscera is usually referred to a somatic structure that has developed from the same embryonic segment or dermatome as the structure in which the pain originates—**dermatomal rule**.

Theories of referred pain are—convergence theory and facilitation theory.

Convergence Theory
- Peripheral nerve fibers from the somatic and visceral structures converge on the same second order neuron present in lamina V of dorsal grey horn.

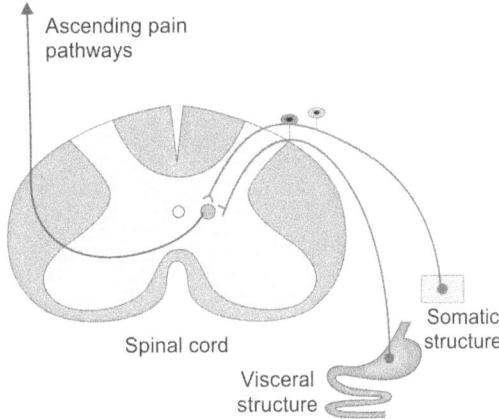

Fig. 38: Convergence theory of referred pain. Note the afferents from somatic and visceral structures converge on the same second order neuron.

- The second order neuron is common for impulses from somatic and visceral structures (*refer* **Fig. 38**).
- So the tract carrying pain sensation from somatic structures also carry pain fibers from visceral structures.
- Cortex sometimes cannot differentiate from somatic and visceral inputs and so pain from visceral structure is referred to the somatic structure.

Facilitation Theory
- The visceral afferent fibers on entering spinal cord give collaterals to afferents coming from the somatic structures.
- So impulses coming from the visceral afferents facilitate and strengthen the impulses coming from the somatic structure (*refer* **Fig. 39**).
- So a minor activity in the somatic afferents is facilitated by the visceral afferents and therefore pain is refers to the somatic structure.

36. Features of shock.

Symptoms are:
- Hypotension
- Rapid thready pulse
- Skin is cold and clammy with greyish tinge
- Intense thirst
- Rapid breathing

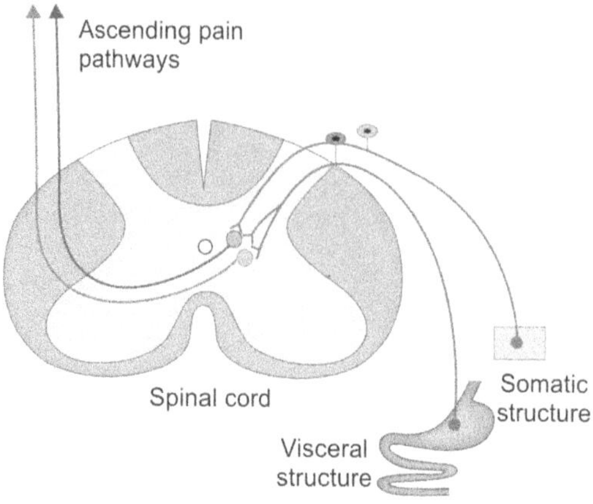

Fig. 39: Facilitation theory of referred pain. Note the visceral afferents give a collateral to second order neurons of somatic structure.

- Restlessness
- Increased lactic acid production

37. Peak expiratory flow rate.

- Peak expiratory flow rate is the maximum velocity of flow in liters per minute with which air is breathed out of the lungs.
- It is a good indicator of patency of airways.
- Normal value is 400–600 L/min or 6 to 10 L/sec.
- It can be recorded by using Wright's Peak flow meter
- The other more sensitive test to measure airway patency is maximum mid expiratory flow rate (MMEFR)

38. Oxygen debt.

- During exercise, there is increase in O_2 consumption to supply the need of O_2 for the exercising muscles.
- But even after the stoppage of exercise there is continuous increase in ventilation.
- This extra O_2 consumed after exercise is used to remove the lactate accumulation, to replenish the ATP and phosphoryl creatinine stores which were depleted and to replace the O_2 that has been removed from the myoglobin.
- The amount of extra O_2 consumed depends on the extra demand of energy consumed during exercise which has exceeded the capacity of aerobic energy synthesis.
- This is said to be the O_2 debt.
- This can be calculated by finding the O_2 consumption after exercise till the basal consumption is reached.

39. Mass reflex.

- This type of reflex is seen in spinal cord lesions.
- In lesions of spinal cord, a single afferent impulse can irradiate from one center to another center of spinal cord.
- Therefore, when a noxious stimulus is applied to the skin, the impulse may radiate to autonomic centers in the spinal cord and produce a **mass reflex** resulting in evacuation of bladder and rectum, sweating, pallor and swings in BP along with withdrawal reflex.
- This reflex may be used to train the paraplegic patients to evacuate bladder and bowels by pinching or stroking the skin on the inner aspect of the thigh.

40. Impedance matching.

- As the sound waves travel from rarer (air in external and middle ear) to denser medium (fluid in the inner ear) they are dampened (by 30 db).
- This loss in sound energy is prevented in the middle ear by impedance matching which is by:
  1. By area differences
  2. By lever action
  3. By buckling factor

1. **Area difference:** Area of tympanic membrane is greater than foot plate of stapes and therefore there is convergence of sound and pressure is increased by 17 times.
2. **Lever action of the ossicles:** Increases pressure by 1.32 times
3. **Buckling factor:** Tympanic membrane is conical in shape and the handle of malleus is attached to the umbo. As the tympanic membrane moves in and out, the buckling of membrane moves the handle of malleus less and this increases the force and decreases the velocity.

41. Dwarfism

Dwarfism is due to deficiency of growth hormone or GRH, deficiency of IGF-1, receptor insensitivity, thyroid hormone deficiency.

Causes for Dwarfism

- Isolated growth hormone deficiency may be due to GRH deficiency or due to abnormalities of GH secreting cells.
- Sometimes the GH levels may be normal or even elevated, but the GH receptors are insensitive to GH due to loss-of function mutation of the genes for GH receptors—this is Laron dwarfism.
- African pygmies are a type of dwarfism and are due to reduction of plasma level of growth-hormone binding protein and there is also absence of rise in IGF-1 at the time of puberty.
- Cretinism is hypothyroidism in children and it results in stunted growth and mental retardation.
- Dwarfism is also seen in conditions of precocious puberty.
- Gonadal dysgenesis is also a cause of dwarfism
- Various bone and metabolic disorders also result in dwarfism.
- **Psychosocial dwarfism:** This type of dwarfism is seen in children who are subjected to chronic abuse and neglect. It is also called as Kaspar Hauser syndrome.
- **Achondroplasia:** It is the most common type of dwarfism. Here the trunk is normal and short limbs. It is an autosomal dominant condition caused by mutation in the gene that code for fibroblast growth factor receptor 3.

Symptoms

- In a hypothyroid dwarf, there is short stature, pot belly, enlarged tongue and delayed sexual maturity. There is definite mental retardation, idiotic facies.
- *In pituitary dwarfism*: There is short stature, proportionated growth retardation, normal mental development, sexual maturation may/may not be delayed and immature facies is seen.

42. Functions of lymphocytes.

Based on the functions the lymphocytes are classified as B lymphocytes, T lymphocytes, and natural killer cells.

B Lymphocytes

These cells are formed in the bone marrow and processed there and are transported to the lymph nodes where they are present till their activation. There are two types of B cells. They are plasma cells and memory B cells.

Plasma Cells

Plasma cells are formed from B cells on antigenic stimulation. Each B cell has a specific receptor for a particular antigen on its membrane. When the antigen is recognized by the specific B cell it undergoes division and differentiation to the specific clone of B cells and transforms into plasma cells. The plasma cells produce the immunoglobulins to destroy that specific antigen. It produces a large quantity of antibodies and release them into circulation.

Memory B Cells

A small proportion of the stimulated B cells stay in the lymph node so that on subsequent exposure to the same antigen they produce a rapid, swift and heightened response.

T Lymphocytes

T cells are formed from the bone marrow and are processed in the thymus gland and are transported to the lymph nodes and stored there till they are activated by the antigen. There are three types of T cells—helper T cells, cytotoxic T cells, and memory T cells.

1. **Helper T cells:** They are also called as CD4 cells as they express CD4 antigen on their cell membrane. They are needed for activation of both cell-mediated and Humoral immunity. There are two types— T_H1 and T_H2 cells.
    - T_H1 cells secrete IL-2 and γ interferon and are needed for cell-mediated immunity.

- $T_H 2$ cells secrete IL-4 and 5 and are needed for humoral immunity.
2. **Cytotoxic T cells:** These cells are also called as CD8 cells as they express CD8 antigen on their cell membrane. On activation by TH_1 cells they bind to the antigen and kill it by inserting pores called perforins on its membrane and it can induce killing by stimulating apoptosis. These cells are responsible for rejection of transplanted tissue, destruction of cancer cells and for delayed allergic reactions.
3. **Memory T cells:** Similar to memory B cells the memory T cells also are a small number of stimulated T cells which remain in the lymph node. On subsequent exposure to the same antigen they get activated immediately to divide and differentiate to a clone of similar cells and they produce a rapid, swift and enormous response to destroy the antigen. They can even live forever in the lymph node if there is no second exposure.

Natural Killer Cells

These cells do not belong to the T or B cell category. They form 10–15% of circulating total lymphocytes.

They are mostly involved in innate defense mechanism. They kill a wide range of microorganisms without any specificity. They do not need the MHC proteins. They kill viruses and antibody-coated viruses. They are the natural first line of defense against viruses. They also destroy the tumor cells.

43. Proximal tubular events.

- The proximal convoluted tubule (PCT) is an important part of the nephron were 67% of Na^+, Cl^-, K^+ and water are reabsorbed from the tubular fluid.
- Na^+ reabsorption in the early part of PCT is along with glucose and amino acid reabsorption and in later part is with Cl^- reabsorption.
- Almost most of the HCO_3^-, K^+, and amino acids are reabsorbed in PCT.
- Glucose is also reabsorbed completely (SGLT1).
- H^+ is also secreted in exchange for Na^+ (Na^+-H^+ exchanger)
- For every H^+ secreted one HCO_3^- and one Na^+ is reabsorbed
- Na^+ reabsorption here is an energy consuming process due to action of Na^+-K^+ ATPase in the basolateral membrane which creates a gradient for Na^+ to move into the cells from the tubule.
- Solute reabsorption is active and water is reabsorbed passively by the osmotic gradient created by solute reabsorption. So the tubular fluid osmolality in PCT is similar to plasma.
- Water reabsorption through epithelial cells is via aquaporin 1 present in cell membrane and also through paracellular routes.

44. Acromegaly.

- Acromegaly is a clinical condition due to excess secretion of growth hormone (GH) in the adults (after the fusion of the epiphyseal plates in the long bones).
- It is usually due to a tumor of the growth hormone producing cells (somatotrophs) in the anterior pituitary gland.
- Rarely, it can also be due to hypothalamic tumors secreting GRH.
- There is no increase in height of the individual.
- But because of the excess levels of GH there is thickening of bones and proliferation of soft tissues like connective tissue and skin.
- This leads to coarse disfigured appearance. "Acro" means extremity and "megaly" is large.

Clinical features are:

Excess GH levels lead to:
- Acromegalic face—jaw and cheek bones become more prominent, lips are thickened, nose is broad and thick, enlarged brows, and coarse skin.
- Prognathism—protrusion of the lower jaw due to elongation and thickening of mandible.
- Enlarged spade, such as hands, broad fingers and large feet.

- Body hair is increased
- Kyphosis—since the vertebral bones continue to grow person has kyphosis.
- They develop osteoarthritis
- Organomegaly—internal organs, such as heart, liver, spleen, and kidneys are enlarged.
- High levels of GH decrease insulin sensitivity in the tissues and the patient has hyperglycemia and are prone to develop diabetes mellitus

Effect of tumor on neighboring structures: The tumor in the anterior pituitary compresses the optic chiasma resulting in visual disturbances.

There will be enlargement of sella turcica and headache.

45. Hormones produced by placenta.

- Human chorionic gonadotropin (hCG)
- Human chorionic somatomammotropin (hCS)
- Placental progesterone
- Placental estrogen
- Relaxin

Human Chorionic Gonadotropin (hCG)

- It is synthesized by syncytiotrophoblasts of placenta
- It is a glycoprotein with α and β subunits
- It starts appearing in the blood of the mother by 6 days after fertilization and reaches a peak by 10-12 weeks.
- Clinically, presence of hCG in urine of a female is "the indicator" of pregnancy.
- It stimulates the corpus luteum to secrete progesterone till the placenta is fully formed.
- hCG helps in sexual differentiation of male fetus.
- It induces hyperemesis in the first trimester.

Human Chorionic Somatomammotropin (hCS)

- It is also secreted from the syncytiotrophoblast of placenta.
- Its secretion starts by 5th week of pregnancy and reaches a peak towards term.
- It is similar to growth hormone and has growth promoting actions, so called as "Maternal growth hormone of pregnancy"
- It stimulates lipolysis, N, K^+, and Ca^{2+} retention and decreases glucose utilization by the mother so that the substrates are diverted to the fetus.
- Amount of hCS secreted is equal to size of placenta and therefore level of hCS indicates placental viability.

Placental Progesterone

- In the early weeks of pregnancy, progesterone is produced by corpus luteum and later the function is taken over by placenta.
- It is produced by coordination between the mother and the fetus—the **fetplacental unit**.
- It makes the endometrium secretory and thereby nourishes the fertilized ovum.
- It keeps the myometrium of the pregnant uterus quiescent which is essential for the survival of the fetus.
- It acts on the alveolar system of the maternal breast and facilitates development of maternal breast.
- It has an immunosuppressive role in protecting the fetus.

Placental Estrogen

- The major estrogen in pregnancy is estriol.
- It stimulates development of the ductular system of the maternal breast
- The levels of estrogen rise during pregnancy but on nearing term estrogen: progesterone ratio rises and estrogen makes the myometrium excitable.
- On decrease of levels of estrogen after delivery of fetus, prolactin stimulates milk secretion from the breast.

Relaxin

- Its level in the early pregnancy is high to relax the uterine wall to favor implantation of fetus.
- In later weeks, it causes relaxation of pubic symphysis and pelvic ligaments to facilitate delivery of fetus.

Other hormones secreted are:

CRH, β endorphin, α-MSH, GnRH, inhibin, prolactin, etc.

46. Stages of deglutition.

Deglutition is the process of swallowing

- It is a reflex response integrated in the medulla in nucleus tractus solitarius (NTS) and nucleus ambiguus (NA).
- Afferents pass through the cranial nerves V, IX, and X
- Efferents come through cranial nerves V, VII, and XII nerves to the tongue and pharynx

There are three phases of deglutition:

1. Oral or voluntary phase
2. Pharyngeal or involuntary phase
3. Esophageal phase

Oral Phase

When food enters mouth, tongue forms it into a bolus and pushes it to the oropharynx by pushing up and against the hard palate.

Pharyngeal Phase

- It starts when food enters pharynx.
- Soft palate is elevated and closes the nasopharynx and prevents food from entering the nose
- Larynx rises, vocal cords approximate and epiglottis closes the laryngeal opening and prevents food from entering the trachea (*refer* **Figs. 40A to D**)
- Deglutition apnea follows.
- Palatopharyngeal folds approximate for selective material to move into the esophagus.
- Cricopharyngeus (upper esophageal sphincter) relaxes and bolus enters upper esophagus.
- On entering of food into esophagus, the cricopharyngeus closes, vocal cords open and air entry is allowed.

Esophageal Phase

- There are two sphincters in the esophagus—upper esophageal sphincter (UES) and lower esophageal sphincter (LES).
- UES is formed by cricopharyngeus muscle which is a skeletal muscle. It opens reflexly at the beginning of swallow.
- LES is made of smooth muscle and its actions are regulated by Vagus nerve and other intrinsic nerves. Its main action is to prevent regurgitation of acids from the stomach
- Food on reaching esophagus is pushed into the stomach by peristalsis—primary and secondary peristalsis.
- Primary peristalsis is initiated by swallowing and is coordinated by vagus nerve.

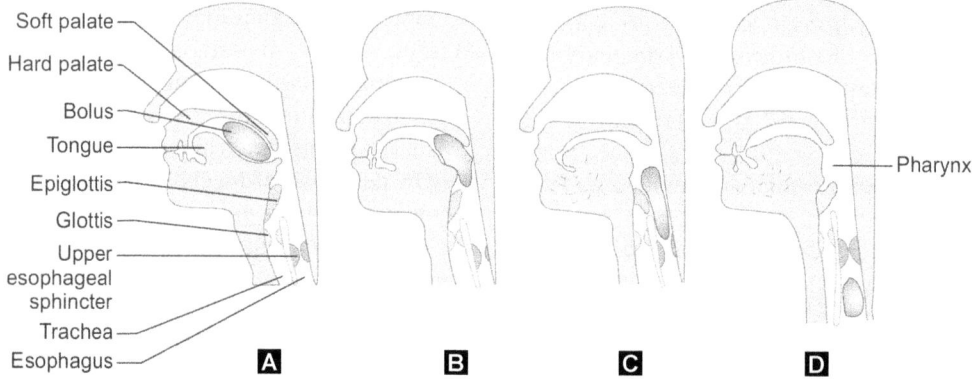

Figs. 40A to D: Phases of deglutition: (A) oral phase; (B) bolus enters the pharynx; (C) pharyngeal phase; (D) esophageal phase.

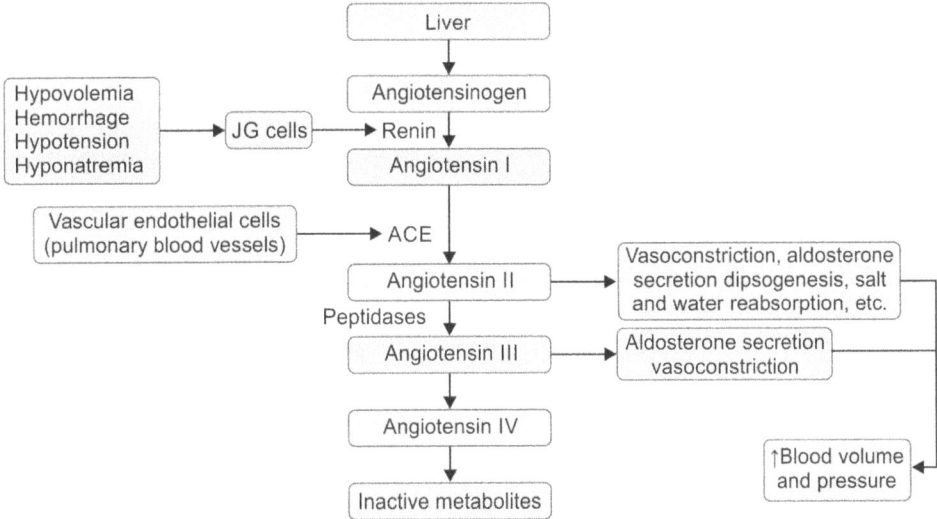

Fig. 41: Renin-angiotensin-aldosterone pathway.

- Secondary peristalsis is initiated by presence of food in the esophagus and it sweeps the food down towards the stomach, coordinated by intrinsic nerves.

47. Renin angiotensin system.

- Renin is an acid protease and is a glycoprotein hormone secreted from the juxtaglomerular cells of kidneys.
- Renin acts on angiotensinogen in plasma and converts it to angiotensin I.
- Angiotensin I is converted to angiotensin II by the angiotensin converting enzyme (ACE).
- ACE is produced by endothelial cells of all blood vessels, especially by the vessels in lungs.
- Angiotensin II is in turn converted to Angiotensin III and IV (*refer* **Fig. 41**).
- The most active form is angiotensin II.
- The major actions of angiotensin II are to regulate blood volume and pressure.

Actions of Angiotensin II

- It is a potent vasoconstrictor
- It acts on the proximal convoluted tubule to increase reabsorption of Na^+ and water.
- It acts on the adrenal cortex to stimulate the secretion of aldosterone and aldosterone in turn increases salt and water reabsorption from the collecting duct.
- It increases release of norepinephrine from sympathetic nerve terminals.
- It also acts on the circumventricular organs in the brain—subfornical organ (SFO) and organum vasculosum of lamina terminalis (OVLT) and increase thirst sensation and thereby increases water intake.
- Increases ADH secretion from posterior pituitary
- It increases secretion of ACTH from anterior pituitary.
- It acts as neurotransmitters in the brain.

Factors Regulating Renin Secretion

Factors that Increase Secretion

- Decreased blood volume
- Decreased blood pressure
- Sympathetic nerve stimulation

Factors that Decrease Renin Secretion

- Increased blood volume and pressure
- ADH
- Increased plasma Na^+ concentration
- Angiotensin II

48. Oral contraceptives.

Oral Contraceptive Pills

- By pills we mean the oral contraceptive pills used for female contraception.
- They are usually synthetic preparation of estrogen, progesterone or combination of both.
- **The pills can be of different types:**
  - Combined pill or classical pill
  - Sequential pill
  - Minipill
  - Postcoital pill

Combined Pill

- It is a combination of estrogen and progesterone pill.
- It contains a strip of 21 tablets and is consumed for 21 days from 5th day of menstrual cycle.
- After 21 days, on stopping the tablets, withdrawal bleeding happens.
- Again from 5th day, next cycle is started.

It Acts by

- Prevents ovulation, as the high estrogen levels disorganize the LH and FSH secretions.
- Prevents implantation of fertilized ovum.
- Progesterone makes the cervical mucus thick and prevents sperm penetration

Sequential Pill

- It has high dose of estrogen and minimal amounts of progesterone.
- It is not used nowadays as the high estrogen may induce endometrial cancer or breast cancer.

Minipill

- It is progesterone only pill.
- It does not affect ovulation but makes the cervical mucus thick and prevents sperm penetration.

Postcoital Pill

- It is used within 72 hours of unprotected intercourse.
- It has high doses of estrogen and is given for 4–6 days.
- High estrogen prevents implantation of the fertilized ovum.

Depot Preparation

- These are implants of progesterone and they are sub dermally implanted and prevent pregnancy for 5 years.
- The only problem is it can cause amenorrhea and irregular cycles.

49. Chronaxie and rheobase.

- Minimal intensity of stimulus acting for a given duration that can produce an action potential is the threshold stimulus.
- **Rheobase:** The weakest strength of current that can excite a tissue when given for an adequate time—**rheobase**. The time for which it is given as **utilization time**.
- **Chronaxiae:** The duration of time for which twice the rheobase strength of current is given to produce a response.
- Chronaxie gives an idea about the excitability of excitable tissues. Excitability and chronaxie are inversely related. The smooth muscles are least excitable and their chronaxie is longer in duration.

50. Significance of glycosylated hemoglobin.

- There are small amounts of hemoglobin A derivatives closely associated with hemoglobin A that represent glycated hemoglobin.
- One of these is Hemoglobin A_{1c} (HbA_{1c}). It has a glucose attached to the terminal valine in each β chain and is of special interest because its quantity increases in poorly controlled diabetes mellitus.
- It gives an idea about the average blood glucose levels for the past 3 months.

51. Phasic changes in coronary blood flow.

- There are phasic changes in blood flow through coronaries. In systole as the myocardium contracts the blood vessels are compressed and there is no blood flow through the coronaries. In diastole

as the myocardium relaxes the vessels dilate and blood flow increases through the vessels.
- The endocardial vessels show the maximum phasic variation in blood flow. Therefore, these areas suffer from hypoxia and are prone for ischemia in compromised states.

52. AV nodal delay.

AV Node
- It is located beneath the endocardium on the right side of lower part of atrial septum near the tricuspid valve.
- The conduction velocity through the AVN is very slow because the fibers are smaller with less number of gap junctions.
- There is a delay of 0.1 s
- The delay provides time for atrial contraction and final ventricular filling.
- It also prevents transmission of all impulses from atria to ventricles in supraventricular tachycardia.
- It is supplied by sympathetic and PS nerves which alter the conduction rate

53. Properties of reflex.
- **Adequate stimulus:** A reflex response can be obtained only when a precise stimulus is applied. The precise stimulus which can initiate the response is the adequate stimulus.
- **Delay:** There is always a delay between application of stimulus and the response due to the presence of synapses in the pathway. More the number of synapses, more will be the delay
- **One way conduction:** The impulses are always transmitted from the receptor→ center → effector.
- **Summation:** Spatial and temporal summation of impulses facilitates responses.
- **Irradiation:** When the stimulus is very strong as that of the noxious stimuli the impulses spread to neighboring neurons and centers and produces a wider response, as in crossed extensor reflex. Mass reflex is an example for irradiation.
- **Final common pathway:** The alpha motor neurons in the spinal cord which supply the extrafusal muscle fibers, is the final pathway through which the excitatory or inhibitory impulses reach the muscles for reflexes.
- **Facilitation:** When repeated stimuli are given there is increased responses in the initial few occasions due to facilitation in the synapse.
- **Inhibition:** During a reflex response, when the agonists are contracting there are inhibitory impulses reaching the antagonists to make them relax. This is because of firing of inhibitory interneurons from the spinal cord which end on the antagonists.
- **After discharge:** When a reflex response is elicited by a strong stimuli, even after cessation of stimulus the response is present. This is said to be after-discharge. It happens due to reverberatory circuits.
- **Rebound phenomenon:** When the reflex activity is inhibited due to some reason and after the inhibition is lifted, the response which we get is a stronger one.
- **Susceptibility to hypoxia:** Reflexes are susceptible to hypoxia
- **Fatigue:** When a reflex is elicited repetitively, gradually the response diminishes and finally disappears due to fatigue. The site of fatigue is usually at the synapse.
- **Occlusion:** The muscles contract forcefully when stimulated directly through motor nerve stimulation rather than the reflex stimulation through the sensory nerve. This is due to property of occlusion when stimulated through sensory nerve.
- **Sensitization:** When a noxious stimulus is applied repeatedly the response gets intensified, this is due to presynaptic facilitation.

54. Splanchnic circulation.

Means Circulation through Abdominal Viscera

- Circulation through GIT
- Circulation through liver
- Circulation through spleen

Intestinal Circulation

- Resting blood flow—20% of cardiac output.
- Increases to 50% after a meal.
- Supplied by 3 main arteries—celiac trunk, superior and Inferior mesenteric arteries.
- Intestinal mucosa receives 60-70% of total intestinal blood flow.
- Arterioles supply the tips of villi.
- Direction of blood flow in arterioles and venules in villi is opposite to each other and form a counter-current system.
- Regulation is by neural and auto regulation (Metabolic-Adenosine, K^+ and Osmolality)

Hepatic Circulation

- Liver is a vital organ performing metabolic activity.
- **Hepatic blood flow:** 28% of cardiac output.
- **Blood flow to liver is through:** Hepatic artery (25%) and portal vein (75%).
- **Normal blood flow:** 1500 mL/min (58 mL/100 g/min).
- Hepatic arterial and portal vein blood flow are reciprocal.
- Regulation is by neural (sympathetic N) and metabolic factors.

Splenic Circulation

- Main blood flow to spleen is through Splenic artery.
- Nerve supply is by sympathetic vasoconstrictor fibers.
- Spleen functions as reservoir for blood especially in animals.
- During circulatory shock, splenic contraction releases blood into circulation.

55. Functions of middle ear.

- **Middle ear:** It is an air-filled cavity in temporal bone. It starts at the tympanic membrane and ends at oval window
- **Contains:** Three ossicles (malleus, incus, and stapes), two small muscles (tensor tympani and stapedius), ligaments, nerves, blood vessels, etc.
- **Functions:**
  1. *Tympanic reflex:* It is a protective reflex. When a loud sound is transmitted through the ossicles in middle ear a reflex is initiated with a latent period of 40-80 milliseconds. Contraction of stapedius and tensor tympani pulls the tympanic membrane medially and membrane covering oval window laterally. This makes the ossicular system rigid and there is reduction in transmission of sounds. This reduces the intensity of sound by 30-40 decibels. It is also called as **attenuation reflex**.
     Functions of this reflex:
     - This reflex protects the cochlea from damaging loud sounds.
     - It filters the low frequency sounds
     - It prevents hearing one's own speech
  2. Transmission of sound waves from external ear to internal ear.
  3. *Impedance matching:*
     - As the sound waves travel from rarer (air in external and middle ear) to denser medium (Fluid in the inner ear) they are dampened (by 30 db).
     - This loss in sound energy is prevented in the middle ear by impedance matching which is by:
       - By area differences
       - By lever action
       - By buckling factor
  4. *Area difference:* Area of tympanic membrane is greater than foot plate of stapes and therefore there is convergence of sound and pressure is increased by 17 times.
  5. *Lever action of the ossicles* increases pressure by 1.32 times
  6. *Buckling factor:* Tympanic membrane is conical in shape and the handle of malleus is attached to the umbo. As the tympanic membrane moves in and out, the buckling of membrane moves the handle of malleus less and this

increases the force and decreases the velocity.

56. Nitrogen narcosis.

N_2 Toxicity or N_2 Narcosis

- At high atmospheric pressure environments, as in deep sea, breathing air under high pressure leads to increased pN_2 and high partial pressure of N_2 dissolves it in body fluids, more easily in fats.
- N_2 dissolves easily in neurons, altering their ionic conductance and decreases their excitability—results in **N_2 narcosis**.
- It starts at a depth of 120 feet below sea level and becomes severe at 250 feet
- **Symptoms:**
  - Symptoms are similar to alcohol intoxication.
  - *Causes euphoria:* Person becomes jovial, carefree, impairment of mental functions, intelligence and poor muscular coordination.
  - This problem can be overcome by breathing mixtures of O_2 and helium, but this also leads to disorders like High pressure nervous syndrome.

57. Effects of positive 'g'.

- Force acting on the body due to acceleration is expressed as 'g' units.
- 1 'g' is the force of gravity acting on earth's surface.
- "Positive g" is force due to acceleration acting in the long axis from head to foot
- During positive 'g' blood is thrown to the lower parts of the body and therefore arterial pressure is high in lower parts and low in the head.
- But as the venous pressure and also intracranial pressures are also reduced there is not much decrease in blood flow to brain.
- The major problem here is decrease in venous return and thereby decrease in cardiac output
- Cardiac output is maintained for some time due to blood being drawn from venous reservoirs.
- At accelerations above 5 'g' there is failure of vision, "Black out" in 5 seconds and unconsciousness immediately after that.
- These effects of positive 'g' can be reduced by wearing 'g suits'.
- These are double-walled pressure suits containing water or air and they compress the abdomen or legs with force equal to the positive g.
- The suit prevents venous pooling and enhances venous return.

58. Papez circuit.

- Hypothalamus along with limbic system participates in the expression of emotions.
- This relation is given as the papex circuit which is responsible for emotions.
- Papez circuit is also responsible for memory and learning.

Papez Circuit

- Hippocampus is connected to mamillary bodies through the fornix.
- Mamillary body is connected to the anterior thalamic nucleus through mammillothalamic tract (*refer* **Fig. 19**).
- Anterior thalamic nucleus is connected to cingulate gyrus and it is in turn connected to hippocampus.

59. Heart sounds.

Heart Sounds can be Recorded by Phonocardiogram

Significance of Heart Sounds

- **1st Sound:** Increased in exercise, hyper-kinetic states, such as anemia and decreased in shock, MI, pericardial effusion.
- **2nd sound:** Loud in hypertension, low in aortic and pulmonary stenosis. Splitting is common.
- **3rd sound:** Increased in MR. Important sign of heart failure.
- **4th sound:** Always seen in abnormal conditions. Seen in left ventricular hypertrophy (*refer* **Fig. 42**).

Heart sounds	Events responsible	Duration	Frequency	Others
First sound (S_1)	Due to vibrations set by sudden closure of AV valves at the onset of ventricular systole	0.15 sec	25–45 Hz In PCG recorded as 9–13 waves	Soft and long, heard as "LUBB"
Second sound (S_2)	Associated with closure of aortic and pulmonary valves after the end of ventricular systole	0.12 sec	50 Hz In PCG recorded as 4–6 waves	Normally S2 can be split due to early closure of aortic valve, heard as "Dup"
Third sound (S_3)	Is heard at 1/3rd of diastole due to rapid filling of ventricle due to vibrations set by inrush of blood		0.1 sec In PCG recorded as 1–4 waves	Normally audible only in children and young adults
Fourth sound (S_4)	Heard just before (S_1) Occurs during atrial contraction Due to ventricular filling		20 cyc/sec In PCG recorded as 1–2 waves	Rarely heard in normal adults Heard in vent hypertrophy and CCF

Fig. 42: Heart sounds; their causes and characteristics.

60. Differentiate REM and NREM sleep.

	NREM sleep	REM sleep
Timing in sleep cycle	Occurs first	Occurs after NREM sleep
Duration in normal adults	75% of total sleep	25% of sleep
Autonomic symptoms	Sympathetic inhibition (low BP, HR, Respiration)	Sympathetic excitation (High BP, HR)
Eyeball movement	No movement	Rapid eye movement occurs
Dreams	Dreams are not memorized	Dreams well memorized
Muscle tone	Is inhibited	Profoundly decreased
Type of sleep	Enters into deep sleep	Sleep lightens
EEG waves	Slow-wave, high amplitude	High frequency, low voltage
Mechanism	Inhibition of RAS	Activation of pontine reticular formation

Answers to 2016 Question Paper

ANSWER ALL QUESTIONS

I. Essay Questions   **(15 Marks each)**

1. What is glomerular filtration rate (GFR)? Enumerate the factors affecting GFR.
2. What is cardiac cycle? Describe the various events in the cardiac cycle.
3. Discuss in detail the stages of erythropoiesis and the factors affecting it. Add a note on polycythemia.
4. Describe the oxygen transport in blood. Add note on fetal hemoglobin.

II. Write Notes on   **(5 Marks each)**

1. Facilitated diffusion.
2. Control of insulin secretion.
3. Golgi tendon reflex.
4. Oxygen-hemoglobin dissociation curve.
5. Neuromuscular junction.
6. Regulation of hydrochloric acid secretion in the gastric parietal cells.
7. Autorhythmicity of heart.
8. Describe the connections and functions of temporal lobe.

III. Short Answers   **(3 Marks each)**

1. Hemophilia.
2. Differentiate between isotonic and isometric contraction.
3. Erythropoietin.
4. Compound action potential.
5. Gastrin.
6. Addisonian crisis.
7. Law of gut.
8. Intestinal phase of pancreatic secretion.
9. Inhibin.
10. Functions of prostate gland.
11. Putamen circuit of basal ganglia.
12. Caisson disease.
13. Hering-Breuer inflation reflex.
14. Einthoven's law.
15. Endocochlear potential.
16. Describe the normal waves in electro-encephalogram (EEG).
17. Presbyopia.
18. Bainbridge reflex.
19. Transpulmonary pressure.
20. Wernicke's and global aphasia.
21. Functions of saliva.
22. Diuretics and their sites of action.
23. Steps in synthesis of thyroid hormones.
24. Enterohepatic circulation.
25. Phagocytosis.
26. Endoplasmic reticulum.
27. Anticoagulants.
28. Functions of estrogen.
29. Importance of Rh typing.
30. Fat absorption.
31. Taste receptors.
32. Functions of utricle and saccule.
33. Sleep-wake theory.
34. Mechanism of accommodation.
35. P-R interval.
36. Trichromatic theory of color vision.
37. Mean arterial pressure.
38. Reward and punishment centers.
39. Changes in cardiac output during exercise.
40. Surfactant.

I. ESSAY QUESTIONS

1. What is glomerular filtration rate (GFR)? Enumerate the factors affecting GFR

❏ GFR refers to the volume of the glomerular filtrate formed each minute by all the

nephrons in both the kidneys. The normal value is 125 mL/min or 7.5 L/hr or 180 L/day.
- Mechanism of filtration across the glomerular capillary is similar to the mechanism of filtration across any of the systemic capillaries.
- So filtration is dependent on the Starling's forces across the capillary membrane and characteristics of the membrane and renal blood flow and arterial blood pressure.
- Filtration across the membrane is decided by the balance of the starling's forces.
- **GFR is expressed as:**

$$GFR = K_f[(P_{GC} - P_T) - (\pi_{GC} - \pi_T)]$$

GFR = Glomerular filtration rate

K_f = Filtration co-efficient of the membrane and it is 12.5 m²/min/mm Hg. It is the product of glomerular capillary wall conductivity and effective filtration surface area.

P_{GC} = Glomerular capillary hydrostatic pressure

P_T = Hydrostatic pressure in Bowman's space

π_{GC} = Glomerular capillary oncotic pressure

π_T = Oncotic pressure in Bowman's space

Factors Regulating GFR

- **Surface area of filtration membrane** is altered by the contraction or relaxation of the mesangial cells. Contraction of mesangial cells decreases the surface area of filtration and relaxation increases it. Contraction is induced by angiotensin II, endothelin, ADH etc. and relaxation is stimulated by ANP, dopamine, cAMP and PGE_2.
- **Permeability of glomerular membrane** for neutral substances of less than 4 nm molecular diameter is favored and neutral substances above 8 nm are not filtered. Between 4 to 8 nm the filtration is inversely proportional to diameter of substances. There are negatively charged sialoproteins lining the glomerular membrane which prevents negatively charged particles like albumin from getting filtered even though it is 6 nm in diameter. Permeability is increased in hypoxia and presence of toxic substances.
- **Hydrostatic pressure in glomerulus:** It is higher than in other capillaries in the body as the efferent arterioles (the outlet of glomerulus) is more constricted and offers more resistance than the afferent arterioles (the inlet for glomerulus) which are short and straight branches. So factors which increase efferent arteriolar constriction will increase the hydrostatic pressure in the glomerulus. Changes in the systemic blood pressure will affect renal perfusion and thereby the filtration. The hydrostatic pressure in the glomerulus at the afferent and efferent end is 45 mm Hg (refer Fig. 1).
- **Hydrostatic pressure in Bowman's space:** This is the pressure exerted by the filtered fluid in the Bowman's space and it opposes filtration. Normally it is 10 mm Hg. It increases in conditions of obstruction of urinary tract as in ureteric calculi blocking the flow of fluid in the tubule.
- **Oncotic pressure in the glomerulus:** GFR is inversely proportional to oncotic pressure. It is exerted by the plasma proteins. The capillary oncotic pressure at afferent end is 25 mm Hg and at

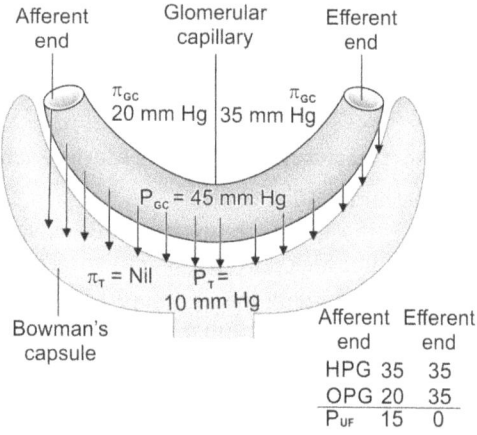

Fig. 1: Mechanism of filtration along the glomerular capillary. In contrast to systemic capillaries filtration happens along the entire capillary.

(P_{GC}: Capillary hydrostatic pressure; P_T: Bowman's space hydrostatic pressure; π_{GC}: Glomerular capillary oncotic pressure; π_T: Osmotic pressure in Bowman's space)

efferent end it is 35 mm Hg. This is because as the fluid leaves the capillary from afferent to efferent ends of capillaries the concentration of plasma proteins increases and thereby oncotic pressure increases. So, in conditions of hyperproteinemia or hemoconcentration oncotic pressure rises and GFR decreases. In hypoproteinemia GFR is increased.

- **Oncotic pressure in Bowman's space:** It is very negligible because no protein is filtered into the Bowman's space.
- **Effective filtration pressure:** It is the net outward pressure which favors filtration and is calculated as the difference between the outward and inward forces
  $GFR = K_f [(P_{GC} - P_T) - (\pi_{GC} - \pi_T)]$
  $GFR = 12.5 (45-10) - (25-0)$
  $= 12.5 \times 10 = 125$ mL/min
- **Other factors affecting GFR:**
  - Sympathetic stimulation of renal vessels leads to marked vasoconstriction and thereby decreases GFR
  - Hormones, such as norepinephrine, endothelin and angiotensin II cause intense vasoconstriction and thereby decrease RBF and GFR. Ang II at low concentrations cause only constriction of efferent arteriole and thereby increases GFR. ANP, dopamine, nitric oxide, prostaglandins cause vasodilatation and increase RBF and GFR.

---

2. What is cardiac cycle? Describe the various events in the cardiac cycle.

Definition

- Cardiac cycle is defined as the cycle of mechanical and electrical events taking place from beginning of one beat to the beginning of next beat.
- It is given as the changes in volume, pressure and flow in different cardiac chambers, the electrical activities occurring (using ECG) and coinciding heart sounds (using PCG) in various phases of cardiac cycle.
- Duration of a cardiac cycle is 0.8 s when heart rate is 75/min.

Phases of Cardiac Cycle and Their Duration:

- Atrial systole—0.1 s
- Atrial diastole—0.7 s
- Ventricular systole—0.3 s
- Ventricular diastole—0.5 s
- Atrial diastole merges with ventricular systole.
- So the phases described here are atrial systole, ventricular systole and diastole.
- **Ventricular systole:** 2 phases—0.3 sec
  1. **Isovolumetric contraction phase—0.05 s**
  2. **Phase of ejection 0.25 s**
     - Phase of rapid ejection—0.1 s
     - Phase of reduced ejection—0.15 s
- **Ventricular diastole:** 0.5 s
  - Protodiastole—0.04 s
  - Isovolumetric relaxation phase—0.06 s
  - Rapid ventricular filling—0.11 s
  - Diastasis—0.19 s
- **Atrial systole:** 0.1 s

Atrial Systole

- Duration is 0.1 sec
- This follows the phase of diastasis
- Begins from peak of "P" wave in ECG to peak of "QRS" complex
- Atria contracts and increases intra-trial pressure. Blood is pumped into ventricles.
- Final filling of ventricle takes place here (Last 25–30%).
- Already the ventricles are in diastole and 75% of filling is complete.
- 4th heart sound is recorded in phonocardiogram.

Ventricular Systole

- **Isovolumic contraction phase:**
  - Starts at peak of 'QRS' complex. Duration is 0.05 sec.
  - Rise in ventricular pressure closes the AV valves and semilunar valves have not yet opened (*refer* **Fig. 2**).
  - 1st heart sound (S1) is heard, due to closure of AV valves.
  - Ventricular pressure rises (>80 mm Hg) steeply and ventricular volume remains same.

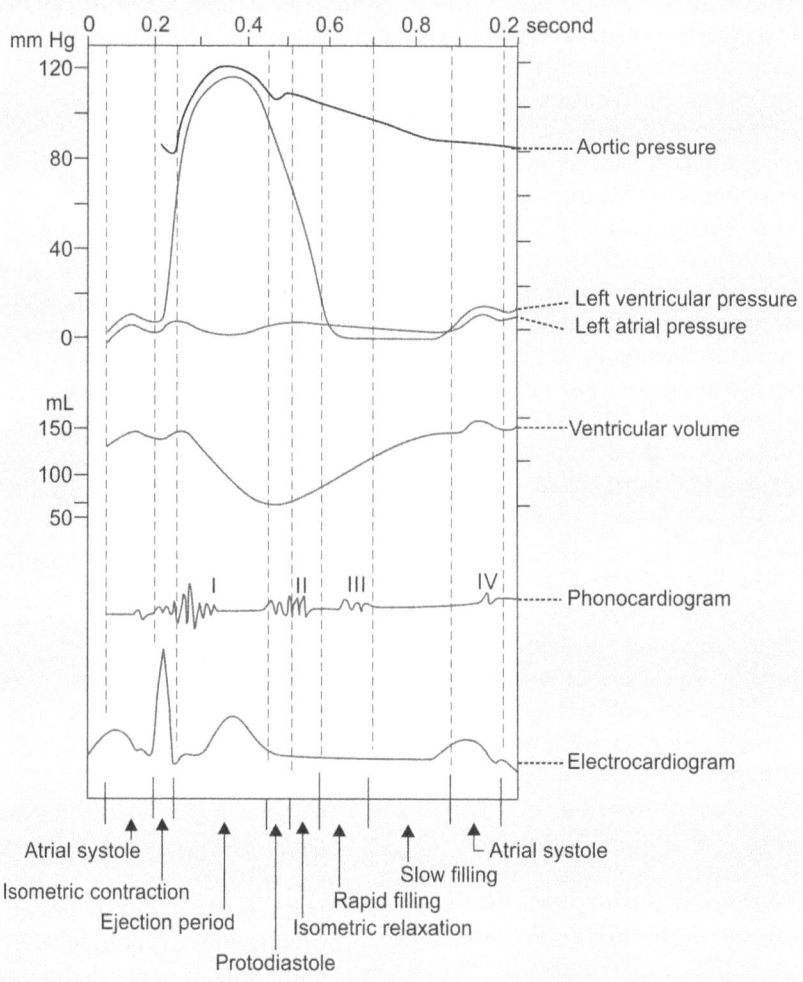

Fig. 2: Cardiac cycle with pressure volume changes in aorta, left ventricle, left atrium, ECG and phonocardiogram.

- There is bulging of AV valves into the atria due to ventricular contraction. This creates 'C' wave in JVP curve.
- Phase ends with opening of semilunar valves and ejection of blood.
☐ **Ventricular ejection**
  - **Rapid ejection phase:** (0.1s)
    - Semilunar valves open and blood is rapidly ejected (2/3rd of stroke volume) into aorta/pulmonary artery.
    - Steep fall in ventricular volume and steep increase in aortic flow
    - Ventricular pressure increases to a peak (120 mm Hg in the left and 25 mm Hg in the right)
    - Aortic pressure also increases.
    - Corresponds to ST segment in ECG
  - **Reduced ejection phase:** (0.15 s)
    - Duration is 0.15 sec
    - Ventricular and aortic pressure decreases but aortic pressure is greater.
    - Aortic blood flow decreases. Only 1/3rd of stroke volume is ejected here.
    - Ventricular volume further decreases.
    - Momentum keeps blood flowing into aorta.
    - 'T' wave appears in ECG

Ventricular Diastole—0.5 s

- Protodiastole—0.04 s
- Isovolumetric relaxation—0.06 s
- Phase of rapid ventricular filling—0.11s
- Phase of reduced filling or diastasis—0.19s
- Phase of second rapid filling—0.1 s

Protodiastole

- Duration is 0.04 sec
- As the reduced filling phase ends, the ventricles start relaxing.
- Intraventricular pressure drops.
- This phase ends when aortic valve closes.

Isovolumetric Relaxation Phase

- Duration is 0.06 sec
- This phase is between closure of semilunar valves and opening of AV valves.
- Second heart sound (S2) appears due to closure of semilunar valves.
- Closure of semilunar valves creates 'Dicrotic Notch' in aortic pressure curve.
- Ventricular volume remains the same and pressure drops steeply as the ventricles relax (2-3 mm Hg).
- When intraventricular pressure drops below atrial pressure, AV valves open.

Rapid Ventricular Filling

- Duration is 0.11 sec
- As the AV valves open there is rapid inrush of blood into ventricles.
- This is because the atria are filled with venous return and pressure is high here.
- This vibration of ventricular wall creates the 3rd (S3) heart sound.
- Major filling takes place here.

Diastasis

- Duration 0.19 sec.
- This is a slow filling phase.
- Ventricular volume rises slowly.
- Ventricular and atrial pressures reduce and remain same (Little >0 mm Hg).
- Nearly 75% of filling has occurred.

Last Rapid Filling

- Duration 0.1 sec.
- Atria contracts and pumps the last 25% of blood into ventricles.
- At rest, this volume is not essential.
- But in tachycardia (as in exercise) when the duration of diastole decreases this volume assumes importance

---

3. Discuss in detail the stages of erythropoiesis and the factors affecting it. Add a note on polycythemia.

- Erythropoiesis is production of RBCs. Life span of RBCs are 120 days.
- Hence continuous destruction and production of RBCs take place at a constant rate.

Site of Erythropoiesis

- **Mesoblastic stage:** In the embryonal stage—yolk sac.
- **Hepatic stage:** Later in the fetal stage up to 5 months—Liver, spleen, thymus and lymph nodes.
- **Myeloid stage:** 3 months before birth—red bone marrow of all bones.
- **Adult life:** Red bone marrow of flat bones and epiphysis of long bones.

Changes During Maturation

- Reduction in size of the cell.
- Cytoplasm increases in amount and nucleus decreases in size.
- Cytoplasm changes from basophilic nature to polychromatophilic and then to acidophilic nature due to hemoglobinization of cytoplasm
- Disappearance of RNA
- Loss of nucleoli and then nucleus

Pronormoblast

- Large cell, diameter—20-25 μm
- Cytoplasm is less.
- High concentration of polyribosomes.
- Large nucleus with multiple nucleoli
- Hemoglobin not formed

Early Normoblast

- Diameter of cell, 15-18 μm
- Cell exhibits mitosis
- Cytoplasm is still less, basophilic
- Nucleus large, occupies 3/4th of cell
- Heterochromatin clumps present.

Intermediate Normoblast

- The cell is smaller in size, 12-15 μm.
- Cytoplasm changes from blue to pink as hemoglobin starts to appear.

- Nucleus small, occupies half the cell. No nucleoli.
- Hemoglobin formation makes the cell acidophilic also—polychromatophilic cytoplasm (*refer* **Fig. 3**).
- Mitosis is sluggish

Late Normoblast

- Cell is smaller in size
- Cytoplasm is deeply eosinophilic—orthochromatic erythroblast.
- Nucleus is small and pyknotic.
- Cart-wheel arrangement of chromatin.
- Hb synthesis increases

Reticulocyte

- Cell size is 7.8 μm
- Nucleus is extruded
- Hemoglobin present
- Chromatin reticulum seen

Mature RBC

- Cell size is 7.5 μm
- RBC is biconcave in shape
- Chromatin reticulum disappears

The whole process of maturation from pronormoblast to reticulocyte takes 7 days. It takes 2 days for reticulocyte to mature as an RBC.

Regulation of Erythropoiesis

There are general and special factors regulating erythropoiesis.

General Factor—Hypoxia

- Major function of RBC is to carry oxygen to the tissues.
- So when there is decrease in tissue oxygen levels, it induces production of RBCs.
- Hypoxia stimulates the interstitial cells of the kidneys to synthesize the hormone **erythropoietin**.
- It acts on bone marrow to stimulate the erythropoietin sensitive stem cells to become proerythroblasts and thereby stimulates formation of RBCs.
- It also increases the release of reticulocytes from the bone marrow.

Factors Increasing Erythropoietin Production

- Hypoxia
- Catecholamines
- Thyroxine
- Testosterone

Special Maturation Factors

Dietary factors:

- Proteins help in globin formation
- Iron helps in heme formation
- Copper, cobalt and nickel also helps in heme formation
- Calcium helps in absorption of iron from GIT
- Vitamin C also helps in iron absorption
- Vitamin B_{12} and folic acid helps in synthesis of nucleic acids and final maturation of RBC

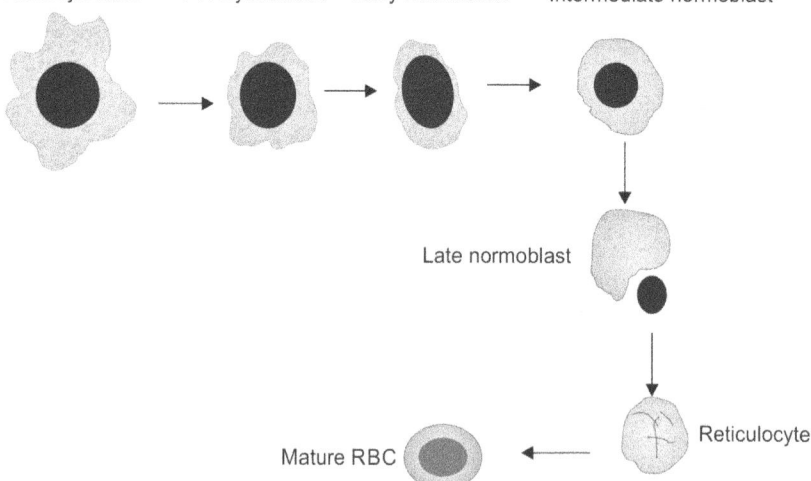

Fig. 3: Stages of erythropoiesis.

- Intrinsic factor synthesized in the stomach by the parietal cells help in absorption of vitamin B_{12}.
- Polycythemia is increase in the RBC count above the normal value. It can be physiological or pathological.

Physiological polycythemia:
- **Age:** At birth the count is high (6-7 million cells/cu mm) and after birth, it starts decreasing due to destruction of RBCs.
- **High altitude:** Hypoxia in high altitude stimulates production of erythropoietin which in turn stimulates RBC production.
- **Excessive** exercise

Pathological polycythemia: 2 types
1. **Primary polycythemia or polycythemia vera:** It is said to be a member of myeloproliferative syndrome and is due to the cancerous condition of the bone marrow. The counts increase more than 10 million cells/cu mm. A high WBC count may also be seen. In this condition erythropoietin levels may be very low.
2. **Secondary polycythemia:** It happens due to hypoxic conditions in the body as in lung (emphysema, COPD) and cardiovascular diseases (Cyanotic heart diseases). The hypoxia stimulates synthesis of erythropoietin and thereby increased production of RBCs.

Complications of Polycythemia

Increase in RBC count, increases the viscosity of blood and thereby increases the peripheral resistance leading to hypertension and left heart failure.

---

4. Describe the oxygen transport in blood. Add note on fetal hemoglobin.

Transport of O_2

- O_2 is transported in blood in 2 forms.
- They are—dissolved form (2%) and as Oxy-Hb (98%)
- As O_2 enters the blood it gets saturated in plasma as dissolved O_2 and then there is a gradient between plasma and RBC → leads to entry of O_2 into RBC → as PO_2 increases inside the RBC, O_2 saturates Hb.

Dissolved O_2

- Dissolved O_2 is measured by the following equation.
- Dissolved O_2 = Solubility of O_2 (0.003 mL/mm Hg) × arterial PO_2 (100 mm Hg)
  = 0.3 mL/dL
- Partial pressure of O_2 (PO_2) in blood is decided by the dissolved O_2 content of blood.

Oxyhemoglobin

- Hemoglobin is an O_2 carrying protein in RBC.
- It increases the O_2 carrying capacity of blood by 70 times.
- Iron in the Hb is in ferrous form (Fe^{2+}) and combines with O_2 in appropriate affinity.
- O_2 + Hb ↔ Hb O_2—Oxygenation reaction (it is not oxidation reaction)
- If Fe^{2+} gets oxidized to Fe^{3+} methemoglobin is formed which does not release O_2
- When the binding of O_2 with hemoglobin happens, affinity of Hb for O_2 increases gradually.
- Initially, Hb is in a tense configuration (T), as one molecule of O_2 combines, the Hb changes to relaxed configuration (R) and the affinity to O_2 increases to maximum when the 3rd O_2 molecule has combined.

O_2 Carrying Capacity of Blood

- Each gram of Hb carries 1.34 mL of O_2.
- Maximum amount of O_2 carried by Hb is the **O_2 carrying capacity of blood.**
- In a healthy individual, it is 20 mL/100 mL of blood. (15 × 1.34 mL = 20.1 mL/dL)
- **O_2 content** is the amount actually bound to Hb.
- % saturation of O_2 (SO_2) = Hb O_2 content/HbO_2 capacity × 100.
- Normally in arterial blood % SO_2 is 98%

O_2-Hb Dissociation Curve

- This curve compares the partial pressure of O_2 and % saturation of Hb with O_2.
- It is sigmoid in shape.
- The shape is sigmoid because of the change in configuration of hemoglobin from T to R state and therefore there is gradual increase in affinity for O_2 and then it gets saturated.

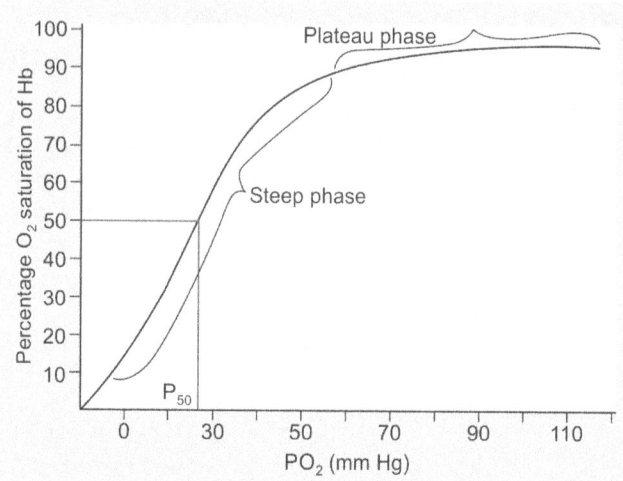

Fig. 4: Oxygen-hemoglobin dissociation curve. P_{50} is the partial pressure of O_2 at which 50% of hemoglobin is saturated with O_2. It is around 27 mm Hg. There are two phases; Steep phase and plateau phase.

- It has a steep and plateau phase (refer **Fig. 4**).
- About 90% saturation of Hb takes place at a PO_2 of 60 mm Hg.
- P_{50} is the partial pressure at which 50% of the hemoglobin is saturated with oxygen.
- P_{50} is inversely related to the affinity of hemoglobin for oxygen.
- The **steep phase** denotes the unloading zone where even a minimum drop in PO_2 results in unloading of large amounts of oxygen to the tissues.
- The **plateau phase** denotes the loading zone, where O_2 is taken up by hemoglobin in the lungs and once all the four sites in Hb are loaded with O_2 there is no further uptake and thereby a plateau phase is reached.
- The curve gets shifted to right are left in conditions of decreased or increase in affinity of hemoglobin for O_2 respectively.

Conditions where O_2-Hb dissociation curve is shifted to right:
- Hypoxia
- ↑ PCO_2
- ↑ temperature
- ↑ 2,3-DPG levels in RBC
- ↑ H^+ concentration (Acidosis)

Conditions where O_2-Hb dissociation curve is shifted to left:
- High PO_2
- Low PCO_2
- Low body temperature
- Presence of fetal hemoglobin
- Alkalosis
- Low 2,3-DPG levels in RBC
- Carbon monoxide poisoning (refer **Fig. 5**)
- **Fetal hemoglobin (HbF)** has 2 alpha chains and 2 gamma chains making up the globin part of Hb.
- About 80% of Hb in the fetus at the time of birth is HbF.
- Disappears by 5th month of age.
- It has greater affinity for oxygen and it shifts the O_2–Hb dissociation curve to the left.
- High affinity is due to its poor binding capacity with 2,3-DPG.
- It is also resistant to action of alkalis. Life span is 1–2 weeks.

II. WRITE NOTES ON

1. Facilitated diffusion.
- Large watersoluble substances (e.g., glucose) are carried by a protein which changes configuration on binding.
- This change in configuration shifts the molecule in or out (refer **Fig. 6**).
- Highly selective and specific
- Types:
  - Uniport
  - Symport
  - Antiport

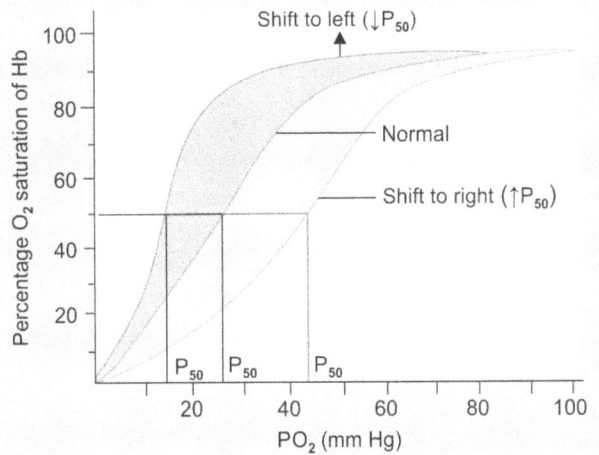

Fig. 5: Right and left shift of O_2-Hb dissociation curve. P_{50}, PO_2 at which hemoglobin is 50% saturated is 27 mm Hg. Right shift denotes decrease in hemoglobin affinity for O_2 and left shift increased affinity for O_2.

- Characteristics:
  - Specificity
  - Saturation
  - Competition

2. Control of insulin secretion.

There are factors which stimulate and inhibit insulin secretion:

Factors stimulating insulin secretion:

- Glucose
- Amino acids (Leucine, arginine)
- Intestinal hormones (GIP, GLP, gastrin, secretin, CCK)
- β-ketoacids
- Acetylcholine
- Glucagon

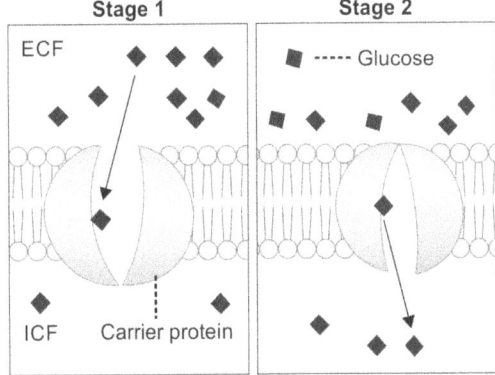

Fig. 6: Facilitated diffusion. A uniport transporting glucose molecules.

- cAMP
- β-adrenergic stimulation
- Sulfonylureas
- Theophylline

Factors inhibiting insulin secretion:

- Somatostatin
- 2-Deoxyglucose
- α-adrenergic stimulation
- β-adrenergic blockers
- Galanin
- Diazoxide
- Thiazide diuretics
- K^+ depletion
- Phenytoin
- Alloxan
- Insulin

Effect of plasma glucose on insulin secretion:

- Blood glucose levels have a direct action on β cells to increase insulin secretion.
- There is an initial rapid increase in secretion followed by a slow rise
- Glucose enters B cells via GLUT 2 transporters. It is phosphorylated by glucokinase and metabolized to pyruvate in cytoplasm
- Pyruvate then enters mitochondria and is metabolized to CO_2 and H_2O via citric acid cycle.
- ATP is produced and it enters cytoplasm and inhibits ATP-sensitive K^+ channels and thereby reduces K^+ efflux.

- This results in depolarization of B cells and causes opening of voltage-gated Ca^{2+} channels. Calcium influx causes exocytosis of secretory vesicles containing insulin.
- Pyruvate metabolism also produces glutamate which in turn causes release of the second pool of secretory granules of insulin (*refer* **Fig. 7**).

Effect of protein and fat derivatives on insulin secretion:
- Insulin stimulates protein synthesis by incorporating amino acids, such as leucine, arginine into proteins.
- It also inhibits fat catabolism.
- Secretion of insulin is stimulated by β-ketoacids like acetoacetate.
- Like glucose, these substrates also induce formation of ATP and close the ATP-sensitive K^+ channels.

Effect of cAMP on insulin secretion:
- Stimuli that increase intracellular cAMP increases insulin secretion by increasing intracellular Ca^{2+}.
- Factors that increase cAMP levels are β-adrenergic agonists, glucagon, phosphodiesterase inhibitors like theophylline.
- Catecholamines while acting through $α_2$-adrenergic stimulation inhibits insulin secretion and while acting on β-adrenergic receptors stimulate insulin secretion. Net effect is inhibition of secretion.

Effect of autonomic stimulation on insulin secretion:
- Stimulation of vagus nerve to pancreatic islets results in secretion of insulin. The neurotransmitter released is acetylcholine which acts on M4 receptors. It stimulates secretion by increasing intracellular calcium.
- Sympathetic nerve stimulation acts through $α_2$-adrenergic receptors and inhibit secretion of insulin.

Effect of intestinal hormones on insulin secretion:
- Elevated plasma glucose levels increase insulin secretion. But it was found that orally administered glucose had a greater effect of increasing insulin secretion.
- This has been identified due to GI hormone effect on insulin secretion, such as: glucagon, secretin, CCK, gastrin, gastric inhibitory peptide (GIP) and glucagon-like polypeptide (GLP).

Effect of plasma K^+ levels on insulin secretion:
- Increase in K^+ levels increase insulin secretion. Insulin decreases plasma K^+ levels
- Insulin is a major hormone which decreases plasma K^+ levels following food intake.
- Thiazide diuretics causes loss of K^+ and Na^+ in urine and thereby decreases K^+ levels and decreases insulin secretion.

3. Golgi tendon reflex.
- When the skeletal muscle is stretched, muscle spindle is stimulated by the stretch and results in muscle contraction.

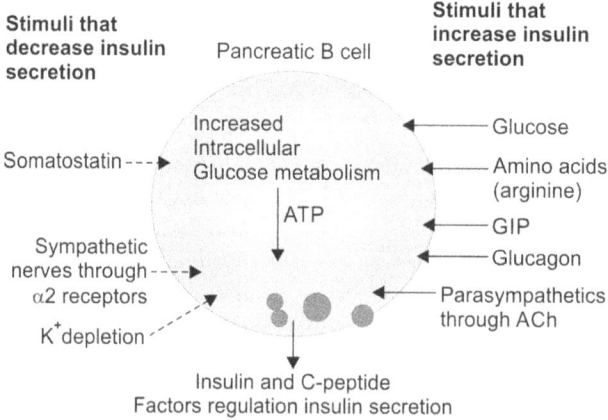

Insulin and C-peptide
Factors regulation insulin secretion

Fig. 7: Regulation of insulin secretion.

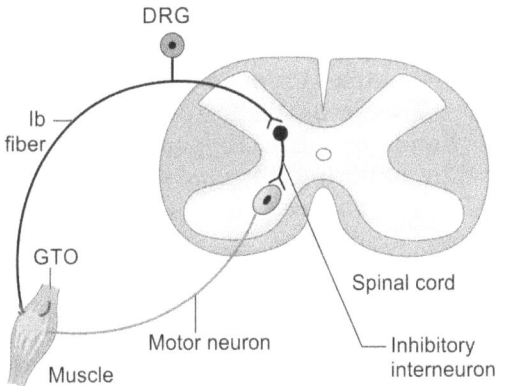

Fig. 8: Golgi tendon reflex or inverse stretch reflex.

- This happens only up to a particular level of stretch.
- If the tension in the muscle is increased beyond a level, the muscle relaxes.
- Relaxation of muscle in relation to strong stretch is called the **inverse stretch reflex** or **autogenic inhibition**.
- The receptor for this reflex is **Golgi tendon organ** (GTO). Therefore, the reflex is also called as **Golgi tendon reflex**.
- Golgi tendon organ, the receptor for this reflex is present in the tendons of the muscles.
- It is stimulated when the extrafusal fibers contract and thereby it induces a stretch to the GTO in the tendon (*refer* **Fig. 8**).
- The afferents from GTO are carried by the Ib fibers.
- Ib fibers end on spinal interneurons and through them they inhibit the motor neurons supplying the same muscles and produces IPSP in them. This causes relaxation of the same muscle.
- This reflex helps in regulation of tension developed in the muscle.

4. Oxygen-hemoglobin dissociation curve.

Refer answer to essay 4.

5. Neuromuscular junction.

It is the junction between the motor neuron and the muscle fiber it supplies.

Structure of NMJ

- The NMJ is formed by the axon terminal of the motor neuron.
- On approaching the muscle fiber, the axon it loses its myelin sheath and divides into many branches and the nerve terminals bulge to form the terminal buttons which approaches the muscle fiber at its center.
- NMJ has a presynaptic membrane, synaptic cleft and postsynaptic membrane.

Presynaptic Terminal

- It is the membrane of the terminal button of the axon.
- It has many ACh vesicles and mitochondria within the membrane.
- The membrane is studded with many voltage-gated Ca^{2+} channels (*refer* **Fig. 9**).

Synaptic Cleft

- It is a space of 50–100 nm width between the presynaptic and postsynaptic membranes.
- It has ECF in it and acetylcholinesterase enzyme is present in it.

Postsynaptic Membrane

- It is the muscle membrane in contact with the nerve terminal and it is thrown into many folds—junctional folds and is thickened and deepened—synaptic trough.
- The muscle membrane here is called as the motor end plate.

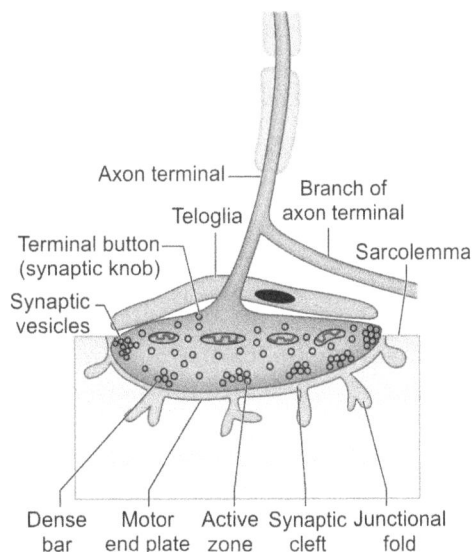

Fig. 9: Neuromuscular junction.

- It contains the nicotinic acetylcholine receptors.

Impulse Transmission in NMJ

Stimulation of nerve fiber
↓
AP generated in nerve fiber
↓
Conduction of AP in nerve fiber
↓
Impulse reaches nerve terminal
↓
Voltage-gated Ca^{2+} channels in nerve terminal open
↓
Ca^{2+} influx into presynaptic membrane
↓
Exocytosis of ACh vesicles and ACh is released into synaptic cleft
↓
ACh moves across the cleft and binds to nicotinic ACh receptors in muscle membrane
↓
The receptor is a nonspecific cation channel which opens on binding with ACh
↓
Influx of Na^+ ions into postsynaptic membrane
↓
Local depolarization of muscle membrane—**end plate potential**
↓
Generation of action potential in the neighboring muscle membrane by the EPP

Drugs Acting on NMJ

Blockers of NMJ

- **Curare:** It binds with the ACh receptors and prevents binding of ACh to their receptors. This blocks the neuromuscular transmission.
- **Bungarotoxin:** This is acquired from snake venom. It also prevents impulse transmission by binding the ACh receptors
- **Succinylcholine:** They act just like ACh and make the muscle membrane depolarized.
- But the choline esterase does not have any effect on these substances and therefore the muscle is continuously depolarized and cannot be stimulated again.
- **Botulinum toxin:** They are derived from the bacteria *Clostridium tetani* and it prevents release of ACh vesicles from terminal buttons.

Stimulators of NMJ

- **Drugs having ACh like action:** Drugs, such as carbachol, nicotine, etc., act on ACh receptors like ACh but cannot be removed or slowly removed by ACh esterase. This makes the muscle to have repeated depolarizations resulting in muscle spasm.
- **Drugs that inhibit choline esterase:** Drugs, such as neostigmine, physostigmine, diisopropyl fluorophosphate (DFP) stimulate the NMJ by inactivating cholinesterase. This results in continuous activation of ACh on receptors and repeated muscle spasm. It takes weeks together for removal of ACh and therefore it has a fatal poisoning effect.

Diseases Affecting NMJ

Myasthenia Gravis

- It is an autoimmune disease.
- Antibodies are formed against the nicotinic ACh receptors in NMJ.
- There is weakness, fatigue and the muscles become weak with use and therefore symptoms worsen towards the evening.
- Antibodies not only combine with ACh receptors, they also flatten the post synaptic membrane and cause endocytosis of ACh into presynaptic membrane.
- Because of these effects, the muscle response to stimulation gradually decreases.
- Symptoms improve after rest and are better on getting up in the morning.
- The extraocular and facial muscles are the first to be affected and ptosis and diplopia are present.

Treatment

- **Acetylcholine esterase (AChE) inhibitors**—AChE inhibitors increase the amount of ACh in the NMJ and they can displace the antibodies and improve functions.
- **Thymectomy:** Decreases the immune response by inhibiting T cell activation.
- **Immunosuppressants**
- **Plasmapheresis**

Lambert-Eaton Syndrome

- It is also an autoimmune disease.
- Antibodies are formed against voltage-gated Ca^{2+} channels in the presynaptic membrane.
- Here the symptoms of muscle weakness improve with repeated stimulation, as Ca^{2+} levels increase with each stimulus.

6. Regulation of hydrochloric acid secretion in the gastric parietal cells.

Regulation of Gastric Secretion

Neural, humoral and reflex regulation of secretion

Factors that Stimulate

1. Vagus N
2. Gastrin
3. Histamine

Factors that Inhibit

1. Low pH in the stomach
2. Somatostatin
3. Prostaglandin E2 (*refer* **Fig. 10**)

Regulation is discussed in terms of:

1. Cephalic phase
2. Gastric phase
3. Intestinal phase

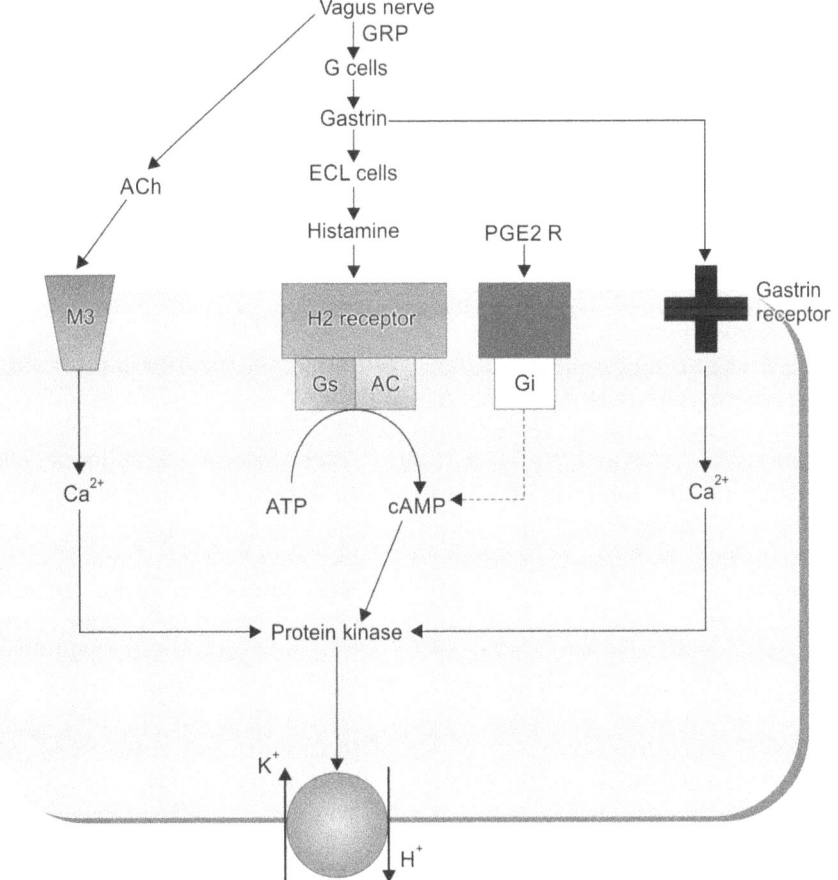

Fig. 10: Parietal cell with the regulating factors for HCl secretion.
(PGE2 R: Prostaglandin E2 receptor; M3: Muscarinic receptor)

Cephalic phase:
- Nearly 500 mL/hr (45% of total secretion)
- Initiated by thought, sight, smell, taste of food through vagus nerve
- Emotions also affect secretion

Gastric phase:
About 50% of total secretion. Food in stomach induces secretion by:
- Distension of body of stomach (through reflexes—vagal reflex)
- Distension of antrum (through gastrin secretion)
- By products of partial digestion of protein (through gastrin secretion)

Intestinal phase:
- It begins when chyme enters the intestine.
- Intestinal influence is inhibitory by:
  - **Enterogastric reflex:** By distension, presence of acid and products of digestion—inhibits secretion.
  - **Hormonal mechanism:** CCK, secretin, GIP, neurotensin, etc.,—**enterogastrone**.

---

7. Autorhythmicity of heart.

- Heart has the capacity to beat even after the nerves supplying the heart are removed. This is because of the presence of the pacemaker tissue in the heart.
- It is called as the pacemaker as it can generate action potentials repeatedly in a rhythmic manner without any neural stimulation.
- The tissues in the heart capable of producing such impulses are; the SA node, AV node, His bundle, Purkinje fibers and the ventricles.
- Even though all the above tissues can function as the pacemaker, SA node is said to be the primary pacemaker of the heart as it generates impulses at a faster rate (60-100/min) than other tissues.
- In case of disease of SA node other pacemakers take up the activity of pacemaking in a hierarchical manner; the AV node, His bundle-Purkinje system and then the ventricle.
- Rhythmicity means the heart beats rhythmically with the intervals between each beat remaining a constant.
- The impulses from SA node are in a rhythmic manner. It contributes to the autorhythmic property of heart.
- The electrical impulses generated in the pacemaker is discussed under the topic of pacemaker potential.

Pacemaker Potential
- The ventricular and atrial muscle cells have a resting membrane potential of -90 mV. On stimulation, the membrane depolarizes and produces an action potential.
- The pacemaker cells are smaller and rounded (P cells) and they do not have a stable resting membrane potential and RMP is around -55 to -60 mV.
- From -60 mV there is a slow depolarization slope which reaches the firing level of -40 mV and there is a rapid depolarization followed by rapid repolarization back to -60 mV and again there is a slow depolarization slope rising to firing level.
- This slope which takes the membrane to firing level is the **pacemaker potential or prepotential**.

Ionic events responsible for pacemaker potential:
- At -60 mV the K^+ channels start closing down thereby preventing K^+ efflux. This is responsible for the first part of pre potential (the slope).
- Next part is due to opening up of **'f'** type Na+ channels (The Na^+ current in this channel is said to be funny current as the channel opens in hyperpolarization)
- Last part of depolarization of the prepotential is due to opening of T-type (transient) Ca^{2+} channels allowing Ca^{2+} influx (*refer* **Fig. 11**).
- Now as the firing level is reached (-40 mV), the long lasting Ca^{2+} channels (L-Type) open and produces a rapid depolarization and the action potential.

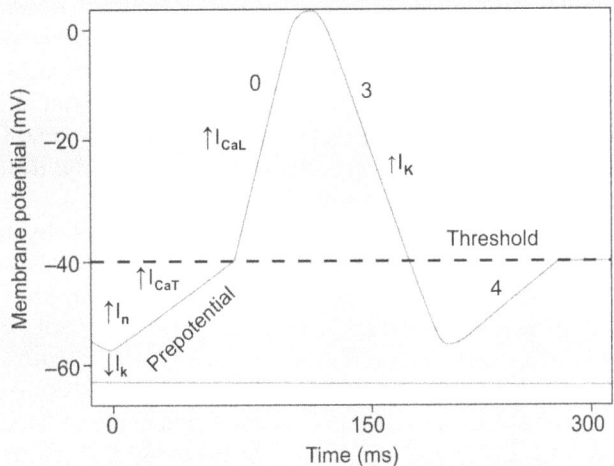

Fig. 11: Pacemaker potential. Slope of pacemaker potential (Phase 4), the prepotential is due to 3 events; first part of depolarization is due to closure of K⁺ channels, 2nd part is due to Na⁺ influx through sodium channel and last part of depolarization is due to Ca²⁺ influx through T-type Ca²⁺ channels. Rapid depolarization (Phase 0) is due to opening of L-type Ca²⁺ channels and repolarization (Phase 3) due to opening of K⁺ channels.

- Then the K⁺ channels open and the K⁺ efflux bring about rapid repolarization and membrane potential reaches –60 mV. Then the next prepotential starts.
- So in the pacemaker cells, it is a Ca²⁺ dependent depolarization rather than Na⁺ dependent depolarization as in ventricular muscles.
- The pacemaker cells are supplied by sympathetic and parasympathetic nerves.
- On stimulation by sympathetic nerves the prepotential slope becomes steeper and the rate of spontaneous discharge increases thereby increasing the heart rate.
- On stimulation by the parasympathetic nerves the slope of the prepotential decreases and spontaneous firing also decreases thereby heart rate decreases.

8. Describe the connections and functions of temporal lobe.

Temporal lobe is located inferior to the lateral sulcus.

It has 3 regions—superior temporal gyrus, inferior temporal gyrus and mediobasal gyrus.

It has the following areas:
- **Brodmann's area 41 and 42:** This is the primary auditory area located in the superior temporal gyrus. Area 42 is below area 41. It receives afferents from medial geniculate body and is concerned with perception of frequency, intensity and location of sound. It projects to area 22 which helps in understanding speech (*refer* **Fig. 12**).
- **Area 22:** It is located below area 42. It also receives inputs from visual areas and projects to frontal lobe, parietal lobe and cingulate gyrus. It is involved in interpretation of

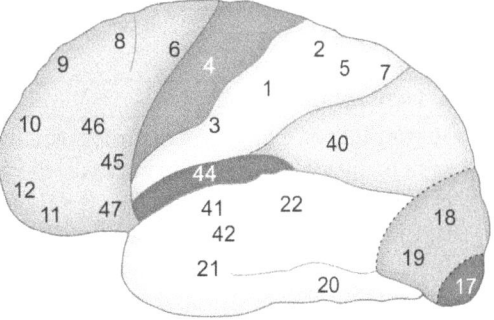

Fig. 12: Lobes of cerebral cortex and Brodmann's areas.

meaning of sound and comprehension of spoken and written words.
- **Wernicke's area:** Posterior part of area 22 is the Wernicke's area. It is the sensory speech area. It is concerned with understanding of spoken and written words and in meaningful word formation for replying back in form of spoken speech or written words.
- **Area 20, 21 and 37:** Present in inferior and middle gyri. It receives inputs from visual areas, thalamus and parietal lobes. It projects to visual areas, amygdala and entorhinal cortex. Area 20 and 21 are concerned with speech and facial recognition. Area 37 is concerned with perception of colors.
- **Areas 28 and 38:** They are located in the medial parts of temporal lobe. They are concerned with speech, limbic functions and olfaction.

Functions of Temporal Lobe

- It perceives sound and has the capacity to discriminate pitch, intensity and localization of sound
- Wernicke's area has a role in comprehension of spoken and written language.
- It has a role in interpretation of sounds.
- Since the areas of limbic system, like hippocampus are located here it has a role in memory and emotions
- Areas 20 and 21 are needed for facial recognition.
- Has a role in color vision
- It has a role in olfaction.

III. SHORT ANSWERS

1. Hemophilia.

- Hemophilia is a bleeding disorder usually seen in the males. In majority of cases there is deficiency of Factor VIII. This is said to be Classical Hemophilia or *Hemophilia A*.
- It is an X-linked recessive disease. Therefore, the males are affected and females are carriers of the disease.
- There are soft tissue hematomas and hem arthrosis which may happen repeatedly resulting in crippling arthropathy.
- Usually there are no spontaneous hemorrhages but there is excessive bleeding after even a mild injury as in tooth extraction.
- Condition is characterized by prolonged clotting time (normal CT = 3–8 minutes) and normal bleeding time. APTT is prolonged.
- Treatment is done by fresh blood transfusion. Factor VIII can also be prepared from fresh frozen plasma and injected.
- Christmas disease or *Hemophilia B* is due to deficiency of factor IX. It is also a sex-linked recessive disease. Symptoms are similar to hemophilia A. Diagnosis is done by the assay of Factor IX.
- *Hemophilia C* is due to deficiency of Factor XI. It affects both males and females.

2. Differentiate between isotonic and isometric contraction.

- Muscle contains both elastic and viscous elements.
- Elastic elements are the connective tissue in the muscle fibers and there are series and parallel elastic elements.
- The parallel ones are in between the muscle fibers and the series are at the ends of the muscles connecting the muscle to the bones.
- The viscous elements are the contractile component of the muscle.
- So, when a muscle contracts there can be differences in the response of the elastic and viscous elements.
- Based on that, the muscle contraction is classified as isometric and isotonic contractions.

Isometric Contraction

- As the name implies, in this type of contraction length of the muscle remains same but tension developed in the muscle is increased.
- The muscle length remains the same because as the contractile components are shortening the series elastic elements are stretched and thereby the tension increases but length remains the same.
- There is no shortening and therefore no movement is happening here.

- Work done = Force X distance and since no distance is changed here, there is no actual work done in isometric contraction.

Examples of Isometric Contraction
- Contraction of arm muscle while pushing against the wall
- Contraction of antigravity muscles of the body

Isotonic Contraction
- In this type of contraction, the muscle length shortens but the tension developed in the muscle remains the same.
- Here the contractile component and parallel elastic elements shorten and series elastic components are not stretched.
- Since the muscle shortens there is work being done in this type of contractions.

Examples are:
- Contraction of upper limb muscles while lifting an object
- Walking
- Swimming

3. Erythropoietin.
- Erythropoietin is a glycoprotein hormone synthesized and secreted from kidneys and liver.
- It is secreted by the interstitial cells in peritubular capillary bed of the kidneys (85%) and by perivenous hepatocytes (15%) in the liver.
- It acts on the bone marrow and increases the number of erythropoietin-sensitive committed stem cells in the bone marrow and converts them into mature RBCs.
- Level of erythropoietin (EPO) is increased in anemia.
- Gene for EPO has been cloned and it can be produced by recombinant technology in animal cells and can be used for treatment of anemia in renal failure.
- It can also be used to stimulate RBC production in people who undergo autologous blood transfusion as in elective surgeries.

Regulation of Secretion
- Hypoxia stimulates EPO secretion. There are O_2 sensors which are heme proteins in the kidneys and liver which are stimulates in its deoxy form and inhibited in their oxy form.
- It is also stimulated by cobalt salts and androgens.
- High altitude alkalosis also stimulates secretion of EPO.
- It is also stimulated by β adrenergic stimulation

4. Compound action potential.
- When a single axon is stimulated, a single peak action potential can be recorded.
- But if a mixed nerve is stimulated there is a multipeaked action potential recorded.
- This is said to be **compound action potential**
- This type of multipeaked action potential is recorded in a mixed nerve due to the differences in the speed of conduction of individual fibers.
- When such a nerve is stimulated, activity in the fast-conducting fibers arrives at the recording electrode sooner than the slower conducting fibers, this creates multiple peaks.
- The number and size of the peaks vary with the type of fibers in the particular nerve being studied.

5. Gastrin.
- Secreted by G cells in stomach in the antrum.
- It is a polypeptide hormone
- 3 types of gastrin—G34, G17 and G 14
- In stomach G 17 is secreted.

Factors Influencing Gastrin Release

Stimuli that Increase Release
- Gastric distension
- Products of protein digestion in stomach
- Increased vagal discharge
- Calcium and epinephrine

Stimuli that Decrease Release
- Low pH in stomach
- Somatostatin
- Secretin
- Vasoactive intestinal peptide
- Calcitonin
- Glucagon

Functions of Gastrin

- Stimulates secretion of HCl and pepsinogen in stomach.
- Stimulates gastric motility and emptying
- Contracts lower esophageal sphincter and prevents reflux gastritis.
- Has a trophic action on gastric and intestinal mucosa.
- Stimulates secretion of pancreatic juice.
- Stimulates insulin and glucagon secretion from endocrine pancreas.
- Responsible for gastro-colic reflex.
- Stimulates histamine from enterochromaffin like cells in GI mucosa and thereby stimulates HCl secretion

6. Addisonian crisis.

- Primary adrenal insufficiency is due to diseases affecting adrenal cortex and is called as **Addison's disease**.
- It is usually seen as a complication of tuberculosis, due to an autoimmune inflammation of adrenal or malignancy of adrenal cortex.
- Here there is deficiency of mineralocorticoids, glucocorticoids and androgens.
- Absence of glucocorticoids—patients are tired, lose weight, nausea, vomiting etc. Fasting results in fatal hypoglycemia and any stress leads to collapse of the patient.
- Mineralocorticoid deficiency—hypotension, hyponatremia, hyperkalemia and acidosis. They have a small heart due to hypotension which results in decrease workload of the heart.
- Adrenal androgen deficiency—loss of hair in females.
- Water excretion is decreased and a water load may lead to water intoxication.
- Low glucocorticoid levels lead to increase in ACTH levels which results in hyperpigmentation. This is because of melanocyte-stimulating hormone (MSH) like action of ACTH.

Addisonian Crisis

- Acute adrenal insufficiency leads to Addisonian crisis.
- It can happen due to major surgery, trauma and sudden withdrawal of glucocorticoid therapy.
- With all the symptoms above they eventually develop severe hypotension and shock which may be fatal.
- It can be treated with fluids, electrolytes, glucocorticoid and mineralocorticoid supplements.

7. Law of gut.

Movement of chyme in intestines by peristalsis is always from oral to aboral direction and never in the opposite direction. Peristalsis is stimulated by distension of the gut which induces a contraction ring in the segment of intestine behind the chyme and a relaxing segment ahead of the chyme. This pushes the food towards the anus.

8. Intestinal phase of pancreatic secretion.

Regulation in Intestinal Phase

- This phase starts when the food enters duodenum and jejunum.
- It stimulates secretion of pancreatic juice rich in bicarbonate.
- It is under the control of intestinal hormones—secretin and CCK.

Role of Secretin

- Secretin is secreted by the 'S' cells of duodenum and jejunum.
- Its secretion is stimulated by presence of acid in the intestine.
- It acts on the pancreatic ductal cells and stimulates secretion of large volume of watery bicarbonate rich pancreatic juice.
- It also stimulates bicarbonate rich bile secretion from hepatocytes in liver.

Role of Cholecystokinin

- It is secreted from 'I' cells of the duodenum and jejunum.
- Its secretion is stimulated by presence of products of amino acids and fatty acids in the intestine.
- CCK is secreted into blood and it acts on the pancreatic acini and stimulates secretion of enzyme rich pancreatic juice.

9. Inhibin.

- Inhibin is secreted both in the males and females.
- Inhibins are present in extracts of testicular fluids and antral fluids of the ovaries
- Inhibins are formed by 3 glycosylated subunits—Glycosylated α subunit and 2 nonglycosylated β subunits, β_A and β_B
- They either form heterodimers or homodimers with α and β subunits.
- They inhibit FSH secretion by acting on anterior pituitary.
- Heterodimers are inhibins and homodimers are called activins.

10. Functions of prostate gland.

- It is an accessory gland of male reproductive system.
- It is present below the urinary bladder and urethra passes through the prostate gland. This part of the male urethra is said to be the prostatic urethra.
- It secretes a milky fluid which forms 20% of semen. It is alkaline in nature.

It contains the following components:
- Spermine
- Citric acid
- Cholesterol
- Phospholipids
- Fibrinolysin, fibrinogenase
- Zinc
- Acid phosphatase

Functions of prostatic fluid:
- Maintains an optimum pH of 6-6.5 in vaginal environment, which is needed for motility of sperm and it favors fertilization.
- It converts fibrinogen from seminal fluid into a coagulum which is needed to hold the sperm in uterine cervix.
- Later, fibrinolysin in prostatic fluid liquifies the coagulum, facilitating sperm motility and activation.

11. Putamen circuit of basal ganglia.

It is the direct pathway in basal ganglia:
Cerebral cortex → striatum (caudate and putamen) → internal segment (IS) of globus pallidus (GP) → thalamus → motor cortex.

Cortex excites striatum
↓
Striatum inhibits IS of GP
↓
IS of GP inhibits the inhibition of thalamus via thalamic fasciculus (goes to VA and VL nuclei of thalamus)
↓
Impulses from thalamus to prefrontal and premotor cortex and the final effect is disinhibition.

Functions of Putamen Circuit

Putamen circuit in connections with the cerebral cortex controls complex patterns of motor activity, such as writing, cutting, hammering nails, vocalization, controlled movements of eyes and all other skilled movements.

12. Caisson disease.

- Also called as "dysbarism, the bends, decompression sickness, Diver's palsy".
- This happens when a person breathing compressed air ascends up rapidly.
- At high pressures, N_2 dissolves in body fluids and stays dissolved.
- When the person ascends up to sea level gradually N_2 is converted to air gradually and is blown out.
- But when he ascends up rapidly the dissolved N_2 does not have enough time to be converted to air and to be blown out and therefor it stays in the tissues as N_2 bubbles.
- N_2 dissolved in tissues forms bubbles while escaping from tissues due to rapid ascent.
- Gas bubbles block the blood vessels and stay in tissues to create symptoms.

Symptoms:
- Pain in joints and muscles of legs or arms.
- Sensation of numbness
- The chokes—shortness of breath, pulmonary edema etc.
- Paralysis of muscles
- Coronary ischemia
- Neurological symptoms

Treatment: Recompression in pressurized chamber followed by slow decompression.

13. Hering-Breuer inflation reflex.

- Hering and Breuer found that over inflation of the lungs results in decreased output through the phrenic nerves to the diaphragm and thereby stimulates expiration.
- This reflex is a protective reflex to prevent over inflation of the lungs.
- The receptors are slowly adapting nerve endings of the myelinated vagus nerves in the airways of the lungs.
- This reflex is stimulated by steady increase in lung volume resulting in immediate and prolonged expiration.
- It is more useful in infants than adults and it regulates the tidal volume in infants.

14. Einthoven's law.

Einthoven's law states that if the electric potentials in any two of the three bipolar limb leads are known at any instance, the potential in the third lead can be known by summing the potentials in the first two leads.

For example:
1. If the right arm is –0.2 mV (negative) with respect to the average potential in the body and the left arm is +0.3 mV (positive).
2. The left leg is +1 mV (positive).
3. Therefore, Lead I record a positive potential of +0.5 mV, Lead III records a positive potential of +0.7 mV and it can be calculated that Lead II will record +1.2 mV positive potential.
4. Therefore, the potential of any wave or complex in Lead II of ECG is equal to the sum of potentials in Leads I and III while recorded at any instant.
5. So using Einthoven's law, amplitude of QRS complex can be calculated in any bipolar limb lead either by summing up or subtracting the amplitude in other two leads.
6. QRS amplitude in Lead II = Lead I + Lead III and amplitude of QRS in Lead III = II – I.

15. Endochlear potential.

- The fluids in the cochlear compartments are responsible for the endocochlear potentials.
- Endolymph in the scala media contains high K^+ concentration than the perilymph in the scala vestibuli and scala tympani.
- There is a potential of + 80 mV due to this difference in ionic concentration.
- This potential is the endocochlear potential.
- It is produced by the stria vascularis lining the lateral wall of scala media.
- Stria vascularis produces this high K^+ concentration in scala media by two mechanisms—High concentration of Na^+-K^+ ATPase and presence of an electrogenic K^+ pump.

16. Describe the normal waves in electro-encephalogram (EEG).

Electroencephalogram

- This is a recording of spontaneous electrical activities generated in the cerebral cortex.
- These waves are recorded by placing electrodes on the scalp at various areas and also on the forehead.
- Neurons are known to generate impulses like AP and graded potentials—collectively called as brain waves.
- Also called as "Berger's rhythm".
- **Waves of EEG:**
  - Alpha waves
  - Beta waves
  - Theta waves
  - Delta waves

Alpha Waves

- Occurs at a frequency of 8–13 per second. Amplitude 50–100 µV
- Present in all normal individuals when they are awake and resting with closed eyes.
- Disappears entirely during sleep.
- It is found in the parietooccipital region.
- Alpha block—alpha rhythm disappears on opening the eyes.
- Also called as desynchronization.
- Alpha rhythm affected by blood glucose levels, body temperature and glucocorticoids.

Beta Waves

- Frequency between 14 and 30 Hz.
- Amplitude 5–10 µV (*refer* **Fig. 13**)

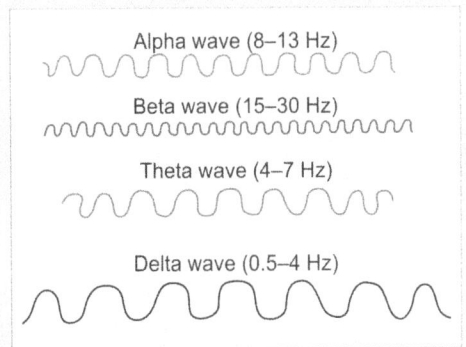

Fig. 13: EEG waves.

- These waves appear when the nervous system is active.
- These waves appear in frontal regions.

Theta Waves
- At a frequency of 4-7 Hz. Amplitude is larger.
- Occurs normally in children and in adults at time of emotional stress.
- Found over parietal and temporal areas.
- Also occurs in many disorders of brain.

Delta Waves
- Frequency of these waves is 1-5 Hz.
- Amplitude is 20-200 μV
- Delta waves occur in sleep in adults but present in infants during wakefulness.
- When present in an awake adult it indicates brain damage.

Uses of EEG
- Used to study normal functions of brain.
- To study the changes in brain activity during sleep.
- To diagnose various brain disorders, such as epilepsy, tumors, sites of trauma, degenerative diseases.

17. Presbyopia.

- It is commonly seen in aged people above the age of 40 years.
- The near point has receded beyond the normal reading distance due to loss of plasticity of lens.
- The loss of plasticity results in loss of accommodation property of the lens.
- It is corrected using convex lens for near work and plain glasses for far work and it is given as the bifocal lenses.

18. Bainbridge reflex.

- In a person with low heart rate when rapid infusion of saline is done there is a rapid rise in heart rate.
- This reflex was described by Bainbridge in 1915 and therefore called as Bainbridge reflex.
- It is a true reflex and the afferents are the vagal afferents. The impulses cause a decrease in vagal tone and thereby increase the heart rate.
- This reflex can be blocked by application of atropine or vagotomy
- The receptors are tachycardia producing atrial receptors.

19. Transpulmonary pressure.

- Transpulmonary pressure (TPP) is the pressure difference across the lung. It is intrapulmonary pressure minus intrapleural pressure.
- There is a difference in intrapleural pressure in the apex and the base of the lung and therefore transpulmonary pressure is different in the apex and the base.
- It is +6 mm Hg in the apex and +1 mm Hg in the base.
- It varies with the phases of respiration.
- At the end of expiration TPP is 2.5 mm Hg and at end of inspiration it is 6 mm Hg.
- Increase in TPP stretches the lungs and therefore it decides the lung volume.

20. Wernicke's and global aphasia
Fluent Aphasia or Wernicke's Aphasia

- Lesion in the sensory speech area—Wernicke's area (Area 22). It can happen due to blockage of vessels supplying the area or injury.
- Also called as fluent aphasia.
- Here the person is able to hear spoken words or identifying written words
- But cannot comprehend spoken or written words.

- Motor speech is intact. So speech is not disturbed. Person speaks excessively.
- Impairment of written words as they are not able to comprehend written words also.

Global Aphasia

- Lesion in both the Wernicke's area and Broca's area results in global aphasia.
- All aspects of speech are impaired.
- The patient is not able to comprehend or repeat words.

21. Functions of saliva.

- Ptyalin (α-amylase) in saliva splits starches. Action of amylase is maximum at a pH of 6.8. Digestion continues in stomach for some time till the pH becomes less than 4.
- **Protective function:** Saliva cleans the mouth after a meal and prevents growth of harmful bacteria.
- Saliva contains lysozyme, IgA and lactoferrin for protection. Lysozymes are bactericidal and lactoferrin is bacteriostatic in action.
- Saliva facilitates speech.
- It helps in taste of food.
- Mucus in saliva helps in lubrication of food, mastication and swallowing
- It buffers the gastric juice in stomach.
- Proline rich proteins in the saliva protect the enamel of tooth.
- Saliva dilutes hot and irritant foods and protects buccal mucosa. It also dilutes regurgitated bile and HCl
- In animals, it helps in temperature regulation.
- Helps in excretion of heavy metals, alcohol, morphine, thiocyanate etc.

22. Diuretics and their sites of action.

Diuretics are chemicals which increase excretion of Na^+ and water and thereby increase urine output.

Site of Action of Diuretics

Drugs Acting in PCT

- Carbonic anhydrase inhibitors like acetazolamide, they inhibit carbonic anhydrase and thereby increases Na^+ excretion, decreases H^+ secretion and bicarbonate reabsorption. Since H^+ and K^+ compete with each other (For secretion) along with reabsorption of Na^+, there is increased K^+ secretion and excretion and therefore K^+ depletion occurs.
- Osmotic diuretics, such as mannitol and isosorbide. They are not reabsorbed in PCT and therefore are retained in the tubule along with water. This in turn alters the gradient for Na^+ reabsorption and therefore it inhibits Na^+ reabsorption.

Diuretics Acting on Loop of Henle

Loop diuretics, such as frusemide, bumetanide and ethacrynic acid: They act by inhibiting Na^+-K^+-$2Cl^-$ transporter. They increase NaCl and K^+ excretion. K^+ depletion occurs while treating with these drugs.

Diuretics Acting on DCT

Thiazides: They act by inhibiting NaCl symport in DCT. They increase excretion of NaCl and K^+.

Diuretics Acting on Late DCT and Collecting Duct

K^+ sparing diuretics, such as spironolactone, triamterene and amiloride act in late DCT and CD by inhibiting actions of aldosterone or epithelial sodium channels (ENacs). They increase excretion of Na^+ and retain K^+ and H^+.

23. Steps in synthesis of thyroid hormones.

Synthesis of Thyroid Hormone

- Synthesis takes place in the follicular cells and the hormone is stored in follicular lumen as colloid.
- Thyroid hormones are iodothyronines, formed by coupling of iodinated tyrosine molecules by ether linkages.

Following are the steps in synthesis of thyroid hormones:
1. Iodide trapping
2. Thyroglobulin synthesis
3. Oxidation of iodide
4. Organification
5. Coupling
6. Storage
7. Release

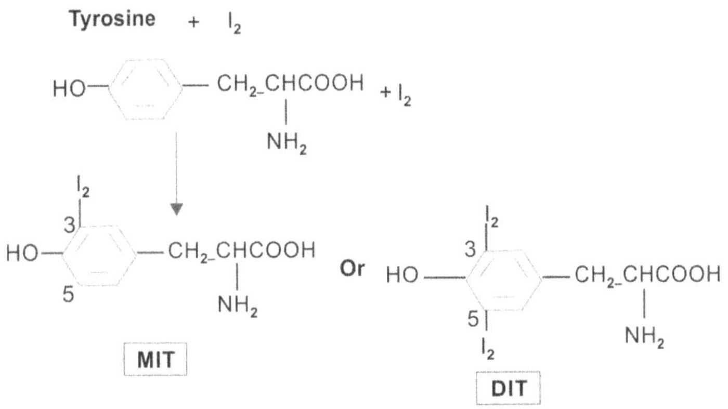

Fig. 14: Organification reaction—I_2 molecule is bound to tyrosine molecules. If it is bound in one position (3) then MIT (monoiodotyrosine is formed). If I_2 is bound in two positions (3 and 5) it is DIT (Diiodotyrosine).

Iodide Trapping

- Iodide is transported from the blood in thyroid capillaries to the follicular cell through sodium-iodide symporter (NIS).
- NIS transports I^- against electrochemical gradient.
- TSH stimulates I^- trapping and concentration in the gland.
- Iodide immediately moves towards the apical membrane of the follicular cell.

Thyroglobulin Synthesis

- As iodide is being trapped, thyroglobulin is also synthesized in the endoplasmic reticulum of follicular cells and transferred to colloid.
- TG is a glycoprotein. Has 131 tyrosine amino acids.

Oxidation of Iodide

- Iodide on reaching the colloid—apical membrane interface is oxidized to iodine.
- This reaction is catalyzed by thyroid peroxidase enzyme (TPO) present in the colloid-membrane interface.
- $2I^- + H_2O_2 \rightarrow I_{2+} 2HO^-$

Organification

- The tyrosine molecules of thyroglobulin get iodinated in the colloid to form iodotyrosines (*refer* **Fig. 14**).
- This is **organification** and is catalyzed by TPO.
- It forms either monoiodotyrosine (MIT) or diiodotyrosine (DIT) depending on the number of iodine attached to tyrosines.

Coupling Reaction

Two DIT molecules couple to form tetraiodotyrosine (T_4) or thyroxine.

Or

One molecule of MIT and DIT couple to form triiodothyronine (T_3)

Or

One molecule of DIT and MIT couple to form reverse T_3 (RT_3), an inactive component formed in the follicular cells.

This is coupling reaction and is catalyzed by TPO (*refer* **Fig. 15**).

Storage

- TG after iodination is stored in the colloid until release.
- In each molecule of thyroglobulin (TG): MIT-7, DIT-6, T_4-2, T_3-0.2 molecules are present.

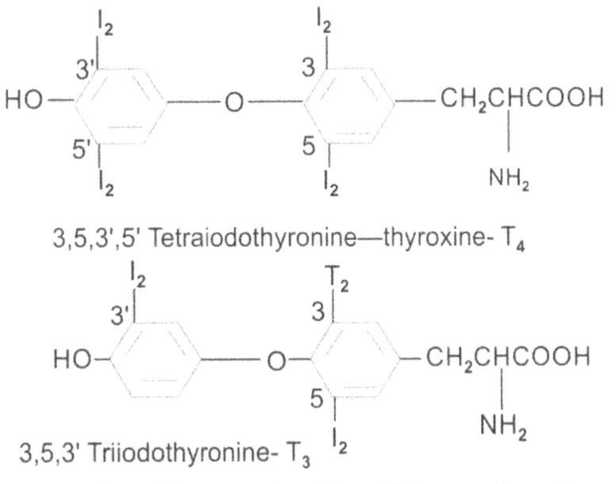

3,5,3',5' Tetraiodothyronine—thyroxine- T_4

3,5,3' Triiodothyronine- T_3

Fig. 15: Coupling reaction. Two MITs couple to form T_4 (thyroxine) and one MIT and one DIT binds T_3 (triiodothyronine) is formed.

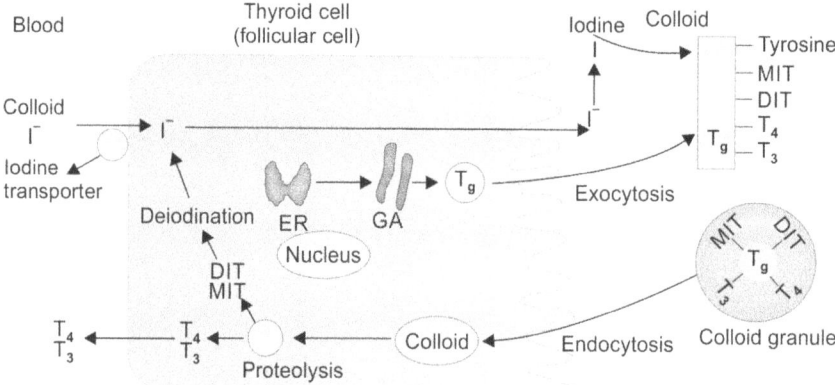

Fig. 16: Synthesis of thyroid hormone in follicular cell.
(DIT: diiodotyrosine; MIT: monoiodotyrosine; ER: endoplasmic reticulum; GA: Golgi apparatus, Tg: thyroglobulin; T4: thyroxine; T3: triiodothyronine)

- The gland is capable of storing secretions needed for 100 days.

Release of the hormone:
- On stimulation by TSH, colloid droplets (with TG and T3 and T4) are endocytosed through megalin into the cell.
- The droplet gets attached to a lysozome and forms a phagosome.
- Proteolytic enzymes of the phagosome break the peptide bonds between thyroid hormone (TH) and TG.
- This releases T3, T4, MIT and DIT.
- Released thyroid hormones enter into the capillaries by diffusion.
- MIT and DIT are deiodinated by the enzyme, **thyroid deiodinases**, which are selective for iodotyrosines and not for iodothyronines.
- Small amounts of TG are also released (*refer* **Fig. 16**).

24. Enterohepatic circulation.

- Bile acids and salts present in the bile on entering the intestine are absorbed from the terminal part of the ileum and reenter the portal vein to be secreted back into the bile from hepatocytes (*refer* **Fig. 17**).
- This process repeats many times—enterohepatic circulation.

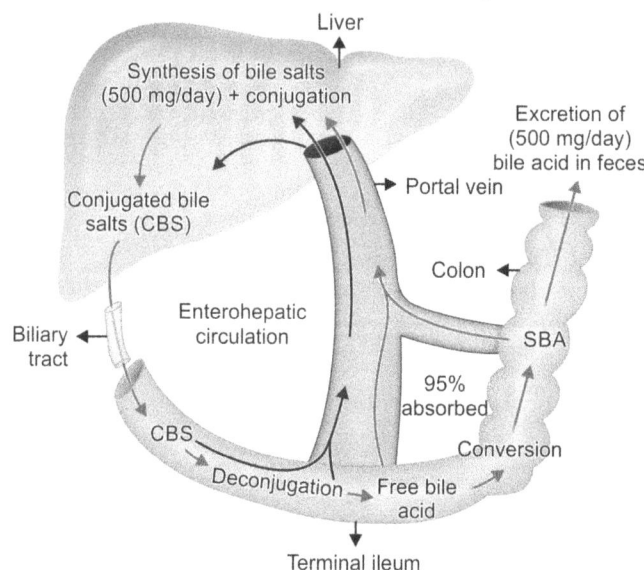

Fig. 17: Enterohepatic circulation. It is the circulation of bile salts following its synthesis from liver in bile and its secretion into duodenum and its reabsorption in terminal ileum and recirculation through portal veins.

- The conjugated bile salts are absorbed and recirculated in the above manner.
- Also, bile salts are unconjugated and some of it is also absorbed.
- Colonic bacteria act on free bile acids and are converted to secondary bile acids and a part of it is also absorbed back into the portal vein.
- About 95% of secreted bile salts are absorbed by the enterohepatic circulation and only 200–500 mg/day are excreted.

Significance of Enterohepatic Circulation
- Only the amount of bile salts which are excreted, are synthesized and replaced daily, to maintain the pool of bile salts in the body which are essential for digestion and absorption of fats.
- The total amount of bile salts is 2–4 g.
- This amount is circulated daily many times to digest and absorb fats in the diet taken.

---

25. Phagocytosis.

It is a process of engulfing and destruction of solid particles/microbes by cells.

Neutrophils and macrophages are the phagocytic cells.

It involves the following stages:
Margination, emigration, diapedesis, chemotaxis, opsonization, engulfing, degranulation and degradation stage.

Steps in Phagocytosis
1. **Margination:** At the site of infection, neutrophils get marginated towards the wall of the vessel and they get attached to the endometrium through proteins called selectins which are present on the endothelial cell membranes.
2. **Emigration and diapedesis:** The marginated neutrophils move out of the capillary wall through the junctions between endothelial cells. Walking out of the WBCs is called as Diapedesis.
3. **Chemotaxis:** It is the process of attraction of neutrophils to site of infection. The chemotactic substances are released by endothelial cells and damaged tissue. They are called chemokines. Leukotrienes and proteins in complementary pathway are some of the chemokines (*refer* **Fig. 18**).

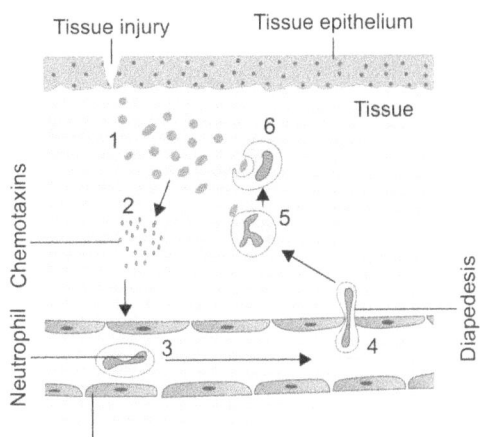

Fig. 18: Steps in phagocytosis; margination of WBCs, diapedesis, chemotaxis and engulfing of microbe: (1) Entry of microorganisms; (2) Chemotaxis; (3) Margination; (4) Diapedesis; (5) Fusion of microbe with lysosome; (6) Formation of phagolysosome.

4. **Opsonization:** It is the process of coating the infective agent with opsonins to make it tastier for neutrophils to engulf it. Some of the opsonins are IgG and complementary proteins.
5. **Engulfment stage:** Once the neutrophils come in contact with the microbe it puts out pseudopodia and engulfs it. The microbe now surrounded by a vesicle (phagosome) enters the neutrophil and is attached to lysososmes to form phagolysosome. The lysosome releases its proteolytic enzymes and destroys the microbe. The phagocytes also have oxidative enzymes in them which form lethal oxidative metabolites, such as—O_2, H_2O_2 and *hypochlorites*. Antimicrobials—*defensins* in phagocytes kill the micoorganisms.
6. **Degradation stage:** The destroyed microbe is now extruded as a residual body from the neutrophil.

---

26. Endoplasmic reticulum.

- Endoplasmic reticulum (ER) are flattened membrane-bound vesicles and tubules. They are continuous with the nuclear membrane (*refer* **Fig. 19**).
- There are two types of ER—Rough ER and Smooth ER.

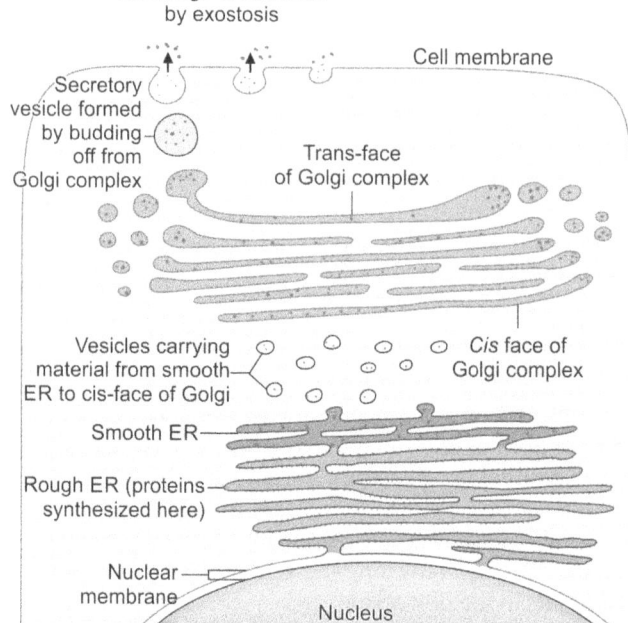

Fig. 19: Structure of endoplasmic reticulum.

Rough ER

- They are flattened membrane-bound tubes
- They appear continuous with nuclear membrane of Golgi complex and cell membrane.
- The membrane is studded with ribosomes.
- It is present in large amounts in cells synthesizing proteins. Their major synthesis is protein synthesis in the cells.

Smooth ER

- It has no ribosomes on the membrane.
- It is the site of lipid and steroid synthesis.
- It is found abundantly in Leydig and adrenal cortical cells.
- In liver it helps in detoxification.
- In skeletal and cardiac muscles it is the site of storage of Ca^{2+}.

27. Anticoagulants.

Anticoagulants are chemicals used to prevent clotting of blood. They are classified as in vitro and in vivo anticoagulants.

In Vitro Anticoagulants

These are chemicals used to prevent clotting of blood while transporting blood to laboratories or while storing blood in blood banks.

They are:

- **Ethylenediamine tetra-acetic acid (EDTA):** This is the anticoagulant of choice in laboratories. It makes Ca^{2+} unavailable for clotting by chelating it. It is used to determine ESR.
- **Trisodium citrate:** This anticoagulant is used for determining clotting disorders and also ESR. This prevents clotting by chelation of Ca^{2+}.
- **Double oxalate mixture:** It is a mixture of ammonium oxalate and potassium oxalate. It prevents clotting by forming insoluble calcium oxalate precipitate.
- **Heparin:** A naturally occurring anticoagulant is used as an in vitro and in vivo anticoagulant. It activates Antithrombin III and antithrombin III prevents clotting of blood.
- Sodium fluoride is an anticoagulant used in the labs for tests to analyze blood glucose levels.

In Vivo Anticoagulants

These are drugs taken to prevent clot formation within the blood vessels. They are:

- **Heparin:** It is isolated from the liver, lungs and granules of basophils and mast cells.

It facilitates action of antithrombin III and thereby inhibits the active forms of IX, X, XI and XII
- **Vitamin K antagonists:** They are—coumarin derivatives, such as warfarin, dicoumarol, etc.

They prevent the action of vitamin K by competitively binding with vitamin K receptors.

Vitamin K is a cofactor for the enzyme which catalyzes the conversion of glutamic acid residues to—γ carboxyglutamic acid residues. Six clotting factors require the conversion of glutamic acid to γ carboxyglutamic acid. They are factors—II, VII, IX and X, protein C and S.

28. Functions of estrogen.

- Estrogen stimulates proliferation of endometrium in 1st half of menstrual cycle.
- It feeds back to regulate LH secretion, positively in the 1st half and negatively in the 2nd half of menstrual cycle.
- It makes the cervical mucus thin and watery, thereby permitting entry of sperm into female reproductive tract.
- It increases size of ovaries and facilitates growth of follicle.
- Induces changes in fallopian tube and increases its motility. Increases the size of internal and external genitalia
- It increases the excitability of uterine myometrium and therefore peaks at the time of parturition.
- Responsible for female behavior and development of secondary sexual characteristics.
- Develops the ducts of mammary gland.
- Lowers plasma cholesterol and rises HDL levels.
- Causes fusion of epiphysis and stops the linear growth, both in males and females.
- Has properties of retaining salt and water and responsible for premenstrual bloating sensation.
- Prevents osteoporosis by inhibiting osteoclastic activity by inhibiting IL-1,6 and TNF-α and stimulating TGF-β.
- Inhibits the formation of acne.
- Makes the skin soft and vascular

29. Importance of Rh typing.

- Rh system is the second most important blood group systems in the body. It was discovered in the rhesus monkey in 1940.
- There are 6 antigens in this system, C, D, E and c, d and e.
- D antigen is highly antigenic and therefore individuals with D antigen on their RBC membrane are Rh positive and persons without D antigen are Rh negative.
- Rh antigen is inherited as a dominant gene.
- Therefore, Rh positive may be homozygous with DD or heterozygous with Dd. Rh negative is homozygous with dd.
- The antibody in Rh system is anti-D antibody.
- There are no naturally occurring antibodies here as in the ABO system.
- But if an Rh negative person receives Rh positive blood his immune system recognizes the Rh antigen as foreign and starts producing antibodies.
- So in first encounter of Rh positive blood there is not much complication. On the next exposure, massive antigen antibody reactions happen resulting in agglutination and hemolysis.
- Therefore, the Rh system does not follow the 2nd law of Landsteiner's which states that "If a particular antigen is absent on the RBC membrane the corresponding antibody will be present in the plasma".
- The **most significant aspect** of Rh incompatibility is the mismatch of Rh factor between the mother and the fetus.
- If the mother is Rh negative and she conceives an Rh positive fetus, at the time of delivery of the fetus, during the placental separation, a small amount of Rh positive blood leaks into mother's circulation.
- As the first baby is already born, it is not affected.
- The mother's immune system starts producing anti-D antibodies.
- If she conceives the next time and that fetus is also Rh positive, the antibodies in the maternal circulation which belongs to IgG type crosses the placenta and attacks the fetal RBCs.

- There is agglutination and hemolysis of fetal RBCs.
- In the subsequent similar pregnancies, the damage to the fetus is severe.
- The child presents with the symptoms of hemolytic disease of the newborn or erythroblastosis fetalis.

The symptoms are:
- **Anemia:** Due to hemolysis the child has anemia.
- **Edema:** The child has generalized edema— hydrops fetalis.
- **Jaundice:** Hemolysis releases bilirubin and results in jaundice.
- **Kernicterus:** The high bilirubin levels in the neonates damages the basal ganglia. In adults the blood-brain barrier prevents the entry of bilirubin into the brain. But in infants blood-brain barrier is not fully developed, so, the bilirubin easily damages the basal ganglia resulting in motor deficits.
- **Erythroblasts appear in the circulation:** Excessive hemolysis induces erythropoiesis and erythroblasts (the precursors) start appearing in the circulation.

Treatment:
- If the hemolysis is mild, no treatment is needed.
- In severe conditions treatment can be given as intrauterine transfusions or after birth, exchange transfusion can be given along with phototherapy.

Prevention:
- After the delivery of the Rh positive fetus by the Rh negative mother, the mother is immunized with anti-D antibodies.
- These antibodies neutralize the antigens which have entered the mother's circulation and prevent formation of further antibodies.

30. Fat absorption.

Absorption of Fats
- It starts in the duodenum and is completely absorbed by the time the fats reach jejunum.
- Absorption of fats is favored by formation of micelles by the bile salts and lecithin.
- The lumen of intestine contains water and therefore movement of digested fats is favored only by micelle formation.
- On reaching enterocytes, fats move out of micelles and enter enterocytes by passive diffusion.
- The rate-limiting step in absorption of fats is formation and movement of micelles from the chyme in the lumen to the brush border.
- The bile salts forming the micelles, are absorbed in the terminal ileum.
- Fate of fats, entering the enterocytes is dependent on their size.
- Fats containing 10-12 carbon atoms, easily pass through the basal side of the enterocytes and enter the portal blood vessels as free fatty acids and are transported.
- Fatty acids with more than 12 carbon atoms are esterified to triglycerides and the absorbed cholesterol is also esterified and they are coated with protein (β lipoprotein), cholesterol and phospholipids to form **chylomicrons.**
- The chylomicrons now exocytosis through the basal side of the enterocytes to enter the lymphatics in the villus, the lacteal.
- They are transported in the lymphatics and are drained into the thoracic duct and finally they enter the blood circulation.
- Absorption of large chain fatty acids are more in the upper parts of the intestine and some amount of absorption happens in terminal parts also.
- In moderate fat intake, nearly 95% of ingested fats are absorbed.

Steatorrhea
- Steatorrhea is malabsorption of fats resulting in excretion of fat in stools.
- The indigested fats appear in stools and the stools are fatty, bulky and claycolored. This is said to be steatorrhea.
- The fecal fat content is more than 40-50 g/day.

- It happens due to either destruction of exocrine pancreas, lipase deficiency or absence of bicarbonate in pancreatic juice which results in acidic environment in the intestine precipitating the bile salts.
- Acids also inhibit pancreatic lipase and therefore patients with gastrin-secreting tumor have steatorrhea.
- It is also seen in conditions with defective absorption of bile salts in terminal ileum.

31. Taste receptors.

- Taste receptors are located in the taste buds.
- There are nearly 10,000 taste buds in a young adult and declines with age.
- Taste buds are present on the tongue and also in soft palate, pharynx and epiglottis.
- Taste buds are present on the papillae of the tongue.
- **Papillae** are elevations on the tongue.

There are four types of papilla:
1. Vallate papilla—has 100-300 taste buds.
2. Fungiform papilla—has 5 taste buds.
3. Foliate papilla—do not have taste buds
4. Filiform papilla—contains tactile receptors and no taste buds.

There are three types of cells in taste buds:
- Type 1 and 2—supporting cells.
- Type 3 cells—receptor epithelial cells and has microvilli projecting (*refer* **Fig. 20**).
- They are replaced constantly in 10 days.
- Taste receptors are elongate, bipolar shaped and extend from the opening of taste bud to its base.
- Through the pore the cilia or hairs project into the oral cavity and come in contact with saliva.
- Tastants when dissolved in saliva stimulate the plasma membrane of the taste hairs.
- Taste hairs are the site of transduction.
- The receptor potential stimulates release of neurotransmitter to trigger nerve impulse in first order neuron.
- Each bud is innervated by 50 nerves at bases of receptor cells.

32. Functions of utricle and saccule.

- The vestibular apparatus in the inner ear consists of—3 semicircular canals and 2 sac like structures—utricle and saccule.
- The receptors for vestibular sensation are the hair cells and they are located in the cristae in the ampulla of semicircular

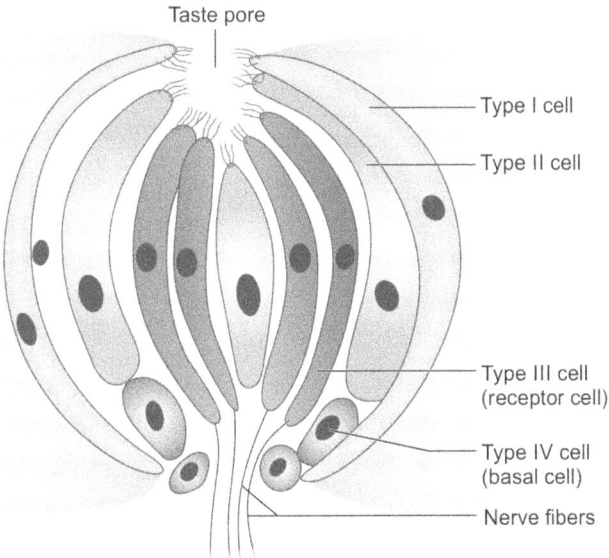

Fig. 20: Taste bud.

canals and the macula or otolithic organ of the utricle and saccule.
- The receptors in the canals and the utricle and saccule are the **hair cells** located in unique structures.
- The hairs of the hair cells are embedded in thick gelatinous substance called the **cupula**.

Receptors in Utricle and Saccule

- The receptor organ in utricle and saccule is called the **macula**.
- Macula in utricle is in horizontal plane and in saccule in vertical plane.
- The macula is an elevation in the sacs.
- It is made of epithelial cells with hair cells interspersed.
- The hair is embedded in the **cupula**.
- Cupula, here is embedded with calcium carbonate crystals—**otoliths**.
- The receptors in utricle and saccule give information about linear acceleration and change in head position in relation to gravity. Saccule responds to vertical acceleration and utricle to horizontal acceleration.
- Saccule detects lateral tilting of head and utricle detects up and down movement of head and they help in maintaining equilibrium during such movements.

33. Sleep-wake theory.

Sleep is a state of temporary unconsciousness from which the individual can be aroused by a sensory stimulus.

Wakefulness

- Wakefulness is a function of reticular activating system (RAS) in the brainstem.
- RAS is a multisynaptic pathway projecting from brainstem to all areas of cerebral cortex. Therefore when stimulated, induces arousal and alertness.
- RAS receives inputs from ascending sensory pathways and RAS inturn sends impulses to cerebral cortex and increases responsiveness to the sensory stimuli.
- When the firing rate of RAS is decreased it results in sleep. When there is damage to RAS it results in coma.

Sleep

There are two types of sleep—nonrapid eye movement sleep or NREM sleep or slow wave sleep and rapid eye movement sleep (REM) or paradoxical sleep.

Control of Sleep-wakefulness

- Sleep-wakefulness is regulated by circadian rhythm. The cycle happens in relation to the day-night variations. It is regulated through the retinohypothalamic pathway and suprachiasmatic nucleus in hypothalamus.
- Pineal gland also plays a role in sleep wakefulness. It secretes the hormone melatonin. Melatonin secretion varies with day-night cycle. It is secreted more in the evening and early part of night. Melatonin acts on neurons of RAS to mediate sleep-wake cycle.
- There are sleep inducing areas in the brain like posterior hypothalamus and intralaminar and anterior thalamic nuclei—diencephalic sleep zone, medullary synchronizing zone—medullary reticular formation and the basal forebrain sleep zone—preoptic area and diagonal band of Broca. These areas when stimulated at low frequency induce slow wave sleep.
- Neurons in pons and midbrain induce REM sleep.
- There are neurotransmitters in the brain which are responsible for sleep and wakefulness.
- **Neurotransmitters for wakefulness:** Serotonin, acetylcholine, histamine, catecholamines and adenosine antagonists like caffeine induce wakefulness.
- **Neurotransmitters inducing sleep:** Adenosine, serotonin antagonists, prostaglandin D_2 and sleep peptides in brain.

Theories of Sleep

There are many theories put forward to explain the transition from wakefulness to sleep. They are:
- **Pavlov's theory** says sleep is a symptom conditioned inhibition of brain activity.

- **Cerebral ischemia:** Sleep may be due to cerebral ischemia. It can be explained by drowsiness following food intake as there is decreased cerebral blood flow after food intake.
- **Biochemical theories:** It is based on action of various chemicals in the brain.
  - Lactic acid accumulation in brain during fatigue can induce sleep
  - Hypnotoxin released from brain of a sleeping animal can induce sleep in another animal
  - Delta sleep inducing peptide released in the brain may induce sleep.

34. Mechanism of accommodation.

- When the eye is focusing on a close object the curvature of the lens increases to get a clear image on retina—accommodation of lens.
- This occurs due to contraction of ciliary muscles
- Results in increase of curvature of lens—adds 12 diopters to the power of the lens, power of lens increases (>70 D)
- Near point—10 cm in young adult.
- Presbyopia—near point increases (83 cm).

Other changes of accommodation are:
- Constriction of pupil
- Convergence of eyeballs

Accommodation Reflex Pathway

Impulses from retina for near vision
↓
Optic nerve
↓
Optic chiasma
↓
Optic tract
↓
Lateral geniculate body
↓
Visual cortex (Area 17)
↓
Frontal eye field
↓
Edinger-Westphal nuclei of both sides (parasympathetic fibers)
↓
Efferents go through the oculomotor nerves → medial rectus → convergence of eyeball
↓
Ciliary ganglion
↓
Supplies the sphincter pupillae and the ciliary muscles
↓
Constriction of pupil and anterior curvature of lens increases
↓
Accommodation of eye

35. PR interval.

PR interval: It is between beginning of P wave to beginning of Q wave.
- The normal duration is 0.12–0.2 sec (average 0.18 sec).
- This denotes atrial depolarization and conduction to AV node.

Prolonged PR interval signifies AV conduction block

36. Trichromatic theory of color vision.

- Trichromatic theory of color vision was put forward by Young and Helmholtz.
- According to this theory, it postulates that there are 3 types of cones with 3 types of photopigments and each one is maximally sensitive to one primary color (Red, green and blue).
- The sensation of a color perceived is based on the frequency of impulses from each cone.

Cone Pigments

- Red sensitive pigment or erythrolabe or long wavelength pigment. It absorbs light maximally in the yellow portion with a peak at 565 nm. The cones with these pigments are L cones.
- Green sensitive pigment or chlorolabe or medium wavelength pigment, and is maximally sensitive in green portion and peaks at 535 nm. The cones with these pigments are M cones.
- Blue sensitive pigment or cyanolabe or short wavelength pigment. It absorbs light maximally in the blue-violet portion

and peaks at 440 nm. The cones with this pigment are S cones.
- Blue, green and red are the primary colors, but cones with maximal sensitivity in yellow portion of the spectrum are sensitive in red portion and responds to red light at a lower threshold than green.
- Based on Young-Helmholtz theory, for perceiving a color at least two cone types are needed.
- The visual cortex compares the relative frequency of action potentials in the activated cone pathways and finds the wavelength and thereby identifies the color.
- Change in intensity is appreciated by change in wavelength
- Gene for rhodopsin is on chromosome 3 and gene for S cone pigment is on chromosome 7 and for green and red pigment it is on X chromosome

37. Mean arterial pressure.

- Mean arterial pressure (MAP) is the average pressure in blood vessels throughout the cardiac cycle.
- Duration of systole is less than diastolic phase and therefore MAP is not the average of systolic and diastolic pressures.
- It is calculated as MAP = Diastolic pressure + 1/3 Pulse pressure = 80 + 1/3 × 40 = 93 mm Hg
- Normal MAP is 75 tp 100 Hg

Significance of MAP: It is the pressure head which is responsible for the tissue perfusion.

38. Reward and punishment centers.

- When we do an act if we are appreciated/rewarded we tend to repeat the act—motivation.
- At the same time when an act has lead to punishment, we tend to avoid the act.
- There are reward and punishment centers in brain which decides our actions.
- There are areas in the brain when electrically stimulated induces a pleasurable feeling and is said to be the **reward center**.
- Certain areas when stimulated induce fear or terror—**punishment center.**

Reward Areas

- It consists of the dopaminergic pathway from the ventral tegmentum to nucleus accumbens.
- Nucleus accumbens is the major reward center and dopamine is the major neurotransmitter.
- This area is also responsible for addiction behaviors.
- The other area is the medial band of tissue extending from frontal cortex through the hypothalamus to the midbrain tegmentum (*refer* **Fig. 21**).

Punishment/Avoidance Area

It includes the lateral portion of posterior hypothalamus, dorsal midbrain and entorhinal cortex.

39. Changes in cardiac output during exercise.

- Cardiac output (CO) increases to supply the extra demand faced by the body.
- It decides the O_2 delivery to the tissues and rise in cardiac output is the rate limiting step for O_2 extraction.
- CO increases from 5 L/min at rest to 25 L/min during exercise.
- CO increase is due to both, increase in HR and stroke volume.
- Increase in stroke volume is due to— increase in myocardial contractility following sympathetic stimulation and increase in EDV due to activation of

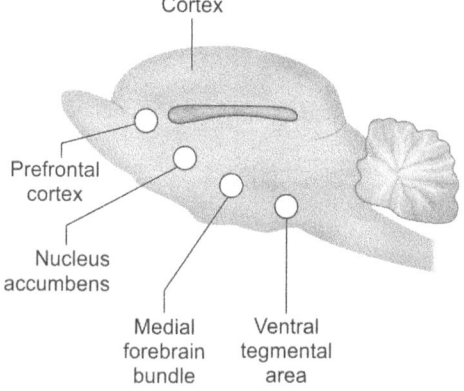

Fig. 21: Reward centers in brain. It extends from Ventral tegmentum to nucleus accumbens.

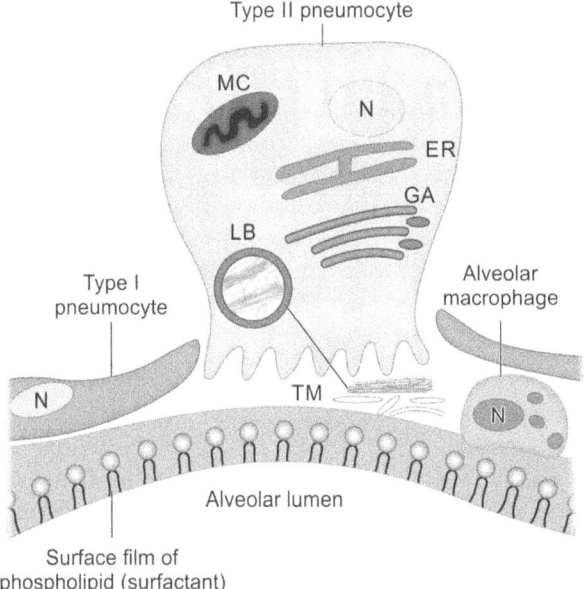

Fig. 22: Arrangement of surfactant molecules in alveolar lumen.
(N: nucleus; MC: mitochondria; ER: endoplasmic reticulum; GA: Golgi apparatus; LB: lamellar body; TM: tubular myelins)

skeletal muscle pump, thoracic pump and abdominal pump.

40. Surfactant.

- It is a protein-lipid complex secreted by the Type II alveolar epithelial cells lining the alveoli (refer **Fig. 22**).
- Surfactant is a mixture of dipalmitoyl-phosphatidylcholine (DPPC), other lipids and proteins—SPA, SPB, SPC and SPD.
- It acts as a detergent to reduce the surface tension of the fluid lining the alveoli and prevent its collapse during expiration.
- The phospholipids have hydrophobic tails and a hydrophilic head. They arrange themselves with the tails facing the alveolar lumen and intersperse between water molecules.
- So during inspiration as the alveoli enlarge the surfactant molecules move apart and surface tension of water increases and during expiration they come closer and the surface tension is lowered.
- Surfactant is important at birth. After birth, the infant tries to breathe and makes inspiratory movements and the lungs expand after which the lung tends to recoil and the presence of surfactant prevents the collapse of the alveoli.
- Surfactant deficiency results in alveolar collapse, which results in infant respiratory distress syndrome (IRDS)
- Maturation of surfactant in the lungs is enhanced by glucocorticoids. During term the fetal and maternal cortisol increases and favors maturation of surfactant.

Other Functions of Surfactant

- Stabilizes the lung alveoli
- It also decreases the effect of surface tension, which if not countered will increase the pulmonary capillary hydrostatic pressure and thereby fluid accumulation in the alveolus. So surfactant prevents pulmonary edema.
- As it prevents alveolar collapse, it decreases the work of breathing
- They help in immunity

Regulation of Secretion of Surfactant

It is regulated by hormones—glucocorticoids, insulin and thyroxine promote secretion of surfactant.

Factors which Affect Surfactant Secretion

- High O_2 content affects surfactant secretion as in O_2 therapy in patients undergoing cardiac surgery using pump oxygenator.
- Occlusion of pulmonary bronchus or pulmonary artery.

Answers to 2017 Question Paper

ANSWER ALL QUESTIONS

I. Essay (15 Marks each)

1. Define immunity. How will you classify immunity? Explain in detail cell-mediated immunity.
2. Define blood pressure. Describe in detail short-term regulation of blood pressure. Add a note on hypertension.
3. Enumerate the hormones secreted by anterior pituitary gland. Discuss the actions and regulation of growth hormone.
4. Define hypoxia. Explain in detail the different types of hypoxia. Add a note on hyperbaric oxygen therapy.

II. Short Notes (5 Marks each)

1. Primary active transport.
2. Excitation-contraction coupling.
3. Stages of deglutition.
4. Micturition reflex.
5. Hyperthyroidism.
6. Compliance.
7. Hypoxic hypoxia.
8. Pacemaker potential.
9. Stages of sleep.
10. Functions of cerebellum.
11. Role of helper T cells.
12. Action potential.
13. Juxtaglomerular apparatus.
14. Achalasia cardia.
15. Fetoplacental unit.
16. Conduction system of heart.
17. Special features of coronary circulation.
18. Vital capacity.
19. Functions of hypothalamus.
20. Properties of synapse.

III. Short Answers (2 Marks each)

1. Positive feedback mechanism.
2. Rigor mortis.
3. Polycythemia.
4. Bombay blood group.
5. Tubuloglomerular feedback.
6. Functions of large intestine.
7. Migrating motor complex.
8. Diabetes insipidus.
9. Features of Cushing syndrome.
10. Male contraception.
11. Triple response.
12. Bainbridge reflex.
13. Residual volume.
14. Artificial respiration.
15. Functions of middle ear.
16. Features of Parkinsonism.
17. Papez circuit.
18. Name to facilitatory and inhibitory neurotransmitters and their sites of action.
19. Saltatory conduction.
20. Sensations carried by posterior column.
21. Reticulocyte response.
22. Clot retraction.
23. Sodium-potassium pump.
24. Name the muscle proteins. What is the role of troponin C in muscle contraction?
25. Role of *H. Pylori* in peptic ulcer.
26. Gastrocolic reflex.
27. Physiological basis of treatment of diarrhea.
28. Anion gap.
29. Radioimmunoassay.
30. List four differences between dwarfism and cretinism.

31. Reynold's number.
32. Jugular venous pulse.
33. Lead II ECG.
34. Bohr's effect.
35. Dead space.
36. Functions of somatosensory area.
37. Stretch reflex.
38. REM sleep.
39. Features of dark adaptation.
40. Stapedial reflex.

I. ESSAY

1. Define immunity. How will you classify immunity? Explain in detail cell-mediated immunity.

Immunity is the response the body develops when challenged by an antigen.

Two types of immunity are present:
1. Innate or nonspecific immunity
2. Acquired or specific immunity

Classification of Immunity

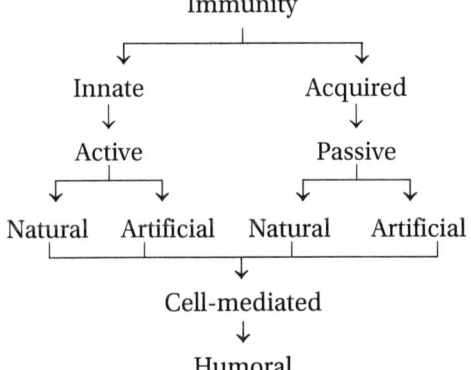

Cell-mediated Immunity

- It is mediated by T lymphocytes.
- T lymphocytes are formed in the bone marrow and they are processed in the thymus.

Stages of Cell-mediated Immunity

1. **Antigen presentation:** Cells like macrophages, mast cells and dendritic cells act as antigen-presenting cells (APCs). Macrophages phagocytose the antigens entering the body and breaks it down to peptide fragments. The antigenic fragment forms a complex with the MHC II protein formed by the macrophages. The antigen and MHC II complex are expressed on the membrane of macrophage.

2. **Antigen recognition by lymphocytes:** The APC with the antigen-MHC II complex is recognized by the T lymphocytes with the receptors for the antigen. T cells become activated if it binds to the antigen and is costimulated with cytokines like IL-2. Once 2 stimulations have happened, the lymphocyte is activated. The activated T cells enlarge and begin to proliferate and differentiate to form a clone of similar T cells. This happens in the secondary lymphoid organs like the lymph nodes.

3. **Types of T cells:** There are 3 main types of T cells—helper T cells (CD4 cells), cytotoxic T cells (CD8 cells) and memory T cells.

- *Helper T cells:* Helper T cells or CD4 cells recognize the antigen presented along with MHC II and cytotoxic or CD8 cells recognize the antigens presented with MHC I.

  After costimulation of helper T cells, they secrete many cytokines. The most important cytokine is IL-2 which is needed for all the immune responses and is the major stimulator for T cell proliferation. IL-2 is also the costimulator for resting helper T cells and cytotoxic T cells. It also enhances activation and proliferation of B cells and natural killer cells.

- *Cytotoxic T cells:* The T cells that express CD8 develop into cytotoxic T cells. They recognize foreign antigens expressed along with MHC I on the membranes of body cells infected by viruses, tumor cells and cells of tissue transplant. But to get activated into a killer cell it needs costimulation by IL-2 produced by helper cells. Therefore, for maximal activation of cytotoxic T cells it needs antigen presentation with MHC I and II (*refer* **Fig. 1**).

- *Memory T cells:* The T cells for a specific antigen which remain in the lymph organ after the immune response is

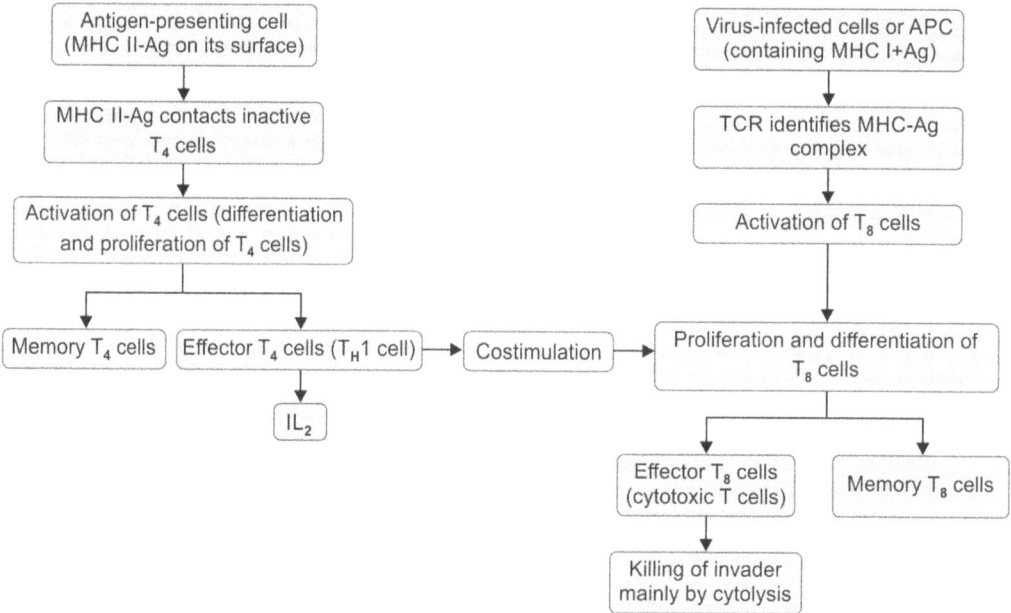

Fig. 1: Mechanism of cell-mediated immunity.

over are termed as memory T cells. If the same pathogen is encountered for the second time, these cells get activated and they initiate a swift and fast immune response. The second response is faster and vigorous and the pathogen is eliminated even before any symptom develops.

- *Elimination of the pathogens:* The killing of the pathogen is done by the cytotoxic T cells.
    - The activated CD8 cells synthesize and secrete proteins called "**Perforins**" which are inserted into the membrane of the pathogen. The perforins are water channels which allow influx of water and thereby swelling of the microbe and cause its lysis.
    - Release of lymphotoxins by activated T cells. These cytokines destroy the microbes.
    - Cytotoxic T cells secrete interferons which will favor the phagocytic activity of the neutrophils and macrophages by promoting opsonization.

Role of Cell-mediated Immunity

- It is activated against intracellular pathogens like viral infections and bacterial infections like mycobacterium tuberculosis.
- It removes the tumor cells.
- It is responsible for rejection of transplanted tissues.
- It is responsible for hypersensitivity reactions.

2. Define blood pressure. Describe in detail short-term regulation of blood pressure. Add a note on hypertension.

BP is defined as the lateral pressure exerted by the moving column of blood on the vessel wall. Normal value = 120/80 mm Hg.

Components of BP

- Systolic BP
- Diastolic BP
- Pulse pressure
- Mean arterial pressure

Neural Regulation of BP

- Regulation by autonomic nerves
- Regulation by medullary control centers

- Regulation by reflexes:
  - Baroreceptor reflex
  - Chemoreceptor reflex
  - CNS ischemic response

Regulation by Autonomic Nerves
- Blood vessels are supplied by sympathetic nerves.
- They are of two types—sympathetic vasoconstrictor and vasodilator fibers.
- Sympathetic VC fibers—in all blood vessels
- Sympathetic VD or cholinergic fibers—blood vessels of skeletal muscles, sweat glands and they originate from frontal cortex to hypothalamus, midbrain medulla and end in the IML of SC.
- **Sympathetic stimulation results in:** Vaso- and venoconstriction, ↑in HR and Contractility and therefore the BP is increased.

Regulation by Medullary Control Centers
- There are two areas in the medulla which control the CVS.
- They are—vasomotor center (VMC) and cardiac vagal center (CVC).
- CVC—nucleus tractus solitarius, nucleus ambiguus
- Vagal center—dorsal motor nucleus of vagus.
- Stimulation of VMC—↑HR, contractility, ↑vaso- and venoconstriction—↑BP and on inhibition vice versa.
- The final pathway from VMC is through sympathetic nerves to heart (*refer* **Fig. 2**).
- Stimulation of CVC—↓HR, decreased vasoconstriction—↓BP.
- Final pathway is through vagus nerve to heart.
- There are inputs to VMC, from limbic centers through hypothalamus which

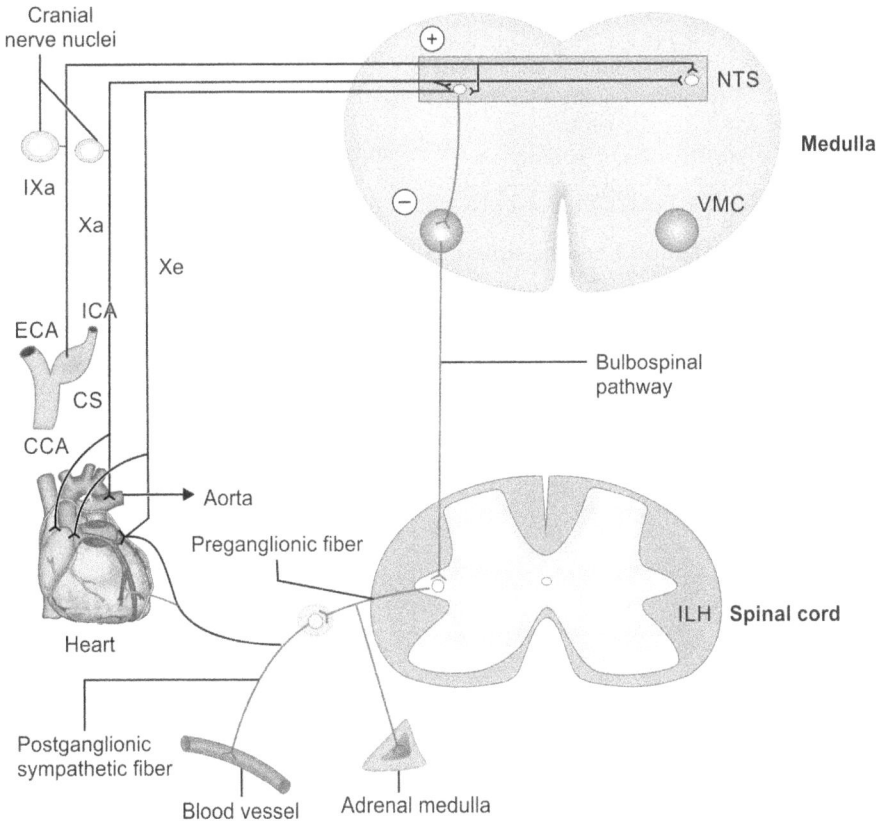

Fig. 2: Medullary cardiovascular centers and baroreceptor reflex pathway.
(CS: carotid sinus; CCA: common carotid artery; ECA: external carotid artery; Xa: afferents of vagus nerve; Xe: efferents of vagus nerve; IXa: afferents of glossopharyngeal nerve; VMC: vasomotor center; NTS: nucleus tractus solitarius; ILH: intermediolateral horn of spinal cord)

are responsible for BP modulation in emotional states like anxiety (Increase in BP and heart rate).

Reflex Regulation of BP

☐ **Baroreceptor reflex:**

Baroreceptors:
- There are two types of baroreceptors (BRs). High pressure and low-pressure baroreceptors.
- High pressure BRs are present in the carotid and aortic sinuses (*refer* **Fig. 3**).
- Low pressure BRs are present in the great veins, right and left atria.
- High pressure BRs are there to monitor and correct the day to day change in BP as in change of posture from supine to standing position.
- They regulate BP maximally when the MAP is between 70 and 110 mm Hg and stops firing when MAP falls < 40 or rises above 150 mm Hg.

The reflex:
- Most important reflex to regulate BP
- Also called as sinoaortic reflex
- Receptor—carotid and aortic sinuses
- Stimulus—stretch of baroreceptors (as in increased BP)
- Afferents—IXth (Supplies carotid sinus) and Xth cranial nerves (Aortic sinus)
- Efferents—sympathetic nerves and vagus nerve
- Effector—heart and blood vessels
- Response—decrease in BP (*refer* **Fig. 4**)

☐ **Chemoreceptor reflex:**
- Chemoreceptors are located in the carotid and aortic bodies.
- They sense the change in PO_2, pH and PCO_2 in arterial blood and stimulate respiration.
- They are supplied by IX and X cranial nerves.
- They usually project to respiratory centers and also to cardiovascular centers in medulla.
- They also send inputs to VMC and CVC and regulate BP
- They are active within a range of 40–100 mm Hg MAP.

Decrease in BP MAP 40–100 mm Hg
↓
Decreased blood flow to chemoreceptors
↓
Stimulation of chemoreceptors
↓
Impulses carried through IXth and Xth cranial nerves to medulla
↓
Respiratory center VMC, cardiac vagal center (CVC)
↓
Release of catecholamines from adrenal medulla
↓
Hyperventilation, tachycardia, vasoconstriction and bradycardia
↓
Release of catecholamines

- **The net effect is mild tachycardia and vasoconstriction → increase in BP**

☐ **CNS ischemic response:** It is activated when MAP falls below 40 mm Hg. It is said to be the "last ditch stand", the last effort put up by the body to try to correct the fall in BP.

Severe hypotension
↓
Decreased cerebral blood flow
↓
Hypoxia and hypercapnia at VMC
↓
Strong stimulation of VMC
↓
Intense vasoconstriction
↓
↑ **BP**

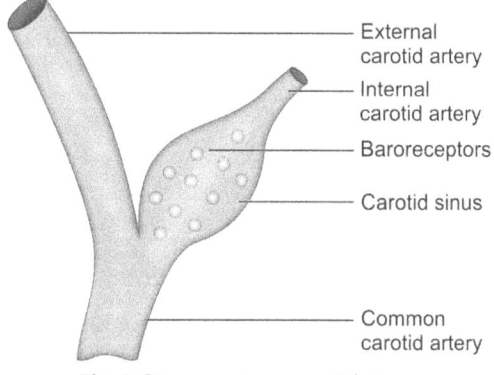

Fig. 3: Baroreceptor—carotid sinus.

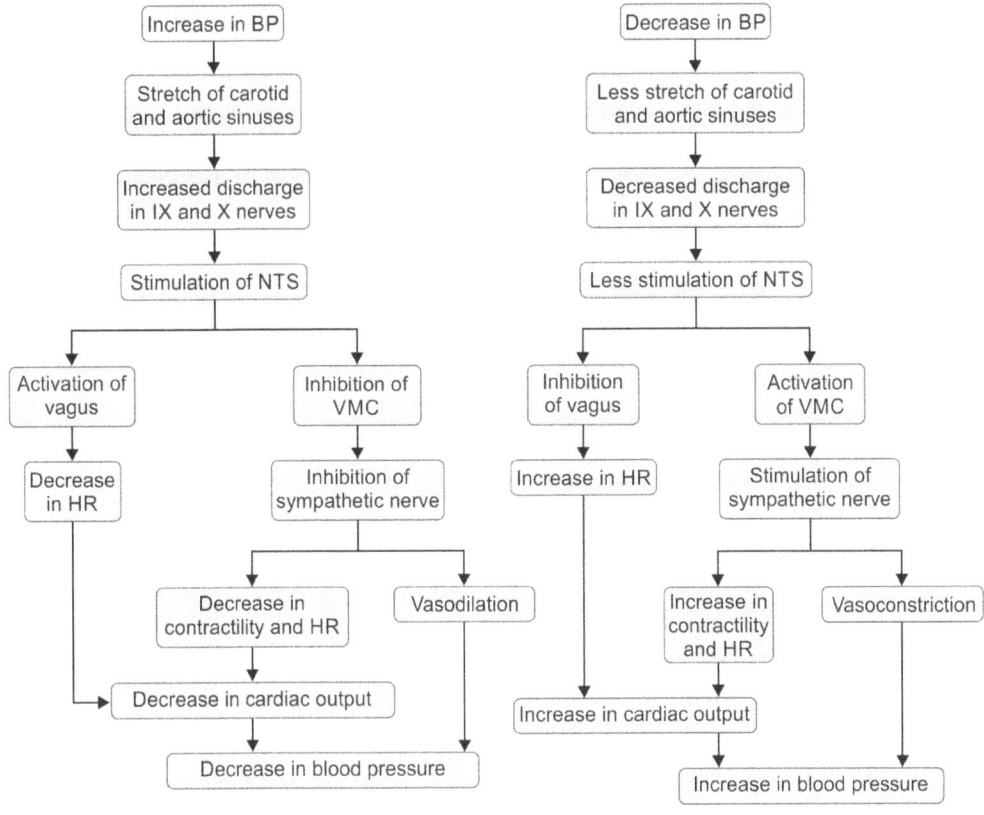

Fig. 4: Regulation of BP by baroreceptors.

Hypertension

- It is defined as the sustained elevation of systemic arterial pressure.
- Blood pressure is determined by cardiac output and peripheral resistance.
- Systolic BP is determined by cardiac output and therefore affected by stroke volume and heart rate. These determinants are subjected to daily activities. Therefore, elevation in systolic BP is not usually considered as hypertension.
- Diastolic BP is determined by peripheral resistance. PR is in turn decided by caliber of blood vessel and viscosity of blood. Sustained elevation of diastolic BP results in hypertension. It is usually associated with elevation of systolic BP also.
- 120/80 mm Hg is normal BP
- 120-139/80-89 mm Hg—prehypertension
- Above 140/90 mm Hg—hypertension

Types of Hypertension (HT)

- Primary or essential hypertension
- Secondary hypertension

Primary or Essential Hypertension

- In over 90% of the individuals with hypertension, the cause is unknown. This is said to be primary HT. It could be due to sympathetic hyperactivity, increased sodium intake, increase in blood volume, etc.
- It can be in the benign form or it can progress to malignant HT.

Benign Form

- There could be moderate or great increase in BP up to 210/110 mm Hg. But there is also fluctuation of systolic BP—So, it is called as labile HT.
- In late stages, systolic BP is increased and fixed and does not come back to normal.
- Antihypertensives are prescribed.
- It causes cardiac hypertrophy, arteriosclerosis of the vessels and increased incidence of myocardial infarction. There are renal changes like albuminuria, hematuria, etc.

Malignant Hypertension

- BP is very much increased even up to 260/150 mm Hg.

- There are arteriolar lesions.
- Patients show symptoms of papilledema, cerebral symptoms and renal failure.
- If patient is not treated, usually death occurs within 6 months to 2 years.

Secondary Hypertension

Blood pressure is increased due to some other underlying disease.
- It can be due to—**renal diseases**, such as glomerulonephritis, pyelonephritis, renal tumors, polycystic kidney disease, etc.
- Goldblatt hypertension—due to renal artery stenosis. They are of two types:
  1. One kidney one-clip Goldblatt hypertension—one kidney is removed and the renal artery of the other kidney is stenosed. Here rise in BP is independent of renin levels.
  2. Two-kidney one-clip Goldblatt hypertension—two kidneys are present and constriction of the renal artery of one kidney. The rise in BP is dependent on increased renin levels.
- **Cardiovascular diseases**, such as atherosclerosis
- **Endocrinal diseases:**
  - Pheochromocytoma
  - Cushing's syndrome
  - Primary hyperaldosteronism or Conn's syndrome
  - Acromegaly
  - Glucocorticoid remediable hyperaldosteronism
  - Myxedema
- **Neurogenic hypertension:** These are done experimentally to demonstrate the role of baroreceptors in regulating blood pressure.
  - Bilateral clamping of the carotid arteries proximal to carotid sinuses results in increase in BP.
  - Similar changes are seen when the carotid sinus nerves (IXth cranial nerve) on each side are cut.
  - The rise is not too high as the aortic sinuses are still functioning.
  - If the vagus nerve from the aortic sinus is also cut it results in rapid rise in BP even up to 300/200 mm Hg.
  - Similar results are seen when the NTS in medulla is bilaterally damaged. This can even be fatal.
  - These forms of hypertension are said to be neurogenic hypertension.
- **Hypertension in pregnancy:** Due to pressor peptides secreted from placenta hypertension is present with pre-eclampsia or eclampsia.
- **Congenital diseases**, such as Liddle's syndrome where there is excessive retention of salt and water.
- **Coarctation of aorta:** Congenital narrowing of the aorta especially the thoracic aorta results in severe hypertension in upper half of the body.
- **Chronic treatment with oral contraceptive pills:**
  - OC pills contain estrogen and progesterone.
  - Estrogen increases production of angiotensinogen resulting in elevated angiotensin II levels.
  - Normally this would decrease renin secretion and that brings Ang II levels to normal.
  - But in consumption of OC pills this feedback is incomplete resulting in hypertension—**pill hypertension**.

Effects of Hypertension

On the Heart
- The consistent increase in peripheral resistance leads to increase in afterload which increases the work of the myocardium resulting in left ventricular hypertrophy.
- Myocardial oxygen requirement increases due to increased ventricular muscle mass.
- So even minimal narrowing of coronary vessels results in ischemia.
- Gradually the ability to compensate for the high peripheral resistance is exceeded and the heart fails.

On the Blood Vessels
- There is increased incidence of atherosclerosis
- High BP also leads to stiffness of vessels and their compliance is lost.

- They are prone for cerebral thrombosis and cerebral hemorrhage.

Kidneys
- Atherosclerosis of renal vessels affects renal functions, such as filtration and tubular functions.
- Renal failure is an important complication in HT.

---

3. Enumerate the hormones secreted by anterior pituitary gland. Discuss the actions and regulation of growth hormone.

Hormones of the anterior pituitary gland are:
- Thyroid stimulating hormone (TSH)
- Adrenocorticotrophic hormone (ACTH)
- Growth hormone (GH)
- Luteinizing hormone (LH)
- Follicle-stimulating hormone (FSH)
- Prolactin

Hormones of the posterior pituitary gland are:
- Antidiuretic hormone (ADH) or vasopressin
- Oxytocin

Hormones of the intermediate lobe are:
- Melanocyte-stimulating hormone
- Lipotropin:
  - GH is a polypeptide hormone.
  - It is a major growth promoting hormone.
  - It has direct and indirect actions.
  - It acts directly to catabolize substrates and to supply energy in starvation.
  - Its anabolic actions are direct on epiphysis and indirect through somatomedins (IGF-1).

Actions of Growth Hormone

Effect on Growth
- Stimulates linear growth by acting on epiphyseal cartilage of long bones.
- It stimulates all aspects of metabolism of chondrocytes as in:
  - Incorporates proline into collagen to form hydroxyproline
  - Promotes cartilage matrix formation.
  - ↑AA uptake and protein synthesis
  - ↑size and number of chondrocytes.
  - Facilitates differentiation of prechondrocytes to chondrocytes.
- All these actions result in growth of epiphyseal cartilage and promote linear growth.

Other Growth Promoting Actions
- **On bone:** Stimulates bone modeling by increasing activity of osteoclasts and blasts, osteoblastic activity predominates.
- **On skeletal muscle:** ↑growth of skeletal muscle by ↑protein synthesis → hypertrophy.
- Increases growth of visceral organs.
- **Induces pubertal growth:** Increase in height and sexual maturation.

Indirect Actions
- Effects of GH on growth, cartilage and protein metabolism is mediated through insulin-like growth factors (IGF)
- Also called as somatomedins
- They are growth factor synthesized in the liver.

Effects on Metabolism

Protein metabolism:
- Protein anabolic
- Positive N_2 and phosphate balance
- ↑Amino acid entry into cells
- ↑RNA and DNA synthesis
- ↑Protein synthesis
- Decreased level of amino acids in blood

Carbohydrate Metabolism
- It is prodiabetogenic
- Releases glucose from liver by facilitating gluconeogenesis
- Decreases glucose uptake by skeletal muscles
- Decreases insulin sensitivity

Lipid Metabolism
- Causes lipolysis and increases FFA in plasma
- Promotes ketogenesis
- Increased FFA and ketones provide the energy during stress

Effect on Water and Electrolyte Metabolism
- ↑plasma Ca^{2+}, by increasing the reabsorption from GIT
- Causes Na^+ retention
- It maintains ECF volume by stimulating renin-angiotensin-aldosterone pathway.
- Also suppresses ANP release

Regulation of Growth Hormone Secretion
- GH secretion is under the control of hypothalamus. There are two hypothalamic hormones regulating secretion of GH—growth hormone-releasing hormone (GRH) and somatostatin (SS) which is GH inhibiting hormone (GIH). It undergoes fluctuations in children and young adults.
- It is under negative feedback control. GH stimulates secretion of IGF-1 from liver which in turn inhibits secretion of GH and stimulates secretion of SS.
- There are various factors which stimulate and inhibit secretion of GH (*refer* **Fig. 5**).

Factors increasing secretion of GH:
1. Hypoglycemia
2. Increase in plasma levels of amino acids
3. Exercise, fasting
4. Stress, emotions
5. Glucagon
6. Puberty
7. Stage IV sleep
8. Enkephalins
9. Drugs, such as, L-Dopa
10. Hormones, such as estrogen, androgen

Factors inhibiting secretion of GH:
1. Increase in glucose
2. Increase in FFA
3. Hormones, such as cortisol, GH
4. REM sleep
5. Medroxyprogesterone
6. Pregnancy

---

4. Define hypoxia. Explain in detail the different types of hypoxia. Add a note on hyperbaric oxygen therapy.

- Hypoxia is defined as deficiency of O_2 at tissue level.
- **Types:**
  a. Hypoxic hypoxia
  b. Anemic hypoxia
  c. Stagnant hypoxia
  d. Histotoxic hypoxia

a. **Hypoxic hypoxia:**
   - Arterial pO_2 is low, therefore tissue pO_2 is less
   - **Mechanism of hypoxia:** pO_2 of arterial blood is low due to either ↓O_2 in inspired air or disease of respiratory apparatus.
   - **Conditions:**
     - Low pO_2 in inspired air (as in high altitude)
     - Hypoventilation as in airway obstruction, paralysis of respiratory muscles
     - Diffusion defects as in pulmonary edema
     - Ventilation/perfusion mismatch
     - A-V shunt as in congenital cyanotic heart disease

b. **Anemic hypoxia:** It is due to decreased O_2 carrying capacity of blood and so → O_2 content in blood. pO_2 is normal.
   - **Conditions:** Anemia, CO poisoning, presence of altered Hb (Methemoglobin), etc.
   - In mild conditions, the 2,3-DPG levels increase in the RBC → Easy dissociation of O_2

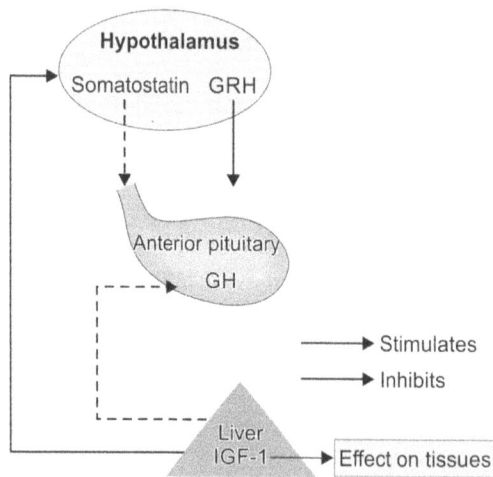

Fig. 5: Regulation of secretion of growth hormone. (GRH: growth hormone-releasing hormone, GH: growth hormone, IGF-1: insulin like growth factor 1)

Table 1: Features of types of hypoxia.

Features	Hypoxic hypoxia	Anemic hypoxia	Stagnant hypoxia	Histotoxic hypoxia
Arterial PO_2	Decreased	Normal	Normal	Normal
% O_2 saturation of hemoglobin	Decreased	Decreased	Normal	Normal
Arterial O_2 content (mL/dL)	Decreased	Markedly decreased	Normal	Normal
A-V PO_2 difference	Decreased	Normal	More than normal	Less than normal
Peripheral chemoreceptor stimulation	Present	Absent	Present	Present
Cyanosis	Present	Absent	Present	Absent

  c. **Stagnant hypoxia:**
   - Hypoxia due to decreased blood flow to tissues. Also called as ischemic hypoxia.
   - **Mechanism:** O_2 content and pO_2 are normal in arterial blood. Hypoxia is due to stagnation of blood → **circulatory hypoxia**.
   - **Seen in:**
     - Heart failure
     - Shock
     - Vascular obstruction
     - Hemorrhage
  d. **Histotoxic hypoxia:**
   - Tissues cannot utilize O_2 in spite of normal O_2 supply as in cyanide poisoning.
   - Venous pO_2 is high (>46 mm Hg)
   - Cyanide poisoning is treated with methylene blue or nitrites → forms methemoglobin → reacts with cyanide → cyanmethemoglobin. It is less poisonous.
   - Hyperbaric O_2 is also used for treatment.
   - **Features of types of hypoxia:** See Table 1.

Hyperbaric Oxygen

- It is administration of O_2 at high pressure.
- Normal O_2 solubility in blood—0.003 mL/100 mL/mm Hg.
- It can be increased to 6 mL/100 mL/mm Hg, when inspired PO_2 is 2000 mm Hg. This is possible when 100% O_2 is given at a pressure of 3 atm.
- O_2 toxicity may appear when 100% O_2 is given at a pressure of 4 atm.

Indications

- CO poisoning
- Radiation-induced tissue injury
- Gas gangrene
- Very severe blood loss anemia
- Diabetic leg ulcers and other wounds those are slow to heal
- Decompression sickness
- Air embolism

Symptoms of O_2 Toxicity

It is due to formation of free radicals (like O_2^-, H_2O_2).
They oxidize PUFA and destroy the cellular enzymes.

Symptoms

- Nausea
- Irritability
- Dizziness
- Disorientation
- Muscle twitching
- Convulsions and in severe cases coma
- Congestion and irritation of airways → tracheobronchial secretions → ↓ surfactant → pulmonary edema

II. SHORT NOTES

1. Primary active transport.

Active Transport

- It is also carrier mediated
- Moves substances uphill against concentration gradient.

- So associated with energy expenditure. Energy is derived from ATP, either directly or indirectly
- **Types:** Primary active transport and secondary active transport.

Primary Active Transport

Here substances are moved uphill across the cell membrane with the help of energy-driven pumps. It involves energy expenditure which is directly derived from break down of ATP.

Example:
- Na^+- K^+ pump
- H^+-K^+ pump
- Ca^{2+} ATPase

Na^+- K^+ Pump

- Sodium-potassium ATPase is a ubiquitous pump.
- It pumps out 3 Na^+ molecules from the cell in exchange for 2 K^+ molecules into the cell.
- Na^+ concentration is more in the ECF and K^+ concentration is more in the ICF.
- So both the ions are pumped against their concentration gradients out and in of the cell respectively.
- The pump is present in all the cells to maintain the cell volume and to maintain the membrane potential.
- It is an electrogenic pump as it pumps 3 Na^+ out of the cell and 2 K^+ into the cell.
- It catalyzes hydrolysis of ATP and uses the energy to move the ions.
- Its activity is inhibited by Ouabain and digitalis used for heart failure.
- It has α and β subunits. Na^+ and K^+ are transported through α subunit.
- α subunit is larger and has intracellular Na^+ and ATP binding sites and a phosphorylation site. When Na^+ binds to α subunit, ATP also binds and is converted to ADP and the P is added to phosphorylation site. This changes the configuration and extrudes Na^+ into ECF. K^+ then binds extracellularly (*refer* **Fig. 6**).
- Dephosphorylating α subunit and comes back to original configuration and releases K^+ intracellularly. β subunit is a glycoprotein and has no transport action but its presence is needed for pump activity.
- Extracellularly there are binding sites for K^+ and ouabain.
- Pump activity is regulated by 2nd messengers and hormones. Thyroid hormone, aldosterone and insulin increase the pump activity, whereas dopamine decreases the pump activity.

Other primary active transporters:
- **Ca^{2+} ATPase:** It is present on the cell membranes, endoplasmic reticulum and sarcoplasmic reticulum of muscles. These pumps help in maintaining a lower concentration of Ca^{2+} in the cytoplasm by pumping it either into ECF or into the SR in muscles.
- **H^+-K^+ ATPase:** These pumps are present on the apical membrane of parietal cells in the gastric mucosa and the luminal side of the 'I' cells of the collecting tubule in the nephron. In the stomach, the pump is the

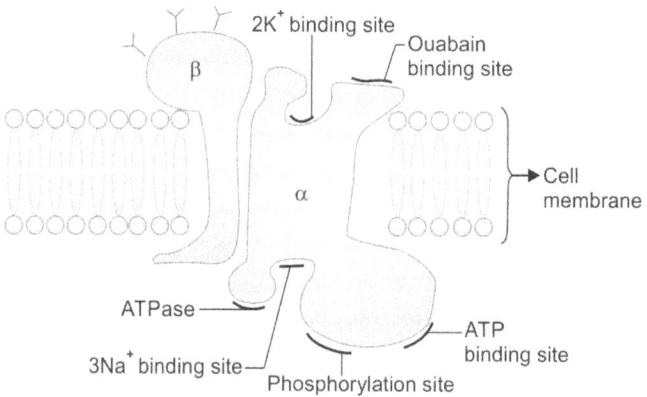

Fig. 6: Sodium-potassium pump; primary active transporter.

primary mechanism of secreting H⁺ into the lumen. In nephron, the pump helps in secreting H⁺ into the tubule and thereby acidification of urine.
- **H⁺ ATPase:** It is present in the luminal membrane of parietal cells of gastric mucosa and also in the 'I' cells of collecting tubule of nephrons. It is also present in the membrane of lysosomes and endoplasmic reticulum. The acidic nature of the lysosomes is essential for its degenerative actions.

---

2. Excitation-contraction coupling.

The process by which the muscle membrane is excited and followed by muscle contraction is given as excitation-contraction coupling.

The steps are given below:
- The action potential generated following the end-plate potential (EPP) moves through the T-tubule and activates the voltage-gated dihydropyridine receptors (DHPRs) which are present in the T tubule membrane.
- The activated DHPRs open the Ca^{2+} channels named as the ryanodine receptors which are located in the terminal cisterns of the sarcoplasmic reticulum (SR).
- This releases Ca^{2+} from the SR into the cytoplasm and the Ca^{2+} concentration in cytosol rises by 2000 times that of the resting state.
- The Ca^{2+} now gets attached to the troponin C subunit.
- Troponin C-Ca^{2+} complex now induce a conformational change in the tropomyosin and the tropomyosin is lifted up, exposing the myosin binding sites on actin molecules.
- So the myosin heads bind to the actin molecules and cross-bridge cycling starts resulting in muscle contraction.

---

3. Stages of deglutition.

Deglutition is the process of swallowing:
- It is a reflex response integrated in the medulla in nucleus tractus solitarius (NTS) and nucleus ambiguus (NA).
- Afferents pass through the cranial nerves V, IX and X
- Efferents come through cranial nerves V, VII and XII nerves to the tongue and pharynx

There are 3 phases of deglutition:
1. Oral or voluntary phase
2. Pharyngeal or involuntary phase
3. Esophageal phase

Oral Phase

When food enters mouth, tongue forms it into a bolus and pushes it to the oropharynx by pushing up and against the hard palate.

Pharyngeal Phase
- It starts when food enters pharynx.
- Soft palate is elevated and closes the nasopharynx and prevents food from entering the nose
- Larynx rises, vocal cords approximate and epiglottis closes the laryngeal opening and prevents food from entering the trachea (*refer* **Figs. 7A to D**)
- Deglutition apnea follows.
- Palatopharyngeal folds approximate for selective material to move into the esophagus.
- Cricopharyngeus (Upper esophageal sphincter) relaxes and bolus enters upper esophagus.
- On entering of food into esophagus, the cricopharyngeus closes, vocal cords open and air entry is allowed.

Esophageal Phase
- There are 2 sphincters in the esophagus— Upper esophageal sphincter (UES) and Lower esophageal sphincter (LES).
- UES is formed by cricopharyngeus muscle which is a skeletal muscle. It opens reflexly at the beginning of swallow.
- LES is made of smooth muscle and its actions are regulated by vagus nerve and other intrinsic nerves. Its main action is to prevent regurgitation of acids from the stomach
- Food on reaching esophagus is pushed into the stomach by peristalsis—primary and secondary peristalsis.

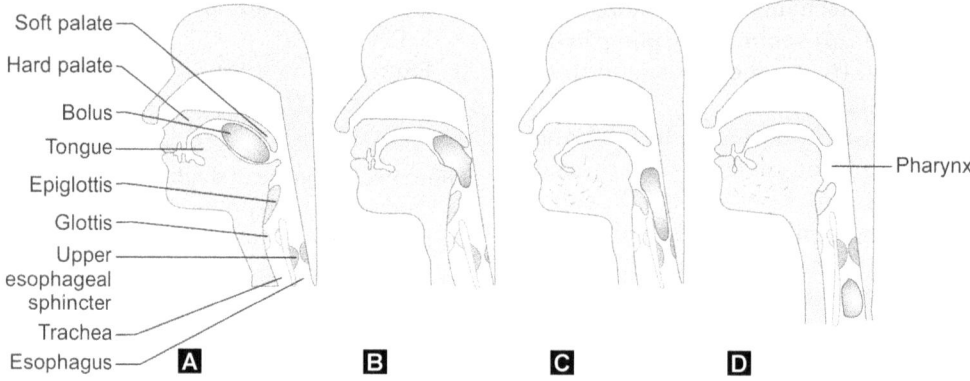

Figs. 7A to D: Phases of deglutition: (A) Oral phase; (B) Bolus enters the pharynx; (C) Pharyngeal phase; (D) Esophageal phase.

- Primary peristalsis is initiated by swallowing and is coordinated by vagus nerve.
- Secondary peristalsis is initiated by presence of food in the esophagus and it sweeps the food down towards the stomach, coordinated by intrinsic nerves.

4. Micturition reflex.

- Micturition is the process of emptying the urinary bladder.
- Two processes are involved:
  a. The bladder fills progressively until the tension in its wall rises above a threshold level, and then
  b. A nervous reflex called the micturition reflex occurs that empties the bladder.
  The micturition reflex is an automatic spinal cord reflex; however, it can be inhibited or facilitated by centers in the brainstem and cerebral cortex (*refer* **Fig. 8**).

The Reflex Pathway

- **Initiation:** Reflex initiated by stimulation of stretch receptors in bladder wall.
- **Stimulus:** Filling of bladder up to 300–400 mL.
- **Afferents:** Through pelvic nerves (PS) to reach S2–S4 segments in spinal cord.
- **Efferents:** PS motor fibers from S2–S4 end in the detrusor muscle (excitatory) and internal sphincter (inhibitory).
- **Response:** Causes contraction of bladder wall and relaxation of internal sphincter. Once it becomes powerful another reflex through pudendal nerve relaxes the ES → voiding.

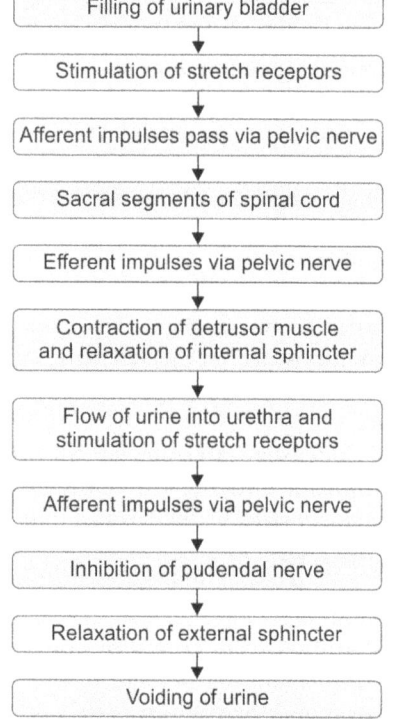

Fig. 8: Micturition reflex.

5. Hyperthyroidism.

Causes

- **Thyroid overactivity:**
  - Graves' disease
  - Solitary toxic adenoma

- Toxic multinodular goiter
- TSH secreting pituitary tumor
- Thyroiditis
- Mutations causing constitutive activation of TSH receptor
- **Extrathyroidal causes:**
  - Administration of T_3 and T_4
  - Ectopic thyroid tissue

Grave's Disease

- Most common cause of hyperthyroidism (60-70%)
- It is an autoimmune disorder with activating Ab to TSH receptor
- More common in women.

Symptoms

Goiter is present.

Symptoms due to action of excess TH on tissues:

- BMR and body temperature
- Heat intolerance
- Nervousness
- Heart rate is increased. Palpitations and fine tremors are present
- Muscle weakness
- Nervousness, irritability and anxiety
- Exaggeration of deep tendon reflexes
- Increased frequency of defecation
- Increased appetite
- Weight loss
- Moist, warm skin
- Bruit over thyroid
- Pretibial myxedema
- Fatigue
- Impotence in males
- Oligomenorrhea or amenorrhea in females

Exophthalmos is present only in Graves' disease and not in other types of hyperthyroidism.

- This is due to increase in retro-orbital contents
- Fibroblasts proliferate and develop into adipocytes, which have receptors for circulating TSH Ab → gets activated → release cytokines → inflammation and edema.

Treatment of Hyperthyroidism

Treated with antithyroid drugs:

- Drugs acting by inhibiting iodide trapping—monovalent anions, such as chlorate, pertechnetate, periodate, biiodate, nitrate, perchlorate and thiocyanate.
- Drugs acting by inhibiting organification and coupling—thioureylenes, such as propylthiouracil and methimazole
- Iodides—large doses inhibit thyroid function.

6. Compliance.

- Stretchability or the recoiling tendency due to the elastic property of the lung is said to be the compliance.
- Compliance of the respiratory system is defined as the change in the lung volume per unit change in the airway pressure.
- It is given as $C = \Delta V/\Delta P$
  C = Compliance
  ΔV = Change in volume
  ΔP = Change in pressure
  It is expressed in $L/cm\ H_2O$

Compliance in respiratory system is given under two headings:

1. Compliance of lungs only
2. Compliance of lungs and thoracic wall

Compliance of lungs and thoracic cavity:

- Both the lungs and thoracic cavity are elastic and viscous in nature and therefore each of them has their own recoiling tendencies.
- Normal value of thoracic cavity and lungs together is $0.13\ L/cm\ H_2O$.
- It means, when there is an increase in airway pressure by 1 cm H_2O the volume of the lungs increase by 0.13 liters.

Compliance of lung alone:

- Normal value is around $0.22\ L/cm\ H_2O$.
- So compliance of lung is twice that of lung and thoracic cavity together.

Measurement of compliance of lungs and chest wall:

- The interaction of recoiling of lung and chest wall is demonstrated in living subjects by using the spirometer.

- After clipping the nose, the subject is asked to breathe in from a spirometer from end expiratory position in increments of volumes.
- There is a valve beyond the mouth piece, through which he breathes and also a pressure recording device is attached to the mouth piece.
- The person inhales a given volume of air and the valve is shut and the person is asked to relax the respiratory muscles and the change in airway pressure is noted.
- This procedure is repeated after inhaling and exhaling various volumes of air and also recording of airway pressures.
- The airway pressures are plotted against the lung volumes to get the relaxation pressure curve of the respiratory system.
- From the curve it is noted that at zero pressure the lung volume is equal to FRC and this volume is said to be the relaxation volume.
- It is the volume at which the recoiling of lungs is exactly balanced by the recoiling of the thoracic wall.
- The measurement of compliance can be made using the curve especially where it is the steepest.
- Above the relaxation volume as the volume increases the pressure also increases and it reaches about + 30 mm Hg (*refer* **Fig. 9**).
- Below the relaxation volume as the volume decreases the pressure also decreases and reaches – 30 mm Hg.

Factors affecting compliance of lungs and chest wall:

- Compliance when decreased shifts the pressure-volume curve to the right and downwards, as in: Pulmonary edema, congestion and pulmonary fibrosis
- Compliance when increased the curve is shifted to the left and above as in: Emphysema and old age.

Measurement of compliance of lungs alone:

- The compliance of lungs alone can be measured by measuring the intrapleural pressures (IPP) at various lung volumes.
- IPP gives an idea about the distensibility of the lungs.
- As the lung expands, the IPP becomes more negative as the recoiling forces are more.
- IPP can be recorded by measuring intra-esophageal pressures.
- The person is asked to breathe in from a spirometer from the end-expiratory

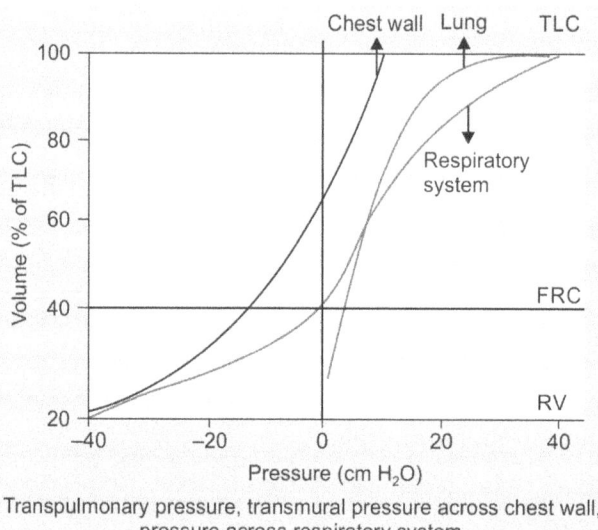

Fig. 9: Relaxation pressure-volume curve of lung and chest wall. It gives the relation between intrapulmonary pressure and volume. Curve in gray color is the curve of total respiratory system. At FRC, the transmural pressure is zero and above it the pressure is positive and below it, negative.

position up to end-inspiratory position and holds the breath.
- The IPP is measured in this manner for various lung volumes inhaled and exhaled and a graph is plotted.
- The observation is that the curves of change in pressure to change in volume is different for inspiration and expiration and is curved.
- The curve depicts that at similar IPP, the lung volume is less in inspiratory phase than in expiratory phase. The curve is said to be the "hysteresis curve" (refer **Fig. 10**).
- The difference in pressure volume-relationship in inspiration and expiration is due to—viscous resistance and airway resistance.
- Compliance is greater when measured during deflation than when measured during inflation.
- Lung compliance is calculated by taking a point on the graph at the end of inspiration when there is no air flow and so there is no viscous and elastic resistance.
- Lung compliance is calculated as $\Delta V/\Delta P = 0.22$ L/cm H_2O.
- This amount of lung compliance is affected by the elastic tissues in the lungs and also the surface tension of the fluid lining the alveoli.
- The contribution of each factor is studied by removing the lungs of an experimental animal and distending them with air and water alternately while measuring the intrapulmonary pressure.
- While distension with air, the pressure-volume curve measures both tissue elasticity and surface tension, whereas while using saline surface tension becomes zero and the curve measures only tissue elasticity.
- In the curve with saline, there is not much difference in inspiratory and expiratory curves. The elasticity due to surface tension is much smaller at small lung volumes than at large lung volumes. This may be due to the effect of surfactant.

Factors affecting lung compliance alone:
- **Lung volume:** A person with one lung, will have the change in volume to change in pressure.
- Compliance is more during deflation of lung than while inflating the lungs.
- Due to effect of gravity in standing position compliance is less in the apex of the lung.

Specific Compliance
- As mentioned above, in a person with one lung (even though compliance of that lung is normal) the compliance is decreased as the lung volume is decreased. To overcome this, compliance can be calculated as a function of FRC.
- Specific compliance = compliance/FRC.

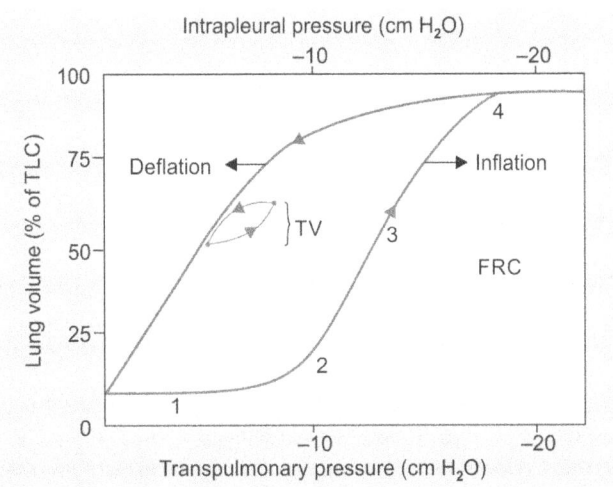

Fig. 10: Pressure-volume relations in the lungs. Pressure changes in inflation and deflation are different.

7. Hypoxic hypoxia.

Refer answer to essay question 4.

8. Pacemaker potential.

- In the mammalian heart, sinoatrial node is the pacemaker. It is said to be the pacemaker as it generates impulses by itself without neural input at a faster rate.
- Other tissues of the heart—AV node, atria and ventricle are also capable of generating impulses but SA node generates impulses at a faster rate and therefore said to be the pacemaker of the heart.

Pacemaker Potential

- The ventricular and atrial muscle cells have a resting membrane potential of −90 mV. On stimulation, the membrane depolarizes and produces an action potential.
- The pacemaker cells are smaller and rounded (P cells) and they do not have a stable resting membrane potential and RMP is around −55 to −60 mV.
- From −60 mV, there is a slow depolarization slope which reaches the firing level of −40 mV and there is a rapid depolarization followed by rapid repolarization back to −60 mV and again there is a slow depolarization slope rising to firing level.
- This slope which takes the membrane to firing level is the **pacemaker potential or prepotential**.

Ionic Events Responsible for Pacemaker Potential

- At −60 mV, the K^+ channels start closing down thereby preventing K^+ efflux. This is responsible for the first part of prepotential (the slope).
- Next part is due to opening up of **'f'** type Na^+ channels (The Na^+ current in this channel is said to be funny current as the channel opens in hyperpolarization)
- Last part of depolarization of the prepotential is due to opening of T-type (Transient) Ca^{2+} channels allowing Ca^{2+} influx (*refer* **Fig. 11**).
- Now as the firing level is reached (−40 mV), the long lasting Ca^{2+} channels (L-type) open and produces a rapid depolarization and the action potential.
- Then the K^+ channels open and the K^+ efflux bring about rapid repolarization and membrane potential reaches −60 mV. Then the next prepotential starts.
- So in the pacemaker cells, it is a Ca^{2+} dependant depolarization rather than Na^+ dependent depolarization as in ventricular muscles.

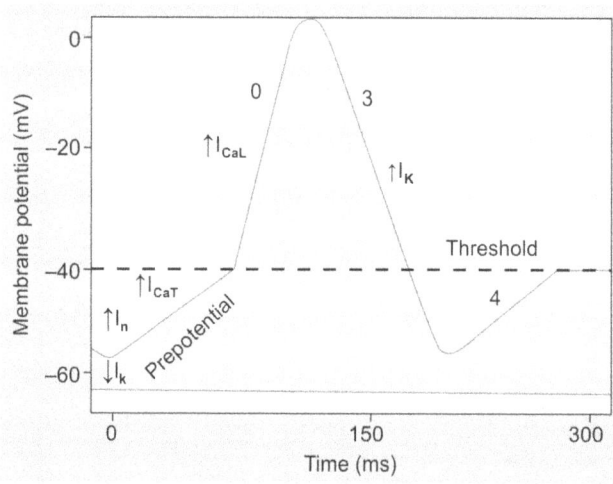

Fig. 11: Pacemaker potential. Slope of pacemaker potential (Phase 4), the prepotential is due to 3 events; first part of depolarization is due to closure of K^+ channels, 2nd part is due to Na^+ influx through sodium channel and last part of depolarization is due to Ca^{2+} influx through T-type Ca^{2+} channels. Rapid depolarization (Phase 0) is due to opening of L-type Ca^{2+} channels and repolarization (Phase 3) due to opening of K^+ channels.

- The pacemaker cells are supplied by sympathetic and parasympathetic nerves.
- On stimulation by sympathetic nerves, the prepotential slope becomes steeper and the rate of spontaneous discharge increases thereby increasing the heart rate.
- On stimulation by the parasympathetic nerves, the slope of the prepotential decreases and spontaneous firing also decreases thereby heart rate decreases.

9. Stages of sleep.

- Sleep is said to be a state of altered consciousness or partial unconsciousness from which a person can be aroused.
- Sleep has two components—nonrapid eye movement (NREM) and rapid eye movement (REM) sleep
- NREM sleep has four stages, each with different EEG activities.

Stage 1

- Stage of transition between wakefulness and sleep.
- Lasts for 1-7 minutes.
- Person is relaxed with eyes closed and fleeting thoughts.
- Alpha waves which were present will diminish.
- People when awakened at this stage will say that they were not sleeping.

Stage 2

- Stage of light sleep.
- It is little more difficult to wake the person.
- Fragments of dreams may be experienced.
- Eyes may role from side to side.
- EEG shows sleep spindles—bursts of sharply pointed waves occurring at a frequency of 12-14 Hz and lasts 1-2 seconds.

Stage 3

- It is a period of moderately deep sleep.
- Body temperature and BP decrease.
- It is difficult to wake the person.
- EEG shows mixture of sleep spindles and large, low frequency waves.

- This stage occurs 20 minutes after falling asleep.

Stage 4 or Slow Wave Sleep

- Deepest level of sleep.
- Brain metabolism drops significantly.
- Body temperature slightly falls.
- Muscle tone is decreased only slightly.
- Reflexes are intact.
- EEG shows slow, large amplitude delta waves.

A person during sleep will go from stage 1-4 in about 1 hour. Then has the REM sleep.

REM Sleep

- In a period of sleep of 7-8 hours, REM and NREM sleep alternate.
- REM sleep occurs 3-5 times during the sleep alternating with NREM sleep.
- Initial episode of REM sleep will be lasting for 10-20 minutes. Then with each episode it prolongs and the final episode is for 50 minutes.
- In adults, REM sleep totals for about 90-120 minutes. With age period of REM sleep decreases.
- About 50% of an infants sleep is REM sleep. 35% for 2-year-old infant, 25% for adults.
- REM sleep is thought to be important for maturation of brain in infants.
- This has been identified by the high percentage of REM sleep in infants.
- Bruxism, erection of penis, twitching of facial muscles.

10. Functions of cerebellum.

Control of Posture and Equilibrium

- Vestibulocerebellum or the flocculonodular lobe controls posture and equilibrium.
- It receives inputs from vestibular apparatus directly and also through vestibular nuclei about position of head and body.
- It sends efferents to vestibular nuclei from which the vestibulospinal tract arises to regulate posture.
- Vestibulocerebellum is also concerned with regulating vestibulo-ocular reflex.

Control of Muscle Tone and Stretch Reflex
- Spinocerebellum influences the muscle tone through its output via fastigial nucleus which in turn controls the vestibulospinal and reticulospinal tract (arising from pontine reticular formation).
- The major influence of cerebellum on tone is facilitatory.
- Vestibulospinal tract is facilitatory to α motor neurons and reticulospinal tract is facilitatory to γ motor neurons.
- Since control of cerebellum is on both α and γ motor neurons it has an important role in α-γ linkage.

Control of Voluntary Movements
- Paravermal portion of spinocerebellum controls skilled voluntary movements.
- It does not initiate movements but it coordinates voluntary movements.
- Coordination of movements is by regulating the time, rate, range, force and direction of movements.
- All three functional divisions of the cerebellum work together as "comparator of servo mechanism".

Comparator Servo Mechanism
- Impulses for voluntary movements are planned and programmed in the premotor cortex and it is sequenced in primary motor area and the command to skeletal muscles is sent through the corticospinal tract.
- A copy of the plan or intended movement is also sent to the spinocerebellum.
- Cerebellum also gets feedback from the proprioceptors about the actual movement performed by the muscles and joints.
- It also receives other sensory inputs from eye, ear and vestibular apparatus.
- Now the cerebellum compares the intended movement and the executed movement along with other sensory inputs mentioned above.
- It thereby modifies appropriately the on-going movement.
- If any corrections have to be done in programming of movements the error signals are sent to the motor cortex.

Control of Body Movements of One Side
- Motor cortex of one side is connected to opposite cerebellum through a closed feedback loop; cerebral-cerebellar-cerebral circuit, the cortico-ponto-dentato-thalamo-cortical pathway.
- So each cerebellar hemisphere controls the opposite cerebral cortex.
- But the corticospinal tract descending down from the motor cortex decussates in medulla and controls the opposite side of the body.
- Since there is double decussation, it is that cerebellum controls same side of the body.

Planning and Programming of Movements
Cerebrocerebellum has extensive connections with motor cortex and therefore is involved in planning and programming of movements.

Learning of Skills
- Cerebellum always tends to make changes in ongoing movements and therefore it improves by learning.
- Another evidence is that there are increased activities in the climbing fibers when a new skill is learnt.
- So cerebellum has a great role in learning skills.

Eyeball Movement
Pyramis of cerebellum is concerned with eyeball movement.

---

11. Role of helper T cells.
There are 4 types of T lymphocytes—Helper T cells, cytotoxic T cells, suppressor T cells and memory T cells.

Helper T cells:
- These are the major types of T cells.
- As the name implies they help the immune system; both cell-mediated and humoral immunity.
- They secrete many interleukins and thereby help the immunity.
- They are also called as CD 4 cells.

Helper T cells are activated in the following mechanisms:
- Antigen which has entered the body is phagocytosed, digested and processed inside the macrophages and the peptide fragment of the antigen in the phagosome combines with the vesicle containing MHC II.
- After fusion of the vesicles, the antigen binds with MHC II and both are incorporated in the cell membrane of antigen-presenting cell (Macrophage).
- The APC with the antigen and MHC II circulate in blood or in lymphatic tissues and the T cells with the receptor for the antigen recognize the antigenic fragment.
- The T cell gets activated and undergoes differentiation and proliferation to form helper T cells.
- Helper T cells secrete interleukin-2 which by autocrine and paracrine influence activate other helper T cells and also activate B cells and cytotoxic T cells.
- As the helper T cells activate cytotoxic T cells and B cells it has an important role in cellular immunity and humoral immunity.

12. Action potential.

- Action potentials are brief, rapid and large changes in the membrane potential (100 mV) following a threshold stimulus, conducted for a long distance along the axon in an all or none fashion with the same shape and amplitude.
- It takes the membrane potential from –70 mV to +35 mV.
- They occur in a small patch of membrane.
- In a motor neuron it originates in the "**initial segment**"
- They are due to opening up of voltage-gated Na$^+$ and voltage-gated K$^+$ channels

Phases of Action Potential

When a stimulus is given there is deflection in the baseline which is due to leakage of current from stimulating electrodes—**Stimulus artifact**.

Latent period: Following the stimulus artifact, there is an isopotential line, the latent period just before the AP.

It is due to the time taken for the impulse to travel from the stimulating to the recording electrode. Its duration is proportionate to the distance between stimulating and recording electrode. It also depends on the type of nerve.

Phase of depolarization: Following latent period there is phase of slow depolarization (*Local response*) due to slow opening of Na$^+$ channels. On reaching –55 mV, the firing level, there is a phase of rapid depolarization.

This is due to the rapid opening of voltage-gated Na$^+$ channels. There is rapid inrush of Na$^+$ ions (5000-fold increase) taking the membrane potential to +35 mV. On reaching this potential, there is inactivation of sodium channels within a fraction of millisecond.

Phase of repolarization: On reaching a potential of +35 mV, the potential reverses and starts falling rapidly to resting level. On completion of 70% repolarization there is decrease in rate of repolarization, it is said to be *after-depolarization* (*refer* Fig. 12).

The repolarization is due to inactivation of voltage-gated Na$^+$ channels and opening of voltage-gated K$^+$ channels and the third reason for repolarization is on reaching +35 mV, there is reversal of electrical gradient for Na$^+$ movement and so no more sodium influx happens.

After-hyperpolarization: On reaching the RMP, the membrane potential hyperpolarizes beyond RMP for a short period. It is called as after-hyperpolarization. It is due to closure of K$^+$ channels after a millisecond delay.

RMP: The membrane potential comes back to –90 mV due to the action of sodium-potassium pump.

Properties of Action Potential

- **All or none law:** When given a threshold stimulus the action potential is produced at the maximum amplitude. If a subthreshold stimulus is given, action potential is not produced and also if a suprathreshold stimulus is given, the amplitude and duration of AP remains the same as the one generated by giving a threshold stimulus.

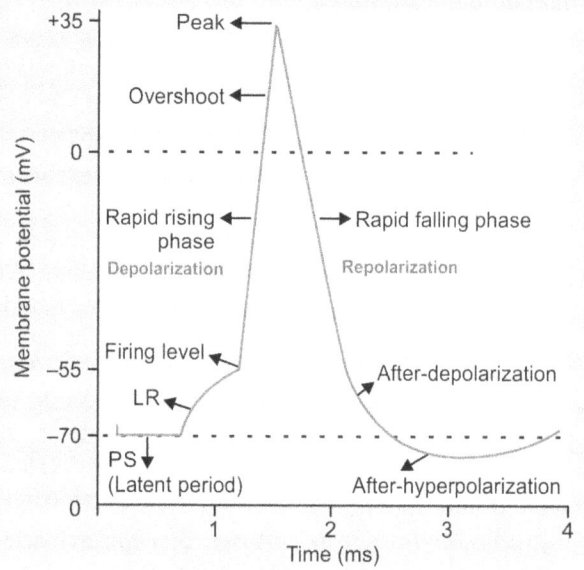

Fig. 12: Nerve action potential.

- **Threshold stimulus:** The minimum intensity of stimulus given for a particular time and can excite a nerve is said to be the threshold stimulus. If a weaker stimulus is given it has to be given for a longer period. The relationship between the strength and duration of the stimulus needed to excite a nerve is given as the Strength-duration curve (*refer* **Fig. 13**).

Rheobase is the minimum strength of a stimulus given for a particular time and is able to excite a tissue. The time for which the rheobase current should be given is said to be the ***Utilization time.*** The time duration for which double the strength of rheobase current should be given to excite a tissue is said to be the ***Chronaxie***. Chronaxie is an indicator of tissue excitability. Shorter the chronaxie for a

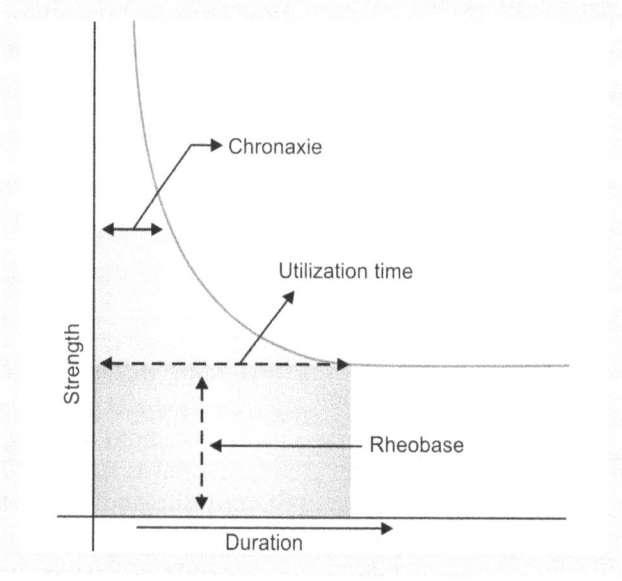

Fig. 13: Strength-duration curve.

tissue, excitability is better. Smooth muscles have the longer chronaxie.

- **Refractory period:** There is a time period during AP, if a second stimulus is given, the stimulated part of the membrane is not excited again. It is said to be the membrane is in a refractory period. The refractory period is divided into absolute refractory period and relative refractory period.

  Absolute refractory period (ARP) is the time period during an AP, application of a second stimulus of how ever strong or for any duration does not excite a nerve. It happens from the firing level to 1/3rd completion of repolarization. It is because of the state of the gates of voltage-gated Na^+ channels.

  Voltage-gated sodium channels: These channels have two gates, inactivation gate (along the exterior of the membrane) and the activation gate (along the interior of the membrane). At **resting state**, the inactivation gates are open and activation gates are closed. During an AP, on reaching the firing level, the activation gates also open and the rapid inrush of Na^+ produces the spike potential (**activated state**). On reaching +35 mV, the inactivation gates close rapidly and the Na^+ influx comes to a halt (**Inactivated state of the channel**). This starts the repolarization phase.

  These voltage-gated channels reach their resting state when the RMP is reached (−90 mV). Only on reaching the resting state, the channels can be reactivated. So during ARP the channels are in the inactivated state, so they are refractory to the second stimulus.

  Relative refractory period (RRP) is the period after ARP when the membrane can be excited by a suprathreshold stimulus. This phase is from the end of ARP to after-depolarization.

  During this phase, some of the channels would have reached the resting state, some may be still in inactivated state. When a suprathreshold stimulus is given it spreads to larger area of membrane and it can activate the channels which have reached the resting state.

- **Conductivity:** The AP in a motor neuron is generated at the initial segment. Once the AP is generated it is conducted towards the axon terminal. The conductivity depends on two factors—Myelination and diameter of the axon.

  Impulse conduction is faster in a myelinated axon and in a larger diameter axon.

  Impulse conduction in unmyelinated axons: The neuronal membrane is polarized at rest with negative charges lined on the interior and positive charges on the exterior. When an AP is generated at a location, the inside of the membrane reverses its polarity and positive charges flow into the depolarized site from either side of the membrane. These are called the "Current sinks". These current sinks excite the membrane ahead of the site of AP and also the site behind the AP. But since the area behind is in refractory period the current sinks travel in one direction only. Now the area excited ahead reaches a threshold and it can fire an AP.

  Impulse conduction in myelinated axon: In a myelinated axon, the voltage-gated Na^+ channels are concentrated in the nodes of Ranvier and the myelin sheath acts as an insulator. So the current sinks move from one node to another node rather than exciting the neighboring area as in unmyelinated axon. This type of impulse conduction is called as Saltatory conduction. Since the impulses jump across nodes it can travel faster (*refer* **Figs. 14A and B**).

  Larger diameter axons: In larger axons as the resistance for movement of ions is less the impulse transmission is faster.

- **Accommodation:** When a stimulus of slow rising nature is given, it does not excite fire the nerve as the nerve adapts to the applied stimulus and it is called as accommodation.

  The cause for this is when there is no rapid depolarization the gradual influx

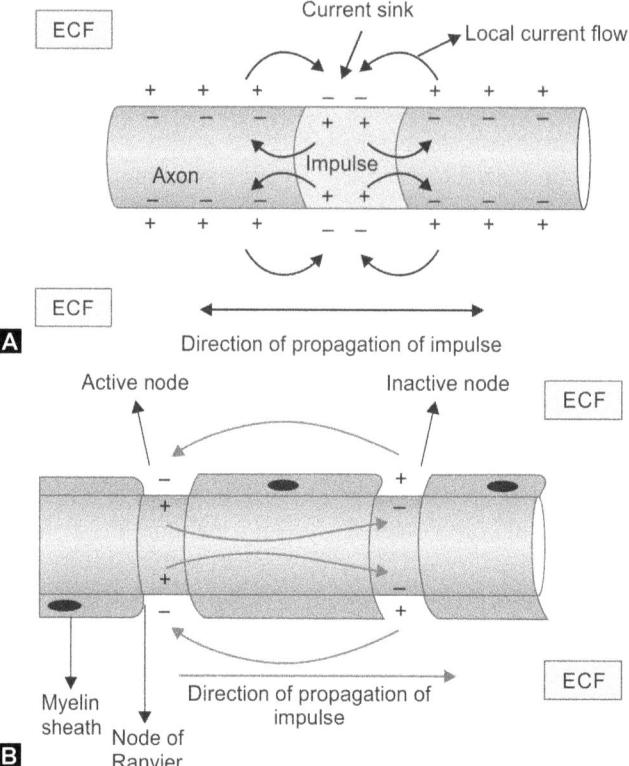

Figs. 14A and B: Conduction of impulses in (A) Unmyelinated neuron and (B) Myelinated neuron.

of sodium is balanced by the efflux of K⁺ through the slow opening voltage-gated K⁺ channels.

13. Juxtaglomerular apparatus.

- Juxtaglomerular apparatus is a combination of tubular cells and vascular cells.
- It is located near the glomerulus where the afferent arteriole enters and efferent arteriole leaves the glomerulus.

It is made up of the following components:
- Juxtaglomerular cells
- Macula densa cells
- Lacis cells (*refer* **Fig. 15**)

Juxtaglomerular Cells

- These are myoepithelial cells lining the afferent arteriole just before it enters the glomerulus.
- These cells are rich in endoplasmic reticulum and they secrete the hormone renin.

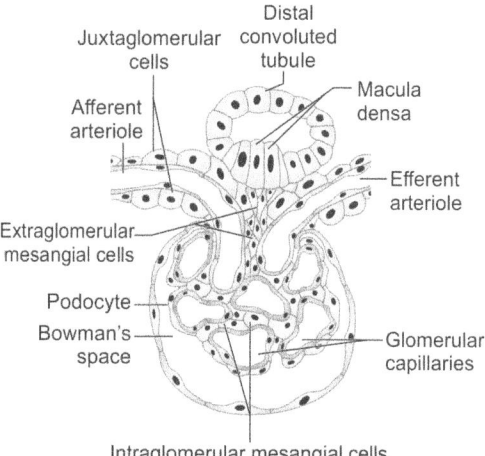

Fig. 15: Juxtaglomerular apparatus. It includes juxtaglomerular cells, macula densa and lacis cells.

- They act as baroreceptors and they sense the change in the renal arterial pressure and respond to the pressure gradient between the afferent arteriole and the interstitium.

- When the renal arterial pressure drops JG cells release renin.
- These cells also sense the ECF volume and respond to hypovolemia by secreting renin.
- They are also supplied by sympathetic nerves and when the stimulation is there it releases renin.

Macula Densa Cells

- They are present in the renal tubules at the junction of thick ascending limb of loop of Henle and the distal convoluted tubule.
- These cells are modified; they are more columnar and densely packed.
- They are in close contact with the mesangial cells and the JG cells.
- They act as chemoreceptors and they sense the NaCl content in the tubular fluid.
- They act through tubuloglomerular feedback and regulate the renal blood flow and GFR.

Mesangial Cells or Lacis Cells

- These are present in between the afferent and efferent arterioles and are in close contact with the JG cells and macula densa cells.
- They are contractile in nature and therefore they regulate GFR.
- They also secrete some amount of renin.

14. Achalasia cardia.

- It is a condition in which the resting tone of the lower esophageal sphincter (LES) is increased and there is improper relaxation of the sphincter on food intake and food does not reach the stomach.
- Food starts accumulating in the proximal esophagus and it starts getting distended.
- This is because of the defect in the myenteric plexus at the LES. There could also be a mismatch of the release of neurotransmitters at the LES.
- Acetylcholine released by parasympathetic nerves, makes the sphincter tonic. Nitric oxide and VIP relax the sphincter.
- Achalasia cardia could be due to increase in the acetylcholine released by the nerves supplying the LES and a decrease in the levels of nitric oxide or VIP. This makes the sphincter to become tonic.
- It can be treated by injecting botulinum toxin which inhibits the release of acetylcholine. Pneumatic dilatation of the sphincter can also be done.
- Myotomy is also done to relax the sphincter

15. Fetoplacental unit.

- Placenta produces steroidal hormones; estrogen and progesterone with the interaction of the fetal adrenals.
- Placenta forms pregnenolone and progesterone from cholesterol.
- Some of this pregnenolone enters the fetal circulation and along with the pregnenolone from fetal liver, forms the substrate for formation of Dehydroepiandrosterone (DHEA) and 16-hydroxy DHEA in fetal adrenals (*refer* **Fig. 16**).
- DHEAS and 16-OH-DHEAS are transported back to the placenta where DHEAS forms estradiol and 16-OH-DHEAS forms estriol.
- Estriol is the major estrogen and since its formation requires fetal adrenals, urinary excretion of estriol by mother is a good indicator of well-being of fetus.

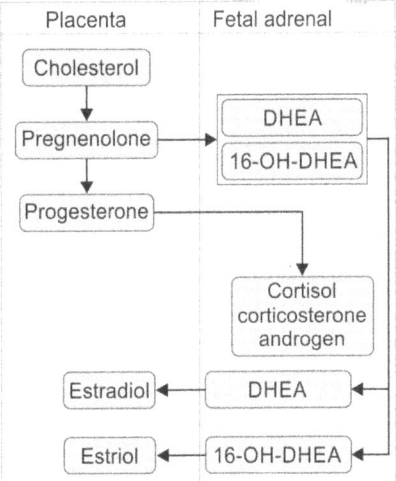

Fig. 16: Fetoplacental unit. Placenta and fetal adrenals, together synthesize progesterone and estrogen.
(DHEA: dehydroepiandrosterone; 16-OH DHEA: 16-hydroxy dehydroepiandrosterone)

16. Conduction system of heart.

- Ability to conduct an impulse (Action potential)
- Conduction of impulse is by sequential depolarization of adjacent membrane.
- In the heart, there is a specialized conducting system.
- It starts in the SA node and reaches the ventricles.
- It consists of the SA node, internodal tracts, AV node, bundle of His, right and left branches of bundle of His, Purkinje fibers and the ventricular muscles.

SA Node

- It is located in the wall of the right atrium close to the opening of SVC.
- It is made up of modified muscle fibers with more rounded cells with indistinct borders and less striations. They are called as P cells.
- Such cells are present in the AV node also.
- In the heart the SA node, AV node, His bundle and ventricles can generate their own impulses.
- But SA node is called the pacemaker as it generates impulses at a faster rate than the other tissues. So it is called the pacemaker.
- The pacemaker cells do not have a stable resting membrane potential.
- They tend to depolarize and repolarize in a continuous fashion in spite of nerve supply.
- The potential developed here is called as the **pacemaker potential**.

Pacemaker Potential

- The RMP in SA node is around –55 to –60 mV.
- But it is not a stable potential. There is a slow depolarization till –40 mV. Once –40 mV is reached there is a rapid depolarization (Phase 0) to +5 mV and there is a rapid repolarization to –55 mV (Phase 3).
- Then it reaches the RMP (Phase 4) (*refer* **Fig. 17**)
- Once again, there is a slow depolarization, the process continues.
- This slow rising phase before the rapid depolarization is called as the **prepotential or pacemaker potential**.

Ionic Events Responsible for Pacemaker Potential

- The prepotential is divided into 3 sections based on the ionic events: The first part of slow depolarization is due to decay of K$^+$ current (Closure of K$^+$ channels), followed

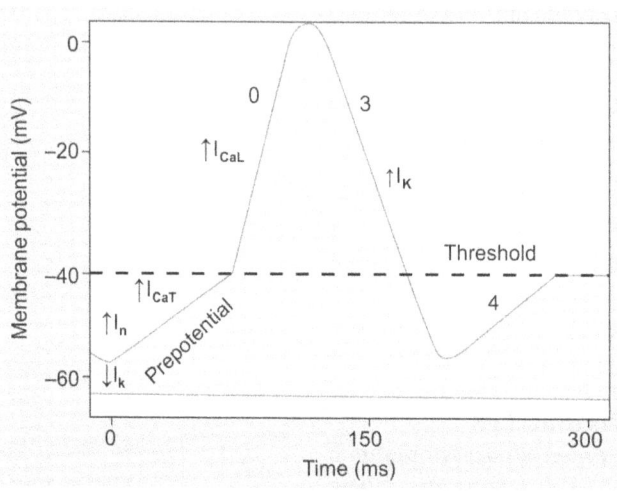

Fig. 17: Pacemaker potential. Slope of pacemaker potential (Phase 4), the prepotential is due to 3 events; first part of depolarization is due to closure of K$^+$ channels, 2nd part is due to Na$^+$ influx through sodium channel and last part of depolarization is due to Ca^{2+} influx through T-type Ca^{2+} channels. Rapid depolarization (Phase 0) is due to opening of L-type Ca^{2+} channels and repolarization (Phase 3) due to opening of K$^+$ channels.

by Na⁺ influx through 'h' or 'f' channels and the last part is due to Ca^{2+} influx through transient type Ca^{2+} (T type) channels.
- The rapid depolarization which starts at –40 mV is due to Ca^{2+} influx through long lasting Ca^{2+} channels (L type).
- Rapid repolarization is due to K⁺ efflux through K⁺ channels resulting in repolarization to –55 to –60 mV.

Conducting Pathway

- These impulses originated in the SA node are conducted down through the specialized conducting system as mentioned above.
- The impulses from SA node are transmitted to the AV node through 3 internodal bundles which are specialized tissues for conduction of impulses from SA node to AV node in a faster way.
- The atrial tissues also conduct impulses but they are slower.

The 3 bundles are:
1. Anterior internodal tract of Bachmann
2. Middle internodal tract of Wenckebach
3. Posterior internodal tract of Thorel
Through these bundles the impulses reach the AV node.

Interatrial Tract of Bachmann
- This bundle starts in the SA node and ends in the left atrium.
- The left atrium is also depolarized simultaneously

AV Node
- It is located beneath the endocardium on the right side of lower part of atrial septum near the tricuspid valve.
- The conduction velocity through the AVN is very slow because the fibers are smaller with less number of gap junctions.
- There is a delay of 0.1 s
- The delay provides time for atrial contraction and final ventricular filling.
- It also prevents transmission of all impulses from atria to ventricles in supraventricular tachycardia.
- It is supplied by sympathetic and PS nerves which alter the conduction rate

Atrioventricular Bundle of His
- This bundle starts in the AV bundle and descends down the fibrous skeleton and divides into right and left branches and they supply the right and left ventricles.
- The bundles divide into many small branches, the Purkinje fibers.

Purkinje Fibers
They are present in the endocardium and reaches all parts of ventricles.

Ventricles
- The spread of depolarization in the ventricular muscles are from the AVN to the His bundle → Purkinje fibers → ventricles.
- The conduction velocity of the AP through ventricular muscles are 0.3–0.4 msec.
- This results in depolarization of both ventricles at the same time and leads to contraction of both ventricles at the same time.
- In ventricle, the spread of depolarization is from endocardium to epicardium.

17. Special features of coronary circulation.

- There are 2 coronary arteries—right and left. Right artery supplies the right atrium and right ventricle and left coronary artery supplies left atrium and ventricles.
- There are no anastomoses between the two arteries and therefore they are end arteries. Therefore blockage of vessels results in ischemia or infarction supplied by those arteries.
- There are phasic changes in blood flow through coronaries. In systole as the myocardium contracts the blood vessels are compressed and there is no blood flow through the coronaries. In diastole as the myocardium relaxes, the vessels dilate and blood flow increases through the vessels.
- The endocardial vessels show the maximum phasic variation in blood flow.

Therefore, these areas suffer from hypoxia and are prone for ischemia in compromised states.
- Metabolic regulation is well-developed in coronary vessels. The blood flow increase is based on the need of the myocardium.
- Coronary circulation is adjustable based on the activities of the myocardium as in exercise the coronary blood flow can increased by 4–5 times to meet the body's demand. So, it has adequate blood flow reserve.
- The myocardium extracts nearly 80% of O_2 from arterial blood and therefore the AV difference of O_2 is high. So, it increases O_2 supply the blood flow should increase.
- The rate of blood flow through the coronary vessels is the second highest next to the renal blood flow. It is 250 mL/min.
- The rate of O_2 consumption is the highest of all the organs in the body. It is about 9.7 mL/100 g of tissue/min.

18. Vital capacity.

- Maximum volume of gas completely expired from the lungs following a maximal inspiration.
- NV—4800 mL (in males) and 3200 mL (in females)
  VC = TLC − RV or VC = IRV + TV + ERV

Factors that Influence VC
- Respiratory muscle power
- Airway patency
- Compliance of the lung
- Elasticity of lung

Conditions Increasing and Decreasing VC

Increased in
- Swimmers and divers
- Trained athletes
- People living in high altitude

Decreased in
- Old age
- Lying posture
- Pregnancy
- Obesity
- Diseases, such as poliomyelitis, pleural effusion, asthma, emphysema, etc.

19. Functions of hypothalamus.

- Regulation of food intake
- Regulation of body temperature
- Regulation of thirst
- Regulation of anterior pituitary hormones
- Regulation of posterior pituitary hormones
- Regulation of sleep wake cycle
- Control of autonomic nervous system
- Control of reproduction
- Control of emotions
- Control of circadian rhythm
- Role in stress
- Role in visceral and somatic function
- Role in reward and punishment

Regulation of Food Intake
- There are 2 groups of neurons involved in food intake:
  1. **Ventromedial N (satiety center)**
  2. **Lateral N (feeding center)**
- Feeding center stimulates appetite and increases food intake and satiety center inhibits feeding center and brings satiety.

Regulation of Food Intake

These are the hypothesis regulating food-intake:
- **Glucostatic hypothesis:** Activity of satiety center is regulated by glucose utilization of the neurons. When the glucose utilization is low their activity is less and vice versa. When satiety center activity is less the feeding center's activity is unchecked and the person feels hungry. When utilization is high, the glucostats activity is unchecked and there is inhibition of feeding center and the person feels sated. Hypoglycemia is an appetite stimulant and the decrease in plasma glucose decreases the utilization of glucose by the cells.
- **Lipostatic hypothesis:** This hypothesis is based on the fact that the adipose tissues send humoral signals like leptin, a hormone secreted by adipose tissue. When fat depots are more, the leptin levels increase and it decreases food intake and increases energy output.
- **Gut-peptide theory:** After food intake, there are hormones released from the

GIT which act on the hypothalamus and thereby inhibits food intake
- **Thermostatic theory:** Food intake is increased in cold weather and decreased in warm weather.

Hormones and NT Regulating Food Intake

- **Hormones increasing food intake:**
  - Neuropeptide Y
  - Orexins
  - Ghrelin
  - MCH
  - AGRP (Agouti-related peptide)
  - Galanin
  - GHRH
- **Hormones decreasing food intake:**
  - Estrogen
  - Dopamine
  - α MSH
  - Cocaine- and amphetamine-regulated transcript (CART)
  - Corticotropin-releasing hormone (CRH)
  - Gut hormones
  - Cholecystokinin
  - Leptin

Temperature Regulation

- Humans need to maintain body temperature at 37°C.
- Preoptic region of anterior hypothalamus has a role in regulation of body temperature in warmth. When body temperature goes above set point it stimulates heat dissipating mechanisms like vasodilation and sweating.
- Posterior hypothalamus acts in cool temperature and involved in heat conserving mechanisms like vasoconstriction, piloerection and sympathetic stimulation.

Regulation of Thirst

- Thirst center is located in the hypothalamus.
- It is located in the lateral hypothalamus.
- It is stimulated by osmoreceptors in increase in tonicity of body fluids.
- A decrease in ECF volume also stimulates thirst center.

Regulation of ECF Volume

Achieved by regulation of ADH, aldosterone and thirst mechanism.

Regulation of Endocrine Functions

- Hypothalamus controls anterior pituitary and through anterior pituitary it regulates secretion of other endocrine glands.
- It secretes posterior pituitary hormones.
- Hypothalamus is considered to be the master of endocrine orchestra.
- It is a part of the brain and therefore is the link between neural and endocrine systems.

Control of Reproduction

- Hypothalamus releases GnRH which regulates the release of FSH and LH from anterior pituitary gland.
- They in turn control reproductive function in males and females.
- They regulate spermatogenesis, development of accessory sex organs in males and menstrual cycle and secondary sexual characteristics in females.
- Also the sexual behavior are influenced by hypothalamus (Preoptic and anterior hypothalamus)

Regulation of Sleep Wake Cycle

- Hypothalamus regulates sleep wake cycle.
- There are 2 sleep centers:
  1. Diencephalic sleep zone
  2. Basal forebrain sleep zone
- Stimulation of these areas at the frequency of 8 Hz induces slow wave sleep

Control of ANS

- Hypothalamus controls and integrates the activities of ANS.
- Through ANS, it is a major regulator of visceral activities.
- Stimulation of posterior hypothalamus- results in increase in HR, BP, pupillary dilatation, piloerection (sympathetic system stimulated).
- Stimulation of anterior hypothalamus results in decreased HR, increased HCl secretion, urination, etc. (Parasympathetic system stimulated).

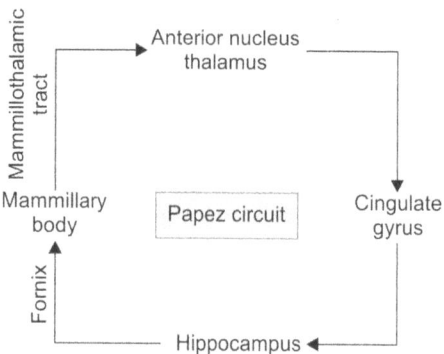

Fig. 18: Papez circuit.

Regulation of Emotional and Behavioral Patterns

☐ With the limbic system it participates in the expressions of emotions.
☐ The circuit given below is responsible for emotions (*refer* **Fig. 18**).

Regulation of Circadian Rhythm

☐ The suprachiasmatic nucleus establishes patterns of awakening and sleep that occur on a circadian (daily) schedule.
☐ This is mediated through retino-hypothalamic tract.

Example:

☐ Cortisol secretion
☐ Body temperature
☐ ACTH secretion
☐ Melatonin secretion
☐ Sleep-wakefulness

Regulation of Reward and Punishment Areas

☐ Hypothalamus along with LS and cortex integrate and bring about smooth responses for reward and punishment.
☐ VM nucleus is associated with reward and posterior and lateral N of hypothalamus with punishment.

---

20. Properties of synapse.

1. Summation—spatial or temporal
2. Convergence and divergence
3. One way conduction of impulses
4. Synaptic delay
5. Facilitation
6. Subliminal fringe
7. Occlusion
8. Synaptic plasticity and learning
9. Synaptic fatigue

1. **Summation:**
   - Summation means adding up of impulses. In the synapse following release of neurotransmitters there could be depolarization or hyperpolarization of the membrane. These are called as postsynaptic potentials and they belong to the category of graded potentials.
   - So these individual potentials from many synapses can summate and excite the membrane and take it to the firing level.
   - There are two types of summations—spatial and temporal summation.
     i. **Temporal summation:** The same input stimulates the postsynaptic neuron repeatedly and thereby excites it.
     ii. **Spatial summation:** Here many inputs stimulate simultaneously to excite it.

2. **Convergence and divergence:** When many presynaptic neurons end one postsynaptic neuron it is convergence and on presynaptic terminal divides and ends on many postsynaptic neurons—divergence.

3. **One way conduction:** Impulse transmission always happen from presynaptic to postsynaptic neurons as the receptors for the neurotransmitter released from presynaptic terminal is present on the postsynaptic membrane.

4. **Synaptic delay:** There are many steps involved in the impulse transmission from the presynaptic neuron to postsynaptic neuron so there is a delay of 0.5 msec in each synapse.

5. **Facilitation:**
   - When a single stimulus is applied to the neuron some response is obtained but if repeated stimuli are given the response is better than the single stimulus response.
   - So the previous stimulus has been facilitatory for the second and third one.

6. **Subliminal fringe:**
   - It is a partially excited stage of the neuron.
   - If two neurons are stimulated simultaneously the response obtained is more than the sum of stimulation of each neuron individually.
   - This is because some neurons are in a subliminal fringe.
7. **Occlusion:**
   - The response obtained by stimulating two presynaptic neurons together is less than the response obtained by stimulating each one individually.
   - This is because of common neurons in both the groups.
8. **Synaptic plasticity and learning:** The changes that occur in a synapse after repeated stimulation is called as synaptic plasticity
9. **Synaptic fatigue:** On repeated stimulation, the synapse goes in for fatigue due to exhaustion of neurotransmitters.

III. SHORT ANSWERS

1. Positive feedback mechanism.

- Most of the control systems in the body are negative feedback regulations.
- There are negative and positive feedback mechanisms.

Positive Feedback Mechanism

- In positive feedback regulation, the output of the control system is enhanced or amplified so that controlled variable continues to move in the direction of the initial change, e.g., parturition reflex (refer **Fig. 19**).
- Positive feedback occurs in only certain instances whereas the negative feedback regulation is the most common one happening in the body.

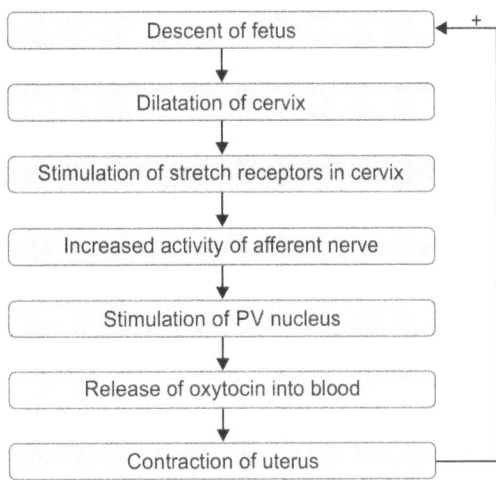

Fig. 19: Parturition reflex (positive feedback regulation).

2. Rigor mortis.

- Rigor mortis is stiffening of muscles after the death of an individual.
- Stiffness is due to sustained attachment of myosin heads to the actin filament due to loss of ATP.
- After myosin cross-bridge attachment to actin filament, removal of the cross-bridge needs attachment of an ATP molecule.
- After death, there is no more ATP synthesized therefore the myosin heads stay attached to actin filament resulting in stiffness of muscle.
- Rigidity disappears after some hours due to release of enzymes from lysosomes which will digest the muscle proteins.
- The appearance and disappearance of rigor mortis is used to identify the time of death.

3. Polycythemia.

Polycythemia is increase in the RBC count above the normal value. It can be physiological or pathological.

Physiological Polycythemia

- **Age:** At birth, the count is high (6–7 million cells/cumm) and after birth it starts decreasing due to destruction of RBCs.
- **High altitude:** Hypoxia in high altitude stimulates production of erythropoietin which in turn stimulates RBC production.
- Excessive exercise

Pathological Polycythemia—2 Types

1. **Primary polycythemia or polycythemia vera:** It is said to be a member of myeloproliferative syndrome and is due to the

cancerous condition of the bone marrow. The counts increase more than 10 million cells/cu mm. A high WBC count may also be seen. In this condition erythropoietin levels may be very low.

2. **Secondary polycythemia:** It happens due to hypoxic conditions in the body as in lung (Emphysema, COPD) and cardiovascular diseases (Cyanotic heart diseases). The hypoxia stimulates synthesis of erythropoietin and thereby increased production of RBCs.

Complications of Polycythemia

Increase in RBC count, increases the viscosity of blood and thereby increases the peripheral resistance leading to hypertension and left heart failure.

4. Bombay blood group.

Antigens of ABO blood group systems are glycoproteins and glycolipids. They are attached to H antigen on the RBC membrane. H antigen is a product of H gene. If N-galactosamine is attached to H antigen, A antigen is derived and the blood group is A. If galactose is attached to H antigen then B antigen is derived and the blood group is B. If both N-galactosamine and galactose are attached the blood group is AB and if only H antigen is present the blood group is O.

In few individuals, there is absence of H antigen due to absence of H gene. If routine blood grouping is done, these individuals will be considered as having O blood group. But their serum will contain anti-A, anti-B and anti-H antibodies. So they have to be transfused only with Bombay blood group.

5. Tubuloglomerular feedback.

- Tubuloglomerular (TG) feedback is an autoregulatory mechanism in the kidneys to regulate the renal blood flow (RBF) and thereby glomerular filtration rate (GFR).
- This feedback mechanism is dependent on the NaCl content in tubular fluid.
- NaCl content in the tubular fluid is sensed by macula densa cells and signals are sent to the afferent arterioles to regulate RBF and GFR.
- Increased renal arterial pressure increases glomerular capillary pressure and thereby increases filtration.
- Increased GFR leads to increased NaCl content in the tubular fluid. This is sensed by Macula densa cells and they send signals to cause vasoconstriction of afferent arterioles and thereby decreases RBF and GFR and NaCl content is brought back to normal.
- If NaCl content is less, it is sensed by the macula densa cells and signals are sent to afferent arterioles resulting in vasodilation followed by increased RBF and GFR.
- The chemicals mediating this feedback may be thromboxane A_2 or adenosine for vasoconstriction and nitric oxide (NO) for vasodilation and they are released by the macula densa cells.

6. Functions of large intestine.

- It acts as a reservoir for undigested food material and they are stored here till they are expelled as feces.
- **Absorption:** The most important components absorbed in the colon are water and electrolytes. The large absorptive capacity of colon can be used to instill certain drugs like anesthetics, analgesics, etc., through the colon.
- **Formation of feces:** The undigested residue of the food substances are made into formed fecal matter in the colon.
- **Colonic bacteria:** Colon has large numbers of beneficial bacteria which helps to form many useful substances like vitamin K, B complex vitamins and folic acid.
- Short-chain fatty acids are also synthesized in the large intestine by action of intestinal bacteria on complex carbohydrates, resistant starch and other dietary fibers.
- Goblet cells in the mucosa of large intestine produce large volume of mucus which helps in smooth passage of feces.
- Alkaline nature (pH 8) of large intestinal secretion neutralizes acids formed by bacteria on feces.

- Undigested cellulose, hemicellulose and some fats are digested by the colonic bacteria.
- Heavy metals, such as lead, mercury, etc., are excreted through feces.

7. Migrating motor complex.

- MMCs are the type of movements seen in the GIT during the interdigestive period. These movements are initiated in the stomach and they migrate to the distal ileum. Each cycle of the MMCs have 3 phases.
  - *Phase I:* It start as a quiescent phase.
  - *Phase II:* The next phase has irregular electrical and mechanical activity
  - *Phase III:* The phase with a regular burst of activity.
- These waves occur at an interval of 90 minutes and they travel at the rate of 5 cm/min. They are accompanied by increased secretion of gastric juice, bile and pancreatic juices.
- MMCs are said to clear the lumen of the stomach and intestines and prepare it for receiving the next meal.
- They are stimulated by the GI hormone motilin secreted from the stomach, small and large intestines.
- These waves come to a halt immediately following intake of food after which peristalsis starts.

8. Diabetes insipidus.

It is of two types—neurogenic or central diabetes insipidus and nephrogenic diabetes insipidus.
1. **Neurogenic diabetes insipidus:** There is defect in synthesis of ADH from hypothalamus
2. **Nephrogenic diabetic insipidus:** Here the synthesis and secretion of ADH is normal but there could be congenital defects of receptors to ADH or mutations of genes for aquaporins and defects in aquaporins, the water channels on the luminal side of principal cells of collecting duct. Symptoms of DI are polyuria, polydipsia.
   They pass a large volume (up to 23 L/day) of hypotonic urine (30 mosm/kg H_2O).

9. Features of Cushing syndrome.

It is due to **hypersecretion of glucocorticoids**.

Causes

- Pharmacological use of exogenous glucocorticoids—ACTH levels are low here.
- ACTH secreting pituitary tumor—Cushing's disease—ACTH levels are high, skin pigmentation present (because of MSH like activity of ACTH).
- Primary hypercortisolism due to adrenal tumor—ACTH levels are low

Symptoms

- Obesity with characteristic centripetal distribution of fat, sparing the limbs.
- Face is rounded and cheeks red due to polycythemia.
- Loss of bone mass → osteoporosis → vertebral fractures and necrosis of hip.
- Increased protein catabolism → atrophy and weakness of skeletal muscles
- Poor wound healing and response to infection due to loss of protein.
- Disturbances in glucose metabolism—blood glucose levels are high resulting in glucose intolerance, insulin resistance, hyperglycemia or even diabetes mellitus.
- Mineralocorticoid activity of glucocorticoids leads to Na^+ and H_2O retention → hypertension.
- Excess androgen secretion in women → hirsutism, male pattern baldness, clitoral enlargement.

10. Male contraception.

Temporary Methods

1. Natural method
2. Barrier method
3. Pills

1. **Natural method or coitus interruptus:** Withdrawal of penis before ejaculation prevents deposition of semen in the vagina. This method needs practice and timing is very important. The disadvantages are that the precoital secretions may contain sperms and it can lead to pregnancy.

2. **Barrier method:** Condoms are the widely used barrier method in males. It is made of fine latex sheet. It prevents deposition of semen in the vagina and prevents fertilization of ovum. It can be used to prevent transmission of sexually transmitted diseases.
3. **Pills:**
   - Drugs are used to inhibit spermatogenesis.
   - Gossypol and testosterone are used.
   - **Gossypol:** It is derived from cottonseed oil. It decreases sperm count.
   - **Testosterone:** High testosterone levels inhibit sperm production.

Permanent Methods

Vasectomy: A small portion of vas deferens is removed after clamping. Both the open ends are ligated and sutured.

---
11. Triple response.

Vascular response of skin to injury with a sharp pointed object—triple response.

Red Reaction
- Occurs within 10 secs when stroked firmly by a sharp object
- Due to capillary dilatation

Wheal
- Swelling within (local edema) few minutes after red reaction.
- There is ↑in permeability of capillaries due to histamine.

Flare
- Spreading out of redness from site of injury
- Due to arteriolar dilatation.
- Due to axon reflex

Axon Reflex
- When there is an injury to skin with a sharp object, impulses from the skin carried by sensory fibers not only go to the spinal cord but also goes antidromically through other branches to the arterioles below the skin (*refer* **Fig. 20**).
- The neurotransmitter released here is Substance P.

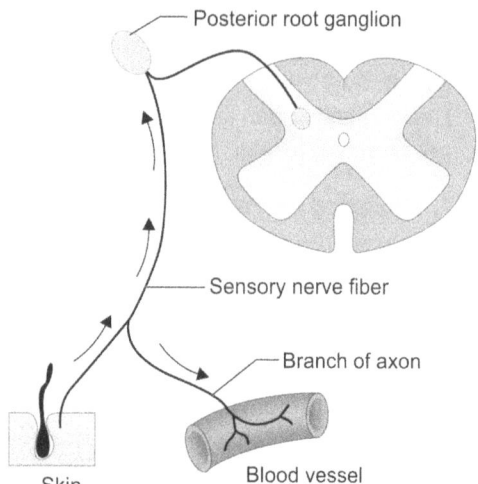

Fig. 20: Axon reflex. Sensory fibers give a branch which travels antidromically to supply arterioles below the skin.

- This causes vasodilatation and extravasation of fluid.

---
12. Bainbridge reflex.
- In a person with low heart rate when rapid infusion of saline is done there is a rapid rise in heart rate.
- This reflex was described by Bainbridge in 1915 and therefore called as Bainbridge reflex.
- It is a true reflex and the afferents are the vagal afferents. The impulses cause a decrease in vagal tone and thereby increase the heart rate.
- This reflex can be blocked by application of atropine or vagotomy
- The receptors are tachycardia-producing atrial receptors.

---
13. Residual volume.
It is the volume of air that remains in the lung after a forceful expiration. Normal value is 1200 mL in males and 1100 mL in females.

---
14. Artificial respiration.
When there is respiratory deficiency or respiratory arrest then artificial respiration is given.

Conditions: Drowning, gas poisoning, electric shock, anesthesia, accidents, etc.

Methods: Instrumental and manual methods.

Instrumental Methods
- Used when there is a need for prolonged support.
- **Three types:**
  1. Positive pressure method
  2. Negative pressure method
  3. Boyles apparatus

Positive Pressure Method
- Used in operation theaters
- Here air or O_2 mixture is used to inflate the lungs at positive pressures either continuously or intermittently.
- It impairs venous return.

Negative Pressure Method
- Achieved by alternate compression and relaxing the chest wall.
- **They are:**
  - Drinker's method (iron lung chamber)
  - Bragg-Paul method—use of hollow elastic rubber bag.
  - Others

Drinker's method (Iron lung method):
- The instrument contains an airtight iron chamber with a bellow on one side of the instrument.
- When the bellow moves in and out it creates a rise and fall of pressure inside the chamber.
- The person is placed inside the chamber with the head and neck outside the chamber.
- When the pressure rises inside the chamber expiration happens for the patient and when the pressure falls in the chamber there is inspiration.

Bragg-Paul Method
- Here an elastic rubber bag is tied around the chest of the patient.
- The bag is connected to a pump which can inflate and deflate the bag.
- When the bag is inflated it compresses the chest and air is expired.
- When the pressure is released, the chest enlarges passively and air is drawn in.

Boyles Apparatus
This apparatus is used in the hospitals for artificial ventilation. It is an automatic instrument in which rate and depth of ventilation and composition of inspired can be altered.

Manual Methods

Holger Nielsen Method
- The subject is made to lie prone and the head is turned to one side **(Fig. 21A)**.
- The shoulder is abducted and flexed at the elbow and the hands are placed under the cheek.
- The operator is in kneeling position at the head of the patient and he places his hands spread on the back of the subject and bends forward to press on his back **(Fig. 21B)**.
- The pressure on the back of the subject and compresses on the chest and expels the air out **(Fig. 21C)**.
- Then he holds the arm above the elbow of the subject and pulls the arm forward **(Fig. 21D)**.
- This enlarges the chest and results in inspiration. It is repeated 12/min. This is an exhaustive method for the examiner.

Eve's Rocking Method
- Here the subject is made to lie prone on board which is rocketed on a pivot so that it can move up and down like a see-saw.
- When the board is tilted head down, the abdominal organs push on the diaphragm resulting decrease in thoracic volume and expiration happens.
- When the board is tilted in the opposite direction the inspiration happens.

Mouth-to-mouth Respiration
- It can be direct or indirect method. In direct method the operator places his mouth directly on the subject's mouth and in indirect method it is done with a small tube.
- The subject is made to lie supine; the airway is kept clean from vomitus, foreign body, etc.

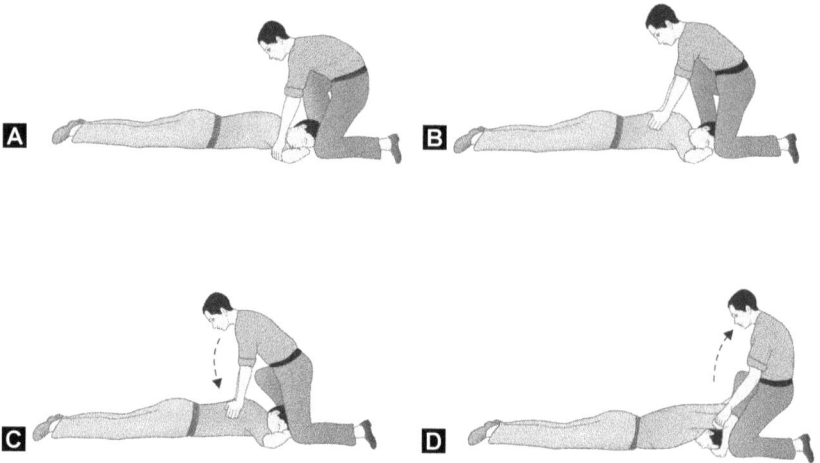

Figs. 21A to D: Holger Nielsen method of artificial respiration.

- The subject's head is extended, the operator sits on the side of the subject holds the lower jaw with his left hand and opens the mouth and with his right hand clips the nostrils.
- The operator then inhales deeply and places his mouth on the subject's mouth or the tube placed in the subject's mouth and blows into the subject's mouth smoothly, volume twice that of the tidal volume.
- This inflates the lungs of the subject and then the examiner removes his mouth from the subject's mouth and the lungs recoil resulting in expiration.
- It is repeated 12 times a minute.
- **Advantages:** Can be applied immediately, can achieve large tidal volumes, CO_2 stimulates respiration, simple technique.
- **Disadvantages:** Infection may spread, volunteer may get exhausted.

15. Functions of middle ear.

- **Middle ear:** It is an air-filled cavity in temporal bone. It starts at the tympanic membrane and ends at oval window.
- **Contains:** 3 ossicles (malleus, incus and stapes), 2 small muscles (tensor tympani and stapedius), ligaments, nerves, blood vessels, etc.
- **Functions:**
  - *Tympanic reflex:* It is a protective reflex. When a loud sound is transmitted through the ossicles in middle ear a reflex is initiated with a latent period of 40–80 msec. Contraction of stapedius and tensor tympani pulls the tympanic membrane medially and membrane covering oval window laterally. This makes the ossicular system rigid and there is reduction in transmission of sounds. This reduces the intensity of sound by 30–40 decibels. It is also called as **attenuation reflex**.

  Functions of this reflex:
  - This reflex protects the cochlea from damaging loud sounds.
  - It filters the low frequency sounds
  - It prevents hearing one's own speech
  - Transmission of sound waves from external ear to internal ear
  - *Impedance matching:*
    - As the sound waves travel from rarer (air in external and middle ear) to denser medium (Fluid in the inner ear) they are dampened (by 30 db).
    - This loss in sound energy is prevented in the middle ear by impedance matching which is:
      - By area differences
      - By lever action
      - By buckling factor
    1. **Area difference:** Area of tympanic membrane is greater than foot-plate of stapes and

therefore there is convergence of sound and pressure is increased by 17 times.
2. **Lever** action of the ossicles increases pressure by 1.32 times
3. **Buckling factor:** Tympanic membrane is conical in shape and the handle of malleus is attached to the umbo. As the tympanic membrane moves in and out, the buckling of membrane moves the handle of malleus less and this increases the force and decreases the velocity.

16. Features of Parkinsonism.

- Also called as **paralysis agitans**.
- Due to destruction of nigrostriatal dopaminergic neurons, to putamen is mostly affected.
- **Causes:**
  - Primary or idiopathic
  - Complication of drugs—phenothiazines
- **Characterized by:**
  - *Hyperkinetic features:*
    - Rigidity—lead pipe or cogwheel
    - Tremors—resting tremors, at 6–8 Hz frequency
  - *Hypokinesia:*
    - Weakness of movements and lack of initiation of movements—**Akinesia**
    - Bradykinesia
  - Lack of automated movements
  - Mask like face without expression
  - Festinant or short shuffling gait—patient walks in an attitude like he is going to catch the center of gravity
- **Treatment:**
  - Treatment with L-Dopa rather than Dopamine as it cannot cross the blood brain barrier
  - Bromocriptine, a dopamine agonist can also be used
  - Anticholinergics like atropine, tries to reduce the acetylcholine levels in basal ganglia and regulates the ratio between dopamine and acetylcholine
  - L-deprenyl
  - Dopamine agonists like bromocriptine
- Transplantation of adrenal medulla in BG
- Implantation of fetal BG

17. Papez circuit.

Papez circuit is responsible for expression of emotions.

It connects the limbic system and thalamus (*refer* **Fig. 18**).

18. Name to facilitatory and inhibitory neurotransmitters and their sites of action.

- Facilitatory neurotransmitters—glutamate and aspartate
- Inhibitory neurotransmitters—glycine and GABA
- Glutamate acts in the cerebral cortex and brainstem. Aspartate acts in the visual cortex.
- Glycine is present in the neurons mediating direct inhibition in spinal cord, brainstem, forebrain and retina.
- GABA acts in cerebellum, basal ganglia, cerebral cortex and neurons mediating presynaptic inhibition.

19. Saltatory conduction.

- In myelinated axons, the action potentials are generated only at the nodes of Ranvier. This part of the axon is exposed to ECF.
- Voltage-gated Na^+ channels are concentrated in the nodes of Ranvier and the myelin sheath in the subsequent area acts as an insulator.
- So the current sinks move from one node to another node rather than exciting the neighboring area as in unmyelinated axon.
- This type of impulse conduction is called as saltatory conduction (*refer* **Fig. 14B**).
- Since the impulses jump across nodes it can travel faster and impulses are conducted 50–100 times faster than the unmyelinated fibers.

20. Sensations carried by posterior column.

- Fine touch
- Conscious proprioception
- Two-point discrimination

- Tactile localization
- Stereognosis
- Pressure
- Vibration sense

21. Reticulocyte response.

It is the rapid increase and release of newly formed red blood cells and reticulocytes into the circulation following treatment for certain types of anemias like vitamin B_{12} deficiency or iron deficiency anemias. Reticulocyte response indicates a favorable response to treatment with vitamin B_{12} or iron.

22. Clot retraction.

- Clot retraction is a function of platelets
- Within 15–30 minutes of formation of clot, the clot shrinks and exudes serum. This process is called clot retraction.
- Platelets have contractile proteins, such as actin and myosin which can change the shape of platelets and make them contractile.
- This shrinking of all the platelets trapped in the fibrin mesh makes the clot a firm structure and also brings the injured walls closer so that healing happens faster.
- Since clot retraction is a function of platelets the clot retraction time is used for assessing platelet function.

23. Sodium potassium pump.

- It is present in all cells of the body.
- It is an electrogenic pump as it pumps 3 Na^+ out of the cell and 2 K^+ into the cell. It catalyzes hydrolysis of ATP and uses the energy to move the ions.
- Its activity is inhibited by ouabain and digitalis used for heart failure.
- It has α and β subunits. Na^+ and K^+ are transported through α subunit. α subunit is larger and has intracellular Na^+ and ATP binding sites and a phosphorylation site.
- When Na^+ binds to α subunit, ATP also binds and is converted to ADP and the P is added to phosphorylation site.
- This changes the configuration of the pump and extrudes Na^+ into ECF. K^+ then binds extracellularly, dephosphorylating α subunit and comes back to original configuration and releases K^+ intracellularly.
- β-subunit is a glycoprotein and has no transport action but its presence is needed for pump activity.
- Extracellularly there are binding sites for K^+ and ouabain.
- Pump activity is regulated by 2nd messengers and hormones.
- Thyroid hormone, aldosterone and insulin increase the pump activity, whereas dopamine decreases the pump activity.
- It pumps out 3 Na^+ molecules from ICF to ECF and takes in 2 molecules of K^+. When Na^+ is pumped out water also move along with it. Thereby it maintains cell volume and prevents rupture of cell.
- It maintains the resting membrane potential of the cell. This is essential for transmission of impulses in nerves and muscles.
- It is the major energy-using process of the cells in the body and therefore it is responsible for the basal metabolic rate.
- It maintains a high intracellular K^+ levels and a high Na^+ concentration in the ECF.

24. Name the muscle proteins. What is the role of troponin C in muscle contraction?

The proteins in skeletal muscles are; contractile proteins—actin and myosin, regulatory proteins are—troponin I, C and T and tropomyosin. Structural proteins are—actinin, titin and desmin.

Troponin C binds with calcium ions and binding of calcium initiates muscle contraction.

25. Role of *H. pylori* in peptic ulcer.

High acid content in the stomach can damage the gastric and duodenal mucosa and cause peptic ulcer. This is prevented by the presence of the 'mucosal barrier'. This barrier is made up of:

- **Mucus** secreted by the neck cells and surface mucosal cells.
- **Prostaglandins** secreted by epithelial cells have antisecretory activity (for HCl) and increases HCO_3 and mucus secretion.

- **Epithelial barrier**—low permeability due to tight junctions between epithelial cells, rapid turnover of lining cells and HCO_3, mucus secretions from there.
- **Bicarbonate secretion** from gastric mucosal cells increases the pH.

When this barrier is disrupted it leads to peptic ulcer. *Helicobacter pylori* disrupts this barrier and thereby is responsible for inducing ulcer. This can be eradicated by giving appropriate antibiotics.

26. Gastrocolic reflex.

Intake of food → distension of stomach with food → contraction of rectum → desire to defecate. This reflex is due to action of gastrin on colon. Because of this reflex defecation after a meal is a regular activity of children. In adults, habits, cultural and social factors play a role in defecation.

27. Physiological basis of treatment of diarrhea.

- Diarrhea is treated with ORS (oral rehydration solution). It helps to replace the salts and water lost. The solution contains a mixture of sodium and glucose.
- Physiological basis of using such a combination is due to the presence of the secondary active transporter sodium-glucose symport (SGLT1) in the luminal membrane of the epithelial cells in the intestinal mucosa.
- The presence of glucose in the intestinal lumen facilitates reabsorption of sodium through SGLT1. This is the reason the ORS contains sodium and glucose
- Following absorption of sodium, water is also reabsorbed.
- Cereals containing carbohydrates can also be used.

28. Anion gap.

- Anion gap refers to the difference in plasma concentration of cations (other than Na^+) and concentration of anions (other than Cl^- and HCO_3^-) and consists mostly of proteins which are anionic, HPO_4^-, SO_4^{2-} and organic acids.
- The normal value is 12 mEq/L. It is used to differentiate between types of metabolic acidosis.

Factors which increase anion gap:
- Decrease in plasma concentration of Ca^{2+}, K^+ or Mg^{2+}.
- Increase in concentration of plasma proteins
- Increase in plasma levels of organic anions like lactate or foreign anions.

Factors which decrease anion gap:
- When the above cation levels are increased in the plasma
- When the plasma albumin levels are decreased

Anion gap is increased in:
- Diabetic ketoacidosis
- Lactic acidosis
- All forms of acidosis

29. Radioimmunoassay.

- It is a highly sensitive method to measure hormone levels in blood.
- First step is to produce an antibody for the hormone to be tested.
- Small quantity of antibody is mixed with the sample to be measured
- Some quantity of antibody is mixed with a standard hormone tagged with radioactive isotope
- There should be too little antibody for the tagged hormone and the hormone in the sample to be assayed to compete for binding sites in antibody.
- After binding of both have reached equilibrium the antibody-hormone complex is separated from the solution and the quantity of radioactive hormone bound is measured by radioactive techniques.
- If large amount of radioactive hormone was bound it is known that the natural hormone levels are low in the assay sample and vice versa.
- To make the test more quantitative, the same procedure is performed for standard solutions of untagged hormone at various concentrations and a standard curve is plotted.

- By comparing the radioactive counts recorded from the unknown sample with the standard curve the concentration of hormone in the sample can be determined with an error of 10–15%

30. List the differences between dwarfism and cretinism.

Features	Dwarfism	Cretinism
Causes	Deficiency of growth hormone in childhood	Deficiency of thyroid hormone in infancy
Height	Short statured	Short statured
Proportionate growth retardation	Yes	Yes
Mental development	Normal	Mental retardation is present
Face	Immature facies	Idiotic face
Sexual maturity	May/may not be absent	Delayed sexual maturity
Organomegaly	Absent	Present, resulting in pot belly, enlarged tongue.

31. Reynolds number.

- The blood flow in a straight vessel is laminar or streamline. The velocity of blood flow in the center of the stream is greatest and lowest immediately below the vessel wall.
- Laminar flow occurs at velocities up to a level called as the **critical velocity**.
- At or above this velocity, the flow becomes turbulent.
- Laminar flow is silent but turbulent flow creates sounds.
- The probability of turbulence is also related to diameter of vessel and viscosity of blood.
- This **is given as the Reynolds number (Re)**
  $Re = \rho DV/\eta$
  ρ = Density of fluid
  D = Diameter of tube
  V = Velocity of flow
  η = Viscosity of fluid
- Higher the value of Re greater is the turbulence
- When D is in cm, V is in cm/s^{-1}, η is in poises, flow is not turbulent if Re is <2000. When Re > 3000 there is always turbulent flow.

32. Jugular venous pulse.

JVP tracing is recorded from internal jugular vein. It reflects the pressure changes in the right atrium as there are no valves in this vein and therefore any pressure change in right atrium is reflected to this vein.

The JVP tracing has three positive waves and two negative waves.

They are:
- **'a' wave:** Atrial contraction
- **'c' wave:** Due to bulging of tricuspid valve into right atrium during onset of ventricular systole
- **'v':** Due to atrial filling
- **'x' descent:** Fall in atrial pressure due to its relaxation
- **'y' descent:** Due to emptying of blood from right atrium to right ventricle (*refer* Fig. 22).

Conditions Altering JVP
- **Increased JVP:**
  - Right heart failure
  - Superior vena caval obstruction
  - Congestive cardiac failure
  - Constrictive pericarditis

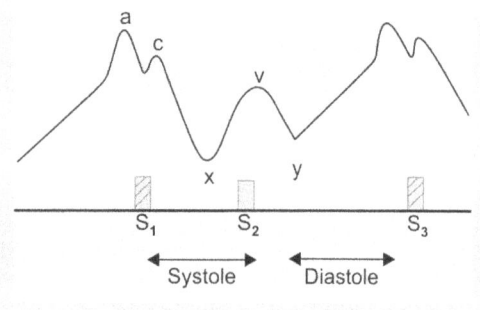

Fig. 22: Jugular venous pulse; a, c and v are positive waves, x and y are negative waves.

☐ **Prominent a wave:**
- Pulmonary stenosis
- Pulmonary hypertension
- Tricuspid stenosis

☐ **Canon wave or giant 'a' wave:** Right atrium contracts with closed tricuspid valve
- Complete heart block

33. Lead II ECG.

Normal ECG in Lead II

☐ Lead II is a bipolar limb lead between right arm (negative electrode) and left arm (Positive electrode.
☐ The ECG tracing in lead II shows both negative and positive deflections equally and therefore used as a standard recording (*refer* **Fig. 23**).
☐ There are intervals and segments in the ECG.

ECG Waves

☐ There are positive and negative waves are deflections in the ECG tracing.
☐ There are 4 waveforms: P wave, QRS complex, T wave and U wave.
  1. *P wave:* This is the first positive wave in ECG and is due to atrial depolarization. Duration is 0.1 second
  2. *QRS complex:* Consists of a negative Q wave, positive R wave and negative s wave. This complex is due to ventricular depolarization. Normal duration is 0.08 seconds.

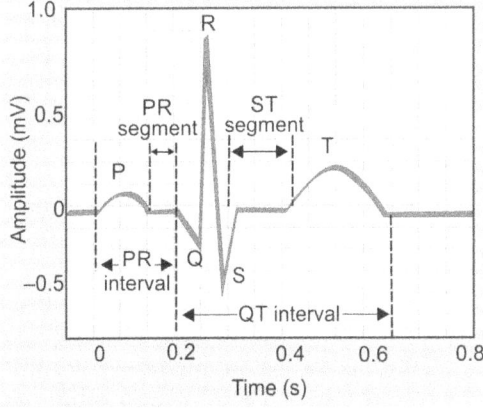

Fig. 23: ECG tracing in lead II.

  3. *T wave:* It is a positive deflection following QRS complex and is due to ventricular repolarization. Normal duration is 0.27 seconds
  4. *U wave:* It is also positive deflection and is normally not seen. It is seen in slow depolarization of the papillary muscle. Duration is 0.08 seconds.

ECG Segments

☐ These are isoelectric lines seen in between the ECG waves.
☐ There are two segments—PR segment and ST segment
  1. *PR segment:* It starts at the end of P wave to beginning of QRS complex.
  2. *ST segment:* It begins in the end of QRS complex and is up to the beginning of T wave.

ECG Intervals

☐ Intervals in ECG include waves and segments.
☐ The intervals are—PR interval, QT interval, ST interval, PP interval and RR interval.
☐ **J point:** This is an indicator of end of ventricular depolarization and start of ventricular repolarization. It is at the end of QRS and is at the isoelectric line.
☐ *PR interval:* It is between beginning of P wave to beginning of Q wave.
☐ The normal duration is 0.12–0.2 seconds (Average 0.18 sec).
  - This denotes atrial depolarization and conduction to AV node.
  - Prolonged PR interval signifies AV conduction block
- *QT interval:* It starts at Q wave and ends with T wave.
  - Normal duration is 0.4 seconds.
  - It denotes the systolic phase of the ventricle
  - It is prolonged in ventricular conduction defects, hypocalcemia and myocardial ischemia.
- *ST interval:* It is from the end of S wave to the end of T wave.
  - Normal duration is 0.32 seconds.
  - It denotes ventricular repolarization

- *PP interval:* It is the interval between two successive P waves.
  - It denotes the diastolic phase of the atria.
- *RR interval:* It is the interval between two successive R waves.
  - It is used to calculate the heart rate

34. Bohr's effect.

- Decrease in O_2 affinity of hemoglobin when pH of blood falls is called the **Bohr's effect**. This signifies that deoxyhemoglobin has more affinity for H^+ than oxyhemoglobin.
- It happens at the tissue level.
- In the tissue level, CO_2 release is more and this increases pCO_2 in blood which shifts the oxygen-Hb dissociation curve to the right (decreases Hb affinity for O_2) and releases O_2.
- The unsaturation of hemoglobin at the tissue level is due to decrease in PO_2 but an extra 1–2% of unsaturation is due to the rise in PCO_2 and thereby shift of curve to right (Bohr effect)

35. Dead space.

- Dead space is the space in the airways in which the volume of air present does not take part in gaseous exchange.
- There are 3 types of dead spaces—anatomical dead space, alveolar dead space and physiological or total dead space.
  1. **Anatomical dead space** is the conducting zone of the respiratory pathway in which the gaseous exchange does not take place and the volume of air is said to be the dead space air.
  2. **Alveolar dead space** is the alveoli which do not have blood supply and the volume of air in these alveoli do not take part in gas exchange and is considered to be wasted ventilation.
  3. **Physiological dead space** is the sum of the above two dead spaces.

Since in normal conditions there are no alveolar dead spaces, physiological dead space is equal to anatomical dead space.

In a normal adult, of the 500 mL of tidal volume inhaled, 150 mL remains in the anatomical dead space, which is also the physiological dead space.

36. Functions of somatosensory area.

Major functions of parietal lobe are somatosensory in nature. It is posterior to the frontal lobe and is posteriorly separated from occipital lobe by the calcarine fissure and laterally from temporal lobe by the Sylvian fissure.

The areas in this lobe are areas 3, 1, 2, 5, 7, SSII, 39 and 43 (*refer* **Fig. 24**).

Functions:
- Perception of somatic sensations, such as touch, pressure, vibration, pain, etc.
- Spatial recognition, two-point discrimination and tactile localization.
- Since taste area is in this lobe, perception of taste is a function
- Area 39 helps in language and speech.
- Area 5 and 7 help in stereognosis and hand-eye coordination
- Also involved in learning and memory
- Helpful in recognition of different intensities of stimuli

37. Stretch reflex.

Stretch Reflex
- It is a monosynaptic reflex integrated at the level of spinal cord and helps in regulating the length of the muscle. The components of the reflex arc are:
- **Stimulus:** Stretch of the muscle
- **Receptor:** Muscle spindle
- **Afferent nerve:** Ia and II sensory fibers
- **Center:** Spinal cord
- **Efferent nerve:** Alpha motor nerve fiber
- **Effector:** Extrafusal muscle fiber
- **Response:** Contraction of extrafusal fibers (*refer* **Fig. 25**).

38. REM sleep.

- Sleep is said to be a state of altered consciousness or partial unconsciousness from which a person can be aroused.
- Sleep deprivation results in impaired attention, learning and performance.
- Sleep has two components—nonrapid eye movement (NREM) and rapid eye movement (REM) sleep

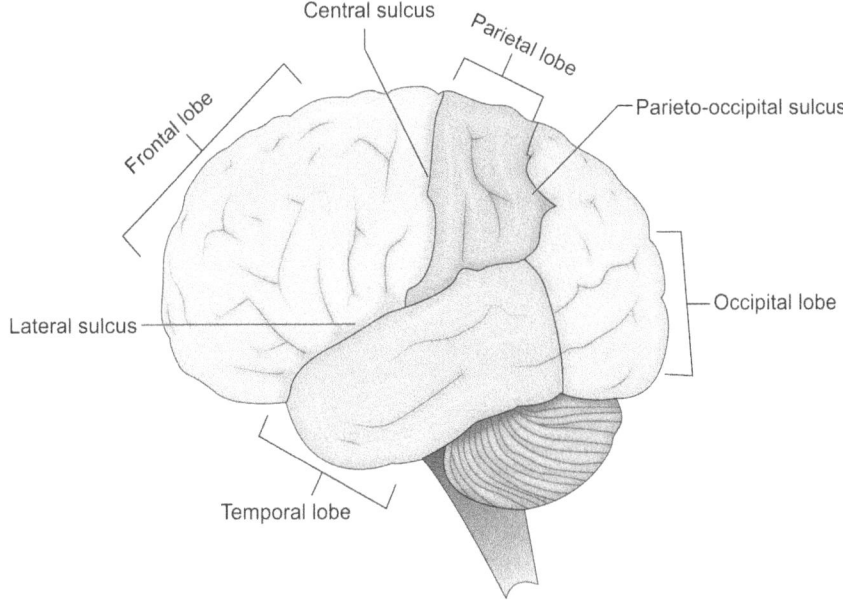

Fig. 24: Parietal lobe.

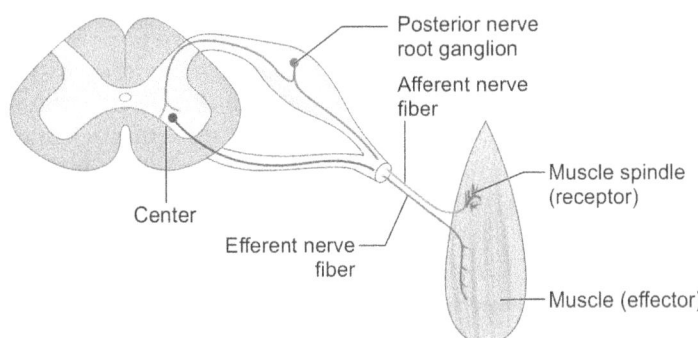

Fig. 25: Stretch reflex pathway.

REM Sleep

- In a period of sleep of 7–8 hours, REM and NREM sleep phases alternate.
- REM sleep occurs 3–5 times during the sleep period alternating with NREM sleep.
- Initial episode of REM sleep will be lasting for 10–20 minutes. Then with each episode, it prolongs and the final episode is for 50 minutes.
- In adults, REM sleep totals for about 90–120 minutes. With increasing age, period of REM sleep decreases.
- About 50% of an infants' sleep is REM sleep. 35% for 2-year-old infant and 25% for adults.
- REM sleep is thought to be important for maturation of brain in infants. This has been identified by the high percentage of REM sleep in infants.

Physiological Changes in REM Sleep

- Most of the dreaming occurs in REM sleep. These dreams can be remembered.
- Eyes move rapidly back and forth under the eyelid.
- Neuronal activities are higher—brain blood flow and O_2 use is high.
- EEG recordings are similar to that of an active and awake person.
- Excepting the motor neurons governing respiration and eye, impulses in most of them are inhibited.
- Inhibition of motor neurons results in loss of muscle tone and even some time paralysis.

- Parasympathetic activity increases and sympathetic activity decreases → decrease in HR and BP.
- Periodically sympathetic activity is also increased.
- Bruxism, erection of penis and twitching of facial muscles are seen in REM sleep.

Control of REM Sleep

- NREM and REM sleep are mediated by different parts of the brain.
- REM sleep—neurons in pons and mid brain.

39. Features of dark adaptation.

- When a person moves from a brightly illuminated place to a dark environment, he is not able to see anything. But gradually the eyes get accommodated to the darkness and his vision improves. This is said to be **dark adaptation**. Complete adaptation happens in 20 minutes.
- The changes happening in the eye in darkness are—dilatation of pupil, shifting of cone vision to rod vision and regeneration of rhodopsin in darkness.
- The changes happening are discussed under neural adaptation and chemical adaptation.

Neural Adaptation

- The dark adaptation happens in two phases.
- The first phase is due to cone adaptation and it happens in the first 5–10 minutes.
- This increases the retinal sensitivity to light 100 times.
- In the second phase of adaptation, the rod sensitivity to light increases and the retinal sensitivity increases by 1000–10,000 times.
- Once rod adaptation has happened even a single photon of light is visible to the eye.

Chemical Adaptation

- When a person stays in bright light, the rod pigment rhodopsin is bleached and is converted to all-trans-retinal and opsin.
- Therefore, rods are insensitive to light and do not respond to light.
- The rod sensitivity can increase only when the rhodopsin is re-synthesized

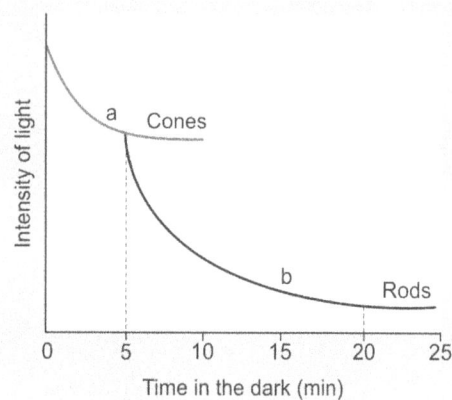

Fig. 26: Dark adaptation curve. There are two curves, curve a shows cone adaptation and curve b shows rod adaptation.

and this takes several minutes to happen.
- That is why the dark adaptation by rods takes 20 minutes (*refer* **Fig. 26**).
- The rods are present in the retina 15–20 degrees away from the fovea. That is the reason there is dilatation of the pupil to expose the retina rich in rods to light.
- The time taken for dark adaptation depends on the degree of brightness of light to which the eye is exposed and for how long it is being exposed.
- Brighter the light and longer the duration later it takes for dark adaptation.

40. Stapedial reflex.

It is a protective reflex. When a loud sound is transmitted through the ossicles in middle ear a reflex is initiated with a latent period of 40–80 msec. Contraction of stapedius and tensor tympani pulls the tympanic membrane medially and membrane covering oval window laterally. This makes the ossicular system rigid and there is reduction in transmission of sounds. This reduces the intensity of sound by 30–40 decibels. It is also called as **attenuation reflex/tympanic reflex**.

Functions of this reflex:

- This reflex protects the cochlea from damaging loud sounds.
- It filters the low frequency sounds
- It prevents hearing one's own speech

Answers to 2018 Question Paper

ANSWER ALL QUESTIONS

I. Essay Questions (10 Marks each)

1. Explain in detail synthesis, secretion, and functions of thyroid hormone. Add a note on cretinism.
2. Describe the classification, connections, and functions of cerebellum.
3. Define hemostasis. Describe the various stages involved in coagulation process.
4. Discuss in detail the neural regulation of respiration.

II. Short Notes (5 Marks each)

1. T lymphocyte
2. Properties of smooth muscle.
3. Counter-current system in kidney.
4. Composition and functions of pancreatic juice.
5. Female contraception.
6. Triple response.
7. Nonrespiratory functions of lungs.
8. Mechanism of receptor potential.
9. Factors regulating cardiac output.
10. Anatomic dead space.
11. Passive transport.
12. Gastric emptying.
13. Peculiarities of renal blood flow.
14. Second messengers.
15. Hypersecretion of growth hormone.
16. Ventricular action potential.
17. Tracts of Goll and Burdach.
18. Venous return.
19. Lung volumes and capacities.
20. Fetal circulation.

III. Short Answers (2 Marks each)

1. Mechanism of action of botulinum toxin and the basis of Botox injection.
2. What is steatorrhea?
3. List out four functions of liver.
4. Draw schematically how HCl is formed.
5. What are renal threshold and tubular maximum for glucose?
6. Give an example of neuroendocrine reflex. Briefly outline its pathway.
7. Name four hormones which increase blood glucose levels. What is the mechanism of action of one of this hormone?
8. Compare the actions of adrenaline and noradrenaline on heart and blood vessels.
9. Explain the mechanism of action of contraceptive pills.
10. How does temperature influence spermatogenesis?
11. Neuromuscular blockers.
12. Na^+- K^+ ATPase.
13. Endocytosis
14. Fibrinolytic agents.
15. Cross matching.
16. Secretin.
17. Enteric nervous system.
18. Mention two substances used for measuring total body water and ECF volume.
19. Loop diuretics.
20. Neuroendocrine reflex.
21. The law of projection.
22. Types of hypoxia.
23. Antegrade amnesia.
24. Draw a normal electrocardiogram. What is Einthoven's triangle?
25. Respiratory exchange ratio.
26. Attenuation reflex.
27. Mean arterial pressure.
28. Reynold's number.

29. Astigmatism.
30. Functions of thalamus.
31. Clinical uses of ECG.
32. P_{50}.
33. Types of deafness.
34. Blood-brain barrier.
35. Anaphylactic shock.
36. Red-green blindness.
37. Reflex arc.
38. Primary taste sensations.
39. Functions of limbic system.
40. Physiological dead space.

I. ESSAY QUESTIONS

1. Explain in detail synthesis, secretion, and functions of thyroid hormone. Add a note on cretinism.

Hormones synthesized from thyroid gland are:
- From follicular cells: Thyroxine (T4) and triiodothyronine (T3). The shape of the follicle varies based on the activity of the gland (*refer* Fig. 1)
- From parafollicular cells: Calcitonin.

Synthesis of Thyroid Hormone
- Synthesis takes place in the follicular cells and the hormone is stored in follicular lumen as colloid.

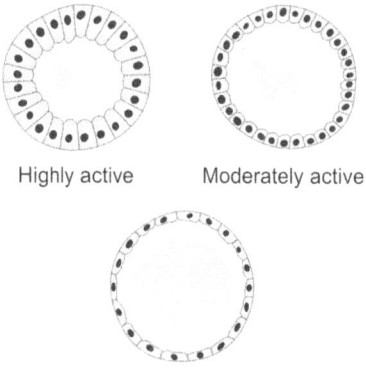

Fig. 1: Thyroid follicle—active follicle, moderately active follicle, and inactive follicle with colloid content. Inactive follicle is lined by flattened epithelial cells and the colloid content is more. In an active follicle the cells are columnar and colloid content is less.

- Thyroid hormones are iodothyronines, formed by coupling of iodinated tyrosine molecules by ether linkages.

Following are the steps in synthesis of thyroid hormones:
1. Iodide trapping
2. Thyroglobulin synthesis
3. Oxidation of iodide
4. Organification
5. Coupling
6. Storage
7. Release

Iodide Trapping
- Iodide is transported from the blood in thyroid capillaries to the follicular cell through **sodium-iodide symporter** (NIS).
- NIS transports I⁻ against electrochemical gradient.
- TSH stimulates I⁻ trapping and concentration in the gland.
- Iodide immediately moves towards the apical membrane of the follicular cell.

Thyroglobulin Synthesis
- As iodide is being trapped, thyroglobulin is also synthesized in the endoplasmic reticulum of follicular cells and transferred to colloid.
- TG is a glycoprotein. Has 131 tyrosine amino acids.

Oxidation of Iodide
- Iodide on reaching the colloid—apical membrane interface is oxidized to iodine.
- This reaction is catalyzed by thyroid peroxidase enzyme (TPO) present in the colloid-membrane interface.
- $2I^- + H_2O_2 \rightarrow I_2 + 2HO^-$

Organification
- The tyrosine molecules of thyroglobulin get iodinated in the colloid to form iodotyrosines.
- This is **organification** and is catalyzed by TPO (*refer* Fig. 2).
- It forms either monoiodotyrosine (MIT) or di-iodotyrosine (DIT) depending on the number of iodine attached to tyrosines.

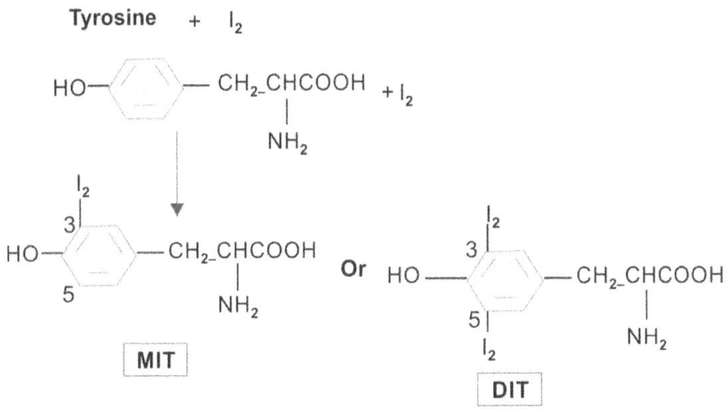

Tyrosine + I₂

$HO-\bigcirc-CH_2CHCOOH \atop NH_2$ + I₂

↓ I₂

$HO-\underset{5}{\overset{3\ I_2}{\bigcirc}}-CH_2CHCOOH \atop NH_2$ **Or** $HO-\underset{5\ I_2}{\overset{3\ I_2}{\bigcirc}}-CH_2CHCOOH \atop NH_2$

[MIT] [DIT]

Fig. 2: Organification reaction—I₂ molecule is bound to tyrosine molecules. If it is bound in one position (3) then MIT (monoiodotyrosine is formed). If I₂ is bound in two positions (3 and 5) it is DIT (di-iodotyrosine).

Coupling Reaction

Two DIT molecules couple to form tetraiodo-tyrosine (T_4) or thyroxine.

Or

One molecule of MIT and DIT couple to form triiodothyronine (T_3)

Or

One molecule of DIT and MIT couple to form reverse T_3 (RT_3), an inactive component formed in the follicular cells.

This is coupling reaction and is catalyzed by TPO (*refer* **Fig. 3**).

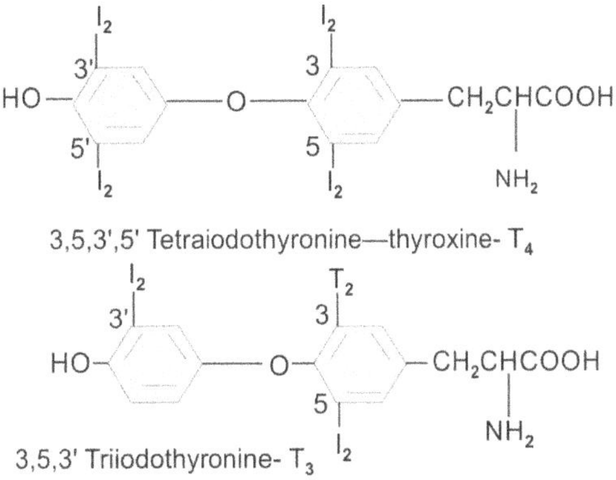

$HO-\underset{5'\ I_2}{\overset{3'\ I_2}{\bigcirc}}-O-\underset{5\ I_2}{\overset{3\ I_2}{\bigcirc}}-CH_2CHCOOH \atop NH_2$

3,5,3',5' Tetraiodothyronine—thyroxine- T_4

$HO-\underset{3'\ I_2}{\bigcirc}-O-\underset{5\ I_2}{\overset{3\ I_2}{\bigcirc}}-CH_2CHCOOH \atop NH_2$

3,5,3' Triiodothyronine- T_3

Fig. 3: Coupling reaction. Two MITs couple to form T_4 (throxine) and one MIT and one DIT binds T_3 (triiodothyronine) is formed.

Storage

- TG after iodination is stored in the colloid until release.
- In each molecule of thyroglobulin (TG): MIT-7, DIT-6, T_4- 2, T_3- 0.2 molecules are present.
- The gland is capable of storing secretions needed for 100 days (*refer* **Fig. 4**).

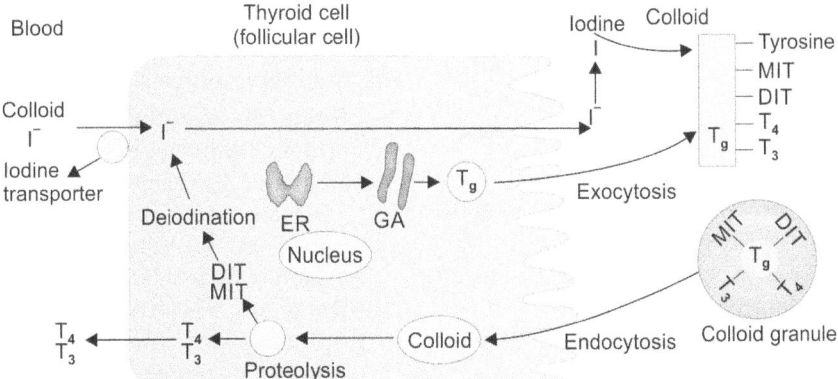

Fig. 4: Synthesis of thyroid hormone in follicular cell.
(DIT: diiodotyrosine; MIT: monoiodotyrosine; ER: endoplasmic reticulum; GA: Golgi apparatus; Tg: thyroglobulin; T4: thyroxine; T3: triiodothyronine)

Release of the Hormone
- On stimulation by TSH, colloid droplets (with TG and T_3 and T_4) are endocytosed through megalin into the cell.
- The droplet gets attached to a lysozome and forms a phagosome.
- Proteolytic enzymes of the phagosome break the peptide bonds between thyroid hormone (TH) and TG.
- This releases T_3, T_4, MIT, and DIT.
- Released thyroid hormones enter into the capillaries by diffusion.
- MIT and DIT are deiodinated by the enzyme, **thyroid deiodinases**, which are selective for iodotyrosines and not for iodothyronines.
- Small amounts of TG are also released.

Functions of Thyroid Hormone
The actions of thyroid hormone are grouped as:
- Metabolic actions
- Developmental effects
- Effects on various systems

Metabolic Actions
- Calorigenesis
- Regulation of intermediary metabolism (of carbohydrate, lipid and protein metabolism).
- Vitamin metabolism.

Calorigenesis:
- It increases heat production
- The major role of thyroid hormone is to increase O_2 consumption and BMR. In hyperthyroidism BMR and O_2 consumption increases 50-100% and in hypothyroidism it decreases by 30-40%.

Effects on protein metabolism:
- Thyroid hormone stimulates protein synthesis and degradation.
- TH increases cellular uptake of amino acids and formation of proteins.
- In hypothyroidism small doses of TH helps in protein anabolism.
- High levels of TH increase protein catabolism

Effects on carbohydrate metabolism:
- Thyroid hormone acts on all aspects of carbohydrate metabolism.
- Increases glucose uptake from GIT.
- Increases insulin resistance and its degradation.
- Glycogen synthesis and degradation is also affected.
- Increases gluconeogenesis.

Effects on lipid metabolism:
- Thyroid hormones affect all aspects of lipid metabolism—lipogenesis, fat mobilization and lipolysis.
- TH increases cholesterol synthesis and also its clearance by increasing LDL synthesis.
- So in hypothyroidism serum cholesterol levels increase and in hyperthyroidism it is decreased.

Effects on vitamin metabolism:
- Thyroid hormones are needed for the conversion of β carotene to vitamin A
- In hypothyroidism carotene accumulate in blood and give yellow discoloration—**carotenemia**.

Effects on Growth, Development, and Maturation
Thyroid hormone has an important action on growth and maturation. This effect has been evidenced in the metamorphosis of tadpoles. Thyroid hormone levels increase sharply just before the major step of metamorphosis.

In hypothyroid humans puberty is delayed or absent. The bone maturation is also delayed.

Effects on Other Systems
- **Effects on skeletal system:** Thyroid hormone stimulates linear growth of bone and maturation of epiphyseal center.
  GH secretion and actions are potentiated by TH. Adequate thyroid hormones are needed for normal growth.
- **Effects on respiratory system:** The respiratory rate, minute ventilation and response to hypercapnia and hypoxia are increased. O_2 carrying capacity is increased by increase in red cell mass.

- **Effects on cardiovascular system:** The main action on CVS is to increase blood supply to tissues to deliver more O_2.

  In hyperthyroidism:
  - Heart rate and stroke volume ↑→↑ cardiac output
  - Systolic BP ↑ and diastolic BP ↓→ widened pulse pressure.
  - Diastolic BP is decreased due to decreased peripheral resistance.

  In hypothyroidism:
  - Heart rate and stroke volume decrease.
  - Peripheral resistance is usually increased.
  - The cutaneous vasoconstriction is responsible for the cold skin in hypothyroids.

- **Effect on nervous system:**
  - Thyroid hormones are important for growth and development of the brain in fetal and neonatal period. So TH deficiency in this period leads to irreversible brain damage and mental retardation.
  - The parts in CNS mostly affected are cerebral cortex, basal ganglia and cochlea.
  - Many actions of excessive TH resemble increased sympathetic activity like: tachycardia, tremor, increase in metabolism.

Hypothyroidism

- Hypothyroidism due to thyroid gland dysfunction is primary hypothyroidism.
- Hypothyroidism may also occur due to disease in the pituitary gland or in hypothalamus.
- Symptoms of hypothyroidism vary in children and adults.
- In children hypothyroidism due to iodine deficiency—**cretinism**.

Symptoms

- **In newborns:** Respiratory distress syndrome, poor feeding, hoarse cry, umbilical hernia, retarded bone age, no visible symptoms detected, so early thyroid screening and TH replacement is essential to prevent mental retardation.
- **In children:** Mental retardation, stunted growth, pot belly, enlarged and protruding tongue, delayed or absent sexual maturity, deaf mutism with rigidity, precocious puberty can also occur.

2. Describe the classification, connections and functions of cerebellum.

Anatomically each hemisphere of cerebellum is divided into three lobes by two transverse furrows into lobes—anterior lobe, posterior lobe, and flocculonodular lobes.

Functional Divisions

- The main functions of cerebellum are to maintain posture and balance and coordinate voluntary movements.
- Based on the functions it is divided into three parts:
  a. **Vestibulocerebellum:** Made up of the flocculonodular lobe.
  b. **Spinocerebellum:** Consists of vermis and the intermediate part of the cerebellar hemispheres (paravermal portion).
  c. **Neocerebellum:** Consists of the lateral parts of the hemispheres (*refer* **Fig. 5**).

Connections and functions of cerebellum:

- Connections include the afferents and efferents to cerebellum which enter cerebellum and leave, through the cerebellar peduncles.
- There are three cerebellar peduncles—superior, inferior and middle cerebellar peduncles.

Afferent Connections

The afferents to cerebellum come through the climbing fibers and mossy fibers (*refer* **Fig. 6**).

Climbing Fibers

- They contain the olivocerebellar tract which arises from the inferior olivary nucleus in medulla.
- The olivary nucleus in turn receives proprioceptive inputs from all over the body.
- The climbing fibers end on the dendrites of Purkinje cells and they make one-to-one

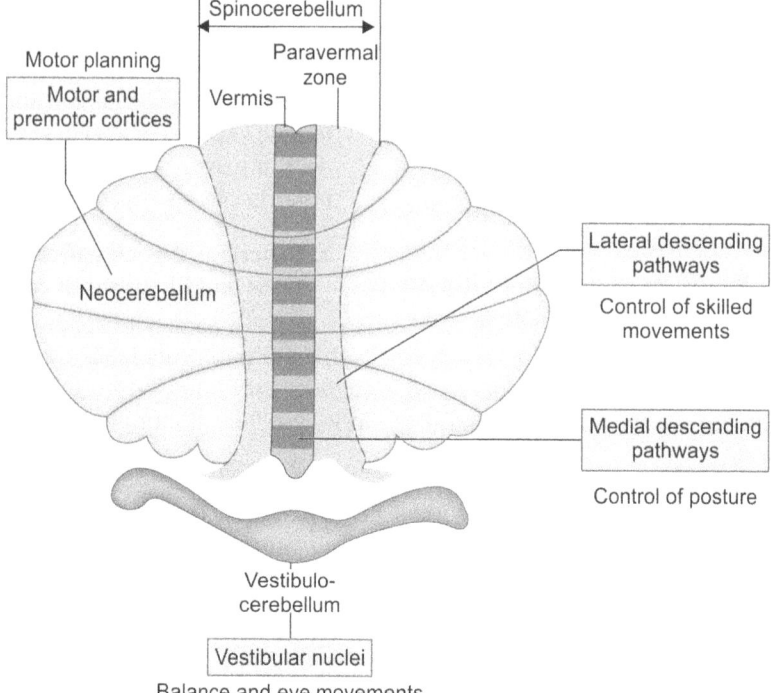

Fig. 5: Functional divisions of cerebellum with their connections and functions.

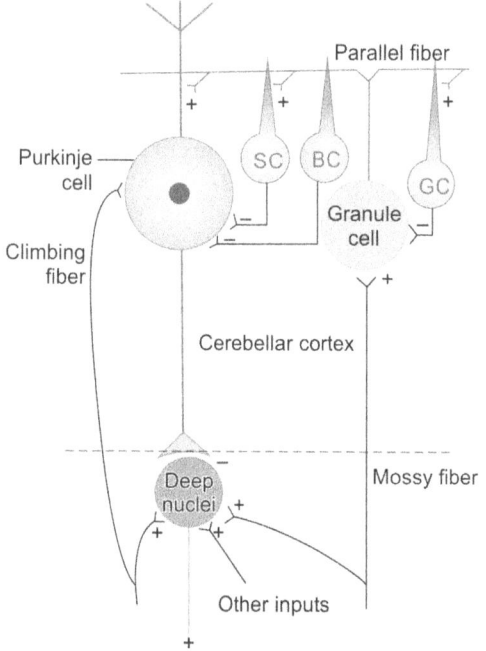

Fig. 6: Afferents to cerebellum through climbing and mossy fibers.
[SC: stellate cells; BC: basket cells; GC: Golgi cells; (−) Inhibition; (+) Stimulation]

connection with the Purkinje cells and excite them.
- Collaterals from climbing fibers also excite the Golgi cells and the deep nuclei of cerebellum.
- Climbing fibers enter the cerebellum through the inferior cerebellar peduncle. This peduncle brings in most of the other afferent fibers to cerebellum.

Mossy Fibers
- Mossy fibers include all the other afferents entering the cerebellum other than olivocerebellar tract.
- **It includes:** Dorsal and ventral spinocerebellar tracts, vestibulocerebellar tract, reticulocerebellar tract, cuneocerebellar tract, tectocerebellar tract, rubrocerebellar tract and pontocerebellar tract.
  - *Dorsal spinocerebellar tract:* It carries unconscious proprioceptive inputs and exteroceptive inputs from same side limbs and trunk of same side and they enter cerebellum through ipsilateral

inferior cerebellar peduncle. It ends on the spinocerebellum.
- *Ventral spinocerebellar tract:* It carries cutaneous and proprioceptive inputs from opposite side of the lower limbs and enters cerebellum through ipsilateral superior cerebellar peduncle and they are distributed to the hind limb area of spinocerebellum.
- *Vestibulocerebellar tract:* It carries impulses from the same side vestibular nucleus about information regarding the position of head in relation to body posture. It enters the cerebellum through ipsilateral inferior cerebellar peduncle. It ends in the flocculonodular lobe (vestibulocerebellum).
- *Reticulocerebellar tract:* It arises from the lateral reticular nucleus and enters through inferior cerebellar peduncle and is distributed to all areas of cerebellar cortex.
- *Cuneocerebellar tract:* It arises from external arcuate nucleus and carries proprioceptive information from head, neck, upper limb and upper part of the body. It enters through ipsilateral inferior cerebellar peduncle and distributed to spinocerebellum.
- *Tectocerebellar tract:* It carries visual and auditory information from superior and inferior colliculi. It enters through superior cerebellar peduncle.
- *Rubrocerebellar tract:* It arises from the red nucleus. It contains information from cerebral cortex. It has both crossed and uncrossed fibers. It enters through superior cerebellar peduncle and ends on dentate nucleus (one of the deep nuclei of cerebellum).
- *Pontocerebellar tract:* These are fibers arising from motor area of cerebral cortex and end on pontine nuclei. From here they arise to form the pontocerebellar fibers. They cross to opposite side and enter through the opposite middle cerebellar peduncle and are distributed to all areas of cerebellar cortex.

Efferent Connections

❏ All the efferents from cerebellar cortex are through the Purkinje fiber output which ends on the deep cerebellar nuclei. Purkinje cell output is inhibitory in nature.
❏ *The deep nuclei are:* Dentate, emboliform, fastigial and globose. Emboliform and globose are together called as nucleus interpositus.
❏ The deep nuclei also receive collaterals from climbing and mossy fibers and both are excitatory in nature.
❏ The net effect of output from deep nuclei is excitatory to brain stem and thalamus.
❏ All parts of cerebellum, except the vestibulocerebellum exit the cerebellum through deep nuclei.
- *Cerebellovestibular pathway vestibulospinal tract:* It leaves the vestibulocerebellum and projects to the vestibular nuclei directly. It controls the activity of vestibulospinal tract
- *Cerebelloreticular pathway reticulospinal tract:* The vermal portion of spinocerebellum projects to pontine reticular formation through fastigial nucleus. From here the reticulospinal tract arises and through this tract cerebellum controls the anterior horn cells.
- *Paravermal portion* of spinocerebellum project to nucleus interpositus and this in turn projects to the red nucleus. Thereby cerebellum controls the rubrospinal tract.
- *Dentato-thalamo-cortical pathway:* Impulses from cerebrocerebellum end on dentate nucleus and from here it goes through thalamus and reaches motor cortex. From motor cortex corticospinal tract arises and ends on alpha motor neurons. Through this pathway cerebellum fine tunes the activity of corticospinal tract (*refer* **Fig. 7**).

Functions of Cerebellum

❏ **Control of posture and equilibrium:**
- Vestibulocerebellum or the flocculonodular lobe controls posture and equilibrium.

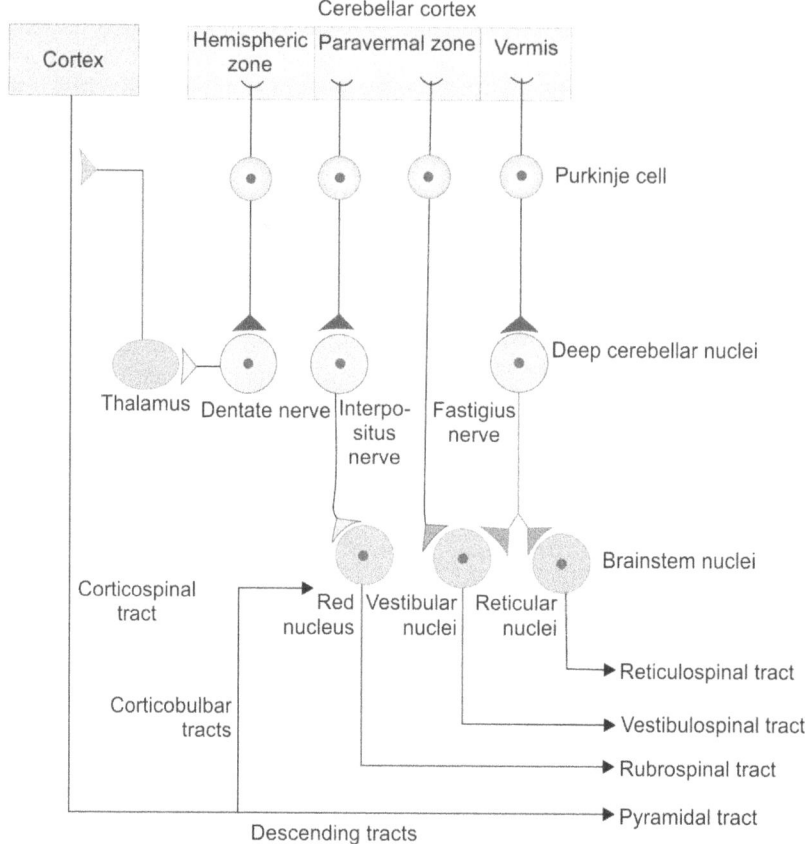

Fig. 7: Efferent connections from cerebellum through deep nuclei to brainstem. They are vestibulospinal tract, reticulospinal tract, rubrospinal tract. Through thalamic connections controls corticospinal tract.

- It receives inputs from vestibular apparatus directly and also through vestibular nuclei about position of head and body.
- It sends efferents to vestibular nuclei from which the vestibulospinal tract arises to regulate posture.
- Vestibulocerebellum is also concerned with regulating vestibulo-ocular reflex.
▫ **Control of muscle tone and stretch reflex:**
- Spinocerebellum influences the muscle tone through its output via fastigial nucleus which in turn controls the vestibulospinal and reticulospinal tract (arising from pontine reticular formation).
- The major influence of cerebellum on tone is facilitatory.
- Vestibulospinal tract is facilitatory to α motor neurons and reticulospinal tract is facilitatory to γ motor neurons.
- Since control of cerebellum is on both α and γ motor neurons it has an important role in α-γ linkage.
▫ **Control of voluntary movements:**
- Paravermal portion of spinocerebellum controls skilled voluntary movements.
- It does not initiate movements but it coordinates voluntary movements.
- Coordination of movements is by regulating the time, rate, range, force and direction of movements.
- All three functional divisions of the cerebellum work together as "comparator of servo mechanism".

Comparator servo mechanism:
- Impulses for voluntary movements are planned and programmed in the premotor cortex and it is sequenced in primary motor area and the command

to skeletal muscles is sent through the corticospinal tract.
- A copy of the plan or intended movement is also sent to the spinocerebellum.
- Cerebellum also gets feedback from the proprioceptors about the actual movement performed by the muscles and joints.
- It also receives other sensory inputs from eye, ear and vestibular apparatus.
- Now the cerebellum compares the intended movement and the executed movement along with other sensory inputs mentioned above.
- It thereby modifies appropriately the ongoing movement.
- If any corrections have to be done in programming of movements the error signals are sent to the motor cortex.

❏ **Control of body movements of one side:**
- Motor cortex of one side is connected to opposite cerebellum through a closed feedback loop; cerebral-cerebellar-cerebral circuit, the cortico-ponto-dentato-thalamo-cortical pathway.
- So each cerebellar hemisphere controls the opposite cerebral cortex.
- But the corticospinal tract descending down from the motor cortex decussates in medulla and controls the opposite side of the body.
- Since there is double decussation, it is that cerebellum controls same side of the body.

❏ **Planning and programming of movements:** Cerebro-cerebellum has extensive connections with motor cortex and therefore is involved in planning and programming of movements.

❏ **Learning of skills:**
- Cerebellum always tends to make changes in ongoing movements and therefore it improves by learning.
- Another evidence is that there are increased activities in the climbing fibers when a new skill is learnt.
- So cerebellum has a great role in learning skills.

❏ **Eyeball movement:** Pyramis of cerebellum is concerned with eyeball movement.

3. Define hemostasis. Describe the various stages involved in coagulation process.

❏ Hemostasis is the spontaneous arrest of bleeding from the damaged blood vessels by physiological processes.
❏ **There are three steps involved in hemostasis:**
   a. Vasoconstriction
   b. Formation of temporary platelet plug
   c. Formation of a definitive clot

Clotting of Blood

❏ Blood while flowing in the vessels is fluid in nature, but when the vessel wall is injured or the blood is removed from the body and collected in a test tube it becomes a jelly like mass—the clot.
❏ Clotting or coagulation of blood involves a series of cascade of events in which many clotting factors (proteins in the plasma) are activated in a serial manner. There are many such clotting factors.

They are:
❏ **Factor I:** Fibrinogen
❏ **Factor II:** Prothrombin
❏ **Factor III:** Thromboplastin
❏ **Factor IV:** Calcium
❏ **Factor V:** Labile factor or proaccelerin
❏ **Factor VI:** Nonexistent
❏ **Factor VII:** Stable factor or proconvertin
❏ **Factor VIII:** Antihemophilic factor
❏ **Factor IX:** Christmas factor or plasma thromboplastic component (PTC) or antihemophilic factor B
❏ **Factor X:** Stuart–Prower factor
❏ **Factor XI:** Plasma thromboplastin antecedent (PTA) or antihemophilic factor C.
❏ **Factor XII:** Hageman factor or glass factor or contact factor
❏ **Factor XIII:** Laki-Lorand factor or fibrin stabilizing factor
❏ HMWK—high molecular weight kininogen or Fitzgerald factor
❏ Pre-Ka (prekallikrein or Fletcher factor)

- Kallikrein-Ka
- **PL:** Platelet phospholipid

The coagulation process involves three major steps:
1. Formation of prothrombin activator
2. Conversion of prothrombin to thrombin
3. Conversion of fibrinogen to fibrin

Formation of Prothrombin Activator is by two Mechanisms

1. Extrinsic pathway
2. Intrinsic pathway

Extrinsic Pathway

The extrinsic pathway is triggered when the injury involves damage to the blood vessels and the surrounding tissues. The damaged tissue releases tissue thromboplastin, a protein-phospholipid mixture which activates factor VII. This triggers the extrinsic pathway (*refer* **Fig. 8**).

- Inactive factor VII is activated to active factor VIIa
- VIIa in the presence of Ca^{++}, platelet phospholipid (PL) and tissue thromboplastin, activates factors IX and X.
- Active factor Xa, Va, Ca^{++}, and PL, forms the prothrombin activator.
- Prothrombin activator converts prothrombin to thrombin.
- Thrombin catalyzes the conversion of fibrinogen to fibrin.

Intrinsic Pathway

This pathway is activated when there is injury to vessel wall and exposure of collagen or blood itself.

Steps involved are:
- Injury to vessel wall exposes collagen activates factor XII to XIIa
- Factor XIIa activates factor XI to XIa
- Factor XIa activates factor IX to IXa
- Factor IXa in the presence of VIII, Ca^{2+} and platelet phospholipids (PPL) activates factor X to Xa.
- The activated factor Xa, platelet phospholipids, factor Va and Ca^{2+} forms the prothrombin activator (*refer* **Fig. 8**).

Conversion of Prothrombin to Thrombin

Prothrombin activator in the presence of Ca^{2+} converts prothrombin to thrombin. This happens at the surface of platelets. Thrombin is a proteolytic enzyme.

Conversion of Fibrinogen to Fibrin

- Thrombin, a proteolytic enzyme removes two pairs of polypeptide chains from each fibrinogen molecule and converts it to fibrin monomer.
- The fibrin monomers now polymerize to form long fibrin threads. The fibrin is initially a loose mesh of interlacing strands. This meshwork traps the blood cells
- It is later converted to a dense tight aggregate by formation of covalent cross-linkages. This is catalyzed by factor XIII and Ca^{2+}. The stabilized fibrin mesh with the trapped blood cells forms the clot.

---

4. Discuss in detail the neural regulation of respiration.

- Breathing is an automatic process occurring throughout life without conscious effort.
- Respiration is a process which is highly regulated.
- Spontaneous respiration is due to rhythmic discharge of neurons from respiratory centers supplying the inspiratory muscles.
- This is under cortical (voluntary) and medullary and pontine control (automatic).
- These centers in turn are regulated by alterations in the PCO_2, PO_2 and pH of arterial blood and other nonchemical influences.

Cortical Control or Voluntary Control of Respiration

Impulses from cerebral cortex
↓
Corticospinal tract
↓
Motor neurons supplying the inspiratory muscles

- Impulses also reach the innervation of expiratory muscles.

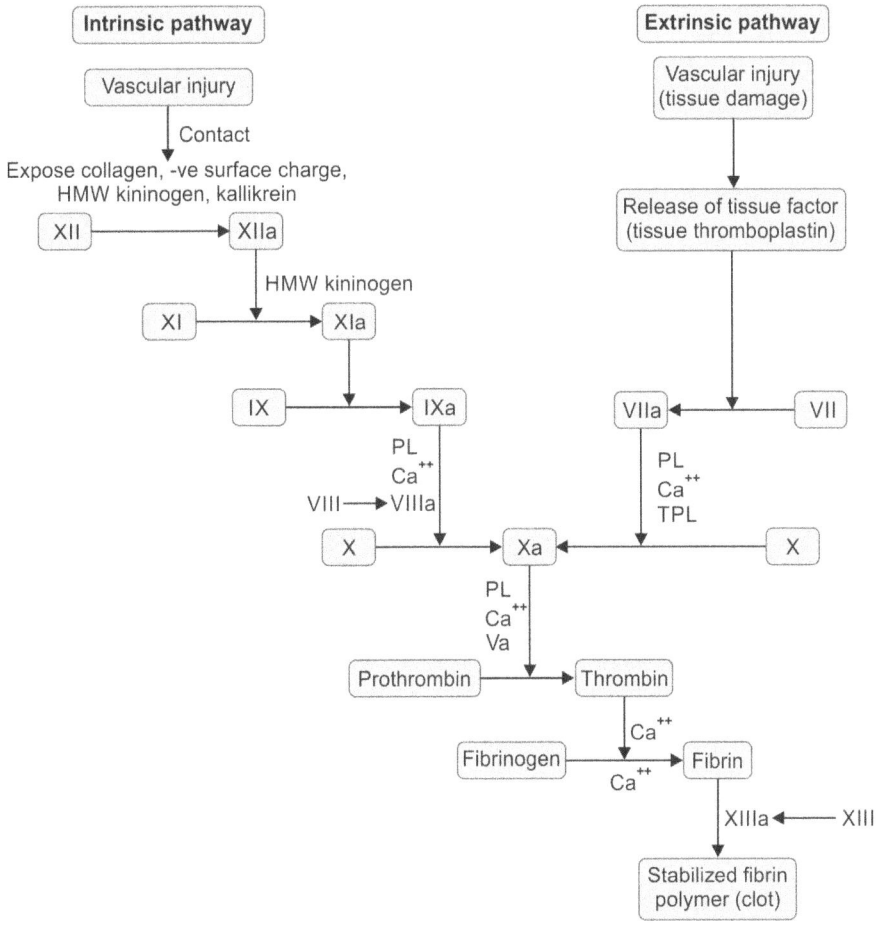

Fig. 8: Mechanism of clotting.
(TPL: tissue phospholipid; PL: platelet phospholipid)

- There is a reciprocal inhibition between the motor neurons supplying the I and E neurons.
- There is an exception for this at the start of expiration were the "I" neurons are active.
- The inspiratory muscles are active for some time during expiration to break the elastic recoil of lungs and make expiration smooth.

Automatic Control of Respiration

Impulses from brainstem respiratory centers in pons and medulla → supplies neurons in intermediolateral horn cells of cervical and thoracic segments → supplies inspiratory muscles.

Medullary Respiratory Centers

- Dorsal respiratory group of neurons (DRG)—has 'I' neurons
- Ventral respiratory group of neurons (VRG)—has 'I' and E' neurons
- Central pattern generator (CPG)—pre-Botzinger complex (*refer* **Figs. 9 and 10**)

Dorsal Respiratory Group of Neurons

- Located near nucleus tractus solitarius (NTS) (*refer* **Fig. 9**)
- Contains only inspiratory neurons
- They project to cell bodies of phrenic nerves in spinal cord.
- Its activity is weaker to start with and gradually increases in a ramp fashion for 2 seconds and abruptly stops for 3 seconds.

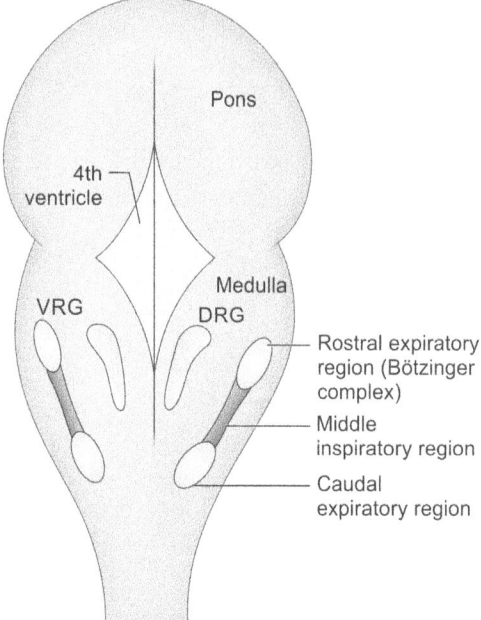

Fig. 9: Respiratory centers in medulla.
[DRG: dorsal respiratory group of neurons (has only inspiratory neurons); VRG: ventral respiratory group of neurons (has both inspiratory and expiratory neurons)]

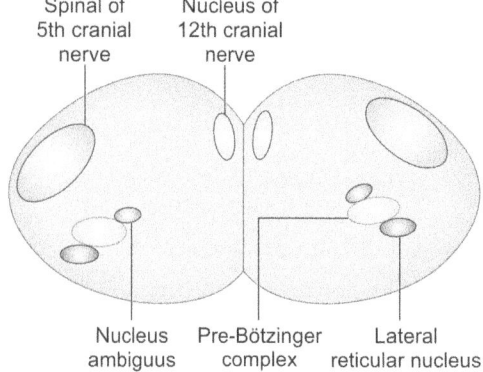

Fig. 10: Location of pacemaker (pre-Bötzinger complex) for rhythm generation in medulla.

- The ramp signal helps in steady increase in lung volume during inspiration
- Receives input from peripheral chemoreceptors through 9th and 10th cranial nerves.

Ventral Respiratory Group of Neurons

- Located in venterolateral medulla in region of nucleus ambiguus (NA) (*refer* **Fig. 9**)
- Contains both inspiratory and expiratory group of neurons
- Three regions—rostral, middle and caudal inspiratory regions
- Middle region—has inspiratory neurons
- Rostral and caudal—has expiratory neurons—supply expiratory muscles.
- They are active only during forceful respiration.
- I and E neurons reciprocally inhibit each other

Pacemaker Cells for Respiration

- Located close to DRG and VRG neurons
- Present in the Pre-Bötzinger complex between nucleus ambiguus and lateral reticular nucleus (*refer* **Fig. 10**).
- They are pacemaker cells and are responsible for generating respiratory rhythm → rhythmically activate phrenic nerves.
- It receives input from higher centers

Pontine Centers

- There are two centers:
  1. Pneumotaxic center:
   - Located in nucleus parabrachialis and Kolliker-Fuse N in the upper part of pons
   - Active during both inspiration and expiration.
   - On stimulation, it shortens the duration of inspiration. When its activity is less, the duration of inspiration is longer.
   - Its major function is to limit inspiration, by inhibiting apneustic center
   - It coordinates switching between inspiration and expiration.

  2. Apneustic center:
   - Present in lower part of pons (*refer* **Fig. 11**).
   - On stimulation → leads to prolonged inspiratory spasms—**apneusis**
   - It sends inputs to DRG to cause a prolonged inspiration
   - It is constantly stimulating DRG.

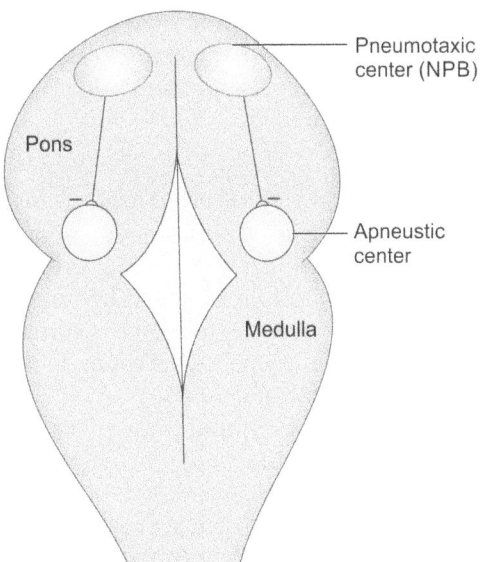

Fig. 11: Respiratory centers in pons, pneumotaxic and apneustic centers.

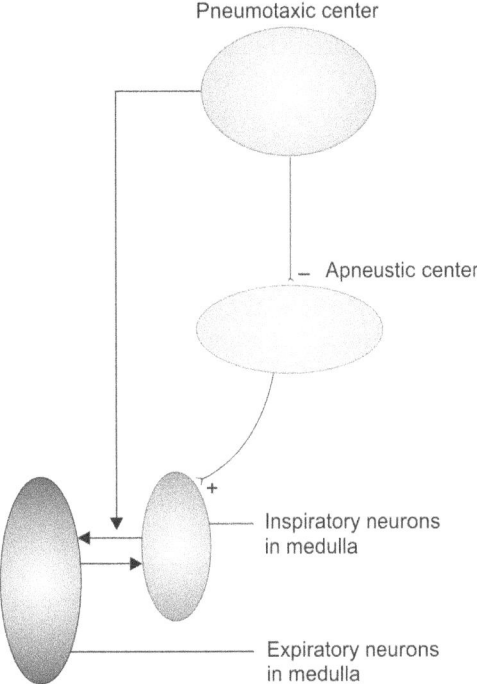

Fig. 12: Interaction of medullary and pontine centers in regulation of respiration.

- But its actions are kept in check by inputs from pneumotaxic center and vagal afferents from airways.

Mechanism of Breathing

- The neurons in DRG discharge steadily and spontaneously in a ramp like fashion for 2–3 seconds.
- Muscles of inspiration contract steadily resulting in expansion of the lung and chest wall resulting in inspiration.
- As the inspiration happens, the stretch receptors in lungs and airways are stimulated and impulses from here travel through vagus nerve to stop the firing of DRG neurons.
- Impulses from pneumotaxic center through inhibition of apneustic center stops the firing of DRG (*refer* **Fig. 12**).
- Inspiratory muscles relax and the lung and chest wall recoils and induces expiration.
- At the end of expiration, the next cycle starts.

Factors Influencing Respiratory Centers

- **Afferents from higher centers:** Cerebral cortex, limbic system, hypothalamus
- **Afferents from peripheral receptors:** Baroreceptors, chemoreceptors, J receptors, pain receptors, proprioceptors, pulmonary stretch receptors and thermoreceptors.
- **Reflexes:** Hering–Breuer reflex, sneezing reflex, swallowing reflex, cough reflex, speech

Afferents from Higher Centers

- Cerebral cortex imparts control over the respiratory centers and therefore voluntary hyperventilation and breath holding is possible
- Limbic cortex sends impulses to respiratory centers and therefore the changes in ventilation in relation to emotions can happen.
- Hypothalamic connections are responsible for respiratory changes associated with body temperature changes.

Afferent Impulses from Peripheral Receptors

- **Baroreceptors:** They regulate blood pressure through the regulation of vasomotor and cardiac vagal centers. But stimulation of baroreceptors also inhibits respiratory center and causes apnea.

- **Chemoreceptors:** There are peripheral and central chemoreceptors. They monitor the PO_2, PCO_2 and pH levels in the arterial blood. Decrease in arterial PO_2 levels will stimulate peripheral chemoreceptors and they will send impulses to DRG to stimulate respiration. Central chemoreceptors are more sensitive to PCO_2 and H^+ levels and when it increases, they stimulate respiration.
- **'J' receptors:** These are endings of unmyelinated C fibers of vagal afferents and are located between the pulmonary capillaries and alveolar walls. They are stimulated in conditions of increase in interstitial fluid between the capillary endothelium and alveolar epithelium as in pulmonary edema, pulmonary congestion, pulmonary embolism, etc. On stimulation, it induces apnea followed by tachypnea, bradycardia and hypotension. In physiological conditions these receptors are stimulated while exercising, especially in high altitude.
  Proprioceptors: While doing exercise, movements in the muscles and joints stimulate the proprioceptors and impulses from here stimulate respiration by stimulating DRG.
- **Pulmonary stretch receptors (Hering-Breuer reflex):** The pulmonary stretch receptors are located in the smooth muscles of the airways and are stimulated by inflation of lungs.

There are two types of reflexes:
1. **Hering-Breuer inflation reflex:** It is activated during inspiration. When the inspiration is more and tidal volume is more than 1 L, the reflex is initiated and it sends impulses to the respiratory centers and inhibits inspiration and stimulates expiration. This reflex is more important in infants to control the tidal volume.
2. **Hering-Breuer deflation reflex:** This reflex is activated during expiration and causes arrest of expiration and stimulates inspiration.

Thermoreceptors: Increase in body temperature stimulates these receptors and send impulses to the cerebral cortex which in turn sends impulses to respiratory centers to increase respiration. Respiration helps to lose body temperature.

Reflexes

- **Sneezing reflex:** Stimulation of nasal mucosa by irritant substances results in sneezing. The act of sneezing involves a deep inspiration followed by forceful expiration with opened glottis initially and later glottis opens to allow air to flow through mouth and nose.
- **Cough reflex:** Stimulation of irritant receptors in the tracheobronchial mucosa leads to deep inspiration followed by forceful expiration against a closed glottis. It is a protective reflex useful for clearing the airway of the irritant substance.
- **Deglutition reflex:** On swallowing there is temporary stoppage of respiration—deglutition apnea. It is a protective reflex which prevents entry of food into the airway.
- **Vomiting reflex:** Apnea happens for a short time during vomiting to prevent aspiration of contents.

II. SHORT NOTES

1. T lymphocyte.

Lymphocytes are produced in the bone marrow and some of them are transported to thymus gland. There they are processed to become T lymphocytes. These cells take part in cell-mediated immunity. They are of three types.

Types of T cells: There are three main types of T cells—helper T cells (CD4 cells), cytotoxic T cells (CD8 cells) and memory T cells.
1. *Helper T cells*: Helper T cells or CD4 cells recognize the antigen presented along with MHC II and cytotoxic or CD8 cells recognize the antigens presented with MHC I. After costimulation, helper T cells secrete many cytokines. The most important cytokine is IL-2 which is needed for all the immune responses and is the major stimulator for T cell proliferation.

IL-2 is also the costimulator for resting helper T cells and cytotoxic T cells. It also enhances activation and proliferation of B cells and natural killer cells.

2. *Cytotoxic T cells:* T cells that express CD8 develop into cytotoxic T cells. They recognize foreign antigens expressed along with MHC I on the membranes of body cells infected by viruses, tumor cells and cells of tissue transplant. But to get activated into a killer cell, it needs costimulation by IL-2 produced by helper cells. Therefore, for maximal activation of cytotoxic T cells it needs antigen presentation with MHC I and II.
3. *Memory T cells:* T cells for a specific antigen which remain in the lymph organ after the immune response is over are termed as memory T cells. If the same pathogen is encountered for the second time, these cells get activated and they initiate a swift and fast immune response. The second response is faster and vigorous and the pathogen is eliminated even before any symptom develops.

Elimination of the Pathogens

The killing of pathogen is done by cytotoxic T cells.
- Activated CD8 cells synthesize and secrete proteins called "**perforins**" which are inserted into the membrane of the pathogen. Perforins are water channels which allow influx of water and thereby swelling of the microbe and cause its lysis.
- Release of **lymphotoxins** by activated T cells. These cytokines destroy the microbes.
- Cytotoxic T cells secrete **interferons** which will favor the phagocytic activity of the neutrophils and macrophages by promoting opsonization.

---

2. Properties of smooth muscle.

The properties of smooth muscles are classified as electrical and mechanical properties.

There are two types of smooth muscles; single-unit or visceral smooth muscles and multi-unit smooth muscles.

The properties differ in these two types of muscles.

Electrical Properties

- Single-unit smooth muscles do not have a stable resting membrane potential, average potential being –50 mV.
- There are pacemaker cells among the single-unit muscles and are capable of generating action potentials by themselves.
- Pacemaker cells generate slow wave potentials which are slow sine-wave like fluctuations of few millivolts in magnitude and if they reach threshold action potentials are fired either in the upstroke or downstroke of the waves.
- Smooth muscle action potentials are of either spike potentials or plateau potential as in cardiac muscle.
- Depolarization is due to Ca^{++} influx and repolarization is due to closure of Ca^{++} channels followed by K^+ efflux.
- Excitation-contraction coupling process is a very slow one in smooth muscles as the muscle starts to contract 200 msec after the start of the spike and 150 msec after the spike is over.

Mechanical Properties

- **Tone of muscle:** Visceral smooth muscles show slow wave potentials which is followed by continuous and irregular contractions. This is maintained state of contraction said to be the tone of muscles.
- **Length-tension relationship; plasticity:** Smooth muscles exert variable tension at any given length. When a piece of visceral smooth muscle is stretched, initially the muscle exerts tension and when the stretch is maintained the tension gradually decreases and may fall below initial tension. Therefore, it is not possible to relate muscle length to tension developed and no resting length is assigned. This property is said to be **plasticity** of smooth muscles.

It is demonstrated in the muscle wall of urinary bladder. As the bladder gets filled there will be little increase in tension initially in the detrusor muscle then the tension decreases but as it reaches its capacity the tension rises to a peak and the bladder contracts forcefully and empties the bladder.

3. Counter-current system in kidney.

Humans have the ability to excrete a dilute urine (30 mOsm/L) or concentrated urine (1400 mOsm/L) to regulate the ECF volume and osmolality.

Concentration of urine involves interaction of two entities, counter-current mechanism and action of ADH on collecting duct of nephron.

Counter-current Mechanism in Kidneys

Counter-current mechanism refers to a system in which the inflow of fluid runs parallel to, counter to and in close proximity to the outflow for some distance in two tubes placed close to each other. An U tube system is used for this counter-current mechanism.

In the kidney it is formed by:
- Counter-current multiplier (loop of Henle)
- Counter-current exchanger (vasa recta)
  - The role of counter-current mechanism is to **create** a hyperosmolar medullary interstitium in the kidneys and to **maintain** the osmolar gradient in medullary interstitium.
  - Hyperosmolarity in the interstitium along with ADH is essential for concentration of urine.

Medullary interstitial osmolarity:
- The medullary interstitial fluid osmolality is important in concentrating the urine, because it provides the driving force for reabsorbing water from both the descending thin limb of loop of Henle and the collecting duct.
- The principal components for creating the hyperosmolarity of the medullary interstitial fluid are NaCl and urea.
- At the junction of medulla with cortex, the interstitial osmolality is approximately 300 mOsm/kg H_2O, with virtually all osmoles attributable to NaCl.
- The concentrations of both NaCl and urea increase progressively as the tubular fluid moves deeper into the medulla to 1,200 mOsm/Kg H_2O with each contributing 600 mos/L.

- NaCl in interstitium is got from its reabsorption in thick ascending limb of LOH (TAL of LOH) through the active transporter, $Na^+ K^+ 2Cl^-$ symport and passive reabsorption from thin descending limb of LOH. This creates a gradient of 200 mOsm/Kg H_2O across the tubular lumen and interstitium, which is called the **single effect**.
- Urea is filtered and reabsorbed in descending and ascending limb of LOH and medullary CD. The last part is favored by ADH. Urea also contributes to hyperosmolarity.
- On excreting dilute urine, urea concentration in the medullary part of CD decreases.

Counter-current Multiplier
- Counter-current multiplier operating in the LOH generates hyperosmolarity and creates osmolar gradient in the interstitium by:
  - Origin of single effect (already mentioned above)
  - Multiplication of the single effect

Multiplication of Single Effect
- Hyperosmolarity of medullary interstitium is generated by multiplication of the single effect.
- **Multiplication happens due to the following characteristic features of the tubule:**
  - High permeability of descending thin segment to water
  - Impermeability to water and active reabsorption of NaCl in TAL of LOH, which creates a osmolar gradient of 200 mOsm/Kg H_2O across the tubule (*refer* **Fig. 13**).
  - In renal medulla, all other tubular structures other than TAL of LOH are in osmotic equilibrium with interstitium.
  - The descending limb acquires the osmolality of the surrounding interstitium.
  - The effect is multiplied when isosmolar filtered fluid enters into descending limb and forces the concentrated fluid to the tip.

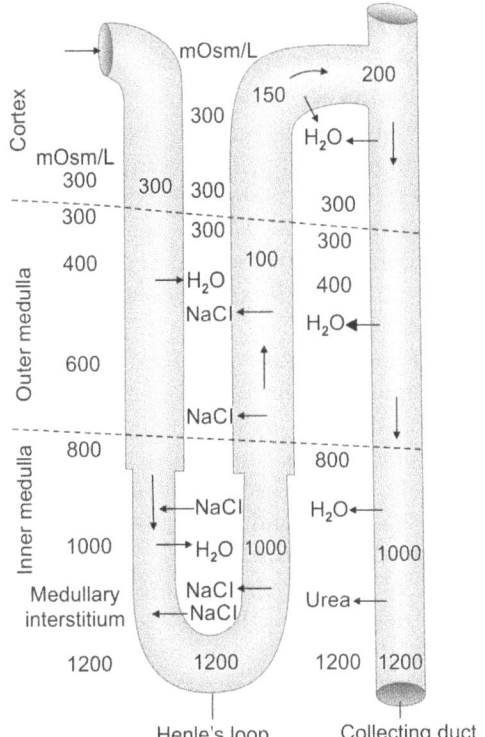

Fig. 13: Counter-current multiplier formed by loop of Henle (descending and ascending limbs) and collecting duct.

Steps in Counter-current Multiplication

- As iso-osmolar fluid passes into PCT, solutes and equal amounts of water are reabsorbed and therefore the osmolality of tubular fluid is unaltered and is 300 mOsm/L.
- In the descending limb as the fluid passes, only water is reabsorbed as the limb is impermeable to solutes, but NaCl enters the tubule.
- Now the tubular fluid concentration increases and as it reaches the tip of the loop, it reaches 1200 mOsm/L.
- Next the hyperosmolar fluid moves into the thin ascending limb where NaCl is reabsorbed passively and in the TAL of LOH the same is reabsorbed by active transport.
- This makes the fluid in TAL hypo-osmolar (200 mOsm/L) and increases the medullary interstitial osmolality to 400 mOsm/L.
- Formation of this 200 mOsm/L gradient is the 'single effect'.
- This segment and DCT are impermeable to water and permeable to NaCl, so the fluid now becomes hypo-osmolar and attains the osmolality of 100 mOsm/L.
- All other segments of the tubule, except TAL of LOH, and the interstitium are all in osmolar equilibrium and their osmolality are the same.
- This is the mechanism by which the hyperosmolar interstitium created.
- By this time more iso-osmolar filtrate enters the PCT and this process repeats and there is multiplication of creation of the gradient.
- Urea also contributes to the osmolality. It is reabsorbed across the CD and LOH and helps in creating the hyperosmolarity in the interstitium. This effect is greater in presence of ADH.

Counter-current Exchanger

- Vasa recta is the counter-current exchanger.
- These are capillaries formed from efferent arterioles and are U shaped resembling the LOH. Because of their U shape, they are able to maintain the solute concentration in medullary interstitium and remove water into general circulation.
- The flow of blood in vasa recta is very slow which also helps to maintain the gradient.
- **Descending limb of vasa recta:** As the descending limb dips into the medulla there is a progressive increase in the osmolality from 300–1200 mOsm/kg H2O.
- Here the solutes move into the capillary and water moves out into the interstitium so that blood in the capillary equilibrates with the interstitium and its osmolality also increases progressively.
- **Ascending limb of vasa recta:** From the point of ascending where the osmolality is 1,200 mOsm/kg H_2O, it starts dropping to 300 mOsm/kg H_2O as water from interstitium enters the ascending limb (*refer* **Fig. 14**).

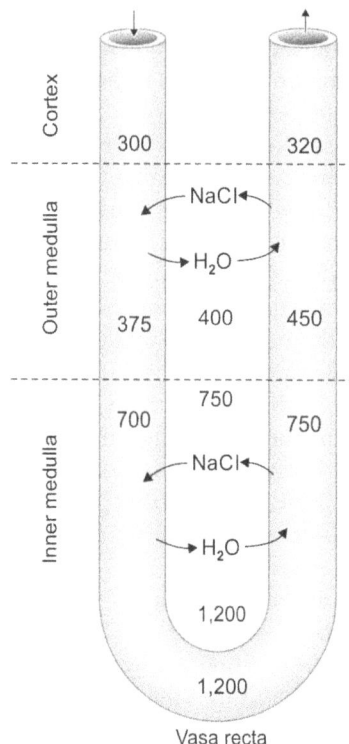

Fig. 14: Counter-current exchanger (vasa recta).

- From this limb, solutes move out into the interstitium and then into descending limb and water moves into the capillary.
- Thus, the water moves from here to the general circulation and solutes are circulating within the medullary interstitium and hyperosmolarity is maintained.

---

4. Composition and functions of pancreatic juice.

Composition of Pancreatic Juice

- Rate of secretion—1,200–1,500 mL/day
- Specific gravity—1.010–1.018
- pH—7.8–8.4, due to high concentration of HCO_3^-
- 99.5% is water and 0.5% solids
- **Organic constituents:** Contains enzymes like amylase, lipase, protease, trypsin inhibitor and traces of albumin and globulin.
- **Inorganic constituents:**
  - *Cations like:* Na^+, K^+, Ca^{++}, Mg^{++} and Zn^{2+}
  - *Anions like:* HCO_3^-, Cl^-, SO_4^{2-} and HPO_4^{2-}

Functions of Pancreatic Juice

Digestive Function of Pancreatic Juice

- **Digestion of lipids:**
  - Pancreatic lipase is the major fat digesting enzyme. It digests triglycerides into monoglycerides and fatty acids
  - **Colipase:** It exposes active sites of pancreatic lipase and facilitates its action
  - **Phospholipase A_2:** It acts on phospholipids and converts it to fatty acids and lysophospholipids.
  - **Cholesterol ester hydrolase** acts on cholesterol esters and splits it into cholesterol and fatty acids.
- **Digestion of proteins:**
  - Proteolytic enzymes are secreted in the inactive forms—trypsinogen, chymotrypsinogen, proelastase and procarboxypeptidase A and B.
  - Trypsinogen on secretion into duodenum is activated to trypsin by the enzyme enterokinase in the intestine.
  - Trypsinogen → trypsin, happens in presence of enterokinase
  - Chymotrypsinogen → chymotrypsin, in presence of trypsin
  - Proelastase and procarboxylase → elastase and carboxylase, in presence of trypsin
  - **Trypsin and chymorypsin** act on proteins and polypeptides and cleaves the peptide bonds in basic and aromatic amino acids.
  - **Elastase** acts on elastin and some other proteins.
  - **Carboxypeptidases** also act on proteins and polypeptides
  - **Nucleases** split ribose and deoxyribose nucleotides
  - Collagenase digests collagen
- **Digestion of carbohydrates:**
  Pancreatic α amylase: It is secreted in active form and just like salivary amylase it hydrolysis glycogen, starch and other complex carbohydrates to form disaccharides.

- **Trypsin inhibitor** secreted from pancreas inhibits activation of trypsinogen and thereby prevents autodigestion of pancreas by trypsin.

  Trypsin if activated initiates a chain of reaction and activates other proteolytic enzymes and can digest the pancreas.

---

5. Female contraception.

Spacing Methods
- Rhythm method
- Barrier method
- Pills
- Intrauterine contraceptive device

Rhythm Method
- This method can be followed in females with regular menstrual cycles of 28-30 days.
- During a normal menstrual cycle, ovulation happens on 14th day of the cycle.
- The ovum stays viable for 48-72 hours after ovulation.
- After ejaculation, sperm stays viable in female reproductive tract for 24-48 hours.
- So pregnancy can happen if intercourse happens within this period.
- This is said to be the "dangerous period".
- So the days are calculated from first day of menstrual cycle and intercourse should be avoided in the dangerous period.
- 5-6 days after the bleeding phase and 5-6 days before the next menstruation is considered to be the "safe period".
- It can be utilized by females with regular cycles and who can keep a record of their time of ovulation by checking basal body temperature.

Barrier Method
- Barriers can be mechanical or chemical barriers. They basically prevent the meeting of sperm and ovum.
- **Mechanical barrier:** Diaphragm and cervical caps
- **Chemical barriers:** Spermicidal agents like nonoxynol, ricinoleic acid in the form of jelly or foam is placed in the female reproductive tract before coitus.

Pills
- By pills we mean the oral contraceptive pills used for female contraception.
- They are usually synthetic preparation of estrogen, progesterone or combination of both.
- **The pills can be of different types:**
  - Combined pill or classical pill
  - Sequential pill
  - Minipill
  - Postcoital pill

Combined pill:
- It is a combination of estrogen and progesterone pill.
- It contains a strip of 21 tablets and is consumed for 21 days from 5th day of menstrual cycle.
- After 21 days, on stopping the tablets, withdrawal bleeding happens.
- Again from 5th day, next cycle is started.

It acts by:
- Prevents ovulation, as the high estrogen levels disorganize the LH and FSH secretions.
- Prevents implantation of fertilized ovum.
- Progesterone makes the cervical mucus thick and prevents sperm penetration

Sequential pill:
- It has high dose of estrogen and minimal amounts of progesterone.
- It is not used nowadays as the high estrogen may induce endometrial cancer or breast cancer.

Minipill:
- It is progesterone only pill.
- It does not affect ovulation but makes the cervical mucus thick and prevents sperm penetration.

Postcoital pill:
- It is used within 72 hours of unprotected intercourse.
- It has high doses of estrogen and is given for 4-6 days.
- High estrogen prevents implantation of the fertilized ovum.

Depot preparation:
- These are implants of progesterone and they are subdermally implanted and prevent pregnancy for 5 years.
- The only problem is it can cause amenorrhea and irregular cycles.

Intrauterine Contraceptive Devices

These are small devices made of plastic or copper and placed in the uterus to prevent implantation of fertilized ovum.

Lippe's loop:
- It is a simple 'S' shaped plastic device with nylon threads.
- Under aseptic precautions, the loop is inserted into the uterus and the thread is present in the vagina.
- The loop is also impregnated with a small amount of barium sulphate for checking its presence by radiographs.

Copper 'T':
- It is a 'T' shaped device made of copper with nylon threads.
- They are inserted during the first 10 days of menstrual cycle.
- Copper prevents implantation of fertilized ovum by stimulating an aseptic inflammation of the endometrium.

Permanent Method

Tubectomy
- It can be done by an open surgery or by laparoscopic surgery.
- Here the fallopian tubes are cut and ligated and buried.

6. Triple response.

Vascular Response of Skin to Injury with a Sharp Pointed Object—Triple Response

Red Reaction
- Occurs within 10 seconds when stroked firmly by a sharp object
- Due to capillary dilatation

Wheal
- Swelling within (local edema) few minutes after red reaction.
- There is ↑in permeability of capillaries due to histamine.

Flare
- Spreading out of redness from site of injury
- Due to arteriolar dilatation.
- Due to axon reflex

Axon Reflex
- When there is an injury to skin with a sharp object, impulses from the skin carried by sensory fibers not only go to the spinal cord, but also goes antidromically through other branches to the arterioles below the skin.
- The neurotransmitter released here is substance P (*refer* **Fig. 15**).
- This causes vasodilatation and extravasation of fluid.

7. Nonrespiratory functions of lungs.

Nonrespiratory Functions
- **Acts as a reservoir for blood:** The pulmonary vessels are highly compliant and therefore can store blood without much increase in pressure. In cases of imbalance in left ventricular output and systemic venous return, the stored blood in the pulmonary circulation helps to regulate cardiac output.

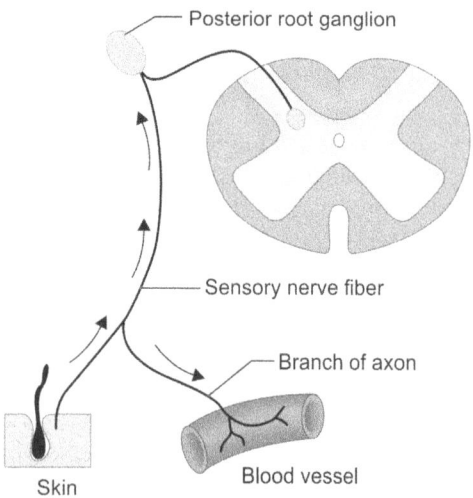

Fig. 15: Axon reflex. Sensory fibers give a branch which travels antidromically to supply arterioles below the skin.

- **Filters** small emboli, particles in blood, detached cancer cells, fat cells, air emboli in blood.
- **Processes inhaled air:** The atmospheric air which enters the airways are hydrated as it passes through the airways.
- **Olfactory function**
- **Metabolic function:**
  - Synthesizes and secretes surfactant
  - Pulmonary capillary endothelial cells secrete angiotensin converting enzyme (ACE) and thereby converts angiotensin I to angiotensin II.
  - Synthesizes, stores and secretes substances like prostaglandins, histamine and kallikrein
  - Partially removes prostaglandin, bradykinin, adenine nucleotides, serotonin, norepinephrine and acetylcholine.
- **Helps in defense:** With the help of pulmonary alveolar macrophages, IgA, mucus secretion, beating of cilia, cough reflex.
- **Helps in speech**
- **Helps in absorption** of drugs like anesthetic gases, aerosols and bronchodilators.
- **Fibrinolytic mechanism** present in the lungs lyses the clot

8. Mechanism of receptor potential.

- Receptor potential is a graded potential.
- The experimental study to identify the receptor potential was done with the pacinian corpuscle.
- It is a receptor for touch and vibration.
- It is quiet larger and therefore can be isolated and studied.
- Each capsule has concentric lamellae of connective tissue surrounding the unmyelinated ending of the sensory nerve fiber.
- Myelin sheath for the terminal starts within the corpuscle.
- The first node of Ranvier is also located inside the corpuscle and the second node is located at the point where the nerve leaves the corpuscle.
- On placing recording electrodes, over the nerve leaving the corpuscle and when graded pressure is applied, a nonpropagated depolarizing potential is recorded.
- It is said to be the generator potential or the receptor potential.
- As the pressure is increased the amplitude of the potential increases and as the potential reaches 10 mV an action potential is fired.
- It has been experimentally identified that the generator potential is generated in the unmyelinated nerve terminal of the sensory nerves.
- The receptor has converted the mechanical energy to electrical energy.
- The generator potential depolarizes the sensory nerve at the first node of Ranvier and generates the action potential there.
- When a weak stimulus is applied to a receptor, a local nonpropagating depolarization potential is produced in the unmyelinated nerve terminal of the receptor (as in pacinian corpuscle). This is the receptor potential.
- If the stimulus intensity is increased, the amplitude of the receptor potential increases to reach a maximum and as it reaches a firing level, current sinks spread to the first node of Ranvier and an action potential is fired here.
- In the receptor studied, the pacinian corpuscle, the receptor or generator potential is produced due to opening of Na^+ channels leading to Na^+ influx.
- In many other receptors also various types of stimuli cause opening of Na^+ channels and are responsible for the receptor potential.

9. Factors regulating cardiac output.

- Cardiac output (CO) is defined as the amount of blood ejected by each ventricle per minute.
  - CO = Stroke volume (SV) × Heart rate (HR)

- NV = 70 mL/beat × 70/min = 4,900 mL/min

Determinants of Cardiac Output
- CO = Stroke volume (SV) × Heart rate (HR)
- So factors affecting either of them will alter CO.

Factors affecting SV:
- Preload
- After load
- Contractility (*refer* **Fig. 16**)

Factors affecting HR:
HR is affected by nerves supplying heart (sympathetic and parasympathetic nerves) and cardiac centers.

Preload
- The initial muscle length is the **preload** (the extent to which the muscle is stretched before contraction).
- Preload is decided by the **end-diastolic volume** (EDV).
- EDV is decided by the **venous return** (VR).
- **Preload affecting stroke volume is based on the Frank-Starling's law:** It states that within physiological limits, the force of contraction is directly proportional to the initial length of the muscle.

Causes for application of Frank-Starling's law:
- Increase in EDV →↑ stretch of muscle fiber → interaction of thick and thin filament increases →↑ force of contraction.
- Stretch of muscle fibers → opens stretch sensitive Ca^{2+} channels on sarcolemma →↑ Ca^{2+} influx →↑ force of contraction.
- ↑Ca^{2+} influx →↑ Ca^{2+} release from SR (CICR) →↑ force of contraction.
- ↑stretch of muscle fiber →↑ affinity of troponin for Ca^{2+}

EDV is dependent on:
- **Venous return, which is dependent on:**
  - *Skeletal muscle pump:* Contraction of limb muscles press on the veins and increases forward movement of blood in the veins
  - *Thoracic pump:* Increase in respiration depresses the diaphragm and decreases intrathoracic pressure and thereby it acts like a suction force to increase VR
  - *Abdominal pump:* During respiration compression of abdominal muscles press on the veins and favors venous emptying
  - *Cardiac pump:* Vis-a-tergo (force from behind), vis-a-fronte (force from front)

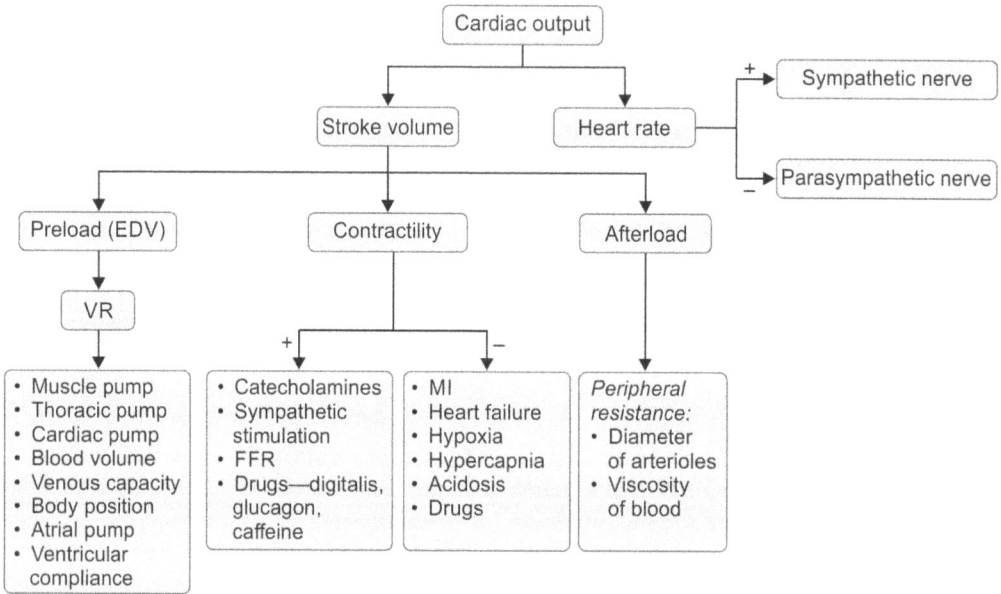

Fig. 16: Regulation of cardiac output.
(FFR: force-frequency relation, MI: myocardial infarction)

- *Total blood volume:* As the blood volume increases VR increases and vice versa
- *Capacity of venous system:* Sympathetic stimulation to the veins causes venoconstriction and thereby increases venous emptying
- *Body position:* On standing there is venous pooling due to gravity and it may decrease the VR.
❏ **Atrial pump activity:** Contributes 20% ventricular filling and stimulated by sympathetic stimulation.
❏ **Ventricular compliance:** Affected by damage to myocardium as in MI, pericardial effusion, cardiac tamponade.

This type of regulation of stroke volume in relation to change in initial length of muscle fiber is said to be **heterometric regulation**.

Contractility

Contractility is increase in force of contraction and there by increase in stroke volume without increase in initial muscle length.
❏ Ventricles are able to do more work per stroke at a given EDV.
❏ Factors which affect contractility—**inotropic agents**.
❏ There are positive and negative inotropic agents.

Contractility is increased by:
❏ Autonomic activity (sympathetics are positively inotropic)
❏ **Muscle mass:** Increase in myocardial mass increases contractility as after regular exercise
❏ Concentration of hormones and chemicals
❏ **Heart rate:** Force frequency relationship

Factors increasing contractility, positive inotropic agents:
❏ Sympathetic stimulation
❏ Circulating catecholamines
❏ Force frequency relationship
❏ Digitalis
❏ Glucagon
❏ Insulin
❏ Thyroxine
❏ Chemicals like xanthine, theophylline

Factors decreasing contractility, negative inotropic agents:
❏ Loss of myocardium as in myocardial infarction
❏ Hypoxia
❏ Hypercapnia
❏ Acidosis
❏ Acetylcholine

Regulation of stroke volume by affecting contractility of myocardium is **homometric regulation**. Here the force of contraction is affected without much change in muscle length.

Afterload

❏ It is the force against which the heart muscle shortens
❏ Cardiac output is inversely proportional to after load
❏ Cardiac output α-1/after load (**Anrep effect**)
❏ It is decided by peripheral resistance
❏ **Peripheral resistance is decided by:**
  - Vessel diameter
  - Viscosity of blood
❏ This is also included in **homometric regulation**.

Regulation of Heart Rate

❏ Heart rate is also a factor affecting CO.
❏ HR is in turn regulated by autonomic nerves.
❏ Sympathetics →↑ heart rate
❏ Parasympathetics →↓ HR
❏ Normally ↑ HR →↑ CO
❏ But in severe tachycardia →↓ duration of diastole →↓ ventricular filling →↓ CO

10. Anatomic dead space.

❏ Dead space is the space in the airways in which the volume of air present does not take part in gaseous exchange.
❏ There are three types of dead spaces—anatomical dead space, alveolar dead space and physiological or total dead space.
❏ **Anatomical dead space** is the conducting zone of the respiratory pathway in which the gaseous exchange does not take place

and the volume of air is said to be the dead space air.
- In a normal adult, of the 500 mL of tidal volume inhaled, 150 mL remains in the anatomical dead space.

---

11. Passive transport.

Here the movement of substances is along the concentration or electrical gradient and there is no energy expenditure.

Types:
1. Simple diffusion
2. Facilitated diffusion
3. Osmosis
4. Filtration
5. Bulk flow
6. Solvent drag

Simple Diffusion

- **Lipid soluble** substances diffuse by dissolving in the membrane and diffuse to either side of membrane—O_2, N_2, steroids, etc.
- **Water soluble** substances move through water filled channel proteins.
- No energy expenditure.
- Moves substances along concentration gradient

Diffusion through Channels

- Channels are water-filled pores.
- This allows water soluble substances to move across the membrane.
- The channels have selective permeability.
- They may be gated or nongated
- Gates could be either change in—voltage, binding ligands or stretch (mechanical) (*refer* **Fig. 17**).

Factors affecting Net Diffusion

- **Cell membrane permeability:**
  - *Thickness of membrane:* Inversely proportional
  - *Lipid solubility:* Directly proportional
  - *Distribution of protein channels in membrane*
  - *Temperature:* Directly proportional
  - *Size of molecule:* Inversely proportional
  - *Area of membrane:* Directly proportional
- **Concentration gradient:** Directly proportional
- **Electrical gradient**
- **Pressure gradient:** Directly proportional

Facilitated Diffusion

- Large water-soluble substances (e.g., glucose) are carried by a protein which changes configuration on binding.
- This change in configuration shifts the molecule in or out (*refer* **Fig. 18**).
- Highly selective and specific
- **Types:**
  - Uniport
  - Symport
  - Antiport
- **Characteristics:**
  - Specificity
  - Saturation
  - Competition

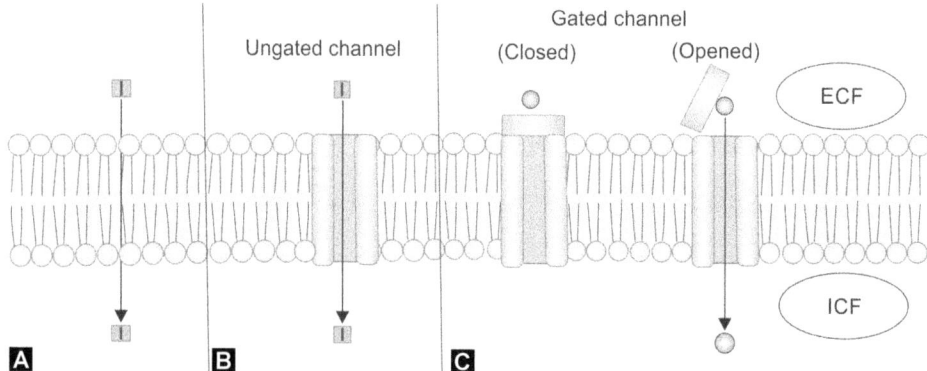

Figs. 17A to C: (A) Simple diffusion through lipid membrane; (B) Simple diffusion through nongated channels; (C) Diffusion through gated channels.

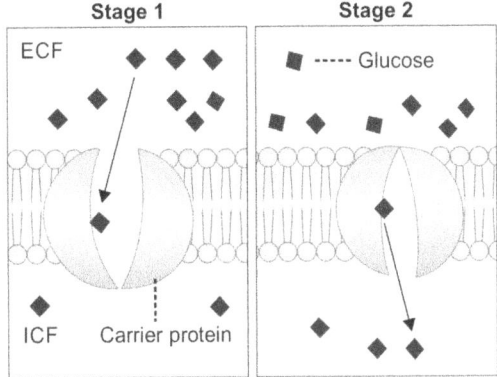

Fig. 18: Facilitated diffusion. A uniport transporting glucose molecules.

Osmosis

Diffusion of water or other solvent molecules through a semi-permeable membrane (i.e., membrane impermeable to solute and not to solvent) from a solution containing lower concentration of solutes to the solution containing higher concentration of solutes— **osmosis**.

Filtration and Bulk Flow

- Filtration or movement of water and solutes through the capillary wall are examples of filtration.
- If filtration involves movement of greater volume of water it is called bulk flow.

Solvent Drag

During bulk flow if solvents are carried along—solvent drag.

---

12. Gastric emptying.

- Gastric emptying is a slow process in which food from stomach is gradually emptied into the duodenum and jejunum.
- There are three mechanisms in gastric emptying:
  a. **Peristaltic contractions:** These are ring like contractions starting in the body of stomach and gradually push the contents towards the antrum. The waves in the proximal part are weak and as it reaches the antrum the waves become stronger and dig into the chyme. So adequate mixing and breaking down of food particles happen in the antrum (*refer* **Fig. 19A**).
  b. **Contractions of antrum:** Antral contractions are very strong and they help in proper mixing of gastric juice with food contents. Not only mixing of food and gastric juice happens but also the force of contraction forces the food towards the pylorus. But the pyloric sphincter ahead is strongly contracted. (*refer* **Fig. 19B**)
  c. **Retropulsion:** Forceful contraction of antrum and closure of pyloric sphincter pushes the food back into the proximal part of the antrum and this continues for few times. The retropulsion helps in mixing and grinding the food particles. The pyloric sphincter opens partially allowing small quantities of chyme at a time to be squirted into the duodenum (*refer* **Fig. 19C**).

Regulation of Gastric Emptying

Regulation is done by neural and humoral mechanisms. Factors which affect emptying are—pH of contents in duodenum, osmotic pressure, products of fat and protein digestion.

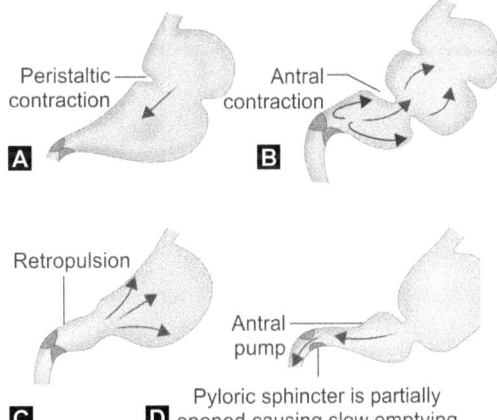

Figs. 19A to D: Gastric emptying; In A, B and C the pyloric sphincter is closed. The contractions in antrum digest the food and is converted to chyme. (C) There is forward movement of chyme and as the sphincter is closed there is retropulsion of chyme which further breaks food particles. (D) Sphincter is partially open allowing small amounts of chyme to be emptied.

- **Low pH:** Acidic content in the duodenum are sensed by receptors in the duodenum and gastric emptying is delayed by secretin released from small intestines.
- **Osmolality of contents:** If the osmolality of the contents entering the duodenum is high it is sensed by osmoreceptors here and hormones are released which inhibit gastric emptying.
- **Products of digestion of fat:** Presence of digested fats and fatty acids are sensed by the duodenum and CCK is released which causes delay in gastric emptying.
- **Products of protein digestion:** Protein products like peptides and amino acids in duodenum cause release of gastrin which in turn causes antral contraction and closure of pyloric sphincter resulting in delaying the gastric emptying.
- **Volume and type of meal:** When volume of meal is more there is delayed emptying. Watery meal hastens the emptying. Carbohydrate emptying is faster and fat emptying is the slowest.
- **Stretch of duodenum:** When duodenal wall is stretched it induces enterogastric reflex which inhibits gastric emptying.
- **Neural factors:** Vagus stimulation promotes emptying and sympathetic stimulation delays emptying.

13. Peculiarities of renal blood flow.

- Rate of renal blood flow is 1,200 mL/min or 400 mL/100 g of tissue per minute
- Renal O_2 consumption is highest next to the heart (6 mL/100 g/min)
- There is a regional difference in blood flow in the cortex and the medulla. Since the glomeruli, where filtration happens, lie in the cortex, cortical blood flow is high (5 mL/g/min) of kidney.
- Medullary interstitial osmolality needs to be maintained and therefore medullary blood flow is low (2.5 mL/g in outer medulla and 0.6 mL/g/min in inner medulla)
- O_2 extraction is less in the cortex (PO_2 is 50 mm Hg) and more in the medulla (PO_2 is 15 mm Hg). AV O_2 difference is also less in the cortex and more in medulla.
- The vasculature is also different in the kidneys. The afferent arterioles break down into glomerular capillaries and they in turn reunite to form the efferent arteriole which again breaks down into peritubular capillaries or vasa recta. Renal circulation is therefore a type of portal circulation.
- The pressure in glomerular capillaries is higher than in any other systemic capillaries as the efferent arteriole is partially constricted than the afferent arteriole. Also the renal artery arises directly from the abdominal aorta.
- Autoregulation of renal blood flow is very well developed in the kidneys. This helps in regulating the GFR.

14. Second messengers.

These are intracellular messengers activated by the membrane bound protein/receptors in the target organs on which the peptide hormones act.

The peptide hormones are said to be the 'First messengers'.

These second messengers are activated through G-proteins which are attached to the receptors on the cell membrane.

The general principle of second messenger activation is:

Binding of the hormone to its receptor on cell membrane
↓
Activates G-proteins and the membrane-bound enzymes
↓
Formation of second messengers
↓
Activation of protein kinase enzymes
↓
Phosphorylation of proteins
↓
Cellular response

The G-proteins are: G_s, G_i, G_q, G_{tl}, G_{13}

The enzymes activated by G-proteins are: Adenylyl cyclase, guanylyl cyclase, phospholipase C, etc.

The second messengers are: cAM P, cGMP, Ca^{2+}, inositol triphosphate (IP3), diacylglycerol (DAG), etc.

Proteinkinases activated by second messengers are:
- cAMP dependent kinases
- cGMP dependent kinase
- Protein kinase C
- Calmodulin dependent kinase
- Tyrosine kinases

G-proteins:
- G-proteins are nucleotide regulatory proteins that bind to GTP.
- GTP is the guanosine analog of ATP.
- There are two types of G-proteins—small G-proteins and large G-proteins.
- When signal reaches a G-protein, the protein exchanges GDP for GTP and brings about the response. On completion of action, the intrinsic GTPase activity of the protein converts GTP to GDP
- Large G-proteins couple cell surface receptors to catalytic units on the membrane that catalyzes formation of intracellular second messengers or couple receptors to ion channels.
- There are three subunits for the G-protein—α, β, and γ (*refer* **Fig. 20**).
- Only α subunit is bound to GDP.
- On binding of the ligand to G-protein coupled receptor, GDP is exchanged for GTP and a subunit is separated from β and γ subunits.
- The intrinsic GTPase activity of the α subunit converts GTP to GDP and the action is terminated.

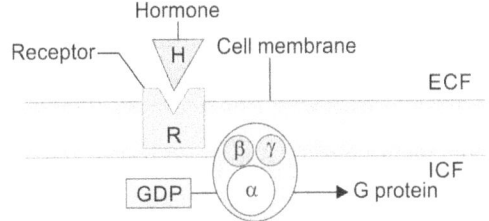

Fig. 20: G-protein: Hormone binds to G-protein bound receptor on the cell membrane; G-protein in inactive form is bound to GDP. There are three subunits for G-protein—α, β, and γ.
(H: hormone; R: receptor)

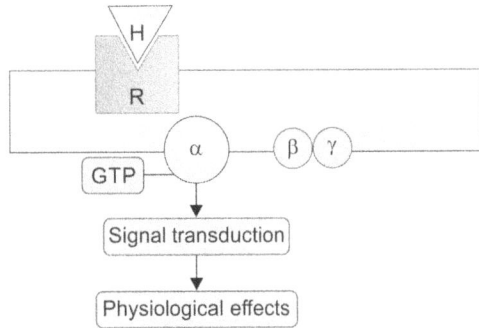

Fig. 21: On binding of hormone to G-protein bound receptor activates G-protein. α-subunit separates and G-protein exchanges GDP for GTP. This induces series of actions and is responsible for hormone action.

Mechanism of action through G-protein-coupled receptors (Gs-adenylyl cyclase-cAMP pathway):
- Ligand (hormone) binds to the G_s protein coupled receptor
- On binding of ligand and receptor, α subunit of G-protein separates from β and γ subunits (*refer* **Fig. 21**)
- On separation of α subunit, the catalytic enzyme—for example, adenylyl cyclase (enzyme) attached to Gs protein is activated (*refer* **Fig. 22**).
- Adenylyl cyclase converts ATP to cAMP.
- cAMP activates the enzyme protein kinase A which phosphorylates proteins and brings about changes in the cell.

15. Hypersecretion of growth hormone.

Acromegaly
- It is a clinical condition due to excess secretion of growth hormone (GH) in adults (after the fusion of the epiphyseal plates in the long bones).
- It is usually due to a tumor of growth hormone producing cells (somatotrophs) in the anterior pituitary gland.
- Rarely, it can also be due to hypothalamic tumors secreting GH releasing hormone.
- There is no increase in height of the individual.
- But because of excess levels of GH, there is thickening of bones and proliferation of soft tissues like connective tissue and skin.

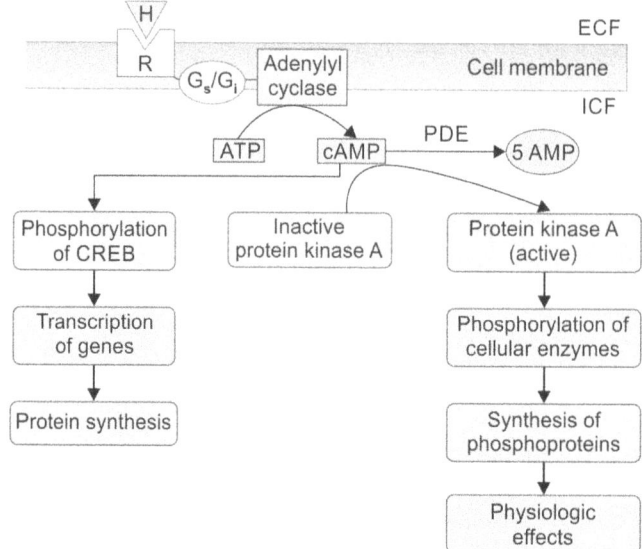

Fig. 22: Mechanism of hormone action through adenylyl cyclase-cAMP pathway.
(H: hormone; R: receptor; Gs/Gi: stimulatory or inhibitory G-protein, PDE: phosphodiesterase, CREB: cAMP-responsive element-binding protein).

- This leads to coarse disfigured appearance. "Acro" means extremity and "megaly" is large.

Clinical Features of Acromegaly
- The tumor in the anterior pituitary compresses the optic chiasma resulting in visual disturbances.
- Enlargement of sella turcica and headache.
- Enlarging tumor may destroy other pituitary cells and decrease in levels of other hormones secreted from anterior pituitary may happen.

Clinical features due to excess GH levels:
- **Acromegalic face:** Jaw and cheek bones become more prominent, lips are thickened, nose is broad and thick, enlarged brows and coarse skin.
- **Prognathism:** Protrusion of the lower jaw due to elongation and thickening of mandible.
- Enlarged spade like hands, broad fingers and large feet.
- Body hair is increased
- **Kyphosis:** Since the vertebral bones continue to grow the person has kyphosis.
- They develop osteoarthritis
- **Organomegaly:** Internal organs like heart, liver, spleen and kidneys are enlarged.
- High levels of GH decreases insulin sensitivity in the tissues and the patient has hyperglycemia and are prone to develop diabetes mellitus

Gigantism

It is due to hypersecretion of GH in children before the closure of epiphysis.

Symptoms
- Abnormal height (7–8 feet tall)
- Enlarged hands and feet
- Gynecomastia
- Loss of libido
- Hyperglycemia which may result in diabetes mellitus
- They also have symptoms similar to acromegaly due to the compression of tumor on neighboring neural structure.

16. Ventricular action potential.

- The resting membrane potential (RMP) of ventricular muscle is –90 mV
- Following the stimulation from the SA node, through the conducting system, the ventricular myocyte, which is a fast muscle

gets excited and it fires an action potential (AP).
- Following the electrical excitation (action potential) the ventricular muscle contracts.
- The ventricular AP has a rapid depolarization followed by a small rapid repolarization and a plateau phase (*refer* **Fig. 23**).
- The plateau is followed by replorization and it reaches the RMP
- The depolarization is for 2 ms, plateau and repolarization is for 200 ms or more. By this time the mechanical contraction is half over. So tetanization is not possible in cardiac muscle.

Ionic Events Responsible for the AP

- The initial rapid depolarization (phase 0) is due to opening of voltage-gated Na⁺ channels and rapid influx of Na⁺. The spike reaches a potential of +20 mV.
- This is followed by an initial rapid repolarization (phase 1) which is due to closure of the Na⁺ channels and opening of K⁺ channels and therefore K⁺ efflux (I_{TO}).
- Initial rapid repolarization is followed by a plateau phase (phase 2) due to influx of Ca²⁺ and efflux of K⁺. The calcium channel opening here is a slower voltage-gated Ca²⁺ channel (L type channels) (*refer* **Fig. 23**).
- Final repolarization (phase 3) is due to closure of Ca²⁺ channels and opening of K⁺ channels (I_{KS}) and K⁺ efflux.
- Phase 4 is the phase of restoration of the RMP.

17. Tracts of Goll and Burdach.

Tracts of Posterior/Dorsal Column

- The posterior or dorsal column consists of the tracts of Goll and Burdach
- They ascend up in two fasciculi—fasciculus gracilis and fasciculus cuneatus.
- They are made up of large myelinated fibers which carry sensations like touch, pressure, vibration, stereognosis, tactile localization, tactile discrimination and proprioception.
- Gracile fasciculus lies medially and carries these sensations from the hind limb and trunk, the cuneate fasciculus lies laterally and carries impulses from the upper half of the body and upper limbs.
- It is also called as the lemniscal system
- First order neurons have their cell bodies in the dorsal root ganglia.
- The peripheral axons of these neurons are nerve fibers from the receptors.
- The central axons from the dorsal root ganglia enter the spinal cord and ascend up in the dorsal column as the dorsal column tract.

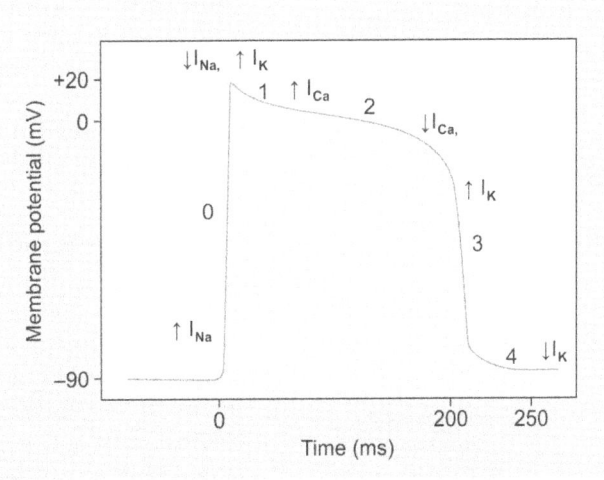

Fig 23: Ventricular action potential.

- Gracile and cuneate fasciculi reach medulla and synapse with ipsilateral nucleus gracilis and nucleus cuneatus respectively (*refer* **Fig. 24**).
- From these nuclei, the second order neurons arise and cross to the opposite side and ascend up as the medial lemniscus.
- Medial lemniscus terminate on the ventroposterolateral nucleus (VPLN) of the opposite side thalamus.
- Third order neuron arises from the thalamus and terminates in the somatosensory area 1 (Broadman's are 3, 1, 2) in postcentral gyrus.

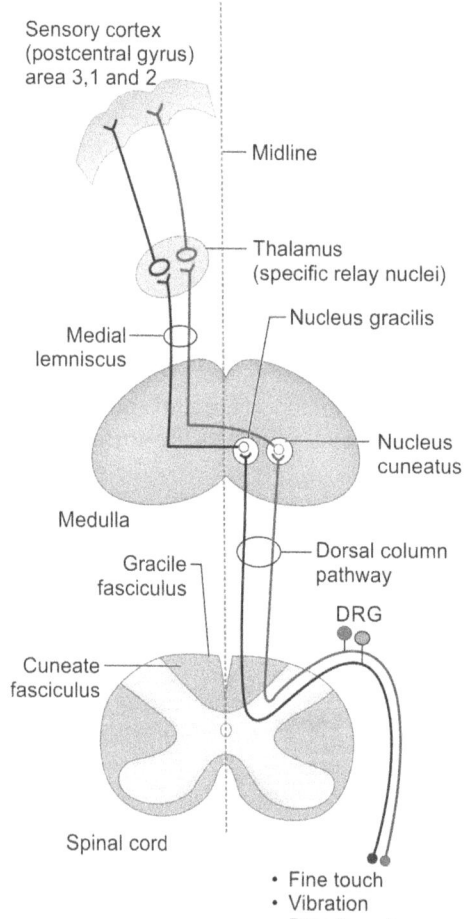

Fig. 24: Pathway of dorsal column tract.

18. Venous return.

- Venous return (VR) is the amount of blood that returns to the right atrium from the periphery through inferior vena cava and superior vena cava.
- VR decides the end diastolic volume (EDV) which in turn decides the stroke volume (SV).
- SV decides the cardiac output and thereby the systolic blood pressure
- So factors affecting venous return will affect the cardiac output.

Venous return is dependent on:
- **Skeletal muscle pump:** Contraction of limb muscles press on the veins and increases forward movement of blood in the veins and thereby increases VR.
- **Thoracic pump:** Increase in respiration depresses the diaphragm and decreases intrathoracic pressure and thereby it acts like a suction force to increase VR
- **Abdominal pump:** During respiration compression of abdominal muscles press on the veins and favors venous emptying
- **Ventricular compliance:** Decrease in ventricular compliance decreases the ventricular filling and thereby decreases EDV
- **Cardiac pump:** Vis-a-tergo (force from behind), vis-A-fronte (force from front)
- **Total blood volume:** As the blood volume increases VR increases and vice versa
- **Capacity of venous system:** Sympathetic stimulation to the veins causes venoconstriction and thereby increases venous emptying
- **Body position:** On standing there is venous pooling due to gravity and it may decrease the VR.

19. Lung volumes and capacities.

- Respiration is the process in which inspiration of atmospheric air is followed by equal volume of air expired out. The measure of quantities of air at different stages of respiration is given as lung volumes and capacities.
- Lung volumes are individual measures of air in the respiratory system at various

stages and capacities are two or more volumes put together.
- Most of the lung volumes and capacities are measured with a spirometer and the recording is said to be the spirogram (*refer* **Fig. 25**). Residual volume and capacities which includes residual volume cannot be measured with spirometer.

Lung Volumes and Capacities

- Lung volumes are—tidal volume (TV), inspiratory reserve volume (IRV), expiratory reserve volume (ERV), residual volume (RV)
- Lung capacities are—inspiratory capacity (IC), functional residual capacity (FRC), vital capacity (VC) and total lung capacity (TLC).

Tidal Volume

- It is the volume of air inspired or expired with each breath during normal breathing.
- Normal volume is 500 mL in adults.
- It is less in children and increases with age. It increases with exercise and muscular activity.

Inspiratory Reserve Volume

- It is the maximal volume of air inspired by forceful inspiration after a tidal inspiration.
- Normal value is 3.3 L in males and 1.9 L in females.

Expiratory Reserve Volume

- It is the maximal volume of air exhaled from the resting end-expiratory level (volume expired by active expiration after passive expiration). 750–1000 mL.
- Normal value is 1 L in men and 700 mL in females.

Residual Volume

- It is the volume of air remaining in the lungs at the end of maximal expiration.
- Normally it is about 1,200 mL in males and 1,100 mL in females.
- Residual volume is the volume remaining in the lung even after forceful and complete expiration.
- This volume cannot be measured by spirometer.
- It can be measured by subtracting ERV from FRC and FRC is measured by helium dilution technique.

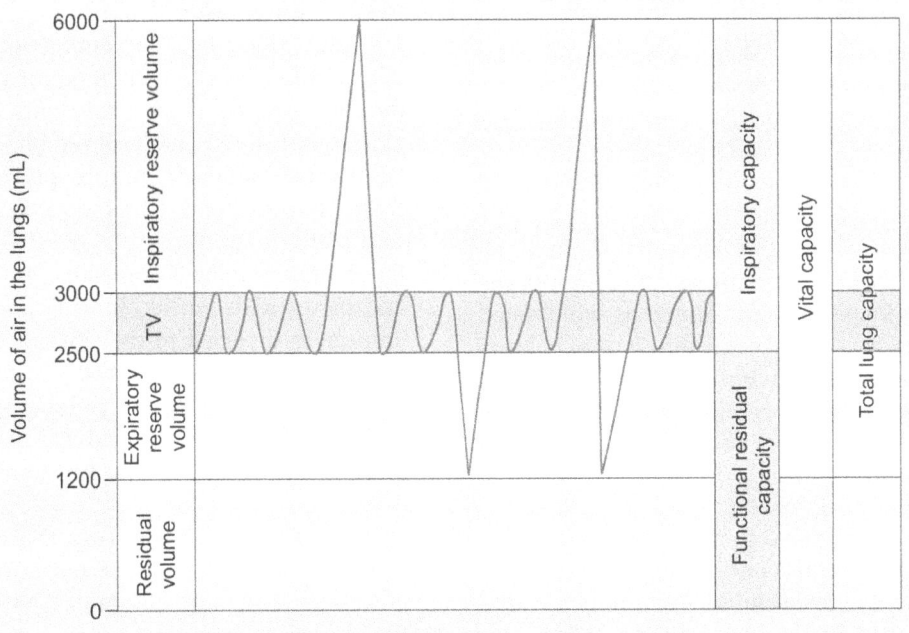

Fig 25: Spirogram.
(TV: tidal volume)

Lung Capacities

Inspiratory Capacity
- It is the maximal volume of air inspired from resting expiratory level.
- Normal value is 3,000–3,500 mL
  IC = IRV + TV.

Functional Residual Capacity
- It is the volume of air remaining in the lungs at the end of resting (normal) expiration.
- Normal value—2,500 mL
- FRC = RV + ERV

Significance of FRC:
- This volume of gas in the lungs helps in continuous exchange of gases even in between the breaths.
- It helps maintain a stable O_2 and CO_2 levels in the alveolus.

Measurement of FRC:
FRC is measured by helium dilution technique.

Helium dilution technique:
- The subject is made to breathe from a spirometer with a known volume of gas mixture with helium of known concentration.
- It is made to breathe from normal end expiration.
- The remaining volume of air in lungs at end expiration will be equal to FRC.
- If it breathes in after forced expiration RV can be measured.
- Now as the subjects breathe through the spirometer many times, the FRC and the gas in spirometer and lung has equilibrated and have equal concentrations of helium. The new concentration of helium is measured and is said to be C2.
- Now the FRC is calculated by using the formula:
  C1 × V1 = C2 × V2.
  - V1 = Initial volume of spirometer
  - C1 = Initial concentration of helium
  - V2 = Final volume of spirometer + FRC
  - C2 = Final concentration of helium
- V2 = V1 × C1/C2

- FRC = V2 − V1
       = V1 (C1 − C2)/C2

Vital Capacity
- Maximum volume of gas completely expired from the lungs following a maximal inspiration.
- Normal value—4,800 mL (in males) and 3,200 mL (in females)
- VC = TLC − RV
  or
  VC = IRV + TV + ERV
- **Total lung capacity (TLC):** It is the total volume of air within the lung after maximum inspiration. It is the maximum volume of air that the lung can contain.
- Normal value—6,000 mL TLC = FVC + RV
  or
  TLC = RV + ERV + TV + IRV
- TLC is increased in airway narrowing with air trapping as in bronchial asthma.

---

20. Fetal circulation.

- Fetal circulation is different from circulation in postnatal life. In postnatal life the circulation between right and left heart is in series and in fetal life it is parallel in many sites.
- The fetal lung is not functioning and the placenta behaves like the fetal lung and the fetus derives O_2 and nutrients from placentas through umbilical vessels.
- Fetus receives blood from the placentas through umbilical veins and is 80% saturated with oxygen.
- Blood from umbilical vein enters the liver and mixes with portal blood and some amount is diverted to the inferior vena cava through 'ductus venosus'.
- The portal and systemic venous blood in fetus is 26% saturated with O_2 and the saturation of mixed blood in IVC is around 67%.
- Most of this blood entering the right atrium through IVC is directed into left atrium through foramen ovale.
- Blood from SVC enters the right ventricle and is sent into the pulmonary artery.

- But the fetal lung is collapsed and therefore resistance in pulmonary artery is higher than in the aorta.
- Most of the blood in pulmonary artery is pushed into the aorta through 'ductus arteriosus'.
- In this fashion relatively unsaturated blood is diverted to the trunk and lower parts of the body and head of the fetus receives better saturated blood from left ventricle.
- From aorta some of the blood is pumped into the umbilical artery and back to the placenta.

Changes Happening at Birth

- At birth placental circulation is cut off and the pressure in aorta rises more than that in the pulmonary artery.
- Since no supply comes from placenta the fetus suffers from asphyxia and it gasps for breath and cries which causes expansion of lungs.
- As the lung expands the pulmonary resistance falls and blood starts flowing into the pulmonary vessels.
- Blood returning to left atrium rises the left atrial pressure and it closes the foramen ovale.
- Ductus arteriosus constricts within few hours after birth and permanent closure happens due to intimal thickening by 24–48 hours.

III. SHORT ANSWERS

1. Mechanism of action of botulinum toxin and the basis of botox injection.

- There are various drugs and toxins acting at the neuromuscular transmission and thereby affect muscle contraction.
- Botulinum toxin is derived from the bacteria *Clostridium botulinum*.
- There are various types in it—toxins A, B, C, D, F and G.
- Toxins B, D, F and G act on the synaptic membrane protein synaptobrevin.
- Toxin C acts on another protein syntaxin and toxins A and B act on the protein SNAP-25.
- By inhibiting these proteins, they prevent the release of neurotransmitter vesicle from presynaptic terminal.
- These toxins act at the neuromuscular junction and they inhibit the release of acetylcholine. This induces flaccid paralysis of the muscles.
- Botox produced from botulinum toxin is used to treat conditions involving muscle hyperactivity as in achalasia cardia to relieve the contraction of lower esophageal sphincter.
- It is also injected into facial muscles to relieve facial wrinkles.

2. What is steatorrhea?

- Excretion of fats in stools is called steatorrhea. Stools in steatorrhea, are fatty, bulky and clay-colored because of impaired digestion and absorption of fats.
- It usually happens following pancreatectomy or damage to exocrine pancreas.
- Indigestion of fats is due to deficiency of lipase, lack of alkaline secretion from the pancreas or lowering of intestinal pH.
- Hypersecretion of gastric acids also causes steatorrhea.
- Other important cause is improper absorption of bile salts and therefore loss of bile salts in stools. Loss of bile salts beyond the capacity for production by liver leads to defective absorption of fats and results in steatorrhea.

3. List out four functions of liver.

- **Storage function:** Liver stores protein, glycogen, vitamins A, D, B_{12} and iron.
- **Synthesis function:** Liver synthesizes albumin, clotting factors (I, II, V, VII, IX and X), lipids, bile salts, cholesterol, heparin and enzymes like SGOT, SGPT, etc.
- **Metabolic functions:** Liver takes part in metabolism of carbohydrates, proteins, lipids and vitamins.
  - *Carbohydrate metabolism:* It takes part in glycogenolysis, glycogenesis and gluconeogenesis
  - *Protein metabolism:* Synthesizes many proteins like albumin. It also converts

ammonia to urea. It is the site of synthesis of urea.
- *Lipid metabolism:* Synthesis of triglycerides from free fatty acids and glycerol, formation of ketones following lipolysis and synthesis of lipoproteins (HDL, LDL)
❏ **Secretory function:** Liver secretes bile acids and bile salts in bile.

4. Draw schematically how HCl is formed.

The steps involved in HCl secretion are:
1. CO_2 in the cell is hydrated in the presence of carbonic anhydrase, $CO_2 + H_2O \rightarrow H_2CO_3$
2. $H_2CO_3 \rightarrow H^+ + HCO_3^-$
3. The H^+ is pumped into the lumen by the H^+-K^+ATPase pump on the apical side. For one H^+ pumped out of cell one K^+ is taken into the cell which later diffuses back into the lumen
4. HCO_3^- is extruded in the basolateral side through an anion exchanger in exchange for one Cl^- (*refer* **Fig. 26**).
5. The Cl^- which enters the cell will diffuse across the apical membrane into the lumen.
6. So for every H^+ secreted, one Cl^- is also secreted into the lumen and one HCO_3^- is absorbed into the blood.

So when gastric secretion is increased after a meal, the HCO_3^- getting added to the blood is increased, thereby raising the pH of blood—*postprandial alkaline tide.*

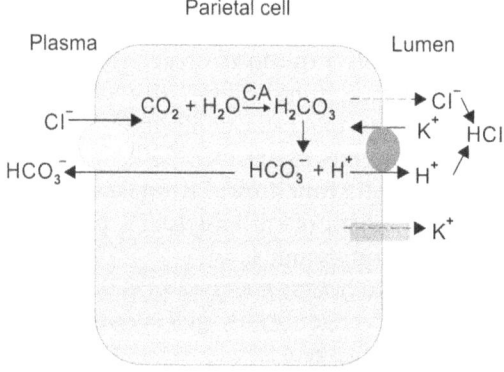

Fig. 26: Mechanism of HCl secretion.
(CA: carbonic anhydrase)

5. What are renal threshold and tubular maximum for glucose?

❏ Transport maximum or tubular maximum (Tm) is the maximum amount of the solute that can be actively transported (reabsorbed or secreted) per minute by the renal tubules.
❏ Tm is the level at which the carrier, transporting the substance, gets saturated and beyond this level, the substances are no more reabsorbed or secreted.
❏ Therefore, the amount of substance transported depends on the amount of the solute present in the tubular fluid up to the Tm for the solute.

Tubular Maximum for Glucose (TmG)

❏ The transporters in the epithelial cells of PCT used for reabsorption of glucose are SGLT2 and GLUT2 on apical and basolateral sides respectively.
❏ The transporter on reaching its Tm, does not reabsorb glucose anymore and it starts appearing in the urine.
❏ Tm for glucose in males is 375 mg/min and 300 mg/min in females.

Renal Threshold

❏ It is the concentration of a solute in plasma at or above which the substance starts appearing in the urine.
❏ Renal threshold for glucose should have been ideally 300 mg/dL (threshold = TmG/GFR, so, 375 mg/min/125 mg/min = 300 mg/dL).
❏ But glucose starts appearing in urine when the plasma concentration reaches 200 mg/dL of arterial plasma and 180 mg/dL of venous plasma.
❏ This is because the TmG differs in different tubules and there is also difference in removal of glucose by the nephrons when the amount filtered is below TmG.

6. Give an example of neuroendocrine reflex. Briefly outline its pathway.

❏ In this type of reflex, the afferent limb of the reflex is neural and the efferent limb is humoral or endocrine.

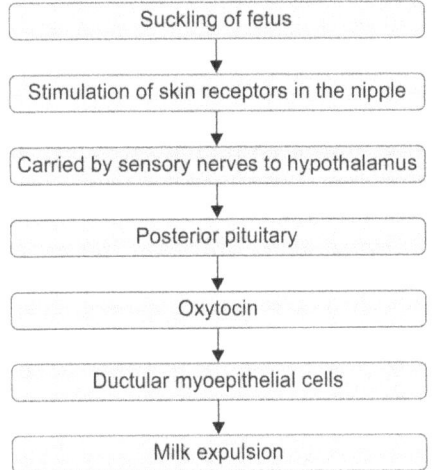

Fig. 27: Milk ejection reflex.

- Examples of this reflex are milk ejection or milk let down reflex and the parturition reflex.

Milk ejection reflex: Oxytocin is a hormone secreted from the hypothalamus and released from posterior pituitary gland. It acts on the myoepithelial cells lining the ducts of breast and expels milk through a reflex.
- The receptors for this reflex are touch receptors around the nipple. When the infant suckles at the breast the touch receptors are stimulated.
- Impulses are relayed through somatic afferent pathways to the supraoptic (SO) and paraventricular (PV) nuclei of hypothalamus.
- These nuclei secrete the hormone oxytocin which is transported through blood and acts on the myoepithelial cells lining the ducts of the breast resulting in expulsion of milk (*refer* **Fig. 27**).

7. Name four hormones which increase blood glucose levels. What is the mechanism of action of one of this hormone?

Hormones which increase blood glucose levels are:
- Glucagon
- Glucocorticoids
- Catecholamines
- Growth hormone
- Thyroid hormones

Mechanism of action of glucagon:
- It increases blood glucose levels by various mechanisms like glycogenolysis and gluconeogenesis.
- In the liver it activates the enzyme phosphorylase and breaks down glycogen.
- Glycogenolysis is favored by activating phospholipase C and increase in cytoplasmic Ca^{2+} in the hepatocytes. It has no glycogenolytic action on muscles.
- It increases gluconeogenesis with the help of pyruvate, lactate, glycerol and amino acids.

8. Compare the actions of adrenaline and noradrenaline on heart and blood vessels.

- Adrenaline and noradrenaline act on the heart and increase the force and rate of contraction.
- They mediate these actions through β1 receptors.
- They also increase the myocardial excitability and thereby increase the heart rate.
- They also decrease the AV nodal delay.
- Norepinephrine produces vasoconstriction in almost all blood vessels via α1 receptors.
- Adrenaline causes vasodilatation in blood vessels in skeletal muscles and liver via β2 receptors.

9. Explain the mechanism of action of contraceptive pills.

- Contraceptive pills are usually synthetic preparation of estrogen, progesterone or combination of both.
- **The pills can be of different types:**
  1. Combined pill or classical pill
  2. Sequential pill
  3. Minipill
  4. Postcoital pill

Combined Pill

- It is a combination of estrogen and progesterone pill.

- It contains a strip of 21 tablets and is consumed for 21 days from 5th day of menstrual cycle.
- After 21 days, on stopping the tablets, withdrawal bleeding happens.
- Again from 5th day, next cycle is started.

It acts by:
- Prevents ovulation, as the high estrogen levels disorganize the LH and FSH secretions.
- Prevents implantation of fertilized ovum.
- Progesterone makes the cervical mucus thick and prevents sperm penetration

Sequential Pill
- It has high dose of estrogen and minimal amounts of progesterone.
- It is not used nowadays as the high estrogen may induce endometrial cancer or breast cancer.

Minipill
- It is progesterone only pill.
- It does not affect ovulation but makes the cervical mucus thick and prevents sperm penetration.

Postcoital Pill
- It is used within 72 hours of unprotected intercourse.
- It has high doses of estrogen and is given for 4–6 days.
- High estrogen prevents implantation of the fertilized ovum.

Depot Preparation
- These are implants of progesterone and they are subdermally implanted and prevent pregnancy for 5 years.
- The only problem is it can cause amenorrhea and irregular cycles.

10. How does temperature influence spermatogenesis?

Spermatogenesis takes place in a temperature less than the inner body temperature. The testes are kept at a temperature of 32°C. If the testis is exposed to higher temperatures the tubular walls degenerate, inhibits spermatogenesis and sterility results.

11. Neuromuscular blockers.

Blockers of NMJ
- *Curare:* It binds with the ACh receptors and prevents binding of ACh to their receptors. This blocks the neuromuscular transmission.
- *Bungarotoxin:* This is acquired from snake venom. It also prevents impulse transmission by binding the ACh receptors
- *Succinycholine:* They act just like ACh and make the muscle membrane depolarized. But the choline esterase does not have any effect on these substances and therefore the muscle is continuously depolarized and cannot be stimulated again. So it is called as depolarizing blockers.
- *Botulinum toxin:* They are derived from the bacteria *Clostridium tetani* and it prevents release of ACh vesicles from terminal buttons and thereby causes flaccid paralysis.
- *Neostigmine and physostigmine*: They are reversible acetylcholine esterase (ACHE) inhibitors. They compete with ACh and prevent the action ACHE and there is continuous action of ACh. It is used to treat diseases like myasthenia gravis.
- *Pesticides like organophosphorus*: They also act by inhibiting ACHE by binding to it and its action is irreversible. It is also present in nerve gases. This type of poisoning leads to respiratory muscle paralysis and death. It can be treated with atropine.

12. Na^+- K_+ ATPase.

- It is an electrogenic pump as it pumps 3 Na^+ out of the cell and 2 K^+ into the cell. It catalyzes hydrolysis of ATP and uses the energy to move the ions across cell membrane.
- It has α and β subunits.
- Na^+ and K^+ are transported through α subunit.
- α subunit is larger and has intracellular Na^+ and ATP binding sites and a phosphorylation site.

- When Na⁺ binds to α subunit, ATP also binds and is converted to ADP and the Pi is added to phosphorylation site.
- This changes the configuration of the pump and extrudes Na⁺ into ECF. K⁺ then binds extracellularly, dephosphorylating α subunit and comes back to original configuration and releases K⁺ intracellularly.
- β-subunit is a glycoprotein and has no transport action but its presence is needed for pump activity.
- Extracellularly there are binding sites for K⁺ and ouabain.
- Pump activity is regulated by 2nd messengers and hormones.
- Thyroid hormone, aldosterone and insulin increase the pump activity, whereas dopamine decreases the pump activity.

Functions
- It is present in all cells of the body.
- It regulates intracellular Na⁺ concentration and thereby the cell volume is maintained.
- It is essential for maintenance of resting membrane potential
- It is needed for regaining the membrane potential following generation of action potential
- Its activity is inhibited by ouabain and digitalis used for heart failure.

13. Endocytosis

It is the process by which substances are internalized within the cell. There are three types:
1. Phagocytosis
2. Pinocytosis
3. Receptor-mediated endocytosis

Phagocytosis: Engulfing of solid substances (cell eating) as that of micro-organisms by the neutrophils

Pinocytosis: Engulfing the liquid components (cell drinking)

Receptor-mediated endocytosis: Here the substances to be internalized get attached to a receptor protein present on the cell membrane and the whole complex is engulfed.

14. Fibrinolytic agents.

- Tendency to form clot in an injured vessel is at the same time balanced by anticlotting or fibrinolytic pathways in the vessel to keep the lumen of blood vessel patent.
- Fibrinolytic system involves an important protease enzyme plasmin which is present in an inactive form as plasminogen in plasma.
- On activation, plasmin lyses the fibrin and fibrinogen to produce fibrin degradation products (FDP) which in turn inhibits thrombin.
- Plasminogen is activated by thrombin, and there are plasminogen activators—the tissue type plasminogen activator (t-PA) and urokinase-type plasminogen activator (u-PA).
- Plasminogen receptors are also located on the endothelial cells and binding to the receptor, plasminogen is activated and prevents clot formation in intact vessels.
- There are also tissue plasminogen inhibitors in plasma which are regulated by protein C and its cofactor protein S.

15. Cross matching.

- Cross matching is done before blood transfusion along with blood grouping.
- There are two types of cross matching—major and minor cross matching.
  a. *Major cross matching:* Here the donor's RBCs are mixed with the recipients plasma and assessed for agglutination. The ABO agglutinogens on RBC membranes are highly antigenic and they may cause agglutination when transfused. So this test confirms the safety of transfusion.
  b. *Minor cross matching:* Here donor's plasma is mixed with recipient's RBCs. This is said to be minor because the plasma of donor will get diluted in recipient's plasma and not much reactions will be produced.

16. Secretin.

- It is the first hormone to be discovered.
- Secreted from S cells in upper SI
- Polypeptide hormone

Functions of Secretin

- Enhances HCO_3 rich pancreatic juice.
- Increases alkaline bile secretion
- Augments action of CCK
- Decreases gastric secretion and motility
- Contracts pyloric sphincter
  Refer answers to 2007 paper (Short Note—Gastrointestinal hormones)

17. Enteric nervous system.

- It includes submucosal and myenteric plexuses
- Neurons of these plexuses are small interneurons that connect afferent and efferent neurons to smooth muscles, secretory cells and epithelial cells. They are involved in the local GI reflexes.
- Submucosal plexuses are present between the submucosal and circular muscle layers. They are also called as Meissner's plexus. They regulate the secretory functions of the GIT.
- Myenteric or Auerbach's plexus is present between the circular and longitudinal muscle layers in the wall of the gut. It regulates the movements of the GIT.
- They are highly connected to sympathetic and parasympathetic nerves supplying the GIT and thereby modulate their actions.
- It is also called as the third division of ANS/mini brain of the gut.
- Neurotransmitters here are—ACh, VIP, serotonin, enkephalins, substance P, norepinephrine, GABA, ATP, NO and CO.

18. Mention two substances used for measuring total body water and ECF volume.

- Substances used to measure total body water—deuterium oxide and aminopyrine
- Substances used to measure ECF volume—inulin and sucrose

19. Loop diuretics.

Diuretics Acting on Loop of Henle

Loop diuretics like frusemide, bumetamide and ethacrynic acid—they act by inhibiting Na^+-K^+-$2Cl^-$ transporter. They increase NaCl and K^+ excretion. K^+ depletion occurs while treating with these drugs.

20. Neuroendocrine reflex.

Refer answer to 6th short answer.

21. The law of projection.

Law of projection: This law codes the location of stimulus in perception. Along the pathway anywhere from the receptor to brain, wherever stimulated, the conscious sensation is referred to the location of receptor. This is one of the causes for phantom limb phenomenon.

22. Types of hypoxia.

- Hypoxic hypoxia
- Anemic hypoxia
- Stagnant hypoxia
- Histotoxic hypoxia

23. Antegrade amnesia.

- Amnesia is loss of memory. It could be retrograde or anterograde amnesia.
- **Retrograde amnesia:** Inability to recall previous events or known facts.
- **Anterograde amnesia:** Inability to learn new facts or acquire new memories. It is seen in lesion of hippocampus which leads to inability to form new long-term memories. They are able to learn things and retain for a very short period and they cannot convert it to long-term memories.

24. Draw a normal electrocardiogram. What is Einthoven's triangle?

- Einthoven's triangle is an imaginary triangle drawn around the heart (*refer* Fig. 28).
- It is formed by the two arms and the left leg forming the apices of the triangle.
- The two apices at the upper part of the triangle represent the points at which the arms connect electrically with the fluid around the heart.
- The lower part of the apex is formed by the left leg connecting with body fluids.

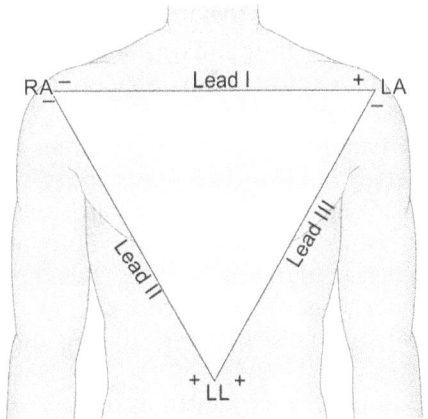

Fig. 28: Einthoven's triangle with placement of bipolar limb leads.

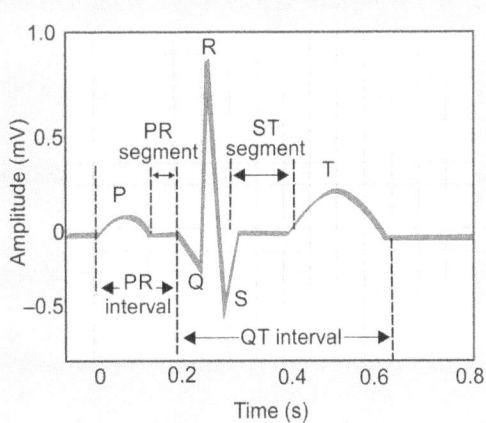

Fig. 29: Normal ECG in lead II with waves, segments and intervals.

There are three bipolar limb leads placed in the three apices of this triangle:
1. **Lead I:** The negative terminal of the electrode is connected to the right arm and the positive terminal is connected to the left arm.
2. **Lead II:** To record limb lead II, the negative terminal of the electrocardiograph is connected to the right arm and the positive terminal to left leg.
3. **Lead III:** To record limb lead III, the negative terminal is connected to the left arm and the left leg is connected to the positive terminal.
Normal ECG recording (*refer* **Fig. 29**).

25. Respiratory exchange ratio.
- Respiratory exchange ratio (R) is the ratio of CO_2/O_2 at any given time whether equilibrium is reached or not.
- Respiratory quotient (RQ) is the ratio of CO_2 produced to O_2 consumed in a steady state per unit of time.
- 'R' is affected by many factors other than metabolism. For example, during hyperventilation CO_2 is blown out and therefore R rises. In severe exercise 'R' rises even to 2.0 as large amount of CO_2 is blown off, CO_2 is produced from lactic acid by anaerobic glycolysis.
- After exercise when O_2 debt is being incurred 'R' falls to 0.5
- In metabolic acidosis, 'R' rises because there is a rise in expired CO_2 levels due to respiratory compensation.
- In metabolic alkalosis 'R' is decreased.

26. Attenuation reflex.
It is a protective reflex. When a loud sound is transmitted through the ossicles in middle ear a reflex is initiated with a latent period of 40–80 msec. Contraction of stapedius and tensor tympani pulls the tympanic membrane medially and membrane covering oval window laterally. This makes the ossicular system rigid and there is reduction in transmission of sounds. This reduces the intensity of sound by 30–40 decibels. It is also called as tympanic reflex/stapedial reflex.

Functions of this reflex:
- This reflex protects the cochlea from damaging loud sounds.
- It filters the low frequency sounds
- It prevents hearing one's own speech

27. Mean arterial pressure.
- Mean arterial pressure (MAP) is the average pressure in blood vessels throughout the cardiac cycle.
- Duration of systole is less than diastolic phase and therefore MAP is not the average of systolic and diastolic pressures.

- It is calculated as MAP = Diastolic pressure + 1/3 pulse pressure
  = 80 + 1/3 × 40 = 93 mm Hg
- Normal MAP is 75 to 100 mm Hg

Significance of MAP:
It is the pressure head which is responsible for the tissue perfusion.

28. Reynold's number.

- The blood flow in a straight vessel is laminar or streamline. The velocity of blood flow in the center of the stream is greatest and lowest immediately below the vessel wall.
- Laminar flow occurs at velocities up to a level called as the **critical velocity**.
- At or above this velocity, the flow becomes turbulent.
- Laminar flow is silent but turbulent flow creates sounds.
- The probability of turbulence is also related to diameter of vessel and viscosity of blood.
- **This is given as the Reynold's number (Re):**
  $Re = \pi DV/\eta$
  π = Density of fluid
  D = Diameter of tube
  V = Velocity of flow
  η = Viscosity of fluid
- Higher the value of Re greater is the turbulence
- When D is in cm, V is in cm/s^{-1}, η is in poises, flow is not turbulent if Re is <2,000.
- When Re >3,000 there is always turbulent flow.

29. Astigmatism.

- It is a condition where curvature of cornea is not uniform.
- The curvature in one meridian is different from the other meridian and light rays in that meridian are refracted to a different focus, so that part of the retinal image is blurred.
- It also happens if the lens curvature is not uniform or if the lens is pushed out of alignment.
- It can be corrected using cylindrical lens.

30. Functions of thalamus.

- Thalamus functions as a major relay station for most sensory impulses reaching the cortex.
- Thalamus acts as a crude center for sense perception like crude touch, pain, crude form of temperature sensation.
- It also contributes to motor function by relaying impulses from cerebellum and basal ganglia to motor cortex.
- Relays impulse between different areas of cortex.
- Contributes to regulation of autonomic activities and maintenance of consciousness.
- Due to the intimate connections of thalamus with frontal cortex and hypothalamus it is involved in various emotions.
- It is an integrating center for sleep, intralaminar nuclei for NREM sleep and lateral geniculate body for REM sleep.
- Concerned with recent memory and emotions due to its involvement in Papez circuit.
- Concerned with language.
- Important role in genesis of synchronization of EEG waves and alertness of the individual. Induces alertness due to its connections with RAS.

31. Clinical uses of ECG.

- It is used to calculate heart rate by using R-R interval
- It is used to detect conduction defects like arrhythmias and bundle branch blocks
- It is used to detect myocardial infarction and ischemia.
- It is used to analyze the cardiac vector
- It is used to detect electrolyte abnormalities
- It is used to detect cardiomyopathies and chamber hypertrophy
- Continuous ECG monitoring is used in theatres during surgeries and intensive care units.
- Holter monitor is an ambulatory continuous monitoring of electrical activity of the heart for 24 hours and the

results are analyzed later for abnormal electrical activities.

32. P_{50}.

- It is the partial pressure of oxygen in the arterial blood at which 50% of the hemoglobin is saturated with oxygen.
- Normal value is 27 mm Hg.
- P_{50} is inversely related to hemoglobin affinity for oxygen

33. Types of deafness.

There are two types of deafness. Conduction deafness and sensorineural deafness

1. **Conductive deafness:** Impaired sound transmission in external or middle ear leading to deafness.

   Causes:
   - Plugging of external auditory canal by wax or foreign body
   - Destruction of ossicles
   - Thickening of ear drum
   - Rigidity of attachment of stapes
   - Otitis media
   - Blockage of pharyngotympanic tube

2. **Neural deafness:** It is due to damage to cochlea, hair cells or neural pathways.

   Causes:
   - Aminoglycoside antibiotics obstruct mechanosensitive channels in stereocilia.
   - Damage to outer hair cells by exposure to prolonged noise.
   - Tumor in vestibulocochlear nerve and cerebellopontine angle.
   - Deafness due to mutation of genes.
   - Degeneration of hair cells in old age
   - Meningitis—viral and bacterial

Test for deafness: The deafness and types of deafness can be assessed with tests like—watch test, tuning fork tests and audiometry.

34. Blood-brain barrier.

- It is a barrier formed between the brain capillaries and brain matter.
- The barrier is formed by tight junctions (TJ) between capillary endothelial cells and TJ between the epithelial cells lining the choroid plexus.
- It is also surrounded by the feet of astrocytes which cover the capillary wall.
- BBB prevents the entry of proteins into brain and allows slow movement of smaller molecules.
- Though passive diffusion is very limited, there are vesicle-mediated transports and other carrier-mediated and active transport mechanisms in cerebral capillaries.
- Lipid-soluble substances like CO_2, O_2 and steroids penetrate brain with ease.
- Water also moves across easily.
- Glucose which is the major source of energy and enters through the glucose transporter GLUT 1.
- There are other transporters like Na^+-K^+-$2Cl^-$ transporter.

Circumventricular Organs (CVO)

- Some of the areas of the brain do not have a BBB.
- They are called as the circumventricular organs. Posterior pituitary is also present out of the BBB.
- It includes small structures in the brainstem—median eminence of the hypothalamus, area postrema, organum vasculosum of the lamina terminalis (OVLT) and subfornical organ (SFO).
- These structures have fenestrated capillaries whose permeability is high and therefore are said to be outside the BBB.
- These organs contain receptors for many peptides and chemicals and they function as chemoreceptor zones in the brain.

For example:
- Area postrema triggers vomiting when exposed to certain chemicals in plasma.
- Angiotensin II acts on SFO and induces thirst
- OVLT is the site of osmoreceptor controlling vasopressin secretion
- Circulating IL-1 induces fever by acting on CVO

Functions of BBB

- It maintains the constancy of environment of the neurons in the CNS
- It maintains the concentrations of K^+, Ca^{2+}, Mg^{2+} and H^+ in the fluid bathing the neurons for their normal functioning.
- Protects the brain from exogenous and endogenous toxins in blood
- Prevents the escape of neurotransmitters from brain

Clinical Aspects

- The knowledge about BBB and the drugs that penetrate it is important for treatment of neurological diseases, as in parkinsonism, the low dopamine level is treated by giving the precursor L-dopa (which crosses BBB) rather than dopamine which cannot cross the BBB.
- BBB breaks in areas of infections and injury.
- It is also broken by marked increase in BP and IV injection of hypertonic fluids.
- In case of brain tumors, there are new vessels formed which lack the BBB and therefore, radioisotopes can be injected to make the tumor identifiable.

35. Anaphylactic shock.

- Anaphylactic shock is a type of distributive shock. It is a warm shock. It develops due to a rapid and severe allergic reaction, especially to an already sensitized antigen and when the person is re-exposed to it.
- The antigen-antibody reaction releases large amounts of histamine. Histamine leads to increased capillary permeability and loss of fluid into interstitial spaces, widespread vasodilation and thereby decrease in venous return and dilatation arterioles and decrease in arterial pressure.
- All the above features decrease the venous return and cardiac output and may lead to a serious shock which may be fatal.
- This can be treated with sympathomimetic drugs like adrenaline and noradrenaline can be given to cause vasoconstriction and to prevent fluid loss.

36. Red-green blindness.

- Red-green blindness is a sex-linked disease and is the commonest type of color blindness.
- It is an X-linked recessive disease and therefore males are affected and females act as carriers.
- The father with color blindness passes on this defect to his female children who are carriers and the daughters pass on the defect to half of the male children.
- Therefore, this disease skips generations and appears in male children.
- This common occurrence of red-green blindness is due to arrangement of genes for green-sensitive and red-sensitive cone pigments on X chromosome.
- They are located near each other on the q arm of X chromosome and are prone for unequal homologous recombination during development of germ cells.
- This produces hybrid pigments with shifted sensitivities.

37. Reflex arc.

- Reflex is defined as the involuntary response to a threshold stimulus obtained by stimulating a sensory receptor.
- The simplest reflex arc has a single synapse.
- **Components of a reflex arc:** Receptor → afferent nerve → integrating center → efferent nerve → effectors (*refer* **Fig. 30**).

38. Primary taste sensations.

Sweet, sour, bitter, salt and umami.

39. Functions of limbic system.

- It controls autonomic functions and thereby regulate visceral activities

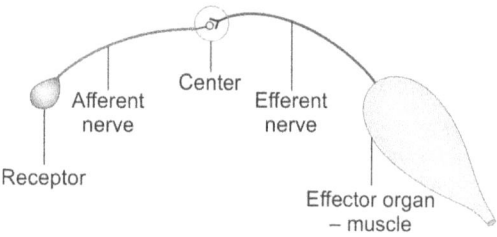

Fig. 30: Reflex arc.

- It has a role in olfaction
- Amygdala and piriform cortex are involved in sexual behavior
- Hippocampus is involved in learning and memory
- Connections with hypothalamus is involved in control of circadian rhythm
- It is the seat of emotions
- Reward and punishment centers are present in limbic system
- Behavioral responses are regulated by amygdaloid nucleus.
- Amygdaloid is responsible for discriminative feeding

40. Physiological dead space.

- Dead space is the space in the airways in which the volume of air present does not take part in gaseous exchange.
- **There are three types of dead spaces:** Anatomical dead space, alveolar dead space and physiological or total dead space.
  a. **Anatomical dead space** is the conducting zone of the respiratory pathway in which the gaseous exchange does not take place and the volume of air is said to be the dead space air.
  b. **Alveolar dead space** is the alveoli which do not have blood supply and the volume of air in these alveoli do not take part in gas exchange and is considered to be wasted ventilation.
  c. **Physiological dead space** is the sum of the above two dead spaces.
- Since in normal conditions there are no alveolar dead spaces, physiological dead space is equal to anatomical dead space.
- In a normal adult, of the 500 mL of tidal volume inhaled, 150 mL remains in the anatomical dead space, which is also equal to the physiological dead space.

Measurement of Physiological Dead Space

It is by using the Bohr's equation or single breath CO_2 technique:

Bohr's equation is used to measure physiological dead space by measuring the CO_2 levels in the alveolar and arterial blood and the tidal volume.

CO_2 gas is used as it is very less in inspired air and all the CO_2 in expired air is got from the alveoli.

Bohr's Equation

- $P_{ECO_2} \times V_T = P_{aCO_2} \times (V_T - V_D) + P_{ICO_2} \times V_D$
- $(V_T - V_D) \times P_{aCO_2} + P_{ICO_2} \times V_D = P_{ECO_2} \times V_T$

Since inspired CO_2 is negligible, $P_{ICO_2} \times V_D = 0$, So:

- $V_T - V_D = P_{ECO_2} \times V_T / P_{aCO_2}$
- $V_D = V_T - [P_{ECO_2} \times V_T / P_{aCO_2}]$
- V_T = Tidal volume
- V_D = Physiological dead space
- P_{ECO_2} = CO_2 in expired air
- P_{ICO_2} = CO_2 in inspired air
- P_{aCO_2} = CO_2 in alveolar air

Answers to 2019 Question Paper

ANSWER ALL QUESTIONS

I. Essay Questions (10 Marks each)
1. Discuss the molecular basis of skeletal muscle contraction. Add a note on Rigor Mortis.
2. Describe the structure of glomerular capillary membrane and the factors affecting glomerular filtration. Add a note on measurement of glomerular filtration rate.
3. Describe the optic pathway from the photoreceptors to the visual cortex. Add a note on visual field defects produced by lesions at various levels of the pathway.
4. Describe the origin, course, termination and functions of pyramidal tract. Write a note on upper motor lesion.

II. Short Notes (4 Marks each)
1. Complement system for antibody action.
2. Nonexcretory functions of kidneys.
3. Glucose transporters.
4. Steps in spermatogenesis.
5. Erythroblastosis fetalis.
6. Monocyte-macrophage system.
7. Genesis of resting membrane potential.
8. Regulation of gastric secretion.
9. Aldosterone escape.
10. Describe the physiological basis of length-tension relationship.
11. Brown-Sequard syndrome.
12. Histotoxic hypoxia.
13. Physiology of fetal circulation before and after birth.
14. Special features of coronary circulation.
15. Caisson's disease.
16. Hypoxic hypoxia.
17. Thalamic syndrome.
18. Surfactant.
19. Sino-aortic reflex.
20. Myocardial infarction.

III. Short Answers (2 Marks each)
1. Apoptosis.
2. Functions of aldosterone.
3. Megaloblastic anemia.
4. Filtration fraction.
5. Gigantism.
6. Atonic bladder.
7. Absorption of carbohydrates in the food.
8. Mast cells.
9. Milk-let down reflex.
10. Shape of erythrocytes.
11. Anticoagulants.
12. Facilitated diffusion.
13. Functions of lymph.
14. Vitamin D deficiency.
15. Enterohepatic circulation.
16. Achalasia cardia.
17. Actions of glucagon.
18. Bartter's syndrome.
19. Female pseudohermaphroditism.
20. Energy sources in muscle.
21. Implicit memory.
22. Stages of sleep cycle.
23. Denervation hypersensitivity.
24. Determinants of force of contraction of heart.
25. Bohr effect.
26. Jugular venous pulse.
27. Endogenous opioids.
28. Mouth to mouth respiration.
29. Heart block.
30. Respiratory distress syndrome of new born.

31. Measurement of dead space.
32. Haldane effect.
33. Ventilation-perfusion ratio.
34. Give two examples of high cardiac output state and low cardiac output state.
35. AV nodal delay.
36. Synaptic plasticity.
37. Prefrontal lobotomy.
38. Accommodation reflex pathway.
39. Traveling wave theory of hearing.
40. Taste pathway.

I. ESSAY QUESTIONS

1. Discuss the molecular basis of skeletal muscle contraction. Add a note on Rigor mortis.

Molecular Mechanism of Muscle Contraction

- Muscle, on excitation by action potential results in contraction.
- So the electrical phenomenon has led to a mechanical response.
- The linking of the electrical event to a mechanical response is given as excitation-contraction coupling.

Excitation–contraction Coupling

When the motor nerve to the skeletal muscle is excited, the neurotransmitter acetylcholine (ACh) is released at the neuromuscular junction.
↓
The ACh binds to **Nicotinic ACh receptors** in the muscle membrane below the nerve—*the motor end plate*.
↓
On binding of ACh with receptor (which by itself is a channel) results in opening of the non specific cation channels followed by influx of sodium ions and there is a local depolarization of motor end plate—*end plate potential (EPP)*.
↓
The EPP excites the neighboring muscle membrane and action potential is generated in the muscle membrane.
↓

The AP spreads to the T-tubule and activates dihydropyridine receptors (DHP) which in turn triggers the calcium release channels called the ryanodine receptors in SR and calcium ions are released.
↓
Calcium diffuses into the cytoplasm and gets attached to the troponin C. Binding of calcium with troponin C triggers many events resulting in muscle contraction.

Muscle Contraction

- Sliding theory or Ratchet theory had been put forward to explain muscle contraction by AF Huxley and HE Huxley in 1954.
- This theory postulates that the actin filament slide over the myosin filament following the formation of actin-myosin complexes and cross-bridge cycling.
- At rest, the myosin binding site on actin is covered by tropomyosin and inhibits binding of actin and myosin.
- On binding of calcium with troponin C, tropomyosin molecule changes its configuration and moves out, exposing myosin binding sites on actin.
- For each tropomyosin molecule moving out, seven actin molecules are exposed.

Cross-bridge Cycling

- Each myosin head has two binding sites.
- One for binding with actin and there one is an ATPase which hydrolysis ATP.
- On attaching with one ATP, the ATPase hydrolyses the ATP molecule and the energy is stored in the head and thereby it is energized.
- ADP and Pi are also attached to the head.
- The energized head is 90° perpendicular to thin filament.
- **Power stroke:** When the troponin C binds with Ca^{2+}, the actin binding sites for myosin are exposed and the perpendicular energized head binds to actin.
- Immediately after binding, the head flexes from 90° to 45° and ADP and Pi are released. This is said to be the power stroke or cross-bridge cycling (*refer* **Fig. 1**).

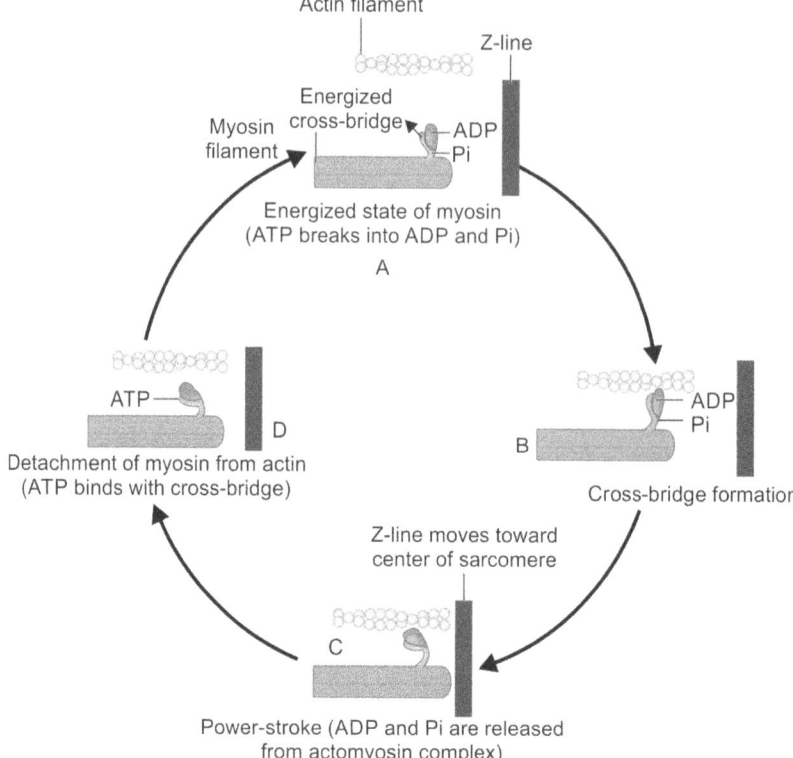

Fig. 1: Cross-bridge cycling in skeletal muscle contraction.

- The bent head is detached from actin molecule when another ATP molecule binds to the myosin head.
- This ATP is again hydrolyzed and the head is re-energized and ready to undergo the next cycle.
- As a result of repeated cross-bridge cycling, the actin filament from either side is moved towards the center of A band and there is muscle contraction.

Muscle Relaxation

- After the excitation process, Ca^{2+} in the cytosol is pumped back into the SR by calcium ATPase pump on SR membrane.
- On removal of Ca^{2+}, Troponin C realigns tropomyosin back to the position of covering of myosin binding sites in actin and the muscle relaxes.

Changes happening in the sarcomere following muscle contraction:
- H zone disappears
- Sarcomere shortens
- A band width remains same
- I band width decreases
- Z lines are brought closer

Rigor Mortis

- Rigor mortis is stiffening of muscles after the death of an individual.
- Stiffness is due to sustained attachment of myosin heads to the actin filament due to loss of ATP.
- After myosin cross-bridge attachment to actin filament, removal of the cross-bridge needs attachment of another ATP molecule.
- Sine after death, there is no more ATP synthesized the myosin heads stay attached to actin filaments resulting in stiffness of muscle.
- Rigidity disappears after some hours due to release of enzymes from lysosomes, which will digest the muscle proteins.
- The appearance and disappearance of rigor mortis is used to identify the time of death.

2. Describe the structure of glomerular capillary membrane and the factors affecting glomerular filtration. Add a note on measurement of glomerular filtration rate.

Formation of urine involves three steps:
1. Glomerular filtration
2. Tubular reabsorption
3. Tubular secretion

Glomerular filtration is ultrafiltration of plasma across the glomerular membrane.

Glomerulo-capillary Membrane

The glomerular membrane is a three layered structure. It includes:
1. The capillary endothelial cell lining
2. Epithelium lining the Bowman's capsule, made of podocytes.
3. Between them, the basement membrane.
   - The total area is 0.8 m^2
   - The capillary endothelial cells are fenestrated with pores of 70-90 nm diameter.
   - The podocytes have filtration slits of 25 nm diameter.
   - So the membrane permits passage of substances up to 4 nm diameter and excludes substances above 8 nm.
   - The presence of sialoproteins in the capillary wall, which are negatively charged substances repel the negatively charged substances from getting filtered.
   - **Plasma** is filtered across the glomerular membrane and all constituents except the proteins are present in the filtrate.
   - The osmolality of the **ultrafiltrate** is 300 mOsm/L.

Glomerular Filtration

Glomerular Filtration Rate (GFR)
- GFR refers to the volume of the glomerular filtrate formed each minute by all the nephrons in both the kidneys. The normal value is 125 mL/min or 7.5 L/hr or 180 L/day.
- Mechanism of filtration across the glomerular capillary is similar to the mechanism of filtration across any of the systemic capillaries.
- So filtration is dependent on the Starling's forces across the capillary membrane and characteristics of the membrane and renal blood flow and arterial blood pressure.
- Filtration across the membrane is decided by the balance of the starling's forces (*refer Fig. 2*).
- **GFR is expressed as:**
  GFR = $K_f[(P_{GC} - P_T) - (\pi_{GC} - \pi_T)]$
- **GFR:** Glomerular filtration rate
- K_f: Filtration coefficient of the membrane and it is 12.5 m^2/min/mm Hg. It is the product of glomerular capillary wall conductivity and effective filtration surface area.
- P_{GC}: Glomerular capillary hydrostatic pressure
- P_T: Hydrostatic pressure in Bowman's space
- π_{GC}: Glomerular capillary oncotic pressure
- π_T: Oncotic pressure in Bowman's space

Factors Regulating GFR
- **Surface area of filtration membrane** is altered by the contraction or relaxation of the mesangial cells. Contraction of mesangial cells decreases the surface area of filtration and relaxation increases it.

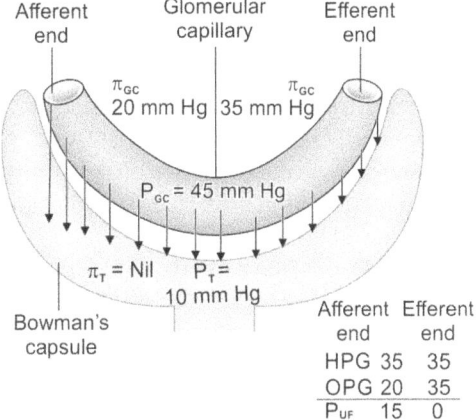

Fig. 2: Mechanism of filtration along the glomerular capillary. In contrast to systemic capillaries filtration happens along the entire capillary.
(P_{GC}: capillary hydrostatic pressure; P_T: Bowman's space hydrostatic pressure; π_{GC}: glomerular capillary oncotic pressure, π_T: osmotic pressure in Bowman's space)

Contraction is induced by angiotensin II, endothelin, ADH, etc., and relaxation is stimulated by ANP, dopamine, cAMP and PGE_2.

- **Permeability of glomerular membrane** for neutral substances of less than 4 nm molecular diameter is favored and neutral substances above 8 nm are not filtered. Between 4 to 8 nm the filtration is inversely proportional to diameter of substances. There are negatively charged sialoproteins lining the glomerular membrane, which prevents negatively charged particles like albumin from getting filtered even though it is 6 nm in diameter. Permeability is increased in hypoxia and presence of toxic substances.
- **Hydrostatic pressure in glomerulus:** It is higher than in other capillaries in the body as the efferent arterioles (the outlet of glomerulus) is more constricted and offers more resistance than the afferent arterioles (the inlet for glomerulus) which are short and straight branches. So factors which increase efferent arteriolar constriction will increase the hydrostatic pressure in the glomerulus. Changes in the systemic blood pressure will affect renal perfusion and thereby the filtration. The hydrostatic pressure in the glomerulus at the afferent and efferent end is 45 mm Hg.
- **Hydrostatic pressure in Bowman's space:** This is the pressure exerted by the filtered fluid in the Bowman's space and it opposes filtration. Normally it is 10 mm Hg. It increases in conditions of obstruction of urinary tract as in ureteric calculi blocking the flow of fluid in the tubule.
- **Oncotic pressure in the glomerulus:** GFR is inversely proportional to oncotic pressure. It is exerted by the plasma proteins. The capillary oncotic pressure at afferent end is 25 mm Hg and at efferent end it is 35 mm Hg. This is because as the fluid leaves the capillary from afferent to efferent ends of capillaries the concentration of plasma proteins increases and thereby oncotic pressure increases. So in conditions of hyperproteinemia or haemoconcentration oncotic pressure rises and GFR decreases. In hypoproteinemia GFR is increased.
- **Oncotic pressure in Bowman's space:** It is very negligible because no protein is filtered into the Bowman's space.
- **Effective filtration pressure:** It is the net outward pressure which favors filtration and is calculated as the difference between the outward and inward forces

  $GFR = K_f[(P_{GC} - P_T) - (\pi_{GC} - \pi_T)]$
  $GFR = 12.5 (45 - 10) - (25 - 0)$
  $= 12.5 \times 10 = 125$ mL/min

- **Other factors affecting GFR:**
  - Sympathetic stimulation of renal vessels leads to marked vasoconstriction and thereby decreases GFR
  - Hormones, such as norepinephrine, endothelin and angiotensin II cause intense vasoconstriction and thereby decrease RBF and GFR. Ang II at low concentrations cause only constriction of efferent arteriole and thereby increases GFR. ANP, dopamine, nitric oxide, prostaglandins cause vasodilation and increase RBF and GFR.

Measurement of GFR

The Best Test to Estimate GFR

- It is done by assessing renal clearance of inulin.
- Renal clearance is defined as the volume of plasma that is cleared of substance in a minute by excretion of the substance in urine.

It is calculated by using the formula: C = UV/P

C = Clearance of the substance
U = Urinary concentration of the substance
V = Rate of urine flow
P = Plasma concentration of substance in plasma

- Inulin is used to measure GFR as it is freely filtered and neither reabsorbed or secreted by the tubules.
- It is biologically inert and nontoxic and is neither metabolized nor stored.

Methodology

- A loading dose of inulin is administered intravenously followed by a continuous infusion to keep the plasma level a constant.
- After the inulin has equilibrated in the body fluids, an accurately timed urine sample of urinary specimen is collected and halfway through plasma sample is obtained.
- Then with the plasma and urinary concentrations the clearance is calculated by using the formula mentioned above.

U_{IN} = 35 mg/mL
V = 0.9 mL/min
P_{IN} = 0.25 mg/mL
$C_{IN} = U_{IN} V/P_{IN}$
= 35 × 0.9/0.25
= 126 mL/min

Routinely used clinical test used to assess renal function:

- A fall in GFR is the first and only clinical sign of kidney disease.
- So measurement of GFR is used to assess kidney diseases.
- Since measurement of GFR by inulin clearance is cumbersome in clinical setting, plasma creatinine is measured and it is level is inversely proportional to GFR.
- But the fall in GFR should be substantial for the rise in plasma creatinine

---

3. Describe the optic pathway from the photoreceptors to the visual cortex. Add a note on visual field defects produced by lesions at various levels of the pathway.

Visual Pathway

- The visual pathway starts in the retina.
- Retina has ten layers. Rods and cones are in the innermost close to choroid.
- The light passes through all the layers and fall on rods and cones.
- The layer close to vitreous chamber is made of ganglion cells. The axons of these cells form the optic nerve.
- The optic nerve leaves the eye through the optic disc, the blind spot.
- The fibers from temporal part of retina receive impulses from nasal field of vision and travels in the lateral half of the nerve and the fibers from nasal part of retina receive impulses from temporal field of vision and travels in medial half of the nerve (*refer* **Fig. 3**).
- The optic nerves cross in the optic chiasma. The medial fibers alone cross over and join the uncrossed fibers of the opposite optic nerve.
- On each side, medial crossed fibers and lateral uncrossed fibers join to form the optic tract.
- The optic tract reaches the lateral geniculate body of the thalamus and relays there.
- The next order of fibers which originate in the LGB is termed the geniculocalcarine fibers and they reach the primary visual area in the occipital cortex (area 17).
- From here impulses reach the visual association areas (area 18 and 19).

Lesions

Injury in the visual pathway leads to visual field defects. The type of lesion depends on the site of lesion.

- Complete loss of vision—**anopia**
- Loss of vision in one half of the visual field—**hemianopia**
  - **Lesion in optic nerve:** There is complete loss of vision (anopia) on the same side visual field.
  - **Lesion** in optic chiasma (crossed fibers): Bitemporal hemianopia
  - **Lesion in optic chiasma (uncrossed fibers):** Damage happens due to carotid artery aneurysm—leads to binasal hemianopia.
  - **Lesion in optic tract:** Lesion in one side will cause homonymous hemianopia of the opposite side, like lesion in left optic tract will cause right homonymous hemianopia.
  - **Lesion** in geniculocalcarine tract: Homonymous hemianopia
  - **Optic radiation (medial fibers):** Homonymous lower quadrantanopia

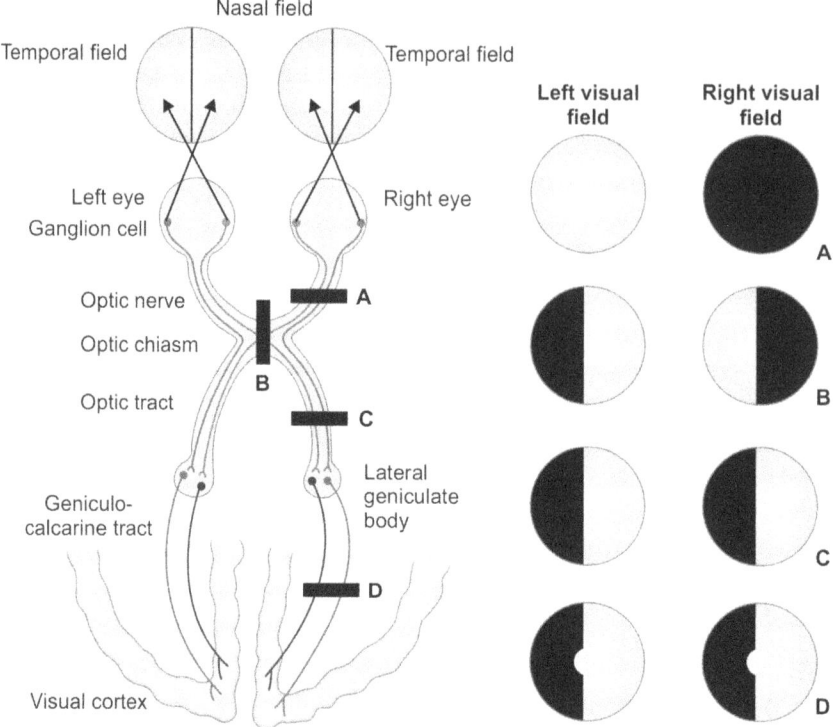

Fig. 3: Visual pathway and lesions.

- **Optic radiation (lateral fibers):** Homonymous upper quadrantanopia.
- **Lesion in visual cortex:** Homonymous hemianopia with macular sparing. Macula is spared because it has a larger area of representation in the visual cortex (*refer* **Fig. 3**).

---

4. Describe the origin, course, termination and functions of pyramidal tract. Write a note on upper motor lesion.

- There are descending tracts arising from cerebral cortex and end on spinal cord motor neurons—**corticospinal tract**. They pass through the pyramid in medulla oblongata, so it is also called as pyramidal tract.

  They are of two types—lateral corticospinal tract and anterior corticospinal tract.
- Fibers originating from cerebral cortex ends on cranial nerves–**corticobulbar tract**.

Pyramidal Tract

Origin of CST

Corticospinal tract (CST) arises from the following areas in the cerebral cortex:
- 30% fibers arise from the primary motor are (area 4)
- 30% fibers arise from premotor area (area 6)
- 40% fibers arise from somatosensory area 1 (area 3, 1, 2)

Course of CST

- The fibers, after originating from the above areas pass through the corona radiata and then pass through the posterior limb of internal capsule.
- In corona radiata, they are spread out and appear fan-like.
- On entering the internal capsule (IC) they are arranged in a very compact manner.

Internal capsule (IC): In IC, CST is present in the anterior 2/3rd of the posterior limb of the capsule. The body is represented here from anterior to posterior aspect.

Midbrain: CST passes through pes pedunculi and occupies the middle 3/5th of it. Here the representation of body is, head in the medial aspect and legs laterally and trunk in the middle.

Pons: In pons, the fibers are dispersed as they pass through the pontine nuclei and pontocerebellar fibers.

Medulla oblongata:
- The split fibers reunite here to form a single bundle which appears as a bulge in the anterior aspect and which is said to be the pyramid. Therefore, it gets the name—pyramidal tract.
- In medulla, 75% of the fibers cross over to the opposite side and forms the lateral corticospinal tract (LCST). 25% of the fibers descend down on the ipsilateral side as the anterior corticospinal tract (ACST).

Spinal cord: The crossed and uncrossed fibers descend down in spinal cord (SC) as the ACST and LCST. The **LCST fibers** end on the internuncial neurons in SC, which in turn synapse with anterior horn cells (α motor neurons) and they supply the distal limb muscles and are responsible for the *fine voluntary movements*.

Uncrossed **ACST fibers** reach the respective spinal segment and they cross over at the segment to opposite side and end on internuncial neurons, which in turn synapse on the anterior horn cells. ACST fibers supply the proximal limb muscles and trunk muscles and are responsible for *regulation of posture and tone*.
- There are many inputs which converge on the spinal motor neurons. These supra segmental inputs come from other spinal segments, brain stem and cerebral cortex. These neurons which converge on the anterior horn cells of spinal cord are the **upper motor neurons**. It includes the pyramidal and extrapyramidal tracts.
- Anterior horn cells and their fibers which supply the muscles form the lower motor neurons. So, they are called as the **"final common pathway"**.

Functions of Pyramidal Tract
- LCST supplies the distal limb muscles and therefore, they control voluntary fine movements, such as writing, stitching, etc.
- VCST supplies axial and proximal limb muscles and they control posture and gross movements, such as balancing, climbing, etc.
- LCST facilitates superficial reflexes and in its lesion, superficial reflexes are lost.
- CST facilitates muscle tone.
- CST also communicates with other areas controlling motor activities, such as basal ganglia, cerebellum and brain stem.
- Some fibers from the cortex also terminate on cranial nerve nuclei (corticobulbar fibers) and therefore, supplies facial muscles.

Upper Motor Neuron Lesion
- Damage to motor tracts above anterior horn cells (from cortical motor areas) is said to be upper motor neuron lesion.
- Common site of lesion is internal capsule
- Muscles are affected in groups
- There will be spastic type of paralysis
- Deep reflexes are exaggerated
- Superficial reflexes are lost
- There is no muscular atrophy
- Muscle tone will be increased
- There will be neo involuntary movements
- Babinski's sign is positive
- Nerve conduction study is normal.

II. SHORT NOTES

1. Complement system for antibody action.

There are certain plasma proteins which take part in both acquired and innate immunity and they complement the antibodies in providing immunity, so they are called the "complement system". There are more than 30 of them and they are named with alphabets and numbers like C1q, C3 and C3b. The principal ones are C1-9, B and D. These proteins are inactive in plasma and they are activated in a cascadic manner by three pathways.

There are three different pathways activated by three enzyme systems:
1. **Classic pathway:** Triggered by immune complexes
2. **Mannose-binding lectin pathway:** Triggered when lectin binds mannose groups in bacteria
3. **Alternative or properdin pathway:** Triggered by contact with various viruses, bacteria, fungi and cancer cells.

Classic Pathway

It is activated by antigen-antibody complexes. When an antibody binds with antigen the constant portion of antibody is exposed to C1 protein and it triggers the rest of the cascadic processes (*refer* **Fig. 1**).

Multiple responses are got which help to protect the body against the microorganisms. They are by:

- C3b coats the microorganisms and make them easy to be engulfed by the phagocytes—opsonization.
- Complement proteins change the surface of the organisms and cause them to adhere to each other and cause agglutination.
- They can make the viruses nonvirulent and thereby they are neutralized.
- C5a promotes chemotaxis and thereby attracts phagocytes towards the antigen
- C5b6789 form a membrane attack complex and insert themselves on the membrane of the microorganisms and induce pores and promotes osmotic lysis.
- Fragments of C3a, C4a and C5a activate mast cells and basophils and release histamine, heparin and several other substances. They increase the local blood flow, leakage of plasma into tissues and thereby immobilize the antigen (*refer* **Fig. 4**).

Alternate Pathway

It is also called as properdin pathway.

Factor 1 recognizes the polysaccharide unit located on the surface of microorganisms

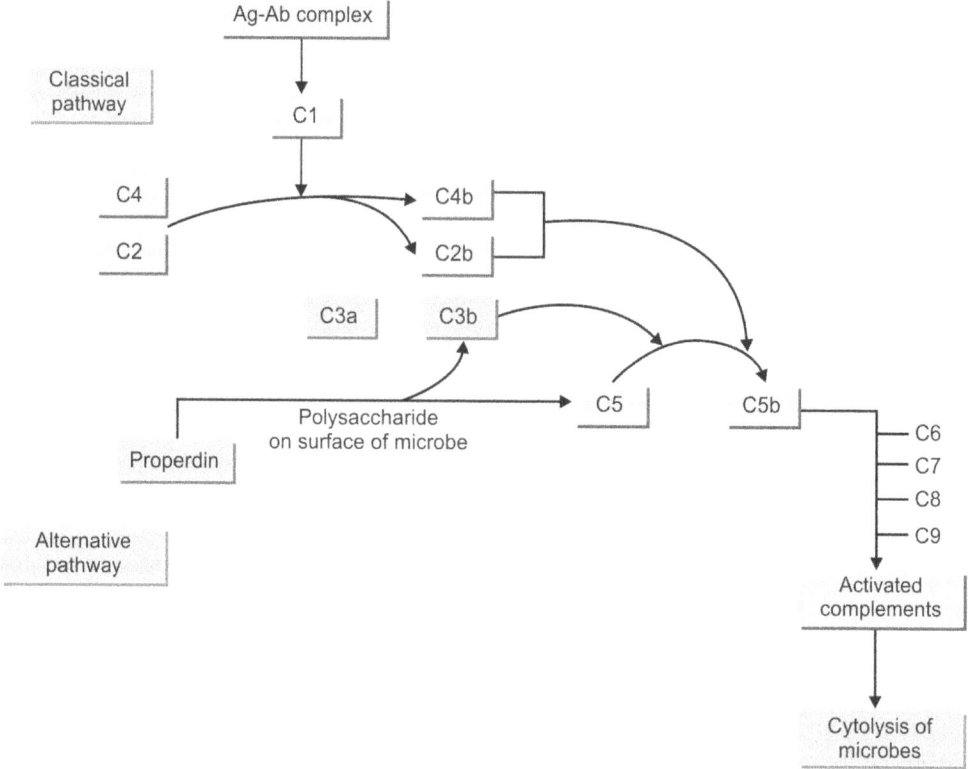

Fig. 4: Pathways of activation of complement system.

and this reaction activates C3 and C5. C3a activates other complement proteins.

2. Nonexcretory functions of kidneys.

- **Regulation of ECF volume:** Kidney is the major organ involved in the regulation of ECF volume. It is through the action of the hormones ADH, aldosterone, angiotensin II and ANP.
- **Regulation of plasma osmolality:** Changes in the plasma osmolality are sensed by the osmoreceptors present in hypothalamus and they stimulate or inhibit the secretion of ADH and thereby regulate the plasma osmolality at 290 mOsm/L.
- **Regulation of blood pressure:** Kidneys play a major role in regulation of blood pressure through regulation of ECF volume by direct mechanism through regulation of GFR and tubular actions. It also regulates BP by indirect mechanism through actions of renin, angiotensin II and aldosterone.
- **Regulation of acid-base balance:** Kidneys play a major role in regulation of acid-base balance. This done by three mechanisms—Reabsorption of HCO_3^-, secretion of H^+ and generation of new HCO_3^-.
- **Regulation of electrolytes in plasma:** Tubular reabsorption and secretion of electrolytes play a major role in regulating the serum electrolyte levels.
- **Endocrine functions of kidneys:** Kidneys secrete the following hormones:
  - *Erythropoietin:* It is secreted by the interstitial cells in the peritubular capillary bed in response to hypoxia. Thereby kidneys have a major role in regulation of erythropoiesis. In chronic renal failure, the patients suffer from anemia.
  - *Renin:* It is a hormone secreted by the juxtaglomerular cells in response to decrease in ECF volume or blood pressure. Renin activates the angiotensin system and thereby corrects the ECF volume and BP.
  - *Calcitriol:* Along with the skin and liver, kidneys synthesize 1,25 dihydroxycholecalciferol.
- **Gluconeogenesis:** It happens in conditions of prolonged fasting

3. Glucose transporters.

There are various types of glucose transporters. Some of them belong to secondary active transporter type and some of them are carrier-mediated transporters by facilitated diffusion.

Secondary Active Transporters

- **SGLT 1:** It is present in epithelial cells of kidneys and small intestine. It is used for glucose absorption and they are sodium and ATP dependent.
- **SGLT 2:** It is present in renal epithelial cells. It is used for glucose reabsorption. It is sodium and ATP dependent.

Facilitated Diffusion

It is through the carrier protein GLUT. There are more than 10 types. But five types are more important:

- **GLUT 1:** They are present in the brain, RBCs, kidneys, colon, heart and blood-brain barrier and they are insulin independent. They are useful for basal glucose uptake
- **GLUT 2:** They are present in liver, B cells of islets, kidneys and small intestine. They act as glucose sensors in the B cells. They transport glucose out of renal and intestinal epithelial cells. They are also insulin independent and they have low affinity for glucose
- **GLUT 3:** They are present in brain, placenta, kidneys and other organs. Their function is for basal glucose uptake.
- **GLUT 4:** Present in skeletal and cardiac muscles and adipose tissues. They are responsible for insulin-stimulated glucose uptake by these cells.
- **GLUT 5:** It is present in jejunum and sperm. They are used for fructose transport
- **GLUT 7:** Present in liver and other tissues. Its function is for transport of Glucose-6-phosphate in endoplasmic reticulum.

4. Steps in spermatogenesis.

- The process of formation of mature sperm is called spermatogenesis.

- It takes place in the seminiferous tubule. It happens in the wall of the tubule from basal lamina towards the lumen.
- The immature cells are present in the basal aspect of the tubule and the maturing cells move toward the adluminal compartment.
- Spermatogenesis involves both mitotic and meiotic divisions and spermiogenesis.

Mitotic Division

- The primitive germ cell, spermatogonia, in the basal lamina of the seminiferous tubule undergoes mitotic divisions to form primary spermatocytes.
- Each spermatogonium divides five times to produce 32 spermatogonia.
- 32 spermatogonia (44+X+Y) reach the adluminal side of the tubule and undergo mitosis to become 64 primary spermatocytes (44+X+Y).
- Primary spermatocytes are large cells with diploid number of chromosomes (2n) (*refer* **Fig. 5**)

Meiotic Divisions

- The primary spermatocytes with diploid number of chromosomes undergo the first meiotic division to form the secondary spermatocyte, which is haploid in nature.
- The second meiotic division results in formation of spermatids (22+X or Y).
- A total of 512 spermatids are derived from single spermatogonia.

Spermiogenesis

- The spermatids do not undergo further divisions but structural changes take place as the spermatids mature into sperm—spermiogenesis.
- This process happens in the deep folds of Sertoli cells.

The changes taking place are:

- The amount of cytoplasm is reduced in spermatids
- The nucleus elongates to become the head of sperm
- The acrosomal cap is formed
- The tail and middle piece are formed.

Spermiation

- After the maturation, the sperms stay attached to the Sertoli cells.
- The release of sperms into the tubule is called spermiation.

Factors Regulating Spermatogenesis

Hormones regulating spermatogenesis are—androgens, gonadotropins and estrogen.

- **Androgens:** A high concentration of testosterone in the tubular fluid is essential for spermatogenesis. LH stimulates Leydig cells to secrete testosterone. Sertoli cells secrete androgen binding protein (ABP) to which testosterone binds and its levels are kept elevated.
  Spermiogenesis is androgen dependent.
- **LH:** It stimulates Leydig cells to secrete testosterone and thereby is needed for spermatogenesis
- **FSH: Stimulates** Sertoli cells and Sertoli cells help in conversion of spermatids to sperms, secretion of ABP and secretion of inhibin. It also increases LH receptors in Leydig cells. It maintains gametogenic function of testis
- **Estrogen** content is high in the fluid in rete testis and estrogen acts to increase fluid reabsorption and spermatozoa

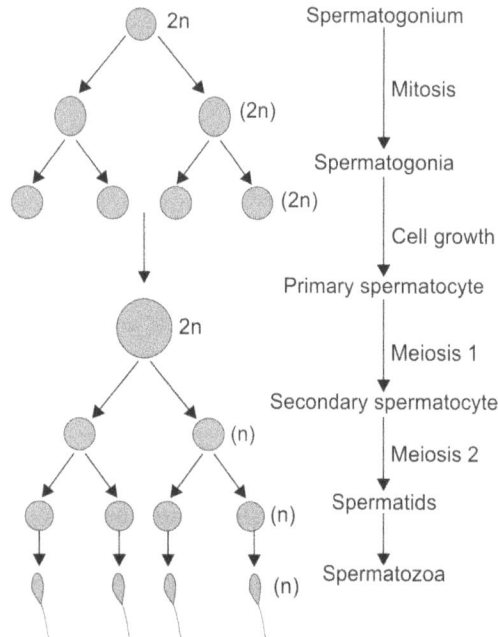

Fig. 5: Steps in spermatogenesis.
(2n: diploid number of chromosomes; n: haploid number of chromosomes)

is concentrated. This is essential for fertility of an individual.
- **Body temperature:** Spermatogenesis takes place in a temperature less than the inner body temperature. The testes are kept at a temperature of 32°C. If the testes are exposed to higher temperatures the tubular walls degenerate and sterility results.

5. Erythroblastosis fetalis.

- It is also called as hemolytic disease of the newborn (HDN).
- This is due to Rh incompatibility between the mother and fetus.
- It happens if the mother is Rh-negative and the fetus is Rh-positive.
- Since Rh system does not follow the 2nd law of Landsteiner's, there are no preformed antibodies in the Rh-negative mother's blood.
- So, in first pregnancy there are no complications.
- At the time of parturition, few fetal RBCs enter the mother's circulation.
- Mother's immune system recognizes the Rh antigen in the fetal RBCs as foreign antigens and starts producing antibodies for D antigen on fetal RBCs.
- These anti-D antibodies belong to IgG type and therefore can cross the placenta.
- If the mother conceives for the second time and if that fetus happens to Rh-positive, the anti-D antibodies from mother crosses the placenta and destroys the fetal RBCs resulting in HDN/EBF.
- As the number of conceptions increase antibody titer increases and causes more damage to the fetus.
- **The symptoms are:**
  - *Anemia:* Due to massive hemolysis, anemia sets in following agglutination
  - *Hemolytic jaundice:* The released hemoglobin, following hemolysis, is converted to bilirubin and the levels may rise very high resulting in jaundice.
  - *Hydrops fetalis:* Generalized edema due to anemia and hypoproteinemia
  - Erythroblasts start appearing in the circulation due to exaggerated erythropoiesis following severe anemia.
  - *Kernicterus:* It happens due to hemolysis and formation of excess bilirubin, and the bilirubin crosses the blood brain barrier (BBB) since the BBB is not fully developed in the fetus. Basal ganglia in the brain, has great affinity for bilirubin and therefore it gets deposited in the basal ganglia. There are motor dysfunctions due to this.

Prevention of EBF

EBF is prevented by administering the mother with anti-D antibodies after delivery of the fetus. Injected antibodies neutralize the antigens which had entered the mother's body and no further antibody production is prevented.

Treatment of EBF

- **Exchange transfusion:** The newborn with the above symptoms are treated with exchange transfusion after birth. This removes sensitized Rh-positive RBCs from the blood and is replaced with Rh negative blood. This is continued till the antibodies are removed from the fetal circulation. The transfused blood should be ABO negative and Rh negative.
- **Phototherapy** can also be given to reduce bilirubin levels.

6. Monocyte-macrophage system.

- Monocytes are formed in the bone marrow. They circulate in blood for 10–20 hours.
- They are the largest blood cells, 12–20 μm in size (2–2.5 times the size of RBCs).
- Nucleus occupies almost 50% of the cell volume and the rest is the cytoplasm. The granules in cytoplasm do not take the regular staining and therefore not visible—so is an agranulocyte
- Monocytes after circulation, enter various tissues through the capillary membrane and swell up to become the **macrophage**.
- They live for months to years as a tissue macrophage.
- They exist as either fixed macrophages or mobile macrophages.
- The monocytes, macrophages and specialized endothelial cells in bone marrow,

spleen and lymph nodes are grouped as **reticulo-endothelial system**.
- They are destroyed once their phagocytic action is over.
- Tissue macrophages are named according to the sites where they are present.

Following are the Tissue Macrophages

- **Pulmonary alveolar macrophage (PAM):** The PAMs are present in the walls of the alveolus. It is one of the routes of entry of microbes from the environment. Macrophages phagocytose the microorganisms and if possible, digests them and release them into the lymph.
- **Kupffer cells in the liver sinusoids:** The other route of entry for microorganisms is through GIT. Bacteria absorbed from ingested food enters the portal circulation and reaches the liver and are phagocytosed and destroyed by Kupffer cells lining the sinusoids.
- **Macrophages in the spleen and bone marrow:** Trabeculae of red pulp and sinuses of the spleen are lined by macrophages and they are very narrow passages and when blood squeezes through this path, unwanted debris and older cells like senile RBCs are phagocytosed and removed by the macrophages.

    In the bone marrow also there are macrophages to take care of microorganisms that enter through other routes of entry into the body.
- **Tissue macrophages in skin and subcutaneous tissues (histiocytes):** Normally skin forms a protective barrier to prevent entry of microorganisms, but in case of breakage of the protective skin barrier infections may enter and they are taken care by the skin macrophages.
- **Macrophages in lymph nodes:** There are macrophages in lymph nodes also.
- **Osteoclasts:** Osteoclasts also belong to the family of monocytes and when they come in contact with stromal cells of bone marrow, they get converted to osteoclasts and they erode the bone and help in its remodeling.
- **Microglia:** Microglia is a type of neuroglial cell and it belongs to the monocyte family and they have the property of scavenging foreign particles in the nervous system.

Functions of Monocyte-Macrophage System

The macrophages have the following functions:
- **Phagocytosis:** As a phagocyte, it is very powerful and it emigrates into the tissues following the bacterial invasion. However, this happens 24 hours after the neutrophil action and therefore it is said to be the **second line of defense**. It engulfs the bacteria and digests it; the process of digestion of bacteria is similar to that of the neutrophils—by producing free radicals—H_2O_2 and lowering the pH. It can also engulf other substances like the cell debris, dead RBCs, foreign bodies, etc.
- **Secretory function:** Monocytes and macrophages secrete many chemicals, such as—interleukins, IL-1, TNF-α, binding proteins, such as transferrin, lysozyme, proteases, acid hydrolase, etc.
    - IL-1 has many important functions—it acts as a WBC growth factor in red bone marrow, it is an endogenous pyrogen, etc. TNF α—it induces shock in septicemia due to gram negative bacterial infections, destroys invading bacteria, etc.
    - Transferrin is an iron-binding protein in plasma to carry iron and also makes it unavailable for bacteria and thereby prevents its multiplication.
- **Role in lymphocyte-mediated immunity:** Macrophages act as antigen presenting cells in immune reactions. It engulfs the microorganism and digests it and attaches the antigenic component to the MHC II molecule in the macrophage. The antigen-MHCII complex now moves towards the membrane of the macrophage and is inserted there. This macrophage moves towards the lymph nodes and the antigen is presented to the lymphocytes. The lymphocytes with the receptor for the

antigen binds to the APC and is activated for further differentiation and division.
- Monocyte-macrophage secretory products also play a key role in healing and repair.

7. Genesis of resting membrane potential.

There is a potential difference across the membrane of all cells and the inside of the cell is more negative than the outside of the cell. This is said to be the membrane potential. The membrane potential at rest in a cell is said to be the resting membrane potential (RMP). The RMP in excitable cells like the nerve and muscle cells are important as the change in the potential makes the cell to become more excited or inhibited.

RMP is due to unequal distribution of ions on either side of the membrane and various forces acting on the membrane. They are:
- Unequal distribution of ions across the cell membrane (*refer* **Fig. 6**)
- Differences in the permeability of the membrane to various ions.
- $Na^+ - K^+$ pump or $Na^+ - K^+$ ATPase

The RMP of various cells:
- RMP of the nerve is –70 mV
- RMP of skeletal membrane is –90 mV
- RMP of cardiac muscle is –90 mV
- RMP of smooth muscles is variable

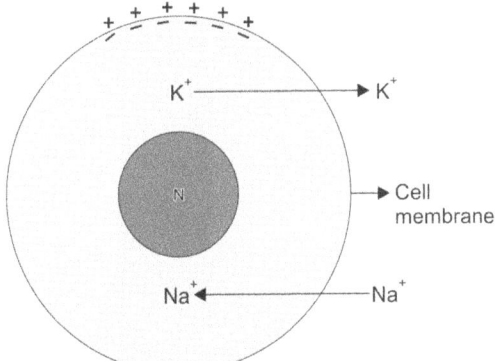

Fig. 6: Genesis of RMP. At rest, an electrical potential difference exists across the membrane of a cell with the inside being negative than the outside of a cell. This is because the cell membrane is more permeable to K^+ at rest than to Na^+. So K^+ efflux is more than Na+ influx. This is responsible for the RMP.

Selective permeability of the membrane to ions:
The membrane allows certain molecules to move freely across and restrict movements of certain ions. It is highly permeable to K^+ and Chloride at rest and only moderately permeable to Na^+. It is totally impermeable to intracellular proteins and phosphates which are anions. The high permeability for K^+ allows it to move out of the cells and the anions are impermeable and they line up along the interior of the membrane to create the negative membrane potential.

There are gated channels for other ions in the membrane, which allows movements of ions in various situations.

Concentration of ions in ICF and ECF:
- **Cations:** Na^+ are high in the ECF (140 mEq/L) and K^+ are high in the ICF (150 mEq/L).
- **Anions:** Cl^- and HCO_3^- are high in ECF and in ICF proteins and PO_4^- are high.

$Na^+ - K^+$ **pump:** This pump, by creating a gradient for Na^+ helps to maintain the RMP. It also contributes minimally for genesis of RMP as the pump extrudes 3 Na^+ ions out of the cell and 2 K^+ ions into the cell. So, a loss of a single positive ion creates a net negativity inside the membrane.

Factors responsible for genesis of RMP:
- **Permeability of membrane to K^+:** Membrane is highly permeable to K^+ at rest and K^+ gradient is outward and the outward movement creates negativity inside the cell.
- **Permeability of membrane to Na^+:** At rest, there is always an inward gradient for Na^+ and the membrane is less permeable to Na^+ than K^+ and therefore the Na^+ influx will not balance K^+ efflux and so inside the cell the potential is negative.
- **Permeability of membrane to anions:** The membrane is totally impermeable to anions and therefore they remain inside the cell to create negativity along the inner aspect of the membrane.
- $Na^+ - K^+$ **pump:** They offer minimum role in genesis of RMP but they help to maintain RMP.

8. Regulation of gastric secretion.

Neural, humoral and reflex regulation of secretion (*refer* **Fig. 7**)

Factors that stimulate:
- Vagus N
- Gastrin
- Histamine

Factors that inhibit:
- Low pH in the stomach
- Somatostatin
- Prostaglandin E2

Regulation is Discussed in Terms of:
- **Cephalic phase**
- **Gastric phase**
- **Intestinal phase**

Cephalic Phase
- Nearly 500 mL/hr (45% of total secretion)
- Initiated by thought, sight, smell, taste of food through vagus nerve.
- Emotions also affect secretion (*refer* **Fig. 8**)

Gastric Phase
- About 50% of total secretion. Food in stomach induces secretion by:
- Distension of body of stomach (through reflexes—vagal reflex)
- Distension of antrum (through gastrin secretion)
- By products of partial digestion of protein (through gastrin secretion)

Intestinal Phase
- It begins when chyme enters the intestine.
- Intestinal influence is inhibitory. By:
- **Enterogastric reflex:** By distension, presence of acid and products of digestion—inhibits secretion.

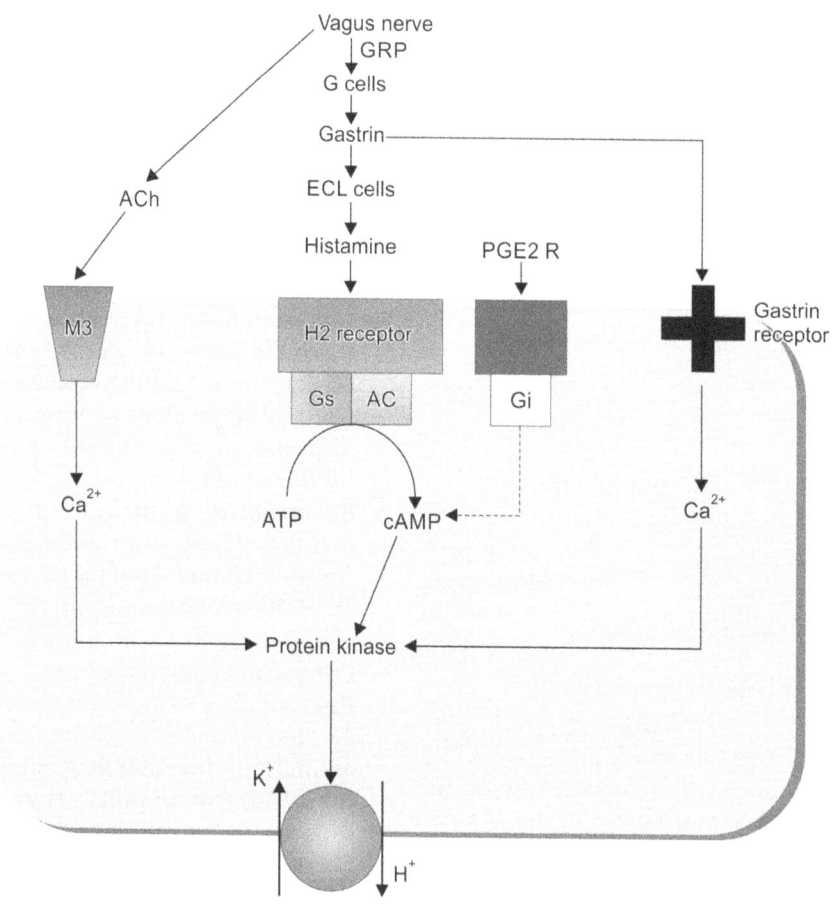

Fig. 7: Parietal cell with the regulating factors for HCl secretion.

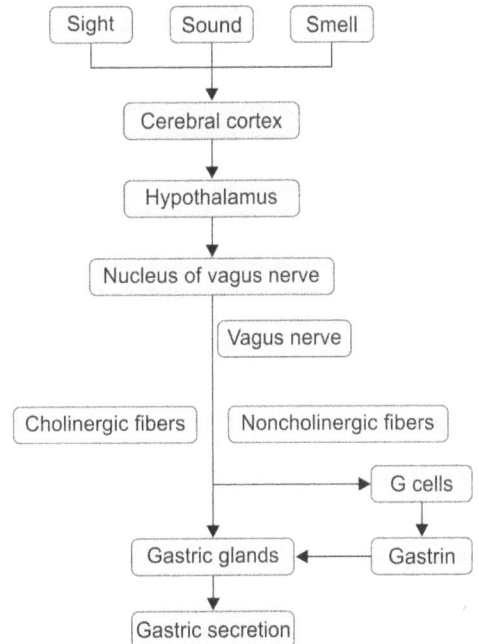

Fig. 8: Cephalic phase of regulation of HCl secretion.

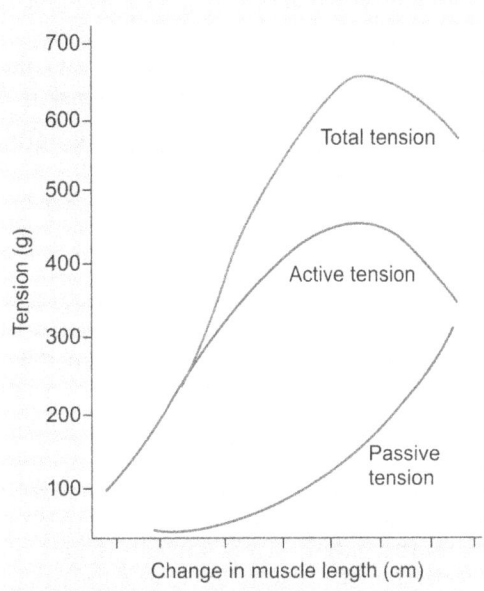

Fig. 9: Length-tension relationship in skeletal muscles.

- **Hormonal mechanism:** CCK, secretin, GIP, neurotensin, etc.,—**enterogastrone**.

9. Aldosterone escape.

Actions of Aldosterone

- Reabsorption of Na^+ and Cl^- from collecting duct which is followed by water reabsorption.
- It also causes secretion of H^+ and K^+ from collecting duct.

Aldosterone Escape

- When there is hyperaldosteronism, there is increased reabsorption of salt and water from the renal tubules.
- This results in increased ECF volume followed by increase in blood pressure.
- But this does not continue indefinitely.
- When ECF volume has increased 10-15% above the normal, there is pressure diuresis
- This phenomenon is called as **aldosterone escape**.
- It is because of secretion of atrial natriuretic peptide (ANP) from the right atrium in response to increase in ECF volume → excretion of water and salt from the body. Therefore, hyperaldosteronism is not associated with edema.

10. Describe the physiological basis of length-tension relationship.

- Length-tension relationship in a whole skeletal muscle is studied by fixing the ends of the muscle to fixed ends and then stimulating the muscle. The tension present in the stretched muscle is the "**passive tension**". The muscle is stretched at various lengths and the passive tension in each length is measured.
- The muscle is then stimulated at each length and the "**total tension**" developed at various lengths are measured.
- The difference between the two values is the "**active tension**" developed in the muscle following its contraction (*refer* **Fig. 9**).
- The recorded values are plotted and it is seen that tension developed is directly proportional to the initial length of the muscle, so as the length increases tension developed also increases.
- The length of the muscle before it starts contracting is the "**initial length**"

- The length of the muscle at which the active tension is maximum is the "**resting length**". It is called as resting length as length of most of the muscles in the body at rest is the length it develops the maximum tension.

Physiological basis of the above length-tension relationship:
- The length-tension relationship is explained by the sliding-filament mechanism of muscle contraction.
- When the muscle contracts isometrically the tension developed is proportionate to the number of cross-linkages between the actin and myosin molecules.
- When the muscle is at the resting length, the cross-bridge linkages are formed optimally and therefore the tension developed is the maximum.
- As the length of the muscle is beyond physiological limits the overlap between actin and myosin are decreased and the cross-linkages are reduced and the tension developed is decreased.
- As the muscle length is reduced than the resting length, the distance the thin filament can move is decreased and thereby cross-linkages are decreased and therefore the tension developed is decreased (*refer* **Fig. 10**).

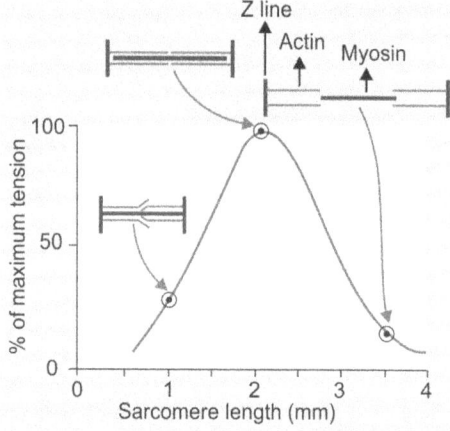

Fig. 10: Active tension developed at different muscle lengths. The maximum active tension developed is at the resting length.

---

11. Brown-Sequard syndrome.

Hemi-section of spinal cord is called Brown-Sequard syndrome. It involves lesion of one lateral half of spinal cord.

Following injury to the spinal cord, there are these following stages:
1. Stage of spinal shock
2. Stage of reflex activity
3. Stage of reflex failure

Immediately after the lesion, there is complete loss of function below the level of lesion. This happens because of sudden removal of impulses from higher centers.

The symptoms of Brown-Sequard are seen in the second stage. Symptoms are explained as the features above the level of lesion, at the level and below the level of lesion, on the same side and opposite side of lesion.

	Sensory		Motor	
	Same side	Opposite side	Same side	Opposite side
Above the level of lesion	Small area of hyperesthesia	Normal	Normal	Normal
At the level of lesion	Complete loss of sensation (anesthesia)	Not affected	Lower motor neuron type of paralysis	Not affected
Below the level of lesion	Damage to dorsal column fibers: Loss of fine touch, tactile localization, two-point discrimination, vibration sense, stereognosis and position sense	Damage to lateral and anterior spino-thalamic tract: Loss of pain, temperature and crude touch sensations. All other sensations are intact	• Upper motor neuron type of paralysis as the inhibition from higher centers is removed. • Temporary loss of vasomotor tone	Not usually affected

12. Histotoxic hypoxia.

- Hypoxia is defined as deficiency of O_2 at tissue level.
- **Types:**
  1. Hypoxic hypoxia
  2. Anemic hypoxia
  3. Stagnant hypoxia
  4. Histotoxic hypoxia
  5. Hypoxia is O_2 deficiency at the tissue level.
  6. Histotoxic hypoxia is a condition in which the amount of O_2 delivered to the tissue is adequate but the tissue is unable to utilize O_2 due to toxic poisoning as in **cyanide poisoning**.
  7. Here tissue oxidative process is affected by inhibition of cytochrome oxidases and other oxidative enzymes.
  8. Arterial PO_2 is normal
  9. Arterial O_2 content is normal
  10. Cyanosis is absent
  11. The arteriovenous difference of oxygen is very low.
  12. It is treated with methylene blue or nitrites which form methemoglobin and this reacts with cyanide to form cyanmethemoglobin, which is a less toxic compound.
  13. Hyperbaric oxygen is also used for treatment.

13. Physiology of fetal circulation before and after birth

- Fetal circulation is different from circulation in postnatal life. In postnatal life, the circulation between right and left heart is in series and in fetal life, it is parallel in many sites.
- The fetal lung is not functioning and the placenta behaves like the fetal lung and the fetus derives O_2 and nutrients from placenta through umbilical vessels.
- Fetus receives blood from the placenta through umbilical veins and is 80% saturated with oxygen.
- Blood from umbilical vein enters the liver and mixes with portal blood and some amount is diverted to the inferior vena cava through 'ductus venosus'.
- The portal and systemic venous blood in fetus is 26% saturated with O_2 and the saturation of mixed blood in IVC is around 67%.
- Most of this blood entering the right atrium through IVC is directed into left atrium through foramen ovale.
- Blood from SVC enters the right ventricle and is sent into the pulmonary artery.
- But the fetal lung is collapsed and therefore resistance in pulmonary artery is higher than in the aorta.
- Most of the blood in pulmonary artery is pushed into the aorta through 'ductus arteriosus'.
- In this fashion relatively unsaturated blood is diverted to the trunk and lower parts of the body and head of the fetus receives better saturated blood from left ventricle.
- From aorta some of the blood is pumped into the umbilical artery and back to the placenta.

Changes Happening at Birth

- At birth, placental circulation is cut off and the pressure in aorta rises more than that in the pulmonary artery.
- Since no supply comes from placenta the fetus suffers from asphyxia and it gasps for breath and cries which causes expansion of lungs.
- As the lung expands the pulmonary resistance falls and blood starts flowing into the pulmonary vessels.
- Blood returning to left atrium rises the left atrial pressure and it closes the foramen ovale.
- Ductus arteriosus constricts within few hours after birth and permanent closure happens due to intimal thickening by 24-48 hours.

14. Special features of coronary circulation.

- There are two coronary arteries—right and left. Right coronary artery supplies the right atrium and right ventricle and left coronary artery supplies left atrium and ventricles.

- There no anastomoses between the two arteries and therefore they are end arteries Therefore, blockage of vessels results in ischemia or infarction supplied by those arteries.
- There are phasic changes in blood flow through coronaries. In systole as the myocardium contracts the blood vessels are compressed and there is no blood flow through the coronaries. In diastole as the myocardium relaxes the vessels dilate and blood flow increases through the vessels.
- The endocardial vessels show the maximum phasic variation in blood flow. Therefore, these areas suffer from hypoxia and are prone for ischemia in compromised states.
- Metabolic regulation is well-developed in coronary vessels. The blood flow increase is based on the need of the myocardium.
- Coronary circulation is adjustable based on the activities of the myocardium as in exercise the coronary blood flow can increased by 4–5 times to meet the body's demand. So, it has adequate blood flow reserve.
- The myocardium extracts nearly 80% of O_2 from arterial blood and therefore the AV difference of O_2 is high. So, it increases O_2 supply the blood flow should increase.
- The rate of blood flow through the coronary vessels is the second highest next to the renal blood flow. It is 250 mL/min.
- The rate of O_2 consumption is the highest of all the organs in the body. It is about 9.7 mL/100 g of tissue/min.

15. Caisson's disease.

- Also called as "Dysbarism, the bends, divers palsy".
- This happens when a person breathing compressed air ascends up rapidly.
- At high pressures, N_2 dissolves in body fluids and stays dissolved.
- When the person ascends up to sea level gradually N_2 is converted to air gradually and is blown out.
- But when he ascends up rapidly the dissolved N_2 does not have enough time to be converted to air and to be blown out and therefore it stays in the tissues as N_2 bubbles.
- N_2 dissolved in tissues forms bubbles while escaping from tissues due to rapid ascent.
- Gas bubbles block the blood vessels and stay in tissues to create symptoms.
- **Symptoms are:**
  - Pain in joints and muscles of legs or arms.
  - Sensation of numbness
  - The chokes—shortness of breath, pulmonary edema, etc.
  - Paralysis of muscles
  - Coronary ischemia
  - Neurological symptoms
- **Treatment:** Recompression in pressurized chamber followed by slow decompression.

16. Hypoxic hypoxia.

- **Hypoxia is defined as deficiency of O_2 at tissue level.**
- **Types:**
  - Hypoxic hypoxia
  - Anemic hypoxia
  - Stagnant hypoxia
  - Histotoxic hypoxia

Hypoxic Hypoxia

- Arterial pO_2 is low, therefore tissue PO_2 is less.
- **Mechanism of hypoxia:** PO_2 of arterial blood is low due to either ↓O_2 in inspired air or disease of respiratory apparatus.
- **Conditions:**
  - Low PO_2 in inspired air (as in high altitude)
  - Hypoventilation
  - Diffusion defects
  - Ventilation/perfusion mismatch
  - A-V shunt
- **Features:**
  - There will be low arterial PO_2
  - O_2 carrying capacity will be normal
  - Arterial O_2 content is decreased
  - Percentage of O_2 saturation of hemoglobin is less
  - Arteriovenous PO_2 difference is less
  - Cyanosis may be present.

17. Thalamic syndrome.

- Thrombosis of the artery supplying thalamus leads to dysfunction of thalamus.
- Signs and symptoms:
  - Alteration of various sense perception
  - Emotional disturbances
  - Ataxia, weakness and tremor
- **Loss of sensations:**
  - Most of the sensations relay in thalamus and therefore in thalamic syndrome there is loss of sensations in contralateral side of body.
  - Loss of tactile localization, tactile discrimination and stereognosis.
  - Loss of kinesthetic sensations → thalamic phantom limb, ameliognosia, sensory ataxia.
  - Hyper-reactivity to pain
- **Damage to motor system:**
  - Hypotonia
  - Choreoathetosis
  - Thalamic hand—moderate flexion of the wrist with hyperextension of fingers.
- Disturbances in sleep-wakefulness cycle.

18. Surfactant.

- It is a protein-lipid complex secreted by the Type II alveolar epithelial cells lining the alveoli (*refer* **Fig. 11**).
- Surfactant is a mixture of dipalmitoyl-phosphatidylcholine (DPPC), other lipids and proteins—SP-A, SP-B, SP-C and SP-D.
- It acts as a detergent to reduce the surface tension of the fluid lining the alveoli and prevent its collapse during expiration.
- The phospholipids have hydrophobic tails and a hydrophilic head. They arrange themselves with the tails facing the alveolar lumen and intersperse between water molecules.
- So, during inspiration as the alveoli enlarge, the surfactant molecules move apart and surface tension of water increases and during expiration, they come closer and the surface tension is lowered.
- Surfactant is important at birth. After birth, the infant tries to breathe and makes inspiratory movements and the lungs expand after which the lung tends to recoil and the presence of surfactant prevents the collapse of the alveoli.
- Surfactant deficiency results in alveolar collapse, which results in infant respiratory distress syndrome (IRDS)
- Maturation of surfactant in the lungs is enhanced by glucocorticoids. During term, the fetal and maternal cortisol increases and favors maturation of surfactant.

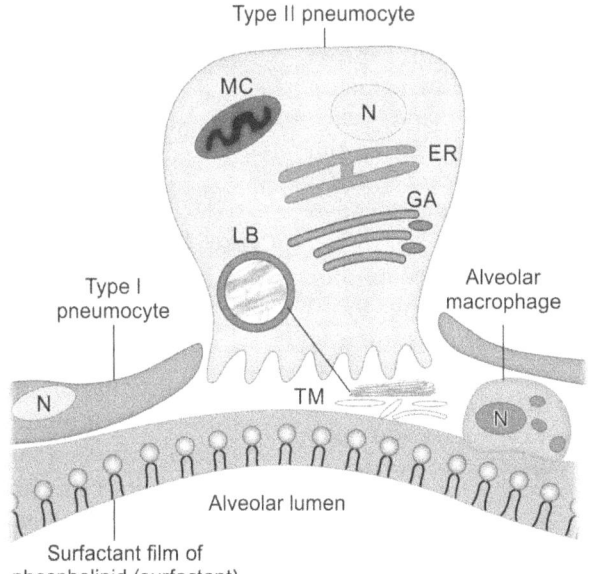

Fig. 11: Arrangement of surfactant molecules in alveolar lumen.
(N: nucleus; MC: mitochondria; ER: endoplasmic reticulum; GA: Golgi apparatus; LB: lamellar body; TM: tubular myelin)

Other Functions of Surfactant

- Stabilizes the lung alveoli
- It also decreases the effect of surface tension, which if not countered will increase the pulmonary capillary hydrostatic pressure and thereby fluid accumulation in the alveolus. So, surfactant prevents pulmonary edema.
- As it prevents alveolar collapse, it decreases the work of breathing
- They help in immunity

Regulation of Secretion of Surfactant

It is regulated by hormones—glucocorticoids, insulin and thyroxine promote secretion of surfactant.

Factors which Affect Surfactant Secretion

- High O_2 content affects surfactant secretion as in O_2 therapy in patients undergoing cardiac surgery using pump oxygenator
- Occlusion of pulmonary bronchus or pulmonary artery
- Long-term inhalation of 100% O_2
- Cigarette smoking

19. Sino-aortic reflex.

It is also called as the baroreceptor reflex

Baroreceptor Reflex

Baroreceptors

- There are two types of baroreceptors (BRs). High pressure and low-pressure baroreceptors.
- High pressure BRs are present in the carotid and aortic sinuses (*refer* **Fig. 12**).
- Low pressure BRs are present in the great veins, right and left atria.
- High pressure BRs are there to monitor and correct the day-to-day change in BP as in change of posture from supine to standing position.
- They regulate BP maximally when the MAP is between 70–110 mm Hg and stops firing when MAP falls <40 or rises above 150 mm Hg.

The Reflex

- Most important reflex to regulate BP
- Also called as sino-aortic reflex

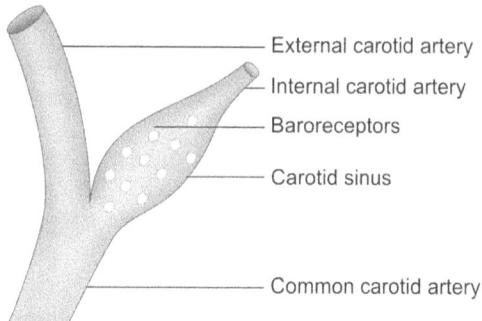

Fig. 12: Baroreceptor—carotid sinus.

- Receptor—carotid and aortic sinuses
- Stimulus—stretch of baroreceptors (as in increased BP) (*refer* **Fig. 13**).
- Afferents—IXth (supplies carotid sinus) and Xth cranial nerves (aortic sinus)
- Efferents—sympathetic nerves and vagus nerve
- Effector—heart and blood vessels
- Response—decrease in BP.

20. Myocardial infarction.

- It is a disease affecting the coronary arteries.
- When blood flow through the coronary artery is decreased it results in hypoxia of the myocardium it supplies. It is myocardial ischemia.
- Hypoxia results in accumulation of "P factor" which induces pain—angina pectoris.
- If the ischemia is severe and prolonged it results in irreversible damage to the myocardium—myocardial infarction (MI).

Causes for MI

- Partially constricted coronary arteries can be further blocked by vasospasm resulting in MI.
- The other important and most common cause for MI is rupture of an atheromatous plaque or hemorrhage into it.
- High dietary intake of cholesterol and hypercholesterolemia
- There has been identified a positive correlation between atherosclerosis and lipoprotein (a) (Lp[a])

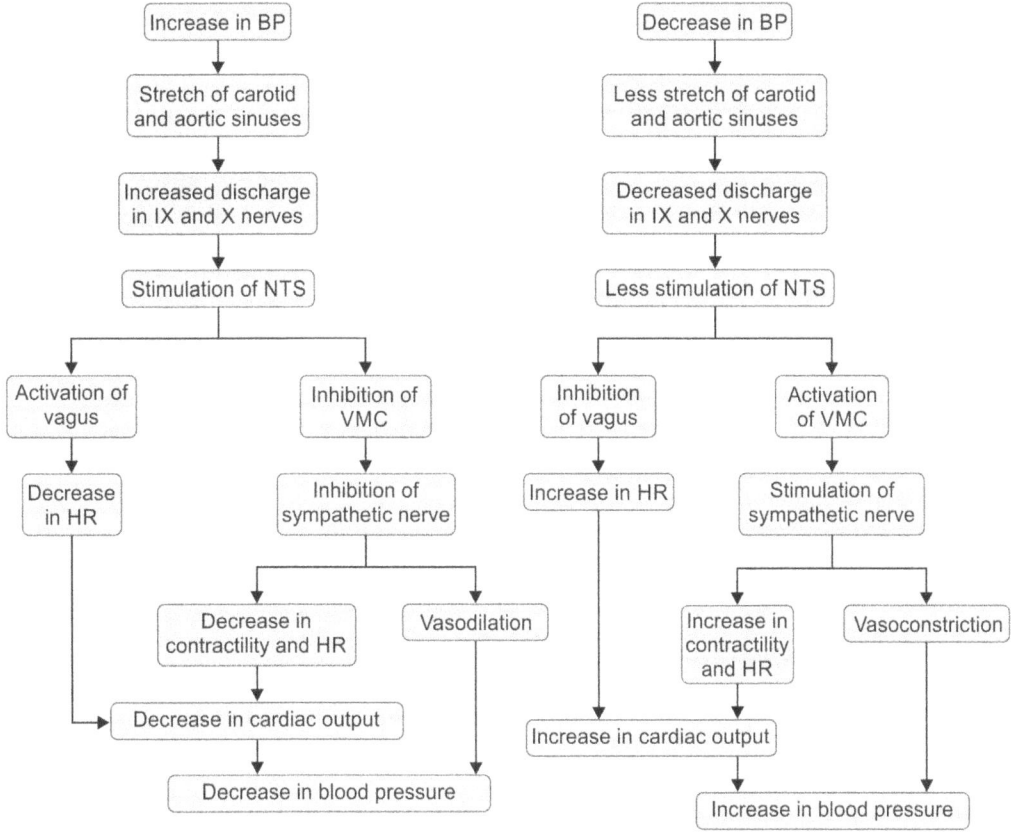

Fig. 13: Regulation of BP by baroreceptors.

- High plasma level of homocysteine is also related to incidence of MI
- Inflammatory markers, such as C-reactive protein also correlates with incidence of MI

Symptoms

- Chest pain is the most common symptom, associated with autonomic symptoms, such as sweating.
- Pain may also radiate along the left arm to the little finger
- It may also present as pain in left shoulder and arm, neck pain or back pain.

Diagnosis of MI

ECG Changes

- The most prominent feature of acute MI in the leads overlying the chest above the infarcted area.
- There will be depression of ST segment in the opposite leads.
- After some days, the ST changes subside and the infarcted tissue transforms into scar tissue and is electrically silent, it is negative in relation to normal tissue.
- This results in Q wave in leads in which it is not initially present or deeper Q waves in which Q wave is present.

Elevation of cardiac enzymes in plasma:

- The infarcted myocardium releases many enzymes and they are elevated following MI.
- The enzymes most commonly measured are—MB isomer of creatine kinase (CK-MB), troponin T and troponin I.
- Coronary angiography can be done to detect the site and extent of occlusion in coronary vessels.

Treatment for MI

- Vasodilators like nitrates provides immediate relief of pain. It also causes vasodilation in systemic vessels thereby

decreases the preload and after load and thereby decrease the work load of the heart.
- Streptokinase, a bacterial enzyme which has fibrinolytic activity is also used for early treatment of MI.
- Tissue-type plasminogen activator (t-PA), another fibrinolytic agent if given intravenously will lyse the clot after the onset of MI. Human t-PA is produced by recombinant technology as alteplase.
- Antiplatelet aggregating agents, such as aspirin in low doses, can be used to prevent further clot formation.
- Coronary angioplasty can be done to dilate the obstructed artery.
- Coronary artery bypass graft (CABG) is the surgical treatment to insert a graft vessel to bypass the blocked vessel.

III. SHORT ANSWERS

1. Apoptosis.
- Apoptosis is "programmed cell death".
- It is also said to be "cell suicide' as the cell's own genes program the cell death.
- It is a common happening in the growth and development and also in adulthood.
- Apoptosis is triggered by fas ligand in the membrane of natural killer cells and T lymphocytes and tumor necrosis factor.
- Fas ligand binds with its receptors triggering apoptosis and it activates an important pathway through the mitochondria which releases cytochrome C and it in turn activates caspases, a cysteine protease.
- It results in DNA fragmentation, cytoplasmic and chromatin condensation and membrane bleb formation and cell break up and removal of debris by phagocytosis.

Examples are:
- In the nervous system development, many neurons are removed by apoptosis while remodeling and formation of synapse.
- In immune system development, apoptosis removes the inappropriate clones of immunocytes and is responsible for the destruction of lymphocytes by glucocorticoids.
- It is responsible for removal of webs between fingers in developmental period of fetal life
- It is responsible for regression of duct system in development of sexual organs
- In adults, cyclical breakdown of endometrium and menstruation is also an example of apoptosis.

2. Functions of aldosterone.
The major actions of aldosterone are:
- Increased reabsorption of Na^+, Cl^- and water in the kidneys, colon and salivary glands. By this mechanism, it regulates ECF volume
- It also stimulates secretion of K^+ and H^+ in exchange of Na^+ reabsorption. Thereby it regulates acid-base balance and serum K^+ levels in blood.

3. Megaloblastic anemia.
- It is a type of nutritional deficiency anemia.
- It is due to deficiency of maturation factors like vitamin B12 and folic acid.
- Vitamin B12 absorption in small intestine is favored by the protein intrinsic factor. It is secreted by parietal cells of stomach.
- Vitamin B12 deficiency due to lack of intrinsic factor results in Pernicious anemia.

Features of megaloblastic anemia are:
- Decrease in all blood cell counts
- RBCs are larger and therefore MCV is increased.
- MCHC is normal
- Peripheral neuropathy may be present
- Subacute combine degeneration of the spinal cord is present
- Glossitis is present
- The condition can be treated by supplementation of vitamin B12 and folic acid.

4. Filtration fraction.
- It is the ratio of GFR to the plasma flow.
- Not all the plasma which flows through the glomeruli gets filtered. So FF is the ratio of plasma getting filtered.

- It is calculated as FF = GFR/renal plasma flow.
- It is = 120 mL/min/7000 mL = 0.16 to 0.20.
- GFR varies less than the renal plasma flow.
- In conditions of decreased arterial blood pressure, the GFR is not much affected due to increase in efferent arteriolar constriction and FF is actually elevated.

5. Gigantism.

- It is due to hypersecretion of growth hormone in children before the fusion of epiphysis.
- It could be due to tumors of somatotrophs in the pituitary or hypothalamic tumors.
- Patients are abnormally tall (7 feet and above) due to elongation of long bones.
- Hyperglycemia leading to diabetes mellitus is a common feature
- Visceromegaly is present
- Visual field defects are present if the gigantism is due to pituitary tumors compressing the optic chiasma.
- Gynecomastia may be present.

6. Atonic bladder.

- Atonic bladder is due to deafferentation of the bladder.
- Destruction of the afferent nerves to bladder results in inhibition of impulses from the bladder due to stretching of the bladder while it is getting filled.
- Loss of afferent impulses results in absence of micturition reflex.
- All bladder reflexes are lost in spite of intact efferent control to bladder.
- Instead of emptying of bladder it gets filled to its capacity and there is overflow dribbling of urine.
- It happens in tabes dorsalis and crush injury to spinal cord.

7. Absorption of carbohydrates in the food

- The sugars are absorbed in the form of hexoses and pentoses in the early parts of the small intestine.
- Along the apical membrane the glucose is transported from the lumen into the enterocytes by the secondary active transporter sodium-glucose transporter 1 (SGLT1) (refer Fig. 14).

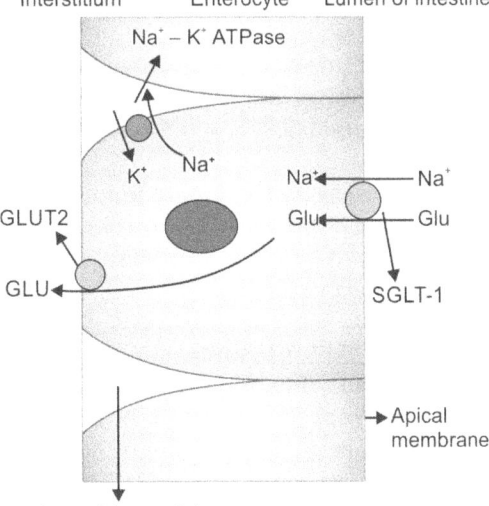

Fig. 14: Absorption of glucose in small intestine.

- There is always a gradient for sodium to move from ECF to ICF and this movement facilitates glucose absorption from the lumen.
- Glucose moves from the ICF into lateral intercellular spaces and then is transported into the interstitium from the basolateral side through the transporter GLUT 2.
- The same transporter is used to transport galactose from the lumen.
- Fructose is absorbed through a sodium-independent mechanism. It is through GLUT 5 on the luminal membrane and GLUT 2 on the basolateral membrane.
- Pentoses are absorbed through simple diffusion.

8. Mast cells.

- These are granulated wandering cells in the connective tissues.
- They are also present abundantly beneath the epithelial surfaces.
- Similar to basophils their granules contain heparin, histamine and other proteases.
- They have receptors for IgE and on binding to the IgE-coated antigens, they

degranulate and release histamine and heparin.
- They are involved in inducing inflammatory responses induced by IgE and IgG.
- The inflammatory response destroys the parasites.
- It also takes part in innate immunity by releasing TNFα
- Massive degranulation may lead to anaphylactic reactions.

9. Milk-let down reflex.

Milk ejection reflex: Oxytocin is a hormone secreted from the hypothalamus and released from posterior pituitary gland. It acts on the myoepithelial cells lining the ducts of breast and expels milk through a reflex.
- The receptors for this reflex are touch receptors around the nipple. When the infant suckles at the breast the touch receptors are stimulated.
- Impulses are relayed through somatic afferent pathways to the supraoptic (SO) and paraventricular (PV) Nuclei of Hypothalamus.
- These nuclei secrete the hormone oxytocin which is transported through blood and acts on the myoepithelial cells lining the ducts of the breast resulting in expulsion of milk.

10. Shape of erythrocytes.
- The RBCs are biconcave disk like structures and with an average diameter of 7.2 µm. The proteins spectrin and actin on the cell membrane are responsible for the biconcave shape.
- Its surface area is 135 µ². Its volume is 80 µ³.
- The center of an RBC is 1 µm thick and the periphery it is 2.2 µm.
- It does not have a nucleus. It does not contain mitochondria, ribosomes and endoplasmic reticulum. It is actually a bag filled with hemoglobin.
- The biconcave shape of RBC and its plasticity allows it to fold itself and move through very narrow capillaries (*refer* Fig. 15).

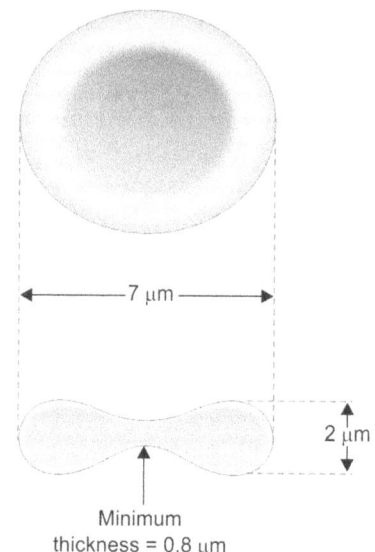

Fig. 15: Shape of RBC.

- The large surface area and the lower thickness in the center helps in easy diffusion of oxygen into the RBCs.
- The cell membrane of RBCs contain the blood group antigens along with other proteins present in other cells.

11. Anticoagulants.
- Anticoagulants are chemicals which are used to prevent blood from clotting. They are classified as in vitro and in vivo anticoagulants.
- In vitro chemicals are used for laboratory purposes
- In vivo anticoagulants are used for treatment of thrombotic disorders

In vitro Anticoagulants
- EDTA
- Double oxalates
- Trisodium citrate
- Heparin
- ACD, CPD

In Vivo Anticoagulants
- Heparin
- Coumarin derivatives—Warfarin

Mechanism of Action of Anticoagulants
- **Ethylenediaminetetraacetic acid (EDTA):** This is the anticoagulant of

choice in the laboratories. It makes Ca^{2+} unavailable for clotting by chelating it. It is used to determine ESR.
- **Trisodium citrate:** This anticoagulant is used for determining clotting disorders and also ESR. This prevents clotting by chelation of Ca^{2+}.
- **Double oxalate mixture:** It is a mixture of ammonium oxalate and potassium oxalate. It prevents clotting by forming insoluble calcium oxalate precipitate.
- **Heparin:** A naturally occurring anticoagulant is used as an in vitro and in vivo anticoagulant. It activates antithrombin III.
- **Sodium fluoride** is an anticoagulant used in the labs for tests to analyze blood glucose levels.
- **ACD and CPD:** Acid citrate dextrose and citrate phosphate dextrose are the anticoagulants used in the blood bank. Dextrose helps in nourishing the blood cells.
- **Coumarin derivatives:** They act as anticoagulants by inhibiting vitamin K. Vitamin K acts as a cofactor in the synthesis of coagulation factor II, VII, IX and X.

12. Facilitated diffusion.

- Large water-soluble substances (e.g., glucose) are carried by a protein which changes configuration on binding (*refer* Fig. 16).

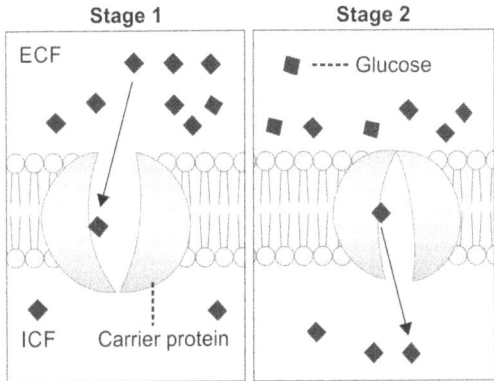

Fig. 16: Facilitated diffusion. A uniport transporting glucose molecules.

- This change in configuration shifts the molecule in or out.
- Highly selective and specific
- **Types:**
  - Uniport
  - Symport
  - Antiport
- **Characteristics:**
  - Specificity
  - Saturation
  - Competition

13. Functions of lymph.

Lymph is a part of the tissue fluid.
It is formed from the excess interstitial fluid which had been filtered in the capillaries

Functions
- It returns the excess fluid remaining in the interstitium, filtered from the capillaries, therefore it helps to maintain the ECF volume.
- It prevents accumulation of fluid in interstitium and thereby it prevents edema.
- It restores the protein content in plasma from the interstitial tissues of liver.
- It helps in absorption of fats and cholesterol from the intestines through "lacteals".
- It removes bacteria and microorganisms as it passes through the lymph nodes and has a protective function.

14. Vitamin D deficiency.

Vitamin D deficiency results in rickets in children and osteomalacia (softening of bones) in adults.

Causes
- Inadequate exposure to sunlight
- Inadequate intake of provitamins on which sunlight can act
- Inactivating mutation of the gene for 1α hydroxylase and there is no response to Vitamin D (Type 1 vitamin D resistant rickets)
- Inactivating mutation of the gene for 1,25 dihydroxycholecalciferol (Type II Vitamin D resistant rickets)
- Hypoparathyroidism

☐ Vitamin D receptor deficiency

Rickets: There is inadequate mineralization of the bones.

Symptoms:
☐ Bowing of weight-bearing bones
☐ Dental defects
☐ Hypocalcemia
☐ Rickety rosary
☐ Pigeon chest

Osteomalacia: There will be softening of bones and the symptoms are very minimal.

15. Enterohepatic circulation.

☐ Bile acids and bile salts present in the bile, on entering the intestine, are absorbed from the terminal part of the ileum and re-enter the portal vein to be secreted back into the bile from hepatocytes (*refer* **Fig. 17**).
☐ This process repeats many times in a day—**enterohepatic circulation**.
☐ The conjugated bile salts are absorbed and recirculated in the above manner.
☐ Also, bile salts are unconjugated and some of it is also absorbed.
☐ Colonic bacteria act on free bile acids and are converted to secondary bile acids and a part of it is also absorbed back into the portal vein.
☐ About 95% of secreted bile salts are absorbed by the enterohepatic circulation and only 200–500 mg/day are excreted.

Significance of Enterohepatic Circulation

☐ Only the amount of bile salts which are excreted, are synthesized and replaced daily, to maintain the pool of bile salts in the body which are essential for digestion and absorption of fats.
☐ The total amount of bile salts is 2-4 g.
☐ This amount is circulated daily many times to digest and absorb fats in the diet taken.

16. Achalasia cardia.

☐ It is a condition in which the resting tone of the lower esophageal sphincter (LES) is increased and there is improper relaxation of the sphincter following food intake and food does not reach the stomach.
☐ Food starts accumulating in the proximal esophagus and it starts getting distended.
☐ This is because of the defect in the myenteric plexus at the LES. There could also be a mismatch of the release of neurotransmitters at the LES.

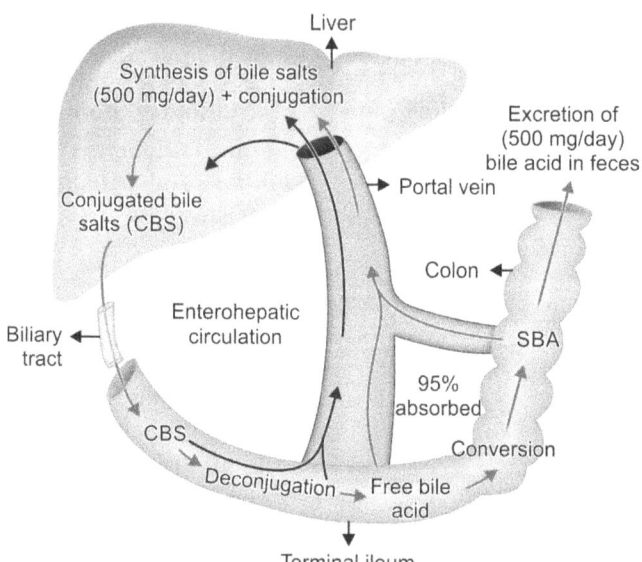

Fig. 17: Enterohepatic circulation. It is the circulation of bile salts following its synthesis from liver in bile and its secretion into duodenum and its reabsorption in terminal ileum and recirculation through portal veins.

- Acetylcholine released by parasympathetic nerves, makes the sphincter tonic and contracted. Nitric oxide and vasoactive intestinal peptide (VIP) relax the sphincter.
- Achalasia cardia could be due to increase in the acetylcholine released by the nerves supplying the LES and a decrease in the levels of nitric oxide or VIP. This makes the sphincter to become tonic.
- It can be treated by injecting botulinum toxin which inhibits the release of acetylcholine. Pneumatic dilatation of the sphincter can also be done.
- Myotomy is also done to relax the sphincter.

17. Actions of glucagon

- It is a polypeptide hormone secreted by the α cells of islets of Langerhans of endocrine pancreas.
- It circulates in plasm unbound and its half-life is 6 minutes.
- Normal fasting level is 100–150 pg/mL

Actions of glucagon: It has metabolic effects on various substrates which are given below:

Effects on carbohydrate metabolism:
- It increases blood glucose levels by various mechanisms, such as glycogenolysis and gluconeogenesis.
- In liver, it activates the enzyme phosphorylase and by activating phospholipase C, it induces glycogenolysis in the hepatocytes
- It has no glycogenolytic action on muscles.
- It increases gluconeogenesis in liver with the help of pyruvate, lactate, glycerol and amino acids.

Effect on lipid metabolism:
- It is lipolytic and ketogenic in nature.
- It stimulates action of lipase in adipose tissue and release of fatty acids and glycerol.
- In the liver, the fatty acids are oxidized resulting in energy production and ketone body formation.

Effect on protein metabolism: It increases amino acid uptake by liver and increases gluconeogenesis.

Other actions:
- It has calorigenic effects.
- It is positively inotropic as it increases myocardial cAMP.
- Stimulates secretion of insulin, growth hormone and pancreatic somatostatin.

18. Bartter's syndrome.

- It is a syndrome due to defective transport of electrolytes in the thick ascending limb of loop of Henle.
- It could be due to loss of function mutation of genes any of the following four transporters—$Na^+K^+2Cl^-$ cotransporter, ROMK K^+ channel, ClC-Kb Cl^- Channel or Bartin, an integral membrane protein which is needed for the function of ClC-Kb Cl^- channels.
- The syndrome is characterized by chronic Na^+ loss in urine, resulting in hypovolemia
- Hypovolemia leads to stimulation of renin-angiotensin-aldosterone system, but without hypertension
- There will be hyperkalemia and alkalosis
- When the defect is due to Bartin, there will be associated deafness.

19. Female pseudohermaphroditism.

- A pseudohermaphroditism is an individual with the genetic constitution of one sex and genitalia of the other sex.
- In a genetic male, external genitalia of a male develop due to the actions of testosterone secreted by the testes.
- But in a genetic female, if male external genitalia develop, it results in female pseudohermaphroditism.
- It can happen if the genetic females are exposed to androgens during the gestational age of 8 to 13 weeks.
- After 13th week if there is exposure to androgens, there will be only clitoral enlargement as the female external genitalia is already formed.
- The causes for exposure to androgens may be due to—congenital adrenal hyperplasia in the fetus or maternal exposure to androgens.

20. Energy sources in muscle.

- Muscle contraction is an energy requiring process.
- The immediate source of energy is from the ATP present in the muscle.
- Hydrolysis of ATP results in formation of ADP, release inorganic phosphate and release of energy which is used for the following purposes:
  - Cross-bridge cycling
  - Detachment of cross-bridges from Actin-binding site
  - Fueling the Ca^{2+}-Mg^{2+} ATPase pump to pump calcium back into the SR
- As the ATP is broken down, it has to be regenerated for contraction to continue.

It is done by the following mechanisms:
- ATP is immediately synthesized from ADP by adding phosphate from the compound, creatinine phosphate (CP). It is present in large amounts in the muscles.
- At rest, some ATP in mitochondria transfers its phosphate to CP and builds the stores and during exercise the CP is broken and phosphate is used to build ATP.
- At rest and during mild exercise, the muscles utilize free fatty acids for energy source. But it is not sufficient to supply the energy needs during continuous exercise.
- Later glucose is utilized for energy supply to form ATP and CP are derived from glucose metabolism to CO_2 and H_2O.
- Glucose for the above processes is derived from the blood stream and from the glycogen stores in the muscle.
- Aerobic glycolysis yields 40 ATP molecules and if O_2 supply is insufficient, anaerobic glycolysis is activated and results in formation of 2 ATP per glucose molecule and lactate is formed.

21. Implicit memory.

- Implicit memory or procedural memory— ability to learn and remember motor skills. There is no need of conscious awareness.
- It is also called as "reflexive or nondeclarative memory".
- It includes—skills, habits, priming and conditioned reflexes.
- Initially explicit memory is needed for certain skills. For example, while learning to ride a bicycle there is need of explicit memory and once it is learnt it transforms to implicit memory.
- The other forms of implicit memory is classified as associative learning and nonassociative learning.
- In nonassociative learning, the organism learns about a single stimulus— habituation, sensitization
- In associative learning, the organism learns about the association of one stimulus to the other—conditioned reflexes.

22. Stages of sleep cycle.

- Sleep is said to be a state of altered consciousness or partial unconsciousness from which a person can be aroused.
- Sleep has two components—non-rapid eye movement (NREM) and rapid eye movement (REM) sleep
- NREM sleep has four stages, each with different EEG activities.
- When a person starts to sleep, he passes through the 4 stages of slow wave sleep and as he moves through each stage, the sleep deepens gradually.
- After stage 4 of NREM seep, it lightens as he enters the REM sleep.
- So, a person moves from stage 1→ stage 2 → stage 3 → stage 4 → REM sleep
- With this, the first cycle of sleep ends and he again goes to the next sleep cycle starting with stage 1 of NREM sleep.
- Each cycle lasts for 70–90 minutes.
- In the initial phases of sleep, the NREM phase is predominant and the in later part of sleep REM sleep duration increases.

23. Denervation hypersensitivity.

- When a nerve is cut and allowed to degenerate the structure supplied by it and close to the cut end shows hypersensitivity or super sensitivity to the neurotransmitter released by that nerve. It is called as denervation hypersensitivity.

- It is seen in skeletal and smooth muscles. If the motor nerve to a skeletal muscle is cut and allowed to degenerate the muscle becomes extremely sensitive to acetylcholine.
- Denervated exocrine glands except sweat glands also become hypersensitive.
- Postganglionic sympathetic nerves to the iris when is cut and norepinephrine is injected intravenously the denervated pupils dilate widely and a minimal response is seen in the normal side.
- The causes for the denervation hypersensitivity are:
- Deficiency of a chemical messenger results in upregulation of its receptors
- Following the release there is lack of reuptake of the neurotransmitter.

24. Determinants of force of contraction of heart

Force of contraction of heart can be increased by homometric and heterometric regulation.

Homometric regulation of contractility: Contractility is increase in force of contraction and thereby increase in stroke volume without increase in initial muscle length.
- Ventricles are able to do more work per stroke at a given EDV.
- Factors which affect contractility—**inotropic agents**.
- There are positive and negative inotropic agents.

Contractility is increased by:
- Autonomic activity (sympathetics are positively inotropic)
- Muscle mass—increase in myocardial mass increases contractility as after regular exercise
- Concentration of hormones and chemicals
- Heart rate—force frequency relationship

Factors increasing contractility, positive inotropic agents:
- Sympathetic stimulation
- Circulating catecholamines
- Force frequency relationship
- Digitalis
- Glucagon
- Insulin
- Thyroxine
- Chemicals, such as xanthine, theophylline

Factors decreasing contractility, negative inotropic agents:
- Loss of myocardium as in myocardial infarction
- Hypoxia
- Hypercapnia
- Acidosis
- Acetylcholine

Heterometric Regulation
- Here the force of contraction is affected with change in muscle length.
- It is achieved by increasing end diastolic volume (EDV), the preload.
- This is based on Frank–Starling's law.
- According to the law the force of contraction is directly proportional to the muscle length within physiological limits.
- As EDV increases, stretch of myocardium increases and results in forceful contraction, within physiological limits.

Causes for application of Frank–Starling's law:
- Increase in EDV →↑stretch of muscle fiber → interaction of thick and thin filament increases →↑ force of contraction.
- Stretch of muscle fibers → opens stretch sensitive Ca^{2+} channels on sarcolemma → Ca^{2+} influx →↑ force of contraction.
- ↑Ca^{2+} influx →↑ Ca^{2+} release from SR (CICR) →↑ force of contraction.
- ↑stretch of muscle fiber →↑ affinity of troponin for Ca^{2+}

25. Bohr effect.

- Decrease in O_2 affinity of hemoglobin when pH of blood falls is called the **Bohr effect**. This signifies that deoxyhemoglobin has more affinity for H^+ than oxyhemoglobin.
- It happens at the tissue level.
- In the tissue level, CO_2 release is more and this increases pCO_2 in blood which shifts the oxygen-Hb dissociation curve to the right (decreases Hb affinity for O_2) and releases O_2.

- The unsaturation of hemoglobin at the tissue level is due to decrease in PO_2 but an extra 1–2% of unsaturation is due to the rise in PCO_2 and thereby shift of curve to right (Bohr effect)

26. Jugular venous pulse.

JVP tracing is recorded from internal jugular vein. It reflects the pressure changes in the right atrium as there are no valves in this vein and therefore any pressure change in right atrium is reflected to this vein.

The JVP tracing has three positive waves and two negative waves (*refer* **Fig. 18**).

They are:
- *'a' wave:* Atrial contraction
- *'c' wave:* Due to bulging of tricuspid valve into right atrium during onset of ventricular systole
- *'v':* Due to atrial filling
- *'x' descent:* Fall in atrial pressure due to its relaxation
- *'y' descent:* Due to emptying of blood from right atrium to right ventricle

Conditions Altering JVP
- **Increased JVP:**
  - Right heart failure
  - Superior venacaval obstruction
  - Congestive cardiac failure
  - Constrictive pericarditis
- **Prominent a wave:**
  - Pulmonary stenosis
  - Pulmonary hypertension
  - Tricuspid stenosis

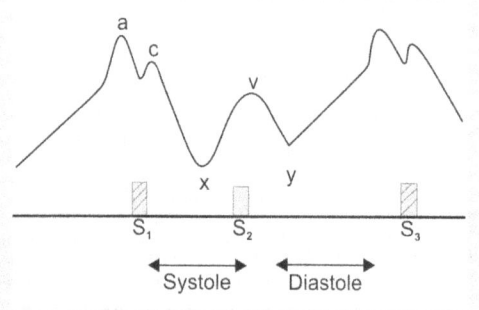

Fig. 18: Jugular venous pulse; a, c and v are positive waves, x and y are negative waves.

- **Canon wave or giant 'a' wave:** Right atrium contracts with closed tricuspid valve
  - Complete heart block

27. Endogenous opioids.

- Presence of opioid receptors in the body has led to the search for endogenous opioids.
- There are precursors identified, which form opioid peptides.

The first one to be recognized is enkephalins:
- Met-enkephalin and leu-enkephalin.
- They are found in the nerve endings of GIT and in brain. They are also present in substantia gelatinosa of spinal cord where gating of pain happens.
- It is also present in the brain stem.
- They bind to the δ and μ opioid receptors

β-endorphin:
- It is an opioid peptide and is a part of proopiomelanocortin produced from the anterior and intermediate lobe of pituitary gland.
- It is has 31 amino acid residues.
- It is present in the brain and the blood coming from the pituitary gland.

The next precursor is prodynorphin:
- It contains dynorphins and α and β neoendorphins.
- Dynorphins are present in the duodenum, posterior pituitary and hypothalamus.
- **Neoendorphins** are also present in the hypothalamus.
- Endorphins bind only to μ receptors whereas other opioids bind to various receptors.

Effect of Stimulation of the Following Opioid Receptors
- **μ receptor:** They get activated on binding to opioids and results in activation of second messengers. This leads to K^+ conductance and thereby hyperpolarizes the neurons.
- **Effects on stimulation are:** Analgesia, respiratory depression, constipation, euphoria, sedation, increased secretion of growth hormone and prolactin and miosis.

- **κ receptor:** Is bound by dynorphins. Activation of these receptors results in closure of Ca^{2+} channels.
- **Effect of stimulation:** Analgesia, diuresis, sedation, miosis and dysphoria.
- **δ receptor:** Bound by all the above types of opioids. Activation of these receptors results in closure of Ca^{2+} channels.
- **Effect of stimulation:** Analgesia

28. Mouth-to-mouth respiration.

- It can be direct or indirect method. In direct method, the operator places his mouth directly on the subject's mouth and in indirect method, it is done with a small tube.
- The subject is made to lie supine; the airway is kept clean from vomitus, foreign body, etc.
- The subject's head is extended, the operator sits on the side of the subject holds the lower jaw with his left hand and opens the mouth and with his right hand clips the nostrils.
- The operator then inhales deeply and places his mouth on the subject's mouth or the tube placed in the subject's mouth and blows into the subject's mouth smoothly, volume twice that of the tidal volume.

29. Heart block.

- Heart block is abnormalities in the conducting system of the heart.
- Normally SA node is the pacemaker and the impulses originating in SA node is conducted to the other parts of the conducting system

Conduction Defects—Heart Block

- Other portions of the conducting system other than the SA node can also generate impulses.
- Since the rate of SA node is faster the impulses discharged here are conducted below at a faster rate and is followed by the other tissues.
- But in disease conditions if there are blocks in conduction, other parts of conduction system can generate electrical activity and they are said to be ectopic pacemakers.
- If there is interruption of conduction of impulses from atria to ventricle it is said to be atrioventricular block (AV Block).
- **There are three types of blocks:** First degree block, second degree block and third degree or complete heart block.
    a. *First degree block:* Conduction between atria and ventricle is slowed as in AV nodal delay and there is no complete interruption of conduction. It is said to be first degree block. Each P wave is followed by a QRS complex, but there is prolongation of PR interval.
    b. *Second degree block:* Here not all the atrial impulses are conducted to the ventricles and there may be a ventricular beat following every second or third atrial beat, 2:1 or 3:1 block. This type is said to be **Mobitz type II block**.
    In another type of incomplete block, there are repeated sequences of beats in which the PR interval lengthens progressively until a ventricular beat is dropped—**Wenckebach phenomenon**. This type is said to be **Mobitz type I** (*refer* **Figs. 19A to D**).
    c. *Third degree or complete heart block:* Here conduction of impulses from atria

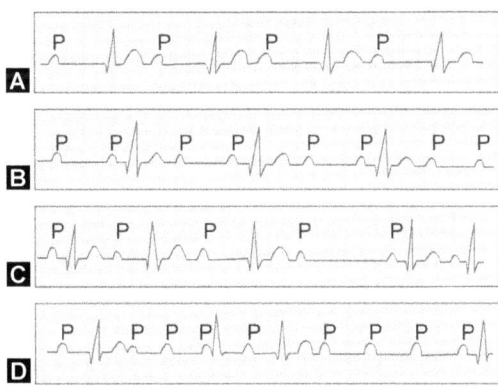

Figs. 19A to D: ECG tracings of heart blocks: (A) First degree heart block; (B) Second degree heart block, Mobitz type II; (C) Second degree heart block, Mobitz type I; (D) Third degree heart block.

to ventricle are completely interrupted and the ventricles beat at a slow rate—**idioventricular rhythm**. It could be a AV nodal block or infranodal block.

The ventricular rate may be lowered to 40–35/min and sometimes there could be a minute of asystole leading to cerebral ischemia and fainting—**Stokes-Adams syndrome**. Causes could be septal MI and damage to His bundle.

d. *Bundle branch block:* Block of one branch of bundle of his—right or left bundle branch block. Ventricular rate is normal, but QRS complex is prolonged and deformed.

e. *Hemiblock or Fascicular block:* Block in anterior or posterior fascicle of the left bundle branch. Left anterior hemiblock leads to left axis deviation and left posterior hemiblock causes right axis deviation.

30. Respiratory distress syndrome of newborn.

- Surfactant is a lipid surface-tension-lowering agent present in the fluid lining the alveoli.
- The presence of surfactant lowers the surface tension of the fluid lining the alveoli and thereby prevents total collapse of alveoli during expiration.
- Surfactant is produced by the Type II alveolar epithelial cells lining the alveoli.
- They also prevent pulmonary edema.
- The presence of surfactant is important at birth.
- The fetus makes respiratory movements in utero but the lungs remain collapsed.
- After birth, the fetus makes respiratory efforts and the lung expands.
- Surfactant prevents the lung from collapsing following the expansion.

In absence of surfactant, as it happens in preterm infants, the lung collapses following the respiratory gasps along with fluid accumulation in the lungs, leading to infant respiratory distress syndrome (IRDS).

31. Measurement of dead space.

- Dead space is the space in the airways in which the volume of air present does not take part in gaseous exchange.
- There are three types of dead spaces—anatomical dead space, alveolar dead space and physiological or total dead space.
  - **Anatomical dead space** is the conducting zone of the respiratory pathway in which the gaseous exchange does not take place and the volume of air is said to be the dead space air.
  - **Alveolar dead space** is the alveoli which do not have blood supply and the volume of air in these alveoli do not take part in gas exchange and is considered to be wasted ventilation.
  - **Physiological dead space** is the sum of the above two dead spaces.
  - Since in normal conditions, there are no alveolar dead spaces, physiological dead space is equal to anatomical dead space.
  - In a normal adult, of the 500 mL of tidal volume inhaled, 150 mL remains in the anatomical dead space, which is also the Physiological dead space.

Measurement of physiological dead space:
It is by using the Bohr's equation or single breath CO_2 technique:
- Bohr's equation is used to measure physiological dead space by measuring the CO_2 levels in the alveolar and arterial blood and the tidal volume.
- CO_2 gas is used as it is very less in inspired air and all the CO_2 in expired air is got from the alveoli.

Bohr's equation:
- $P_{ECO2} \times V_T = P_{aCO2} \times (V_T - V_D) + P_{ICO2} \times V_D$
- $(V_T - V_D) \times P_{aCO2} + P_{ICO2} \times V_D = P_{ECO2} \times V_T$

Since inspired CO_2 is negligible, $P_{ICO2} \times V_D = 0$,
So:
- $V_T - VD = P_{ECO2} \times V_T / P_{aCO2}$
- $V_D = VT - [P_{ECO2} \times V_T / P_{aCO2}]$
- V_T = Tidal volume

- V_D = Physiological dead space
- P_{ECO2} = CO_2 in expired air
- P_{ICO2} = CO_2 in inspired air
- P_{aCO2} = CO_2 in alveolar air

32. Haldane effect.

- The effect of PO_2 or oxyhemoglobin saturation on CO_2 content is known as **Haldane effect**.
- The relationship between PO_2 and CO_2 content is inverse.
- When blood passes through pulmonary capillaries, O_2 diffuses into blood, binds to hemoglobin and forms Oxy-Hb.
- Oxygenation of Hb shifts the CO_2 dissociation curve to the right and Hb gives out CO_2.
- So in the lungs, loading of O_2 helps in unloading of CO_2.
- In the tissues, low PO_2 increases the capacity of Hb for carrying CO_2.

33. Ventilation-perfusion ratio.

- It is the ratio of ventilation to the lungs to the blood flow through pulmonary circulation.
- Alveolar ventilation (V_a) is 4000 L/min and perfusion (Q) is equal to cardiac output, 5 L/min
- So V_a/Q ratio = 4/5 = 0.8
- Ventilation as well as perfusion increases from the apex to the base of the lungs due to the effect of gravity.
- But rate of increase of perfusion is more than the increase in ventilation
- So V_a/Q ratio is more in the apex (3.3) than the base (0.63)
- The high O_2 content in the apex favors the growth of TB bacilli there
- The V_a/Q ratio can get altered in conditions of uneven ventilation and nonuniform blood flow to alveoli as in certain disease conditions.

Decreased V_a/Q Ratio

- In conditions where there is inadequate ventilation to the alveoli and normal perfusion, the oxygenation of blood and removal of CO_2 are not normal.
- So alveolar PO_2 falls and PCO_2 rises.
- So, it is like the deoxygenated blood empties directly into the left atrium
- So, it is like a physiological shunt (*refer* **Fig. 20**)

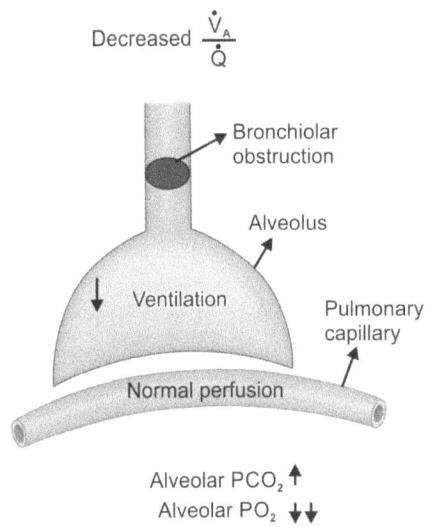
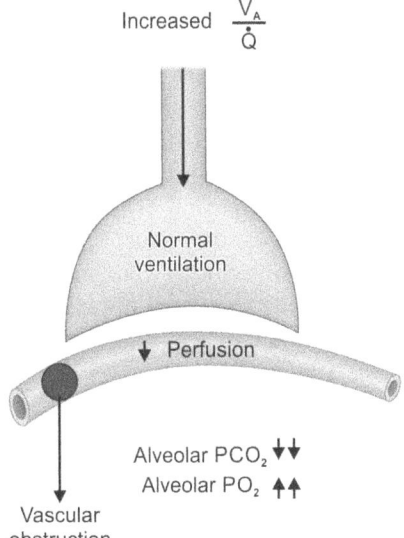

Fig. 20: V_a/Q ratio in complete airway obstruction and complete circulatory obstruction conditions.

Causes
Bronchial asthma, pneumothorax, emphysema, pulmonary fibrosis.

Increased Va/Q Ratio
- When perfusion through pulmonary capillary is decreased in relation to alveolar ventilation the ratio increases.
- Alveolar PCO_2 falls and PO_2 increases.
- As the alveolus is under-perfused, it is like wasted ventilation and is like increased physiological dead space (*refer* **Fig. 20**)

Causes
- Anatomical shunts in the heart like Fallot's tetralogy
- Decrease in vascular bed as in emphysema
- Pulmonary embolism

34. Give two examples of high cardiac output state and low cardiac output state.

High Cardiac Output State
- Thyrotoxicosis
- Anemia

Low Cardiac Output State
- Cardiomyopathy
- Aortic stenosis

35. AV nodal delay.
- Impulses originating from the SA node travels through the three bundles of internodal tracts and atrial musculature to reach the AV node (AVN).
- AV node is located beneath the endocardium on the right side of lower part of atrial septum near the tricuspid valve.
- The conduction velocity through the AVN is very slow because the fibers are smaller with less number of gap junctions.
- There is a delay of 0.1 s
- The delay provides time for atrial contraction and final ventricular filling.
- It also prevents transmission of all impulses from atria to ventricles in supraventricular tachycardia.
- It is supplied by sympathetic and PS nerves which alter the conduction rate

36. Synaptic plasticity.
- The changes that occur in a synapse after repeated stimulation is called as synaptic plasticity.
- It may be facilitatory or inhibitory inputs.
- It is involved in learning and memory.
- It is usually a property of chemical synapse
- When stimulated for short-term, there are physiological changes in the synapse and they disappear when the stimulus is eliminated. This helps in short-term memory.
- Continued stimulation for longer periods results in physiological and anatomical changes in the synapse and this help in long-term memory.
- Physiological changes can be increase or decrease in release of neurotransmitters.
- Anatomical changes can be either appearance or disappearance of the connections in the synapse.

37. Prefrontal lobotomy.
- It is a procedure in which the connections between the frontal lobe and deeper portions of the brain.
- It is done in some patients in whom the tensions resulting from true or imagined failure caused by delusions, compulsions and phobias are incapacitating.
- Lobotomy decreases the tension and the delusions or phobias no longer bother the patient.
- It is also used in intractable pain, where the patient does not feel the emotional upset of pain.
- But the prefrontal lobotomy leads to lack of concern with other aspects of life also.
- It results in prefrontal lobe syndrome.

The features are:
- Hypermotility
- Lack of concern
- Flight of ideas
- Impairment of moral and social sense

- Impairment of learning capacity and loss of recent memory

38. Accommodation reflex pathway.

- When the eye is focusing on a close object, the curvature of the lens increases to get a clear image on retina—accommodation of lens.
- This occurs due to contraction of ciliary muscles
- Results in increase of curvature of lens—adds 12 diopters to the power of the lens, power of lens increases (>70 D)
- Near point—10 cm in young adult.
- Presbyopia—near point increases (83 cm).

Other changes of accommodation are:
- Constriction of pupil
- Convergence of eyeball

Accommodation Reflex Pathway

Impulses from retina for near vision
↓
Optic nerve
↓
Optic chiasma
↓
Optic tract
↓
Lateral geniculate body
↓
Visual cortex (area 17)
↓
Frontal eye field
↓
Edinger-Westphal nuclei of both sides (parasympathetic fibers)
↓
Efferents go through the oculomotor nerves → medial rectus → convergence of eyeball
↓
Ciliary ganglion
↓
Supplies the sphincter pupillae and the ciliary muscles
↓
Constriction of pupil and anterior curvature of lens increases
↓
Accommodation of eye

39. Traveling wave theory of hearing.

Von Bekesy's Traveling Wave Theory

- Von Bekesy studied the nature of basilar membrane and he showed that the membrane was narrow and stiff at the base and wide and flexible at the apex.
- He also showed that the sound with high frequency, displaced the membrane at the base and the rest of the membrane at lower frequency.
- When the stapes moves with the sound waves it creates pressure waves in scala vestibuli and the wave moves through the cochlea from base to apex.
- The pressure wave displaces the basilar membrane.
- The membrane at the base is first displaced down along with the stapes and it moves towards the apex. These waves are the "Traveling waves".
- The area of displacement is dependent on the frequency of sound.
- High frequency sounds displace the membrane maximally near the base and low frequencies displace the other areas of the membrane.

40. Taste pathway.

The taste receptors are present in the taste buds, which are located on the tongue in the papillae.
- There are 10,000 taste buds.
- Taste buds are located in—fungiform, foliate and vallate papillae.
- Cells in taste buds—type 1 and 2—supporting cells.
- Type 3 cells—receptor epithelial cells have microvilli projecting into taste pore.
- They are receptors are replaced constantly in 10 days.

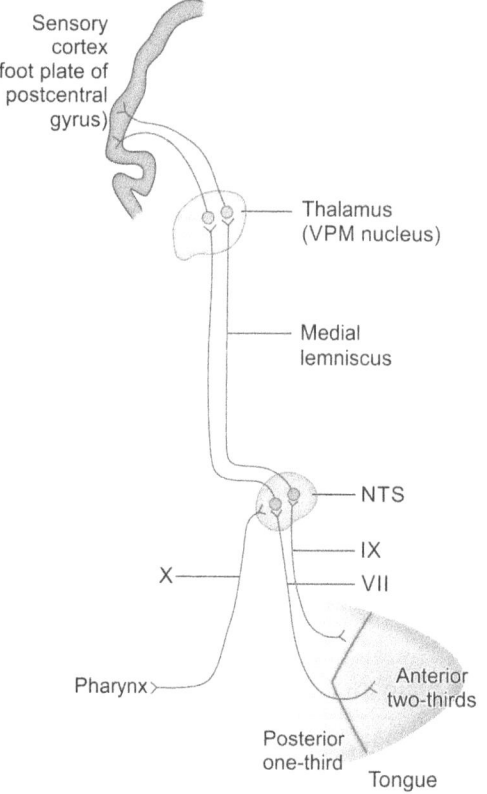

Fig. 21: Taste pathway.

- Each bud is innervated by 50 nerves at bases of receptor cells.
- Each nerve innervates five taste buds.
- The sensory fibers from the taste buds travel through three nerves—chorda tympani branch of facial nerve (from anterior two-thirds of the tongue), glossopharyngeal nerve (from posterior one-third of the tongue) and vagus N from epiglottis, pharynx and palate (*refer* **Fig. 21**).
- They all reach the medulla and terminate on the same side nucleus tractus solitarius of the same side.
- From here the second order neurons travel along with medial lemniscus to reach ventral posteromedial nucleus of ipsilateral thalamus.
- Some fibers from medulla go to the vomiting center, hypothalamus, limbic system and salivary nucleus.
- The 3rd order neurons arise from the thalamus and they reach the foot of post central gyrus on the same side (area 43).
- From there impulses are also transmitted to the insula and lateral orbitofrontal cortex.

Answers to 2020 Question Paper

ANSWER ALL QUESTIONS

I. Essay Questions   **(10 Marks each)**
1. Describe in detail the mechanism of clotting of blood.
2. Define immunity. Discuss in detail about various types of immunity. Add note on autoimmune disease.
3. Describe the neural regulation of respiration. Add a note on periodic breathing.
4. Describe the structure and function of the conducting system of the heart. Add a note on pacemaker potential.

II. Short Notes   **(4 Marks each)**
1. Factors affecting glomerular filtration rate.
2. Micturition reflex.
3. Functions of growth hormone.
4. Negative feedback mechanism.
5. Peptic ulcer.
6. Functions of plasma proteins.
7. Various stages of nerve action potential.
8. Functions of stomach.
9. Conn's syndrome.
10. Heat production in skeletal muscles.
11. Factors affecting cardiac output.
12. Pacemaker potential.
13. ECG–Lead II.
14. Auditory pathway.
15. Functions of cerebellum.
16. Nonrespiratory functions of the lung.
17. Oxyhemoglobin dissociation curve.
18. Heart sounds.
19. Functions of basal ganglia.
20. Four properties of synapse.

III. Short Answers   **(2 Marks each)**
1. Refractory period.
2. Enteric nervous system.
3. Name four GI hormones.
4. Cretinism.
5. Diuretics.
6. Functions of placenta.
7. LH surge.
8. Gallstones.
9. Functions of platelets.
10. Motor unit.
11. Functions of neutrophils.
12. Endocytosis.
13. Free water clearance.
14. Actions of parathyroid hormone.
15. Thyroid function tests.
16. Composition of semen.
17. Pregnancy test.
18. Disseminated intravascular coagulation.
19. Laws of blood grouping.
20. Law of gut.
21. Lung compliance.
22. Exchange vessels.
23. Functions of parietal lobe.
24. Waves of EEG.
25. Referred pain.
26. Circadian rhythm.
27. Aphasia.
28. Kluver-Bucy syndrome.
29. Homunculus.
30. Sensation carried by posterior column.
31. Receptor potential.
32. Reynolds number.
33. Artificial respiration.
34. Vital capacity.
35. Errors of refraction.
36. Functions of thalamus.
37. Papez circuit.
38. Functions of cerebrospinal fluid.
39. Bell-Magendie Law.

I. ESSAY QUESTIONS

1. Describe in detail the mechanism of clotting of blood.

- Blood while flowing in the vessels is fluid in nature, but when the vessel wall is injured or the blood is removed from the body and collected in a test tube, it becomes a jelly like mass—The clot.
- Clotting or coagulation of blood involves a series of cascade of events in which many clotting factors (proteins in the plasma) are activated in a serial manner. There are many such clotting factors.

They are:
- **Factor I:** Fibrinogen
- **Factor II:** Prothrombin
- **Factor III:** Thromboplastin
- **Factor IV:** Calcium
- **Factor V:** Labile factor or proaccelerin
- **Factor VI:** Nonexistent
- **Factor VII:** Stable factor or proconvertin
- **Factor VIII:** Antihemophilic factor
- **Factor IX:** Christmas factor or plasma thromboplastic component (PTC) or antihemophilic factor B
- **Factor X:** Stuart-Prower factor
- **Factor XI:** Plasma thromboplastin antecedent (PTA) or antihemophilic factor C.
- **Factor XII:** Hageman factor or glass factor or contact factor
- **Factor XIII:** Laki-Lorand factor or fibrin stabilizing factor
- **HMW-K:** High molecular weight kininogen or Fitzgerald factor
- **Pre-Ka** (Prekallikrein or Fletcher factor)
- **Kallikrein:** Ka
- **PL:** Platelet phospholipid

The coagulation process involves three major steps:
1. Formation of prothrombin activator
2. Conversion of prothrombin to thrombin
3. Conversion of fibrinogen to fibrin

Formation of Prothrombin Activator is by Two Mechanisms

1. Intrinsic pathway
2. Extrinsic pathway

Intrinsic Pathway

This pathway is activated when there is injury to vessel wall and exposure of collagen or blood itself (*refer* **Fig. 1**).

Steps involved are:
- Injury to vessel wall exposes collagen activates factor XII to XIIa
- Factor XIIa activates factor XI to XIa
- Factor XIa activates factor IX to IXa
- Factor IXa in the presence of VIII, Ca^{2+} and platelet phospholipids (PPL) activates factor X to Xa (*refer* **Fig. 1**).
- The activated factor Xa, platelet phospholipids, factor Va and Ca^{2+} forms the **prothrombin activator.**

Extrinsic Pathway

The **extrinsic pathway** is triggered when the injury involves damage to the blood vessels and the surrounding tissues.

The damaged tissue releases tissue thromboplastin, a protein-phospholipid mixture which activates factor VII. This triggers the extrinsic pathway.
- Inactive factor VII is activated to active factor VIIa
- VIIa in the presence of Ca^{2+}, platelet phospholipid (PL) and tissue thromboplastin, activates factors IX and X.
- Active factor Xa, Va, Ca^{2+} and PL, forms the prothrombin activator.
- This pathway involves fewer steps in the clot formation and therefore is a faster pathway than the intrinsic pathway.

Conversion of Prothrombin to Thrombin

Prothrombin activator in the presence of Ca^{2+} converts prothrombin to thrombin. This happens at the surface of platelets. Thrombin is a proteolytic enzyme.

Conversion of Fibrinogen to Fibrin

- Thrombin, a proteolytic enzyme removes two pairs of polypeptide chains from each fibrinogen molecule and converts it to fibrin monomer.
- The fibrin monomers now polymerize to form long fibrin threads. The fibrin is initially a loose mesh of interlacing

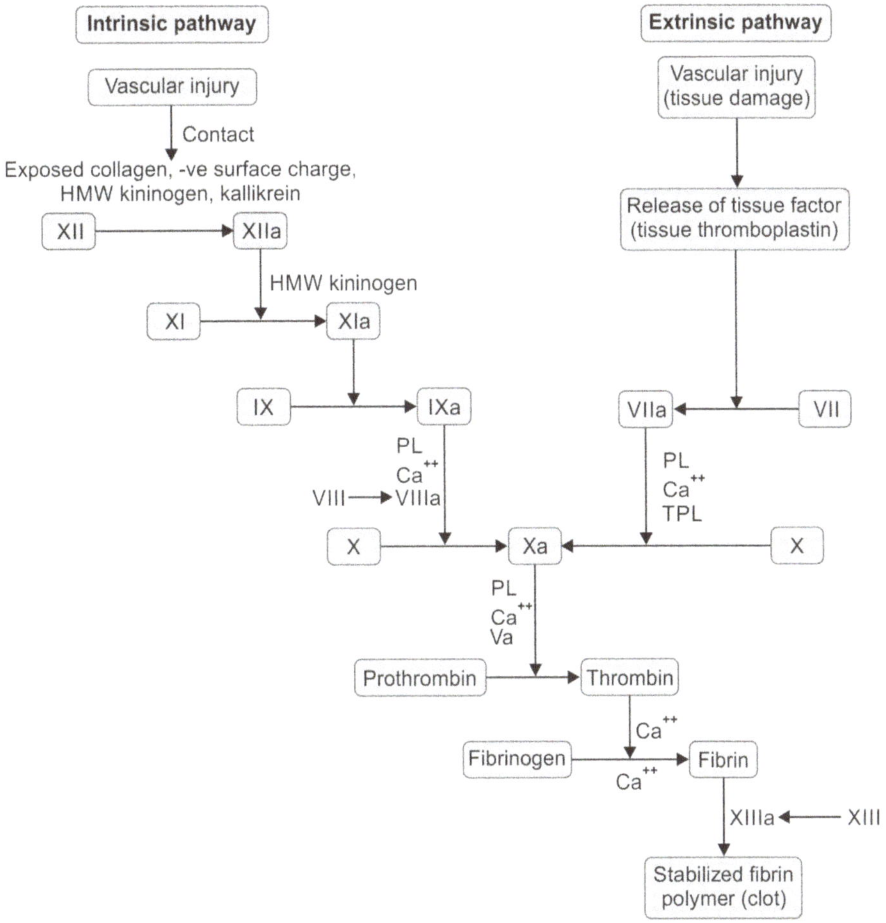

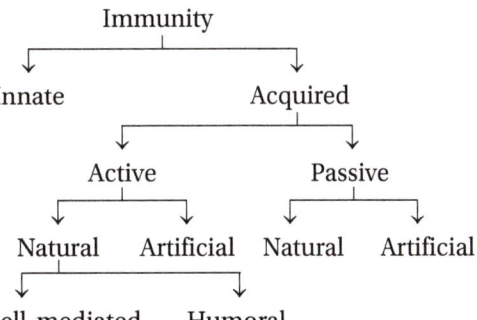

Fig. 1: Mechanism of clotting.
(TPL: tissue phospholipid; PL: platelet phospholipid)

strands. This meshwork traps the blood cells
- It is later converted to a dense tight aggregate by formation of covalent cross-linkages. This is catalyzed by factor XIII and Ca^{2+}. The stabilized fibrin mesh with the trapped blood cells forms the **clot**.

2. Define immunity. Discuss in detail about various types of immunity. Add note on autoimmune disease.

Immunity is the response the body develops when challenged by an antigen.

Two types of immunity are present:
1. Innate or nonspecific immunity
2. Acquired or specific immunity

Classification of Immunity

```
                    Immunity
                   /        \
                Innate      Acquired
                            /      \
                         Active    Passive
                         /    \    /     \
                   Natural  Artificial Natural Artificial
                   /    \
            Cell-mediated  Humoral
```

Innate or nonspecific immunity is present since birth and offer protection against wide variety of pathogens and foreign substances. Nonspecific means there is no specific response for specific invaders; protective mechanisms function the same way regardless of the type of invaders.

They are:
- **External barriers provided by skin and mucous membranes:** Skin has the keratinized layer of cells in epidermis which offers protection. Mucus membrane forms thick mucus, has hair and cilia which aids protection. Secretions, such as saliva, tears, sweat, sebum, vaginal secretions, gastric juice, flow of urine also help in protection.
- **Antimicrobial proteins:** Interferons, complement proteins, transferrin
- **Natural killer cells:** They are a type of lymphocytes. They protect against various infections, such as bacterial and viral and also against cancer cells. They kill cells by inducing **perforins** and causing **apoptosis** of the target cells.
- **Phagocytosis:** By Neutrophils and monocyte-macrophage system
- Inflammation
- Fever

Acquired immunity or specific immunity, the ability of the body to defend against specific invading agents, such as bacteria, toxins, viruses, and foreign tissues, is called as specific resistance or immunity and it develops after exposure to the antigen.

It has two properties—specificity and memory.

Specificity for particular antigen which involves distinguishing self from nonself-molecules.

Memory for previously encountered antigen is present and when a second encounter happens there is a swift and rapid response.

It includes two types:
1. Cell-mediated
2. Humoral immunity

Cell-mediated Immunity
- It is mediated by T lymphocytes.
- T lymphocytes are formed in the bone marrow and they are processed in the thymus.

Stages of Cell-mediated Immunity
- **Antigen presentation:** Cells, such as macrophages, mast cells, and dendritic cells act as antigen presenting cells (APCs). Macrophages phagocytose the antigens entering the body and breaks it down to peptide fragments. The antigenic fragment forms a complex with the MHC II protein formed by the macrophages. The antigen and MHC II complex are expressed on the membrane of macrophage.
- **Antigen recognition by lymphocytes:** The APC with the antigen-MHC II complex is recognized by the T lymphocytes with the receptors for the antigen. T cells become activated if it binds to the antigen and is co-stimulated with cytokines like IL-2. Once two stimulations have happened, the lymphocyte is activated. The activated T cells enlarge and begin to proliferate and differentiate to form a clone of similar T cells. This happens in the secondary lymphoid organs like the lymph nodes.
- **Types of T cells:** There are three main types of T cells—helper T cells (CD4 cells), cytotoxic T cells (CD8 cells), and memory T cells.
  a. *Helper T cells:* Helper T cells or CD4 cells recognize the antigen presented along with MHC II and cytotoxic or CD8 cells recognize the antigens presented with MHC I.

   After costimulation of helper T cells, they secrete many cytokines. The most important cytokine is IL-2 which is needed for all the immune responses and is the major stimulator for T cell proliferation. IL-2 is also the costimulator for resting helper T cells and cytotoxic T cells. It also enhances activation and proliferation of B cells and natural killer cells.

  b. *Cytotoxic T cells:* The T cells that express CD8 develop into cytotoxic T cells. They recognize foreign antigens expressed along with MHC I on the membranes of body cells infected by viruses, tumor cells, and cells of tissue transplant. But to get activated into a killer cell it

needs costimulation by IL-2 produced by helper cells. Therefore, for maximal activation of cytotoxic T cells it needs antigen presentation with MHC I and II (*refer* **Fig. 2**).
c. *Memory T cells:* The T cells for a specific antigen, which remain in the lymph organ after the immune response is over, are termed as memory T cells. If the same pathogen is encountered for the second time, these cells get activated and they initiate a swift and fast immune response. The second response is faster and vigorous and the pathogen is eliminated even before any symptom develops.

Elimination of the pathogens: The killing of the pathogen is done by the cytotoxic T cells.
a. The activated CD8 cells synthesize and secrete proteins called "perforins" which are inserted into the membrane of the pathogen. The perforins are water channels which allow influx of water and thereby swelling of the microbe and cause its lysis.
b. Release of lymphotoxins by activated T cells. These cytokines destroy the microbes.
c. Cytotoxic T cells secrete interferons, which will favor the phagocytic activity of the neutrophils and macrophages by promoting opsonization.

Role of Cell-mediated Immunity
- It is activated against intracellular pathogens, such as viral infections and bacterial infections, such as *Mycobacterium tuberculosis*.
- It removes the tumor cells
- It is responsible for rejection of transplanted tissues
- It is responsible for hypersensitivity reactions.

Humoral Immunity
- B lymphocytes mediate humoral immunity.
- Humoral immunity provides protection against extracellular pathogens, takes part in immediate hypersensitivity reactions type I, II, and III.

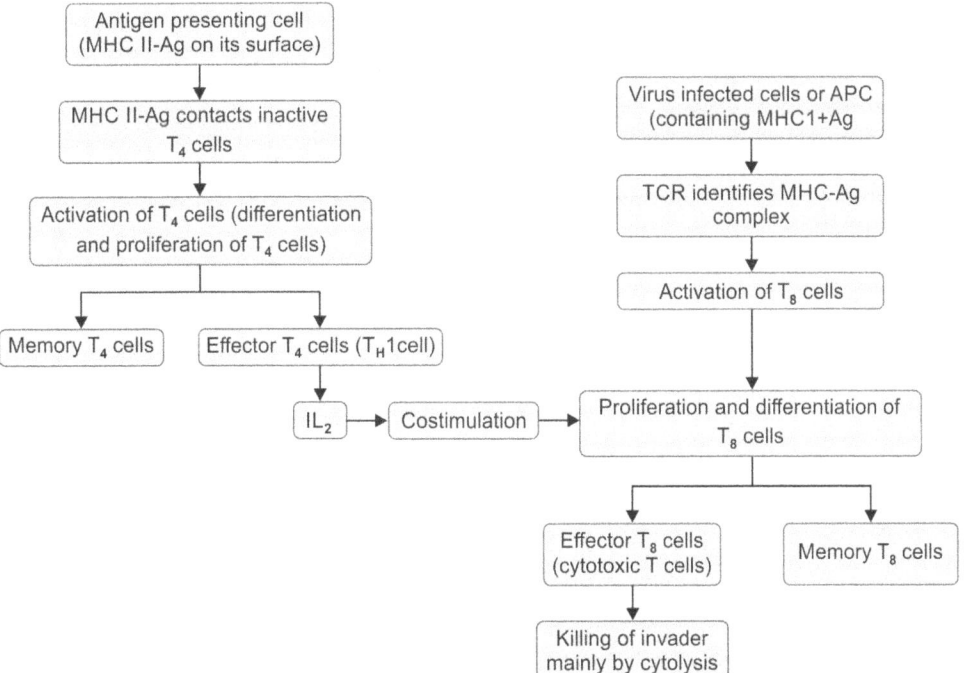

Fig. 2: Mechanism of cell-mediated immunity.

Stages of Humoral Immunity Include

1. Antigen processing and presentation
2. Activation of B cells
3. Differentiation of B cells to plasma cells
4. Proliferation of plasma cells
5. Formation of antibodies by plasma cells
6. Destruction of pathogens by antibodies
7. Formation of memory B cells

1. **Antigen processing and presentation:** Antigen on entering the body is engulfed by macrophages and is broken to fragments and the antigenic fragments are attached to the MHC II protein and inserted on the cell membrane of macrophage. Macrophage with the antigen and MHC II are presented to the lymphocytes—antigen presentation.
2. **Activation of B cells:** B cells in the lymph nodes which have the receptor for the antigen recognizes it and binds with the receptor. This is said to be antigen recognition and activation. Activation is further stimulated when it is co-stimulated by helper T cells. T helper cells secrete interleukin—2, 4, and 5 which stimulates B cells.
3. **Differentiation of B cells to plasma cells:** Activated B cells become enlarged and looks like a blast cell. It then gets transformed into plasma cells. Plasma cells are larger and have lot of endoplasmic reticulum and they secrete antibodies. Costimulation by T helper cells help in transformation.
4. **Proliferation of plasma cells:** Activated plasma cells undergo proliferation to form millions of similar cells. This is called clonal selection of plasma cells.
5. **Formation of antibodies:** The plasma cells secrete antibodies which are called as immunoglobulins. Each cell can form 2000 **Immunoglobulins** (Ig) in a second. The Igs formed are very specific to the antigen which stimulated the B cells.
6. **Destruction of pathogens:** Antibodies do the killing of antigens by the following mechanisms:
   a. Neutralization of antigens
   b. Precipitation of antigens
   c. Activation of complementary pathway
   d. Opsonization of antigens and facilitates phagocytosis
   e. Prevent mobilization of microbes
7. **Formation of memory B cells:** Some of the plasma cells get differentiated into memory B cells and they stay inactive in the lymph nodes till the second encounter with the same pathogen. On exposure for the second time, they produce a rapid, swift and strong response to the antigen—secondary immunological response.

3. Describe the neural regulation of respiration. Add a note on periodic breathing.

- Breathing is an automatic process occurring throughout life without conscious effort.
- Respiration is a process which is highly regulated.
- Spontaneous respiration is due to rhythmic discharge of neurons from respiratory centers supplying the inspiratory muscles.
- This is under cortical (voluntary) and medullary and pontine control (automatic).
- These centers in turn are regulated by alterations in the PCO_2, PO_2, and pH of arterial blood and other Nonchemical influences.

Cortical Control or Voluntary Control of Respiration

Impulses from cerebral cortex
↓
Corticospinal tract
↓
Motor neurons supplying the inspiratory muscles

- Impulses also reach the innervation of expiratory muscles.
- There is a reciprocal inhibition between the motor neurons supplying the I and E neurons.
- There is an exception for this at the start of expiration were the "I" neurons are active.
- The inspiratory muscles are active for some time during expiration to brake the

elastic recoil of lungs and make expiration smooth.

Automatic Control of Respiration

Impulses from brainstem respiratory centers in pons and medulla → supplies neurons in intermediolateral horn cells of cervical and thoracic segments → supplies inspiratory muscles.

Medullary Respiratory Centers
- Dorsal respiratory group of neurons (DRG)—Has 'I' neurons
- Ventral respiratory group of neurons (VRG)—Has 'I' and 'E' neurons
- Central pattern generator (CPG)—pre-Botzinger complex

Dorsal respiratory group of neurons:
- Located near nucleus tractus solitarius (NTS)
- Contains only inspiratory neurons (*refer* **Fig. 3**)
- They project to cell bodies of phrenic nerves in spinal cord.
- Its activity is weaker to start with and gradually increases in a ramp fashion for 2 seconds and abruptly stops for 3 seconds.
- The ramp signal helps in steady increase in lung volume during inspiration
- Receives input from peripheral chemoreceptors through 9th and 10th cranial nerves.

Ventral respiratory group of neurons:
- Located in ventrolateral medulla in region of nucleus ambiguus (NA)
- Contains both inspiratory and expiratory group of neurons
- Three regions—rostral, middle, and caudal inspiratory regions
- Middle region—has inspiratory neurons
- Rostral and caudal—has expiratory neurons—supply expiratory muscles.
- They are active only during forceful respiration.
- I and E neurons reciprocally inhibit each other

Pacemaker cells for respiration:
- Located close to DRG and VRG neurons (*refer* **Fig. 4**).
- Present in the pre-Bötzinger complex between nucleus ambiguus and lateral reticular nucleus.
- They are pacemaker cells and are responsible for generating respiratory rhythm → rhythmically activate phrenic nerves.
- It receives input from higher centers

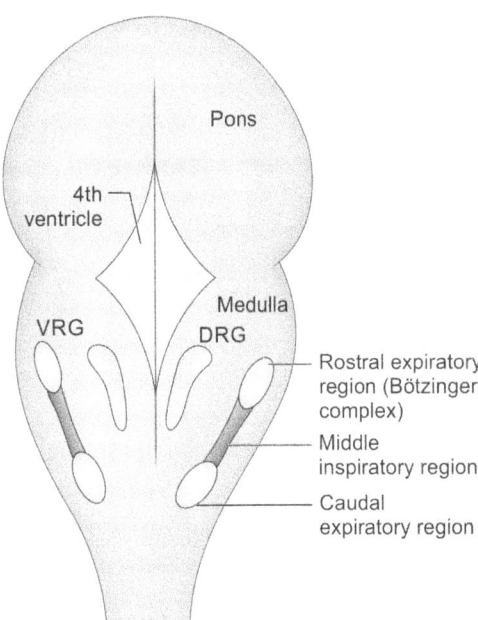

Fig. 3: Respiratory centers in medulla.
(DRG: dorsal respiratory group of neurons (has only inspiratory neurons); VRG: ventral respiratory group of neurons (has both inspiratory and expiratory neurons)

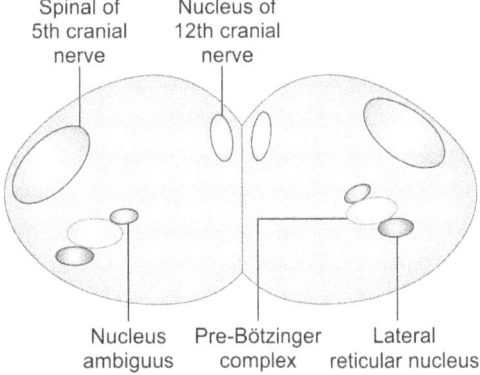

Fig. 4: Location of pacemaker (pre-Bötzinger complex) for rhythm generation in medulla.

Pontine Centers

There are two centers:

- **Pneumotaxic center:**
  - Located in nucleus parabrachialis and Kolliker-Fuse N in the upper part of pons
  - Active during both inspiration and expiration.
  - On stimulation, it shortens the duration of inspiration. When its activity is less, the duration of inspiration is longer.
  - Its major function is to limit inspiration, by inhibiting apneustic center
  - It coordinates switching between inspiration and expiration.
- **Apneustic center:**
  - Present in lower part of pons
  - On stimulation → leads to prolonged inspiratory spasms—**apneusis**
  - It sends inputs to DRG to cause a prolonged inspiration
  - It is constantly stimulating DRG.
  - But its actions are kept in check by inputs from pneumotaxic center and vagal afferents from airways (*refer* **Fig. 5**).

Mechanism of Breathing

- The neurons in DRG discharge steadily and spontaneously in a ramp like fashion for 2–3 seconds.
- Muscles of inspiration contract steadily resulting in expansion of the lung and chest wall resulting in inspiration.
- As the inspiration happens, the stretch receptors in lungs and airways are stimulated and impulses from here travel through vagus nerve to stop the firing of DRG neurons.
- Impulses from pneumotaxic center through inhibition of apneustic center stops the firing of DRG.
- Inspiratory muscles relax and the lung and chest wall recoils and induces expiration.
- At the end of expiration, the next cycle starts (*refer* **Fig. 6**).

Factors Influencing Respiratory Centers

- **Afferents from higher centers:** Cerebral cortex, limbic system, hypothalamus
- **Afferents from peripheral receptors:** Baroreceptors, chemoreceptors, J receptors, pain receptors, proprioceptors, pulmonary stretch receptors, and thermoreceptors.

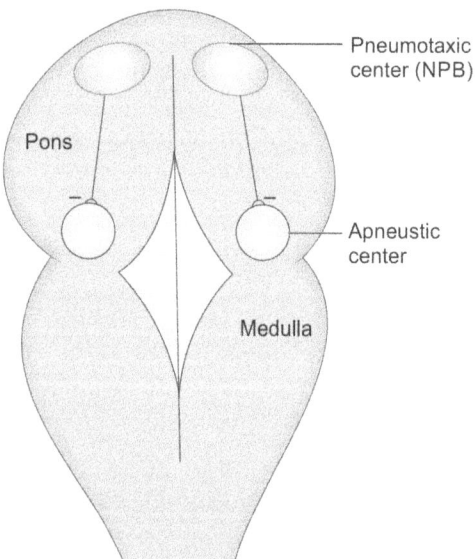

Fig. 5: Respiratory centers in pons, pneumotaxic, and apneustic centers.

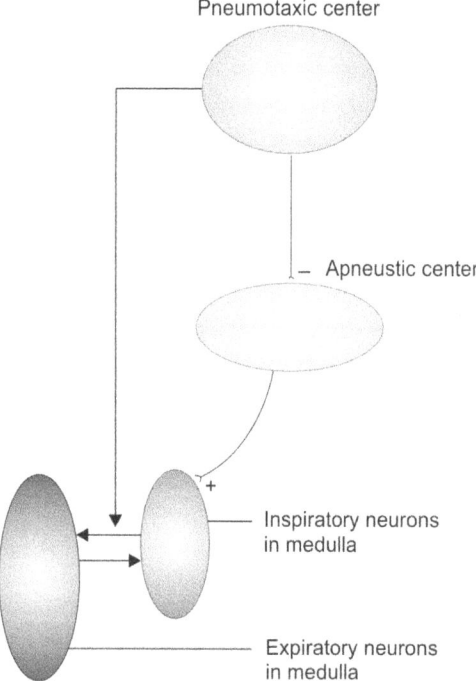

Fig. 6: Interaction of medullary and pontine centers in regulation of respiration.

- **Reflexes:** Hering-Breuer reflex, sneezing reflex, swallowing reflex, cough reflex, speech

Afferents from higher centers

- Cerebral cortex imparts control over the respiratory centers and therefore voluntary hyperventilation and breath holding is possible
- Limbic cortex sends impulses to respiratory centers and therefore the changes in ventilation in relation to emotions can happen.
- Hypothalamic connections are responsible for respiratory changes associated with body temperature changes.

Afferent Impulses from Peripheral Receptors

- **Baroreceptors:** They regulate blood pressure through the regulation of vasomotor and cardiac vagal centers. But stimulation of baroreceptors also inhibit the respiratory center and causes apnea.
- **Chemoreceptors:** There are peripheral and central chemoreceptors. They monitor the PO_2, PCO_2, and pH levels in the arterial blood. Decrease in arterial PO_2 levels will stimulate peripheral chemoreceptors and they will send impulses to DRG to stimulate respiration. Central chemoreceptors are more sensitive to PCO_2 and H levels and when it increases, they stimulate respiration.
- **'J' receptors:** These are endings of unmyelinated C fibers of vagal afferents and are located between the pulmonary capillaries and alveolar walls. They are stimulated in conditions of increase in interstitial fluid between the capillary endothelium and alveolar epithelium as in pulmonary edema, pulmonary congestion, pulmonary embolism, etc. On stimulation, it induces apnea followed by tachypnoea, bradycardia, and hypotension. In physiological conditions these receptors are stimulated while exercising, especially in high altitude.
- **Proprioceptors:** While doing exercise, movements in the muscles and joints stimulate the proprioceptors and impulses from here stimulate respiration by stimulating DRG.
- **Pulmonary stretch receptors (Hering-Breuer reflex):** The pulmonary stretch receptors are located in the smooth muscles of the airways and are stimulated by inflation of lungs.

There are two types of reflexes:
1. **Hering-Breuer inflation reflex:** It is activated during inspiration. When the inspiration is more and tidal volume is more than 1 L, the reflex is initiated and it sends impulses to the respiratory centers and inhibits inspiration and stimulates expiration. This reflex is more important in infants to control the tidal volume.
2. **Hering-Breuer deflation reflex:** This reflex is activated during expiration and causes arrest of expiration and stimulates inspiration.

Thermoreceptors: Increase in body temperature stimulates these receptors and send impulses to the cerebral cortex, which in turn sends impulses to respiratory centers to increase respiration. Respiration helps to lose body temperature.

Reflexes

- **Sneezing reflex:** Stimulation of nasal mucosa by irritant substances results in sneezing. The act of sneezing involves a deep inspiration followed by forceful expiration with opened glottis initially and later glottis opens to allow air to flow through mouth and nose.
- **Cough reflex:** Stimulation of irritant receptors in the tracheobronchial mucosa leads to deep inspiration followed by forceful expiration against a closed glottis. It is a protective reflex useful for clearing the airway of the irritant substance.
- **Deglutition reflex:** On swallowing, there is temporary stoppage of respiration—deglutition apnea. It is a protective reflex which prevents entry of food into the airway.
- **Vomiting reflex:** Apnea happens for a short time during vomiting to prevent aspiration of contents.

Periodic Breathing

Periodic breathing means respiratory activity alternating with apnea.

- **Cheyne-Stokes respiration:**
  - It is an abnormal respiratory pattern with waxing and waning of respiration separated by periods of apnea.
  - Duration of each cycle is 1 minute
  - Arterial PO_2 and PCO_2 levels fluctuate in different phases of respiration.
  - Seen in conditions, such as drug overdosage, brain diseases, congestive cardiac failure, uremia and hypoxia due to other causes.
  - It is also seen in physiological conditions, such as—sleep and during voluntary hyperventilation, also in persons with increased sensitivity to CO_2.
  - There is usually disruption of neural pathways that inhibit respiration.
- **Cheyne-Stokes respiration in voluntary hyperventilation:** Following hyperventilation there is apnea → accumulation of CO_2 → stimulation of respiratory center → gradual increase in respiration → as PCO_2 decreases → CO_2 is blown out → apnea.
- **Cheyne-Stokes respiration in congestive cardiac failure (CCF):**
  - In patients with heart failure the circulation time of blood is longer (as the pumping of heart is inefficient).
  - So it takes a longer time for the changes in blood PCO_2 to reach the respiratory centers.
  - As these patients hyperventilate the PCO_2 levels are lowered and since the circulation time is prolonged it takes time for this lowered PCO_2 levels to be detected.
  - By the time, the PCO_2 levels are further lowered in pulmonary capillaries and when this blood reaches the brain, the low PCO_2 inhibits respiratory center producing apnea.
  - Therefore, the respiratory control system oscillates because the negative feedback loop between brain and lungs is lengthened (*refer* **Fig. 7**).

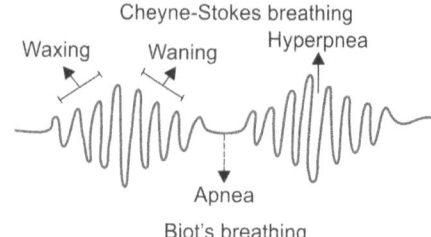

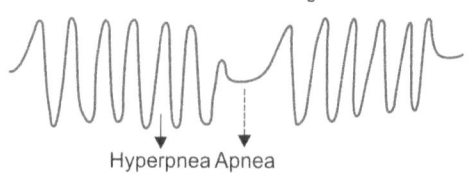

Fig. 7: Periodic breathing; Cheyne-Stokes breathing and Biot's breathing.

- **Biot's breathing:**
  - Has one or more large tidal volumes separated by apnea.
  - It is seen in irregular intervals
  - It is seen only in pathological conditions
  - Present in diseases ↑ intracranial tension—tumors, meningitis, pontine hemorrhage, central medullary lesions.

---

4. Describe the structure and function of the conducting system of the heart. Add a note on pacemaker potential.

- Conductivity is a property of cardiac muscle.
- It is the ability to conduct an impulse in the myocardium (action potential)
- Conduction of impulse is by sequential depolarization of adjacent membrane.
- In the heart, there is a specialized conducting system.
- It starts in the SA node and reaches the ventricles.
- It consists of the SA node, internodal tracts, interatrial tract, AV node, Bundle of his, right and left branches of bundle of his, Purkinje fibers, and the ventricular muscles.

SA Node

- It is located in the wall of the right atrium close to the opening of SVC.
- It is made up of modified muscle fibers with more rounded cells with indistinct

borders and less striations. They are called as P cells.
- Such cells are present in the AV node also.
- In the heart the SA node, AV node, His bundle, and ventricles can generate their own impulses.
- But SA node is called the pacemaker as it generates impulses at a faster rate than the other tissues. So, it is called the pacemaker.
- The pacemaker cells do not have a stable resting membrane potential.
- They tend to depolarize and repolarize in a continuous fashion in spite of nerve supply.
- The potential developed here is called as the **pacemaker potential**.

Pacemaker Potential

- The RMP in SA node is around –55 to –60 mV.
- But it is not a stable potential. There is a slow depolarization till –40 mV. Once –40 mV is reached there is a rapid depolarization (Phase 0) to +5 mV and there is a rapid repolarization to –55 mV (Phase 3).
- Then it reaches the RMP (Phase 4)
- Once again there is a slow depolarization, the process continues.
- This slow rising phase before the rapid depolarization is called as the **prepotential** or **pacemaker potential** (*refer* **Fig. 8**).

Ionic Events Responsible for Pacemaker Potential

- The prepotential is divided into three sections based on the ionic events – The first part of slow depolarization is due to decay of K^+ current (closure of K^+ channels), followed by Na^+ influx through 'h' or 'f' channels and the last part is due to Ca^{2+} influx through transient type Ca^{2+} (T type) channels.
- The rapid depolarization which starts at –40 mV is due to Ca^{2+} influx through long lasting Ca^{2+} channels (L type).
- Rapid repolarization is due to K^+ efflux through K^+ channels resulting in repolarization to –55 to –60 mV.

Conducting Pathway

- These impulses originated in the SA node are conducted down through the specialized conducting system as mentioned above.
- The impulses from SA node are transmitted to the AV node through three internodal bundles which are specialized tissues for conduction of impulses from SA node to AV node in a faster way (*refer* **Fig. 9**).
- The atrial tissues also conduct impulses but they are slower.

The three bundles are:
1. Anterior internodal tract of Bachman
2. Middle internodal tract of Wenckebach
3. Posterior internodal tract of Thorel

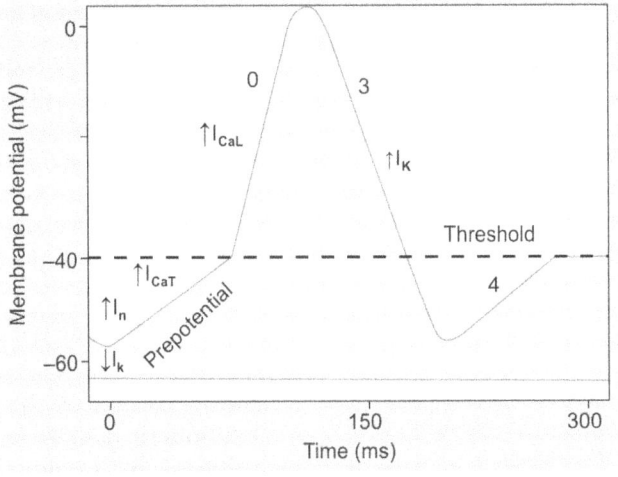

Fig. 8: Pacemaker potential.
(I_K: potassium current; I_{CaT}: calcium current through T type calcium channel; I_{CaL}: calcium current through L type calcium channel)

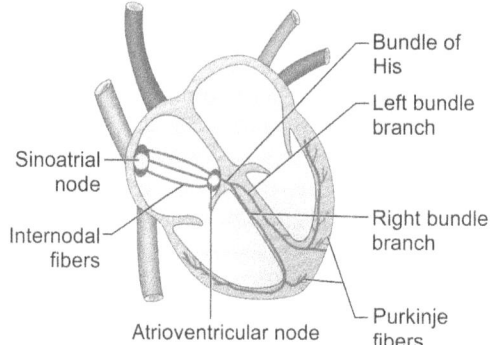

Fig. 9: Conducting system of the heart.

4. Through these bundles the impulses reach the AV node.

Interatrial tract of Bachman

- This bundle starts in the SA node and ends in the left atrium.
- The left atrium is also depolarized simultaneously.

AV Node

- It is located beneath the endocardium on the right side of lower part of atrial septum near the tricuspid valve.
- The conduction velocity through the AVN is very slow because the fibers are smaller with less number of gap junctions.
- There is a delay of 0.1 s.
- The delay provides time for atrial contraction and final ventricular filling.
- It also prevents transmission of all impulses from atria to ventricles in supraventricular tachycardia.
- It is supplied by sympathetic and PS nerves which alter the conduction rate.

Atrioventricular Bundle of His

- This bundle starts in the AV bundle and descends down the fibrous skeleton and divides into right and left branches and they supply the right and left ventricles.
- The bundles divide into many small branches, the Purkinje fibers.

Purkinje Fibers

They are present in the endocardium and reaches all parts of ventricles.

Ventricles

- The spread of depolarization in the ventricular muscles are from the AVN to the His bundle → Purkinje fibers → Ventricles.
- The conduction velocity of the AP through ventricular muscles are 0.3–0.4 msec.
- This results in depolarization of both ventricles at the same time and leads to contraction of both ventricles at the same time.
- In ventricle, the spread of depolarization is from endocardium to epicardium.
- Repolarization starts in the epicardium and spreads towards endocardium.
- Ability to contract follows the excitation of atrial and ventricular myocardium.

In humans the ventricular depolarization starts in the left side of interventricular septum
↓
Then moves to the right side across the midportion of the septum
↓
Then the wave spreads downwards to the apex of the ventricle
↓
Then it turns back along the ventricular muscle towards the AV-groove from endocardium to epicardium
↓
The last part to be depolarized are the posterobasal part of left ventricle, pulmonary conus and uppermost portion of the septum
↓
Repolarization proceeds from epicardium to endocardium in the ventricle

- The function of conducting system is to excite the myocardium following which intracellular calcium is increased and thereby contraction of the muscle follows.

II. SHORT NOTES

1. Factors affecting glomerular filtration rate.

Glomerular Filtration Rate (GFR):

- GFR refers to the volume of the glomerular filtrate formed each minute by all the nephrons in both the kidneys. The normal value is 125 mL/min or 7.5 L/hr or 180 L/day.
- Mechanism of filtration across the glomerular capillary is similar to the

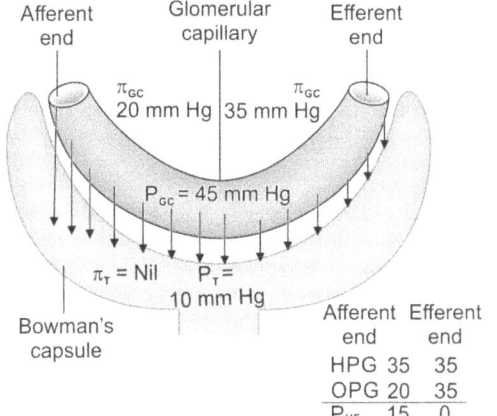

Fig. 10: Mechanism of filtration along the glomerular capillary. In contrast to systemic capillaries filtration happens along the entire capillary.
(P_{GC}: capillary hydrostatic pressure; P_T: Bowman's space hydrostatic pressure; π_{GC}: glomerular capillary oncotic pressure; π_T: osmotic pressure in Bowman's space)

mechanism of filtration across any of the systemic capillaries.
- So filtration is dependent on the Starling's forces across the capillary membrane and characteristics of the membrane and renal blood flow and arterial blood pressure.
- Filtration across the membrane is decided by the balance of the starling's forces (*refer* **Fig. 10**)
- **GFR is expressed as:** $GFR = K_f [(P_{GC} - P_T) - (\Pi_{GC} - \Pi_T)]$
  - **GFR:** Glomerular filtration rate
  - **K_f:** Filtration co-efficient of the membrane and it is 12.5 m/min/mm Hg. It is the product of glomerular capillary wall conductivity and effective filtration surface area.
  - **P_{GC}:** Glomerular capillary hydrostatic pressure.
  - **P_T:** Hydrostatic pressure in Bowman's space.
  - **Π_{GC}:** Glomerular capillary oncotic pressure.
  - **Π_T:** Oncotic pressure in Bowman's space.

Factors Affecting GFR:

- **Surface area of filtration membrane** is altered by the contraction or relaxation of the mesangial cells. Contraction of mesangial cells decreases the surface area of filtration and relaxation increases it. Contraction is induced by angiotensin II, endothelin, ADH, etc., and relaxation is stimulated by ANP, dopamine, cAMP, and PGE_2.
- **Permeability of glomerular membrane** for neutral substances of less than 4 nm molecular diameter is favored and neutral substances above 8 nm are not filtered. Between 4 to 8 nm the filtration is inversely proportional to diameter of substances. There are negatively charged sialoproteins lining the glomerular membrane, which prevents negatively charged particles like albumin from getting filtered even though it is 6 nm in diameter. Permeability is increased in hypoxia and presence of toxic substances.
- **Hydrostatic pressure in glomerulus:** It is higher than in other capillaries in the body as the efferent arterioles (the outlet of glomerulus) is more constricted and offers more resistance than the afferent arterioles (the inlet for glomerulus) which are short and straight branches. So factors which increase efferent arteriolar constriction will increase the hydrostatic pressure in the glomerulus. Changes in the systemic blood pressure will affect renal perfusion and thereby the filtration. The hydrostatic pressure in the glomerulus at the afferent and efferent end is 45 mm Hg.
- **Hydrostatic pressure in Bowman's space:** This is the pressure exerted by the filtered fluid in the bowman's space and it opposes filtration. Normally it is 10 mm Hg. It increases in conditions of obstruction of urinary tract as in ureteric calculi blocking the flow of fluid in the tubule.
- **Oncotic pressure in the glomerulus:** GFR is inversely proportional to oncotic pressure. It is exerted by the plasma proteins. The capillary oncotic pressure at afferent end is 25 mm Hg and at efferent end it is 35 mm Hg. This is because as the fluid leaves the capillary from afferent to efferent ends of capillaries the concentration of plasma proteins increases and thereby oncotic pressure increases. So in conditions of hyperproteinemia or hemoconcentration oncotic pressure rises

and GFR decreases. In hypoproteinemia GFR is increased.
- **Oncotic pressure in Bowman's space:** It is very negligible because no protein is filtered into the Bowman's space.
- **Effective filtration pressure:** It is the net outward pressure which favors filtration and is calculated as the difference between the outward and inward forces.

$$GFR = K_f [(P_{GC} - P_T) - (\Pi_{GC} - \Pi_T)]$$
$$GFR = 12.5 (45-10) - (25-0)$$
$$= 12.5 \times 10 = 125 \text{ mL/min}$$

- **Other factors affecting GFR:**
  - Sympathetic stimulation of renal vessels leads to marked vasoconstriction and thereby decreases GFR.
  - Hormones like norepinephrine, endothelin and angiotensin II cause intense vasoconstriction and thereby decrease RBF and GFR. Ang II at low concentrations cause only constriction of efferent arteriole and thereby increases GFR. ANP, dopamine, nitric oxide, prostaglandins cause vasodilatation and increase RBF and GFR.

2. Micturition reflex.

- Urinary bladder is a triangular-shaped sac like structure. The bladder extends down as the urethra.
- The bladder wall is made of detrusor, a smooth muscle and there are two sphincters—internal and external urethral sphincters.
- Internal sphincter is at the neck of the bladder and is made of smooth muscle. It is supplied by sympathetic and parasympathetic nerves.
- External sphincter is made of skeletal muscle and is supplied by somatic motor nerve (pudendal nerve).
- The bladder wall is also supplied by sympathetic and parasympathetic nerves.
- Parasympathetic nerves (pelvic nerve) have both afferents and efferents to bladder wall and internal sphincter. They arise from S2–S4 segments of spinal cord. When they are stimulated they cause contraction of bladder wall and relaxation of internal sphincter and therefore emptying of bladder.
- The sympathetic nerves (hypogastric nerve) also have afferents and efferents and they arise from L1–L3 segments of spinal cord. They also supply the bladder wall and internal sphincter. When stimulated, they cause relaxation of bladder wall and contraction of internal sphincter and therefore filling of bladder (*refer* **Fig. 11**).

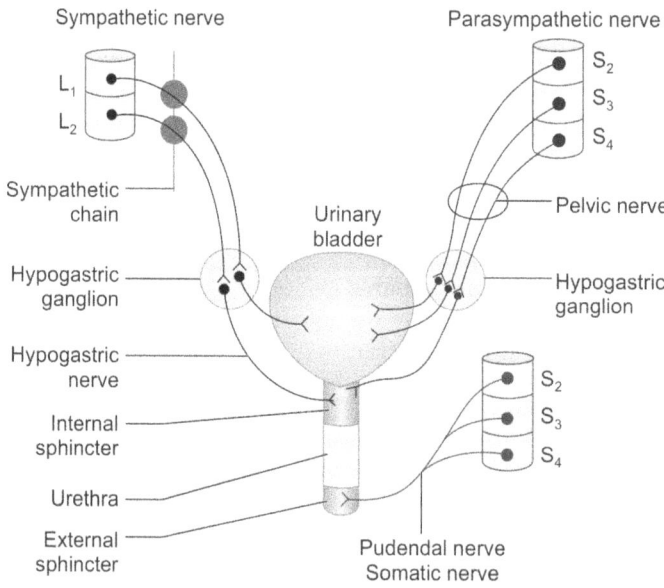

Fig. 11: Nerve supply of urinary bladder.

- Somatic nerve (pudendal nerve) to external sphincter arises from S2–S4 segments of spinal cord and have control from higher centers. It is under voluntary control.
- Once urine enters the renal pelvis, it flows through the ureters and enters the bladder, where urine is stored.
- **Micturition is the process of emptying the urinary bladder.**
- **Two processes are involved:**
  a. The bladder fills progressively until the tension in its wall rises above a threshold level, and then
  b. A nervous reflex called the micturition reflex occurs that empties the bladder.
    The micturition reflex is an automatic spinal cord reflex; however, it can be inhibited or facilitated by centers in the brainstem and cerebral cortex.

The reflex pathway:
- **Initiation:** Reflex initiated by stimulation of stretch receptors in bladder wall.
- **Stimulus:** Filling of bladder up to 300–400 mL.
- **Afferents:** Through pelvic nerves (PS) to reach S2–S4 segments in spinal cord.
- **Efferents:** PS motor fibers from S2–S4 end in the detrusor muscle (excitatory) and internal sphincter (inhibitory).
- **Response:** Causes contraction of bladder wall and relaxation of internal sphincter. Once it becomes powerful another reflex through pudendal nerve relaxes the ES → voiding (refer **Fig. 12**).

3. Functions of growth hormone.

- GH is a polypeptide hormone.
- It is a major growth promoting hormone.
- It has direct and indirect actions.
- It acts directly to catabolize substrates and to supply energy in starvation.
- Its anabolic actions are direct on epiphysis and indirect through somatomedins (IGF-1).

Effect on Growth

- Stimulates linear growth by acting on epiphyseal cartilage of long bones.

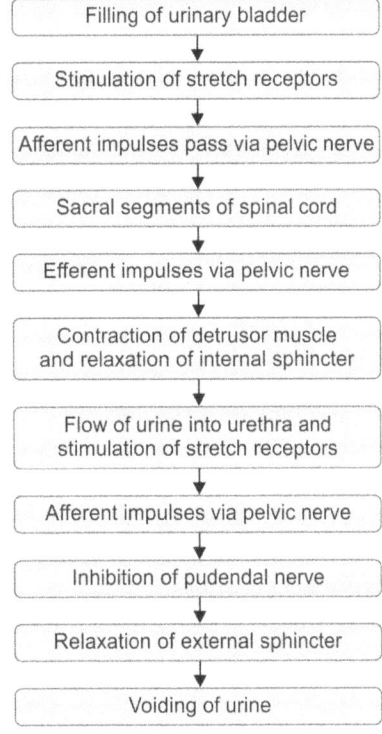

Fig. 12: Micturition reflex.

- It stimulates all aspects of metabolism of chondrocytes as in:
  - Incorporates proline into collagen to form hydroxyproline.
  - Promotes cartilage matrix formation.
  - ↑ AA uptake and protein synthesis
  - ↑ Size and number of chondrocytes.
  - Facilitates differentiation of prechondrocytes to chondrocytes.
- All these actions result in growth of epiphyseal cartilage and promote linear growth.

Other Growth Promoting Actions

- **On bone:** stimulates bone modeling by increasing activity of osteoclasts and blasts, osteoblastic activity predominates.
- **On skeletal muscle:** ↑ growth of skeletal muscle by ↑ protein synthesis → hypertrophy.
- Increases growth of visceral organs.
- **Induces pubertal growth:** Increase in height and sexual maturation.

Indirect Actions
- Effects of GH on growth, cartilage and protein metabolism is mediated through insulin-like growth factors (IGF).
- Also called as somatomedins.
- They are growth factor synthesized in the liver.

Effects on Metabolism
Positive Nitrogen and Phosphate

Protein metabolism:
- Protein anabolic
- Positive N_2 and phosphate balance
- ↑ Amino acid entry into cells
- ↑ RNA and DNA synthesis
- ↑ Protein synthesis
- Decreased level of amino acids in blood

Carbohydrate metabolism:
- It is prodiabetogenic
- Releases glucose from liver by facilitating gluconeogenesis
- Decreases glucose uptake by skeletal muscles.
- Decreases insulin sensitivity.

Lipid metabolism:
- Causes lipolysis and increases FFA in plasma
- Promotes ketogenesis
- Increased FFA and ketones provide the energy during stress

Effect on water and electrolyte metabolism:
- ↑ Plasma Ca^{2+}, by increasing the reabsorption from GIT
- Causes Na^+ retention
- It maintains ECF volume by stimulating renin-angiotensin-aldosterone pathway.
- Also suppresses ANP release.

4. Negative feedback mechanism.
- Most of the control systems in the body are negative feedback regulations.
- In negative feedback regulation, if a particular activity is increased or decreased, the control system initiates a chain of actions by which the activity returns back to normal.
- So the control system has a sensor to sense the change, a control center that receives signals from the sensor and sends command to the effector which will bring about the change.

Examples:
Body temperature regulation, regulation of pH, regulation of blood glucose levels, regulation of thyroid hormone secretion.

Blood pressure regulation:

Increase in mean arterial pressure
↓
Sensed by baroreceptors
↓
Impulses are carried by IXth and Xth cranial nerves
↓
Inhibits vasomotor center and stimulates cardiac vagal center
↓
Decreases heart rate and stroke volume
↓
Decreases cardiac output
↓
Decreases mean arterial pressure

5. Peptic ulcer.
There are two types of ulcers:
1. **Duodenal ulcer**
2. **Gastric ulcer:** Ulcer is due to disruption of the mucosal barrier or excess secretion of gastric juice.

Acid or pepsin in gastric juice digests the mucosa leading to ulcer.

Mucosal barrier is formed by:
- **Mucus secreted** by the neck cells and surface mucosal cells in the mucosal lining. It also contains mucin, phospholipid, HCO_3^- and water.
- **Prostaglandins** secreted by epithelial cells have antisecretory activity (HCl) and increases HCO_3^- and mucus.
- **Epithelium of mucosa**—low permeability, rapid turnover and HCO_3^-, mucus secretions from there.
- **Bicarbonate secretion** from gastric mucosal cells increases the pH.

Factors which Impair Mucosal Defense
- Defective mucus secretion
- Drugs like NSAIDs, cortisol, etc.—they inhibit secretion of mucus and bicarbonate

- Alcohol
- Type of food
- Smoking—↓ mucus and pancreatic secretions. Causes reflux of duodenal contents.
- Stress
- Reflux of gastric contents
- Delayed gastric emptying
- H pylori infection—causes local inflammation in antral mucosa and disrupts the barrier.

Factors which Increase Secretion

- Genetic factors—increased parietal cell mass, increased postprandial gastrin response.
- Psychosomatic factors—anxiety increases secretion.
- Food—alcohol, tea, coffee, spicy food.
- Rapid gastric emptying.
- Zollinger-Ellison syndrome—It is a gastrin secreting tumor of pancreas.

Symptoms of Peptic Ulcer

- The most common symptom is upper abdominal pain especially in empty stomach and is relieved after food intake.
- If the ulcer becomes erosive there will be features of hematemesis or melena (dark colored stools).
- If there is perforation of ulcer it can lead to peritonitis.

Physiological basis of Treatment of Peptic Ulcer

- Antacids can be used and they coat the mucosal layer.
- H_2 receptor blockers like ranitidine, cimetidine, and famotidine are used to block the actions of histamine. Histamine is a potent stimulator of parietal cells for HCl secretion.
- Proton-pump blockers like omeprazole, pantoprazole, and rabeprazole are the various generations. They block the H^+-K^+ pump and thereby decrease HCl secretion.
- Sucralfate, forms a coating over the ulcer and prevents further erosion.
- Atropine antagonists are used to inhibit its action on the muscarinic receptors.
- Proglumide a gastrin inhibitor blocks the actions of gastrin.
- In *H. pylori* infections antibiotics can be used.
- NSAID-induced ulcers can be treated by stopping the usage of NSAIDs and administering prostaglandin antagonists like misoprostol.
- Gastrinomas can be removed surgically.
- Vagotomy—truncal, selective or highly selective vagotomy can be done to decrease secretion from the parietal cells.

6. Functions of plasma proteins.

Albumin, globulin, and fibrinogen are the plasma proteins.

Functions

- Fibrinogen helps in blood coagulation.
- Albumin helps in maintaining colloidal oncotic pressure which is around 25–30 mm Hg. Oncotic pressure is related inversely to molecular shape, size and directly proportional to concentration of molecules. Therefore 80% of oncotic pressure is contributed by albumin.
- Maintains acid-base balance in blood. Plasma proteins act as buffers and they are amphoteric in nature. Therefore, they buffer both acids and base and maintain pH at 7.4.
- Maintains the viscosity of blood. Since 80% of the total plasma proteins is contributed by albumin they regulate the viscosity of blood.
- Diastolic blood pressure is regulated by peripheral resistance which in turn is regulated by viscosity of blood and therefore plasma proteins regulate BP.
- Immunoglobulins provide immunity
- Transport function - plasma proteins combine with the following substances and transport them - hormones, drugs, metals, bilirubin, etc.

7. Various stages of nerve action potential.

- Resting membrane potential of a neuron is -70 mV.
- On excitation of a neuron the change in RMP can be of two types—graded potential and action potential.

- Action potentials are brief, rapid and large changes in the membrane potential (100 mV) following a threshold stimulus, conducted for a long distance along the axon in an all or none fashion with the same shape and amplitude.
- It takes the membrane potential from –70 mV to +35 mV.
- They occur in a small patch of membrane.
- In a motor neuron it originates in the "initial segment".
- They are due to opening up of voltage-gated Na⁺ and voltage-gated K⁺ channels.

Phases of Action Potential

- When a stimulus is given there is deflection in the baseline which is due to leakage of current from stimulating electrodes—stimulus artifact.
- **Latent period:** Following the stimulus artifact, there is an iso-potential line, the latent period just before the AP.
- It is due to the time taken for the impulse to travel from the stimulating to the recording electrode. Its duration is proportionate to the distance between stimulating and recording electrode. It also depends on the type of nerve.
- **Phase of depolarization:** Following latent period there is phase of slow depolarization (local response) due to slow opening of Na⁺ channels. On reaching –55 mV, the firing level, there is a phase of rapid depolarization (*refer* **Fig. 13**).
- This is due to the rapid opening of voltage-gated Na⁺ channels. There is rapid inrush of Na⁺ ions (5000 fold increase) taking the membrane potential to +35 mV. On reaching this potential there is inactivation of sodium channels within a fraction of millisecond.
- **Phase of repolarization:** On reaching a potential of +35 mV, the potential reverses and starts falling rapidly to resting level. On completion of 70% repolarization, there is decrease in rate of repolarization, it is said to be after-depolarization.
- The repolarization is due to inactivation of voltage-gated Na⁺ channels and opening of voltage-gated K⁺ channels and the third reason for repolarization is on reaching +35 mV, there is reversal of electrical gradient for Na⁺ movement and so no more sodium influx happens.
- **After-hyperpolarization:** On reaching the RMP, the membrane potential hyperpolarizes beyond RMP for a short period. It is called as after-hyperpolarization. It is due to closure of K⁺ channels after a millisecond delay.
- **RMP:** The membrane potential comes back to –90 mV due to the action of sodium-potassium pump.

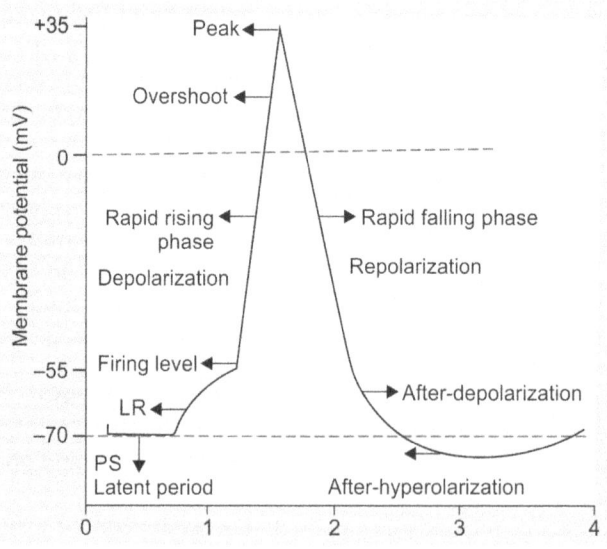

Fig. 13: Nerve action potential.
(LR: local response; PS: point of stimulation)

8. Functions of stomach.

- **Storage function:** It temporarily stores large volume of food and therefore serves as a reservoir of food.
- Secretes gastric juice. It contains:
  - *HCl:* Secreted from parietal cells, protects against microbes ingested with food, maintains low pH which is essential for activation of pepsinogen to pepsin and converts iron from ferric to ferrous form which is essential for its absorption.
  - *Intrinsic factor:* Secreted by parietal cells, essential for absorption of Vitamin B_{12}. Absence of IF results in pernicious anemia.
  - *Pepsinogen,* secreted by chief cells, gets converted to pepsin and helps in initial digestion of proteins.
  - *Mucus* secreted from gastric glands help in lubrication of food and also protects stomach mucosa from its digestion by HCl.
  - *Bicarbonate* secreted by neck cells maintains optimum pH in mucosa.
- Gastric motility (retropulsion) helps in mixing and grinding of food particles into smaller molecules.
- Gastric emptying is a controlled process which allows chyme to enter the duodenum in very small quantities thereby prevents damage of duodenal mucosa and gradual digestion and absorption of chyme.

9. Conn's syndrome.

- Hyperaldosteronism can be primary or secondary.
- **Primary hyperaldosteronism is Conn's syndrome.**
- The cause of excess secretion of aldosterone could be due to an adenoma in the adrenal cortex, adrenal hyperplasia or carcinoma of adrenal gland.
- Conn's syndrome is due to a tumor in the adrenal cortex, in the zona glomerulosa layer.
- Actions of aldosterone are Na^+ reabsorption in the kidneys along with Cl^- and water reabsorption and K^+ and H^+ secretion in exchange for Na^+ reabsorption.
- So in hyperaldosteronism the symptoms are due to Na^+ retention and K^+ and H^+ depletion.
- Patient presents with hypertension, which is due to salt and water retention without edema.
- Hypokalemia leads to muscle weakness.
- Loss of H^+ leads to alkalosis.
- Tetany can be present due to alkalosis induced hypocalcemia.
- They also present with polyuria due to impairment of concentrating ability of kidneys.
- Due to salt and water retention and increase in ECF volume, renin levels are low.
- Edema is absent in spite of water retention due to aldosterone escape phenomenon.

10. Heat production in skeletal muscles.

- During muscle contraction energy output in a muscle is in the form of work done, for generation of heat and for building up of ATP stores.
- The overall mechanical efficiency of muscle during lifting a weight is around 50% (Isotonic contraction) and is 0% in isometric contraction as there is no work done.
- The heat generated can be measured by thermocouples.
- **Heat generated in the muscles are as follows:**
  - *Resting heat,* is the heat generated by the muscle at rest and is a manifestation of basal metabolism.
  - Initial heat is the heat generated in excess of the resting heat. It consists of *activation heat,* which is generated when the muscle is contracting and *shortening heat* is proportional to the shortening distance of the muscle. It is due to change in structure of muscle during its shortening.
  - *Recovery heat* is the heat liberated by the metabolic process in which the muscle returns to the precontraction state. Recovery heat is equal to the initial heat, i.e., the heat produced during recovery is equal to heat produced during contraction.

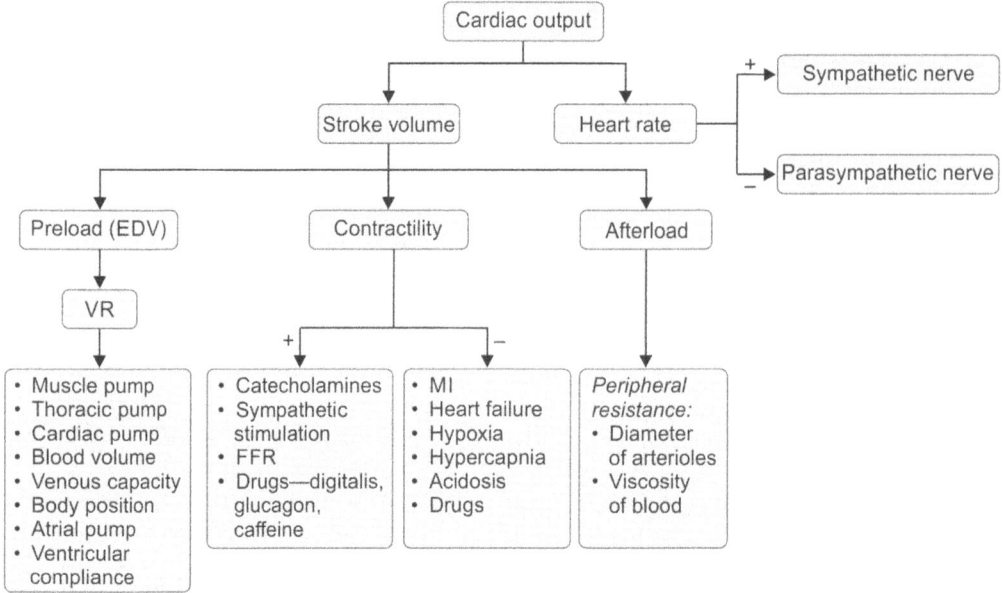

Fig. 14: Regulation of cardiac output.
(FFR: force-frequency relation; MI: myocardial infarction)

11. Factors affecting cardiac output.

Cardiac output (CO) is defined as the amount of blood ejected by each ventricle per minute.
- CO = Stroke volume (SV) × Heart rate (HR) (*refer* **Fig. 14**)
- NV = 70 mL/beat × 70/min = 4900 mL/ min.

Determinants of Cardiac Output
- CO = Stroke volume (SV) × Heart rate (HR)
- So factors affecting either of them will alter CO (*refer* **Fig. 6**).

Factors Affecting SV
- Preload
- Afterload
- Contractility

Factors Affecting HR
HR is affected by nerves supplying heart (sympathetic and parasympathetic nerves) and cardiac centers.

Preload
- The initial muscle length is the **preload** (the extent to which the muscle is stretched before contraction).
- Preload is decided by the **end-diastolic volume (EDV)**.
- EDV is decided by the **venous return (VR)**.

Preload affecting stroke volume is based on the Frank-Starling's law: It states that within physiological limits, the force of contraction is directly proportional to the initial length of the muscle.

Causes for application of Frank-Starling's law:
- Increase in EDV →↑ stretch of muscle fiber → interaction of thick and thin filament increases →↑ force of contraction.
- Stretch of muscle fibers → opens stretch sensitive Ca^{2+} channels on sarcolemma →↑ Ca^{2+} influx →↑ force of contraction.
- ↑Ca^{2+} influx →↑ Ca^{2+} release from SR (CICR) →↑ force of contraction.
- ↑ Stretch of muscle fiber →↑ affinity of troponin for Ca^{2+}.

EDV is Dependent on
- **Venous return, which is dependent on:**
  - *Skeletal muscle pump:* Contraction of limb muscles press on the veins and increases forward movement of blood in the veins.
  - *Thoracic pump:* Increase in respiration depresses the diaphragm and decreases

intrathoracic pressure and thereby it acts like a suction force to increase VR.
- *Abdominal pump:* During respiration compression of abdominal muscles press on the veins and favors venous emptying.
- *Cardiac pump:* Vis A Tergo (force from behind), Vis A Fronte (force from front).
- *Total blood volume:* As the blood volume increases VR increases and vice versa.
- *Capacity of venous system:* Sympathetic stimulation to the veins causes venoconstriction and thereby increases venous emptying.
- *Body position:* On standing there is venous pooling due to gravity and it may decrease the VR.

❏ **Atrial pump activity:** Contributes 20% ventricular filling and stimulated by sympathetic stimulation.

❏ **Ventricular compliance:** Affected by damage to myocardium as in MI, pericardial effusion, cardiac tamponade.

This type of regulation of stroke volume in relation to change in initial length of muscle fiber is said to be **heterometric regulation**.

Contractility

Contractility is increase in force of contraction and thereby increase in stroke volume without increase in initial muscle length.

❏ Ventricles are able to do more work per stroke at a given EDV.
❏ Factors which affect contractility—inotropic agents.
❏ There are positive and negative inotropic agents.

Contractility is increased by:
❏ Autonomic activity (sympathetics are positively inotropic).
❏ **Muscle mass:** Increase in myocardial mass increases contractility as after regular exercise.
❏ Concentration of hormones and chemicals.
❏ **Heart rate:** Force frequency relationship.

Factors increasing contractility, positive inotropic agents:
❏ Sympathetic stimulation
❏ Circulating catecholamines

❏ Force frequency relationship
❏ Digitalis
❏ Glucagon
❏ Insulin
❏ Thyroxine
❏ Chemicals like xanthine, theophylline.

Factors decreasing contractility, negative inotropic agents:
❏ Loss of myocardium as in myocardial infarction
❏ Hypoxia
❏ Hypercapnia
❏ Acidosis
❏ Acetylcholine

Regulation of stroke volume by affecting contractility of myocardium is **homometric regulation**. Here the force of contraction is affected without much change in muscle length.

Afterload

❏ It is the force against which the heart muscle shortens
❏ Cardiac output is inversely proportional to afterload.
❏ Cardiac output $\propto$ 1/afterload (**Anrep effect**)
❏ It is decided by peripheral resistance.
❏ **Peripheral resistance is decided by:**
  - Vessel diameter
  - Viscosity of blood
❏ This is also included in **homometric regulation**.

Regulation of Heart Rate

❏ Heart rate is also a factor affecting CO.
❏ HR is in turn regulated by autonomic nerves.
❏ Sympathetics →↑heart rate
❏ Parasympathetics →↓ HR
❏ Normally ↑ HR →↑ CO
❏ But in severe tachycardia →↓ duration of diastole →↓ ventricular filling →↓ CO.

---

12. Pacemaker potential.

❏ In the mammalian heart, sino-atrial node is the pacemaker. It is said to be the pacemaker as it generates impulses by itself without neural input at a faster rate.

- Other tissues of the heart—AV node, atria and ventricle are also capable of generating impulses but SA node generates impulses at a faster rate and therefore said to be the pacemaker of the heart.

Pacemaker Potential

- The ventricular and atrial muscle cells have a resting membrane potential of -90 mV. On stimulation the membrane depolarizes and produces an action potential.
- The pacemaker cells are smaller and rounded (P cells) and they do not have a stable resting membrane potential and RMP is around -55 to -60 mV.
- From -60 mV there is a slow depolarization slope which reaches the firing level of -40 mV and there is a rapid depolarization followed by rapid repolarization back to -60 mV and again there is a slow depolarization slope rising to firing level.
- This slope which takes the membrane to firing level is the **pacemaker potential or prepotential** (*refer* **Fig. 15**).

Ionic Events Responsible for Pacemaker Potential

- At -60 mV the K^+ channels start closing down thereby preventing K^+ efflux. This is responsible for the first part of prepotential (the slope).
- Next part is due to opening up of 'f' type Na^+ channels (The Na^+ current in this channel is said to be funny current as the channel opens in hyperpolarization).
- Last part of depolarization of the prepotential is due to opening of T-type (transient) Ca^{2+} channels allowing Ca^{2+} influx.
- Now as the firing level is reached (-40 mV), the long lasting Ca^{2+} channels (L Type) open and produces a rapid depolarization and the action potential.
- Then the K^+ channels open and the K^+ efflux bring about rapid repolarization and membrane potential reaches -60 mV. Then the next prepotential starts.
- So in the pacemaker cells, it is a Ca^{2+} dependent depolarization rather than Na^+ dependent depolarization as in ventricular muscles.
- The pacemaker cells are supplied by sympathetic and parasympathetic nerves.
- On stimulation by sympathetic nerves the prepotential slope becomes steeper and the rate of spontaneous discharge increases thereby increasing the heart rate.
- On stimulation by the parasympathetic nerves the slope of the prepotential decreases and spontaneous firing also decreases thereby heart rate decreases.

13. ECG –Lead II.

- Lead II is a bipolar limb lead between right arm (negative electrode) and left arm (positive electrode).

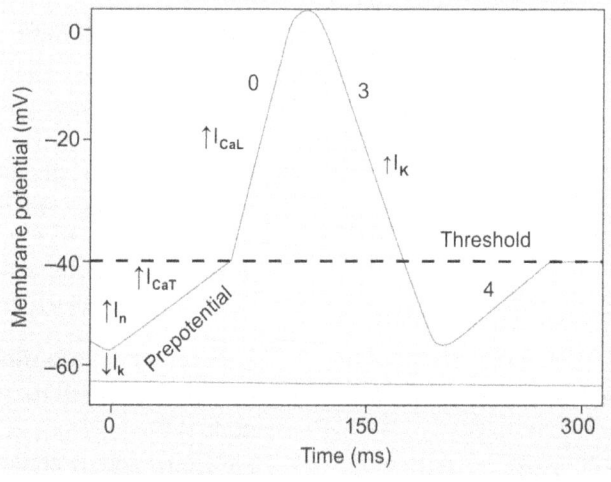

Fig. 15: Pacemaker potential.

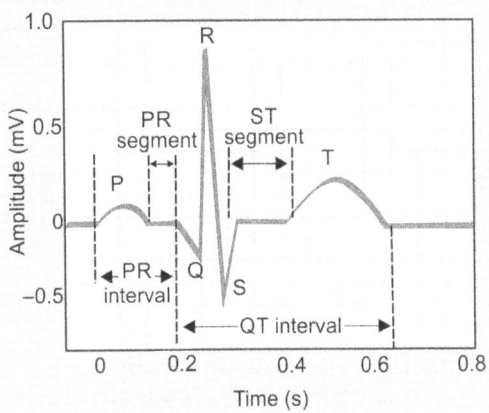

Fig. 16: Normal ECG in lead II.

- The ECG tracing in Lead II shows both negative and positive deflections equally and therefore used as a standard recording (*refer* **Fig. 16**).
- There are intervals and segments in the ECG.

ECG Waves

- There are positive and negative waves are deflections in the ECG tracing.
- There are four waveforms—P wave, QRS complex, T wave, and U wave.
  a. *P wave:* This is the first positive wave in ECG and is due to atrial depolarization. Duration is 0.1 second.
  b. *QRS complex:* Consists of a negative Q wave, positive R wave, and negative S wave. This complex is due to ventricular depolarization. Normal duration is 0.08 seconds.
  c. *T wave* is a positive deflection following QRS complex and is due to ventricular repolarization. Normal duration is 0.27 seconds.
  d. *U wave* is also positive deflection and is normally not seen. It is seen in slow depolarization of the papillary muscle. Duration is 0.08 seconds.

ECG Segments

- These are isoelectric lines seen in between the ECG waves.
- There are two segments—PR segment and ST segment:
  a. *PR segment:* It starts at the end of P wave to beginning of QRS complex.
  b. *ST segment:* It begins in the end of QRS complex and is up to the beginning of T wave.

ECG Intervals

- Intervals in ECG include waves and segments.
- The intervals are—PR interval, QT interval, ST interval, PP interval, and RR interval.
- **J point:** This is an indicator of end of ventricular depolarization and start of ventricular repolarization. It is at the end of QRS and is at the isoelectric line.
  - *PR interval:* It is between beginning of P wave to beginning of Q wave.
    - The normal duration is 0.12–0.2 seconds (average 0.18 seconds).
    - This denotes atrial depolarization and conduction to AV node.
    - Prolonged PR interval signifies AV conduction block.
  - *QT interval:* It starts at Q wave and ends with T wave.
    - Normal duration is 0.4 seconds.
    - It denotes the systolic phase of the ventricle.
    - It is prolonged in ventricular conduction defects, hypocalcemia, and myocardial ischemia.
  - *ST interval:* It is from the end of S wave to the end of T wave.
    - Normal duration is 0.32 seconds.
    - It denotes ventricular repolarization.
  - *PP interval:* It is the interval between two successive P waves.
    - It denotes the diastolic phase of the atria.
  - *RR interval:* It is the interval between two successive R waves.
    - It is used to calculate the heart rate.

14. Auditory pathway.

The action potentials generated in the cochlear division of VIII cranial nerve travels in the following path as the auditory pathway (*refer* **Fig. 17**).

Organ of Corti
↓
Bipolar cells of spiral ganglion
↓
Cochlear nuclei (dorsal and ventral) in brainstem
↓
Superior olivary nuclei of both sides
↓
Lateral lemniscus (both sides)
↓
Inferior colliculus (both sides)
↓
Medial geniculate body in thalamus (both sides)
↓
Primary auditory cortex (area 41) (both sides)
↓
Auditory association areas (areas 42, 22) (both sides)

15. Functions of cerebellum.

Vestibulocerebellum

Connections

- **Afferents:** Receive input from vestibular nuclei and primary vestibular apparatus.
- **Efferents:** Projects to the vestibular nucleus → vestibulospinal tract and medial longitudinal fasciculus → motor neurons of anterior horn.

Functions

- Fixing the body during skilled movements.
- Maintains the equilibrium of body.
- Controls ocular movement.
- Modulates the muscle tone.

Spinocerebellum

This part receives afferents from:

- The spinal cord, about position of limbs, and degrees of muscle contraction.
- Visual, auditory and vestibular apparatus, sensory cortex.

Functions

- **Primary motor cortex:** Gives information about the intended movements.
- With all these information the cerebellum **constantly compares** the intended movements and the actual movement of the muscles.
- Correction of purposeful movements—**comparator-servo action**—constantly

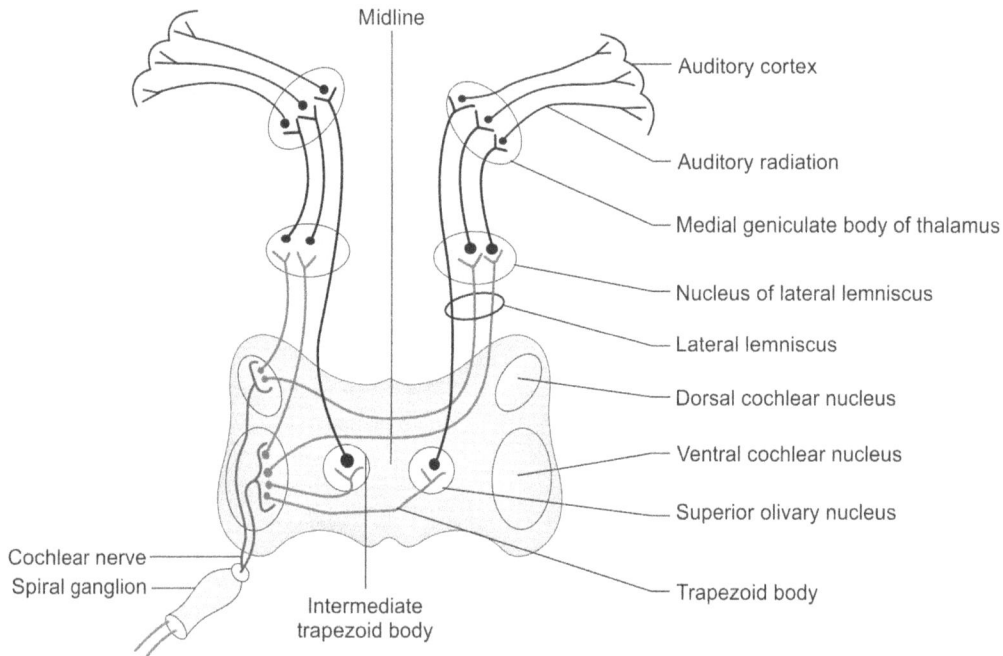

Fig. 17: Auditory pathway from right cochlea. There is bilateral route through brainstem and bilateral cortical representation.

compares the intended and executed movements.
- Thereby detects the errors and makes **continuous corrections.**
- This makes **movements smooth**.
- Also it helps in making **movements accurate.**
- All these are done by sending efferents to motor cortex, red nucleus, reticular formation.
- Controls synergistic activity of agonists and antagonists—smooth activity.
- Helps in skilled movements.
- Learning of motor skills.

Cerebrocerebellum

Connections
- **It receives afferents from:** Sensory cortex, primary motor cortex, premotor cortexz and posterior parietal cortex.
- **It sends efferents to:** Thalamus, premotor cortex, and primary motor cortex.

Functions
- Planning and programing of voluntary movements.
- Learning of special motor skills.
- Cognitive function.

16. Nonrespiratory functions of the lung.

Nonrespiratory Functions
- **Acts as a reservoir for blood:** The pulmonary vessels are highly compliant and therefore can store blood without much increase in pressure. In cases of imbalance in left ventricular output and systemic venous return, the stored blood in the pulmonary circulation helps to regulate cardiac output
- **Filters** small emboli, particles in blood, detached cancer cells, fat cells, air emboli in blood.
- **Processes inhaled air:** The atmospheric air, which enters the airways are hydrated as it passes through the airways.
- **Olfactory function**
- **Metabolic function:**
  - Synthesizes and secretes surfactant
  - Pulmonary capillary endothelial cells secrete angiotensin-converting enzyme (ACE) and thereby converts angiotensin I to angiotensin II.
  - Synthesizes, stores and secretes substances like prostaglandins, histamine and kallikrein.
  - Partially removes prostaglandin, bradykinin, adenine nucleotides, serotonin, norepinephrine and acetylcholine.
- **Helps in defense:** With the help of pulmonary alveolar macrophages, IgA, mucus secretion, beating of cilia, cough reflex.
- **Helps in speech**
- **Helps in absorption** of drugs like anesthetic gases, aerosols and bronchodilators.
- **Fibrinolytic mechanism** present in the lungs lyses the clot.

17. Oxyhemoglobin dissociation curve.

- Oxygen is transported in blood in two forms—as dissolved O_2 and in combination with hemoglobin as oxyhemoglobin.
- This curve compares the partial pressure of O_2 and % saturation of Hb with O_2.
- It is sigmoid in shape (*refer* **Fig. 18**).
- The shape is sigmoid because of the change in configuration of hemoglobin from T to R state and therefore there is gradual increase in affinity for O_2 and then it gets saturated.
- It has a steep and plateau phase.
- 90% saturation of Hb takes place at a PO_2 of 60 mm Hg.
- P_{50} is the partial pressure at which 50% of the hemoglobin is saturated with oxygen.
- P_{50} is inversely related to the affinity of hemoglobin for oxygen.
- The steep phase denotes the unloading zone where even a minimum drop in PO_2 results in unloading of large amounts of oxygen to the tissues.
- The plateau phase denotes the loading zone, where O_2 is taken up by hemoglobin in the lungs and once all the four sites in Hb are loaded with O_2 there is no further uptake and thereby a plateau phase is reached.
- The curve gets shifted to right are left in conditions of decreased or increase in affinity of hemoglobin for O_2 respectively (*refer* **Fig. 19**).

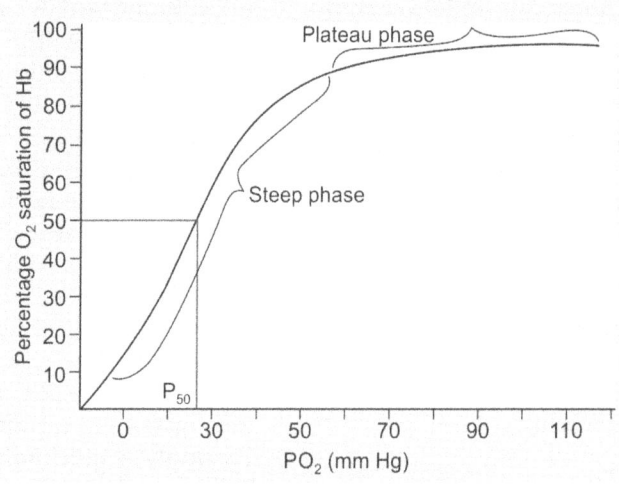

Fig. 18: Oxygen-hemoglobin dissociation curve.

Conditions where O_2-Hb dissociation curve is shifted to right:
- Hypoxia
- ↑PCO_2
- ↑temperature
- ↑2,3-DPG levels in RBC
- ↑H^+ concentration (acidosis)

Conditions where O_2-Hb dissociation curve is shifted to left:
- High PO_2
- Low PCO_2
- Low body temperature
- Presence of fetal hemoglobin
- Alkalosis (*refer* **Fig. 4**)
- Low 2,3-DPG levels in RBC
- Carbon monoxide poisoning.

18. Heart sounds.

- Heart sounds are heard over the precordium.
- There are four heart sounds heard—S1, S2, S3, and S4
- The causes, features and significance of the four heart sounds are mentioned in the **Figure 3**.
- Heart sounds can be recorded by phonocardiogram.

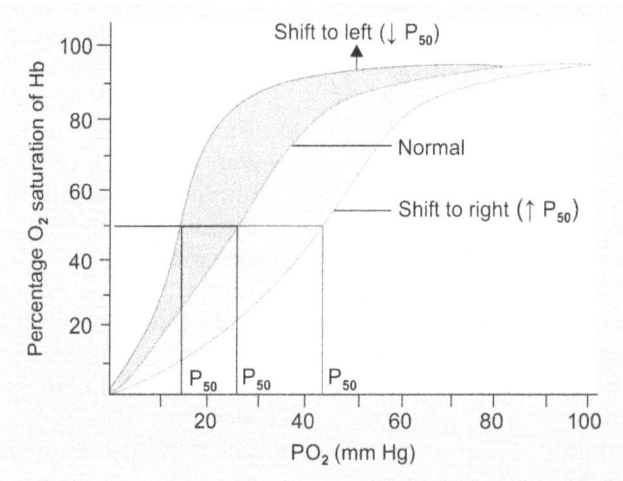

Fig. 19: Right and left shift of O_2-Hb dissociation curve. P_{50}, PO_2 at which hemoglobin is 50% saturated is 27 mm Hg.

Heart sounds	Events responsible	Duration	Frequency	Others
First sound (S_1)	Due to vibrations set by sudden closure of AV valves at the onset of ventricular systole	0.15 sec	25–45 Hz In PCG recorded as 9–13 waves	Soft and long, heard as "LUBB"
Second sound (S_2)	Associated with closure of aortic and pulmonary valves after the end of ventricular systole	0.12 sec	50 Hz In PCG recorded as 4–6 waves	Normally S2 can be split due to early closure of aortic valve, heard as "Dup"
Third sound (S_3)	Is heard at 1/3rd of diastole due to rapid filling of ventricle due to vibrations set by inrush of blood		0.1 sec In PCG recorded as 1–4 waves	Normally audible only in children and young adults
Fourth sound (S_4)	Heard just before (S_1) Occurs during atrial contraction Due to ventricular filling		20 cyc/sec In PCG recorded as 1–2 waves	Rarely heard in normal adults Heard in vent hypertrophy and CCF

Fig. 20: Heart sounds; their causes and characteristics.
(CCF: congestive cardiac failure; PCG: phonocardiogram)

Significance of Heart Sounds

- **1st sound:** Increased in exercise, hyperkinetic states like anemia and decreased in shock, MI, pericardial effusion.
- **2nd sound:** Loud in hypertension, low in aortic and pulmonary stenosis. Splitting is common.
- **3rd sound:** Increased in MR. Important sign of heart failure.
- **4th sound:** Always seen in abnormal conditions. Seen in left ventricular hypertrophy (*refer* **Fig. 20**).

19. Functions of basal ganglia.

- Basal ganglia is involved in planning and programing of voluntary movement. The neurons of basal ganglia fire impulses even before the movements starts. Caudate loop is involved in planning of movements (direct pathway through caudate nucleus).
- Controls muscle tone through inhibition of motor cortex and inhibitory medullary RF. The pathway involved is cortex – striatum – GP – SN– medullary RF – spinal cord via reticulospinal tract. In lesion of BG there is hypertonia.
- Controls the limb movements. In diseases of BG unpurposeful limb movements appear.
- Controls automated associative limb movements like swinging of arms while walking. Putamen circuit (direct pathway through putamen nucleus) is involved in control of subconscious movements.
- Timing the movements is also a role of BG.
- BG exerts an inhibitory effect on spinal reflexes which help to regulate posture.
- Somatic movements associated with emotions are controlled by BG.
- Provides muscle tone for skilled movements.
- Functions in motivated behavior.
- Caudate nucleus plays a role in cognition because of its connections with associative cortex. Lesion leads to deficits of performance-based learning.
- Because of its connections with RF, GP has a role in arousal mechanism.
- Lesion of head of left caudate nucleus leads to dysarthric aphasia.

20. Four properties of synapse.

Properties of Synapse

- Summation—spatial or temporal
- Convergence and divergence
- One way conduction of impulses
- Synaptic delay
- Facilitation
- Subliminal fringe

- Occlusion
- Synaptic plasticity and learning
- Synaptic fatigue.

Summation
- Summation means adding up of impulses. In the synapse following release of neurotransmitters there could be depolarization or hyperpolarization of the membrane. These are called as postsynaptic potentials and they belong to the category of graded potentials.
- So, these individual potentials from many synapses can summate and excite the membrane and take it to the firing level.
- There are two types of summations—spatial and temporal summation.
    - *Temporal summation:* The same input stimulates the postsynaptic neuron repeatedly and thereby excites it.
    - *Spatial summation:* Here many inputs stimulate simultaneously to excite it.

Convergence and Divergence
When many presynaptic neurons end one postsynaptic neuron it is convergence and on presynaptic terminal divides and ends on many postsynaptic neurons divergence.

One Way Conduction
Impulse transmission always happens from presynaptic to postsynaptic neurons as the receptors for the neurotransmitter released from presynaptic terminal is present on the postsynaptic membrane.

Synaptic Delay
There are many steps involved in the impulse transmission from the presynaptic neuron to postsynaptic neuron so there is a delay of 0.5 msec in each synapse.

III. SHORT ANSWERS

1. Refractory period.

- **Refractory period:** There is a time period during AP, if a second stimulus is given, the stimulated part of the membrane is not excited again. It is said to be the membrane is in a refractory period. The refractory period is divided into absolute refractory period and relative refractory period.
- **Absolute refractory period (ARP)** is the time period during an AP, application of a second stimulus of how ever strong or for any duration does not excite a nerve. It happens from the firing level to 1/3rd completion of repolarization. It is because of the state of the gates of voltage-gated Na^+ channels.
- **Voltage-gated sodium channels:**
    - These channels have two gates, inactivation gate (along the exterior of the membrane) and the activation gate (along the interior of the membrane).

    At **resting state**, the inactivation gates are open and activation gates are closed. During an AP, on reaching the firing level, the activation gates also open and the rapid inrush of Na^+ produces the spike potential (**activated state**). On reaching +35 mV, the inactivation gates close rapidly and the Na^+ influx comes to a halt (**inactivated state of the channel**). This starts the repolarization phase.

    These voltage-gated channels reach their resting state when the RMP is reached (-90 mV). Only on reaching the resting state, the channels can be reactivated. So, during ARP the channels are in the inactivated state, so they are refractory to the second stimulus.
- **Relative refractory period (RRP)** is the period after ARP when the membrane can be excited by a suprathreshold stimulus. This phase is from the end of ARP to after-depolarization.
  During this phase some of the channels would have reached the resting state, some may be still in inactivated state. When a suprathreshold stimulus is given, it spreads to larger area of membrane and it can activate the channels which have reached the resting state.

2. Enteric nervous system.

- GIT is innervated by autonomic nerves and the enteric nervous system.

- Sympathetic nerves arise from prevertebral and paravertebral ganglia. It is usually inhibitory to GIT and inhibits motor activity and secretions.
- Parasympathetic supply is by the vagus nerve and is stimulatory to the GIT. It increases motility and secretions. But PS nerves inhibit the sphincters and thereby relax it and favors emptying.

Enteric Nervous System

- This is the intrinsic nervous system of the GIT; it includes neurons and nerve fibers.
- There are two plexuses—submucosal or meissner's plexus and myenteric or auerbach's plexus. Meissner's plexus regulates secretory functions of GIT and myenteric plexus regulates motility of GIT (*refer* **Fig. 21**).
- Submucosal plexus lies between submucosal and circular muscle layer and myenteric plexus is between circular and longitudinal muscle layers of the wall of GIT.
- They are connected with the extrinsic nerves and function as interneurons.
- These neurons can regulate GI motility and their actions can be modified by the extrinsic nerves.
- The sympathetic and parasympathetic nerves project to both the plexuses.
- The vagus nerve which is cholinergic terminates on intrinsic nerve plexuses and stimulates secretion and motility.
- Sympathetic nerves which are noradrenergic they terminate on the intrinsic neurons and thereby inhibits secretions and motility.

3. Name four GI hormones.

Gastrin, secretin, somatostatin, and cholecystokinin.

4. Cretinism.

Hypothyroid children from birth or from in utero are called cretins and the disease is said to be cretinism.

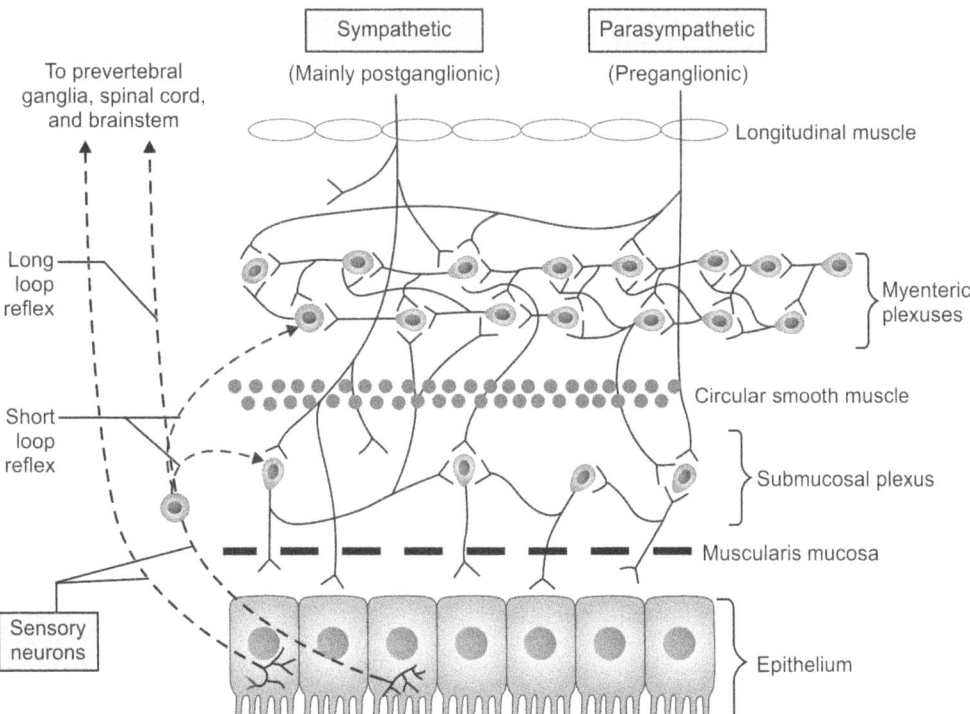

Fig. 21: Enteric nervous system; submucosal plexus is present between mucosa and circular muscle layers. Myenteric plexus is present between circular and longitudinal layers.

The main causes for cretinism are:
- Maternal iodine deficiency
- Fetal thyroid dysgenesis
- Inborn error of thyroid hormone synthesis
- Maternal antithyroid antibodies that cross the placenta and damage fetal thyroid
- Fetal hypopituitary hypothyroidism.

If the mother's thyroid status is normal, mother's T4 can cross the placenta and thereby the fetal growth and development are normal till birth.

The child with cretinism has the following symptoms:
- Stunted growth
- Mental retardation
- Potbelly
- Enlarged and protruding tongue
- Hoarse cry
- Poor feeding
- Umbilical hernia
- Retarded bone age
- Deaf mutism and rigidity
- Respiratory distress syndrome.

Prevention of Cretinism
- Worldwide congenital hypothyroidism is the most common cause of preventable mental retardation.
- So, if the thyroid screening is done immediately after birth and thyroid hormone replacement is done early the prognosis for normal growth and development is good and mental retardation can be prevented.
- If the mother is hypothyroid as in iodine deficiency the mental development is further affected and response to treatment is less after birth.
- This can be prevented by using iodized salts by the mothers.

5. Diuretics

Diuretics are chemicals which increase excretion of Na^+ and water and thereby increase urine output.

Site of Action of Diuretics

Drugs Acting in PCT
- **Carbonic anhydrase** inhibitors like acetazolamide, they inhibit carbonic anhydrase and thereby increases Na^+ excretion, decreases H^+ secretion and bicarbonate reabsorption. Since H^+ and K^+ compete with each other (for secretion) along with reabsorption of Na^+, there is increased K^+ secretion and excretion and therefore K^+ depletion occurs.
- **Osmotic diuretics** like mannitol and isosorbide. They are not reabsorbed in PCT and therefore are retained in the tubule along with water. This in turn alters the gradient for Na^+ reabsorption and therefore it inhibits Na^+ reabsorption.

Diuretics Acting on Loop of Henle
Loop diuretics like furosemide, bumetanide, and ethacrynic acid—they act by inhibiting Na^+-K^+-$2Cl^-$ transporter. They increase NaCl and K^+ excretion. K^+ depletion occurs while treating with these drugs.

Diuretics Acting on DCT
Thiazides: They act by inhibiting NaCl symport in DCT. They increase excretion of NaCl and K^+.

Diuretics Acting on Late DCT and Collecting Duct:
K^+ sparing diuretics like spironolactone, triamterene and amiloride act in late DCT and CD by inhibiting actions of aldosterone or ENacs. They increase excretion of Na^+ and retain K^+ and H^+.

6. Functions of placenta.

- Synthesis of hormones (endocrine function of placenta).
- Transport of substances across the placenta between the mother and fetus.
- Protection of fetus.

Hormones Synthesized by Placenta
- Human chorionic gonadotropin (hCG)
- Human chorionic somatomammotropin (hCS)
- Placental progesterone
- Placental estrogen
- Relaxin.

Human Chorionic Gonadotropin (hCG)
- It is synthesized by syncytiotrophoblast of placenta.

- It is a glycoprotein with α and β subunits.
- It starts appearing in the blood of the mother by 6 days after fertilization and reaches a peak by 10–12 weeks.
- Clinically, presence of hCG in urine of a female is "the indicator" of pregnancy.
- It stimulates the corpus luteum to secrete progesterone till the placenta is fully formed.
- hCG helps in sexual differentiation of male fetus.
- It induces hyperemesis in the first trimester.

Human Chorionic Somatomammotropin (hCS)

- It is also secreted from the syncytiotrophoblast of placenta.
- Its secretion starts by 5th week of pregnancy and reaches a peak towards term.
- It is similar to growth hormone and has growth promoting actions, so called as "Maternal growth hormone of pregnancy".
- It stimulates lipolysis, N, K$^+$ and Ca^{2+} retention and decreases glucose utilization by the mother so that the substrates are diverted to the fetus.
- Amount of hCS secreted is equal to size of placenta and therefore level of hCS indicates placental viability.

Placental Progesterone

- In the early weeks of pregnancy, progesterone is produced by corpus luteum and later the function is taken over by placenta.
- It is produced by co-ordination between the mother and the fetus—the **fetoplacental unit**.
- It makes the endometrium secretory and thereby nourishes the fertilized ovum.
- It keeps the myometrium of the pregnant uterus quiescent which is essential for the survival of the fetus.
- It acts on the alveolar system of the maternal breast and facilitates development of maternal breast.
- It has an immuno-suppressive role in protecting the fetus.

Placental Estrogen

- The major estrogen in pregnancy is estriol.
- It stimulates development of the ductular system of the maternal breast.
- The levels of estrogen rises during pregnancy but on nearing term estrogen: progesterone ratio rises and estrogen makes the myometrium excitable.
- On decrease of levels of estrogen after delivery of fetus, prolactin stimulates milk secretion from the breast.

Relaxin

- Its level in the early pregnancy is high to relax the uterine wall to favor implantation of fetus.
- In later weeks it causes relaxation of pubic symphysis and pelvic ligaments to facilitate delivery of fetus.

Other hormones secreted are:
CRH, β endorphin, α-MSH, GnRH, inhibin, prolactin, etc.

Transport Functions of Placenta

- **Transport of nutrients:** Placenta transports nutrients from the mother to the fetus. The nutrients transported are glucose, fats, amino acids and Ca^{2+}, inorganic phosphates, K$^+$, Na$^+$.
- **Transports of waste products** from the fetus to the mother—substances transported are urea, uric acid, and creatinine.
- **Transport of gases:** Dissolved O$_2$ is transported from maternal side of placenta to the fetus along the pressure gradient. Fetus receives its O$_2$ from maternal venous sinuses and therefore is living in an hypoxic environment. But the fetal Hb with 2α and 2γ chains has higher affinity for O$_2$. CO$_2$ is also eliminated from fetal circulation into maternal blood by diffusion across the placenta.
- **Transport of antibodies:** Maternal antibodies are transferred to the fetus and are responsible for innate immunity.

Protection of Fetus

- It acts as a barrier for prevention of transport of toxic substances from the mother to fetus.
- Progesterone produced by placenta helps to maintain pregnancy.

7. LH surge.

- It is the rise in LH levels in plasma just before ovulation.
- From day one of the menstrual cycle the FSH and LH levels are increasing. This results in stimulation of the growth of a crop of follicles in the ovary.
- Except one follicle, the rest gets atrophied by 7–8 days.
- The dominant follicle secretes estrogen and the estrogen levels increases.
- Estrogen has a positive feedback effect on LH secretion in the first half of the menstrual cycle.
- Therefore, as estrogen levels rise, LH levels also rise.
- LH levels reach a peak 9 hours before ovulation—this is the LH surge.
- High LH level is necessary for the final maturation and rupture of graafian follicle.
- LH acts on the granulosa and theca cells and make them secrete progesterone.
- Now progesterone levels rise just before ovulation and estrogen levels decrease.
- All the above hormonal changes results in ovulation.
- So, without the LH surge ovulation does not happen.

8. Gallstones.

- Cholelithiasis is the presence of gallstones.
- There are two types of gallstones—calcium bilirubinate stones and cholesterol stones.
- 85% of the stones are cholesterol stones.
- Normally the cholesterol in bile is kept as micelles by bile salts and lecithin.
- If the cholesterol levels are high or the bile salts levels are low the balance is deranged resulting formation of gallstones.

Factors involved in the formation of Gallstones

- *Bile stasis*: Gallstones are formed in bile stored in the gallbladder rather than bile flowing in the ducts.
- Supersaturation of bile with cholesterol, as mentioned above.
- Presence of nucleation factors which favor formation of gallstones along with the supersaturated bile.

Symptoms

- When the gallstones are in gallbladder not much symptoms are present.
- On moving through the bile ducts if they block the ducts there will be severe colicky pain in the abdomen.
- Obstructive jaundice may also be a presenting feature.

Diagnosis

- Plain X-ray abdomen can detect the stones
- Ultrasound abdomen can be done
- CT abdomen
- Nuclear cholescintigraphy can be done.

Treatment

Cholecystectomy can be done to remove the gallbladder with stones.

9. Functions of platelets.

- **Role in primary hemostasis or temporary platelet plug formation:** Damage to the endothelial lining of the blood vessels exposes collagen which activates the platelets and results in adhesion and aggregation of platelets to the injured vessel and thereby seals the injured vessel. Platelets have receptors for collagen, ADP and VWF which favor adhesion of platelets.
- **Role in secondary hemostasis:** Formation of clot is said to be the secondary hemostasis. The platelets release platelet phospholipid and platelet factor II which activates prothrombin to thrombin.
- **Role in clot retraction:** Platelets have contractile proteins actin, myosin, and thrombosthenin. Once the platelets and other blood cells are trapped in the fibrin mesh, these contractile proteins contract and the clot shrinks. This squeezes out the serum from the clot. Clot retraction happens only in the presence of functional platelets and it helps in sealing the wound in the blood vessel.
- Platelets store and release serotonin (5HT) which is a potent vasoconstrictor.
- Platelets also stores and release platelet derived growth factor which multiplies endothelial cells and fibroblasts and thereby help in wound healing.

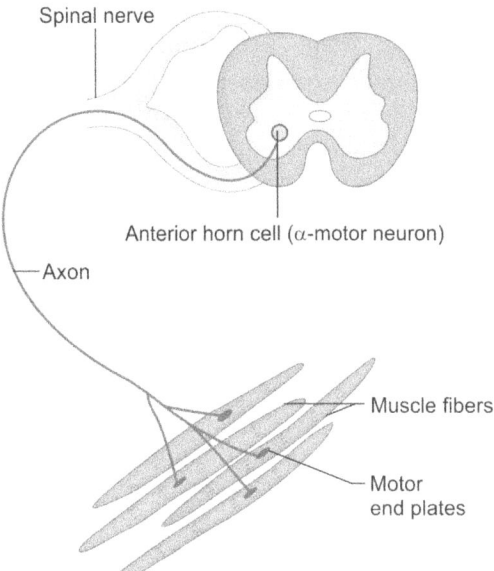

Fig 22: Motor unit.

- Platelets are also involved in mild phagocytosis. They ingest carbon particles, immune complexes and viral particles.

10. Motor unit.
- Motor unit is a single motor neuron with all its branches and all the muscle fibers supplied by it (*refer* **Fig. 22**).
- The size of the motor unit is decided by the muscle fibers supplied by it.
- The ones which supply the intrinsic muscles of the hand supply only less than 10 fibers and produce less tension but the ones which supply back muscles are large motor units and have hundreds of fibers.
- All the muscle fibers in a single motor unit are of the same type, i.e., either oxidative type or glycolytic type.
- Based on this, the motor units may be classified as either oxidative or slow and glycolytic or fast motor units.

11. Functions of neutrophils.
The major function of neutrophils is phagocytosis. The granules of neutrophils contain many chemicals which are antimicrobial and bactericidal in nature. They migrate to the site of infection and phagocytose the microbes and destroy them by the release of these granules. It is considered as the "First line of defense".

12. Endocytosis.
Vesicle-mediated Transport
- Large polar molecules—like protein hormones in endocrine glands are transported across the cell as membrane wrapped vesicles.
- Types—endocytosis, exocytosis.

Endocytosis
It is the process by which substances are internalized within the cell.
 The substance to be transported and a part of the membrane surrounding it are pinched off to form a vesicle and it is internalized.

It occurs by two mechanisms: Constitutive and clathrin-mediated.

Constitutive endocytosis: It is a simple process which does not need a special stimulus.

Clathrin-mediated endocytosis:
- This process takes place in the membrane where clathrin accumulates.
- Clathrin is a protein having the shape of a triskelion.
- The clathrin forms a geometric array and surrounds the endocytic vesicle.
- A protein called dynamin, GTPase protein pinches off the vesicle from its attachment. This protein is called as pinchase.
- Once the vesicle is internalized the clathrin falls off and is recycled to the membrane to form another vesicle.
- The vesicle then fuses with the lysosome to form an early endosome and releases its chemicals (proteases) and thereby degrades the internalized particle.
- Clathrin-mediated endocytosis is responsible for internalizing many receptors and ligands bound to them, like the nerve growth factor and its receptor and LDL.

There are three types of endocytosis:
1. Phagocytosis
2. Pinocytosis
3. Receptor mediated endocytosis
1. **Phagocytosis:** Engulfing of solid substances (cell eating) as that of microorganisms by the neutrophils.

2. **Pinocytosis:** Engulfing the liquid components (cell drinking).
3. **Receptor-mediated endocytosis:** Here the substances to be internalized get attached to a receptor protein present on the cell membrane and the whole complex is engulfed.

13. Free water clearance.

- It is a test done to quantitate the gain or loss of water by excreting the concentrated or dilute urine.
- The free water clearance (C_{H_2O}) is calculated by finding the difference between the volume of urine and the clearance of osmoles (C_{osm}).
- $C_{H_2O} = V - U_{osm}V/P_{osm}$
- V = Urine flow rate
- U_{osm} and P_{osm} = Urine and plasma osmolality
- Cosm is the amount of water necessary to excrete the osmotic load in a urine that is isotonic with plasma.
- Therefore, C_{H_2O} is negative when the urine is hypertonic and is positive when it is hypotonic.
- This test is used to differentiate the polyuria between diabetes mellitus, diabetes insipidus and due to excessive water intake.

14. Actions of parathyroid hormone.

- Parathormone is a polypeptide hormone with 84 AA secreted by the chief cells of the parathyroid gland.
- The main actions of PTH are to increase blood calcium levels and decrease phosphate levels.

Effect on Bones

- It increases activity of both osteoclasts and osteoblasts.
- But the osteoclastic activity is the major effect resulting in resorption of bone and release of calcium and phosphates into the ECF.
- **Action on osteoclasts:** This effect comes into action after a few days of exposure to PTH. The number and activity of osteoclasts are increased. Osteoclasts increase bone resorption and thereby increases calcium and phosphate levels in the blood. Also, levels of hydroxyproline and hydroxylysine are increased.
- **Action on osteoblasts:** At low doses PTH increases osteoblastic activity but in high doses it inhibits action of osteoblasts.

Action on Kidneys

There are three major actions on the kidneys:
1. Increased reabsorption of calcium in the thick ascending limb of loop of Henle and DCT. 25-30% of the filtered Ca^{2+} is reabsorbed in the DCT and loop of Henle by the action of PTH. 65% of filtered Ca^{2+} is reabsorbed in the PCT.
2. Decreases reabsorption of phosphate in the kidneys by its action on the PCT and induces phosphaturia. Serum phosphate levels are lowered by the action of PTH.
3. Stimulates the formation of 1, 25 dihydroxycholecalciferol (calcitriol) by the kidneys. PTH stimulates the 1a hydroxylation of 25 hydroxycholecalciferol to form the active form of vitamin D3. calcitriol in turn increases reabsorption of calcium from GIT and kidneys.

15. Thyroid function tests.

- Thyroid function tests help us to identify the status of thyroid gland activity.
- It includes, estimation of hormone levels, basal metabolic rate, radioactive iodine uptake, thyroid antibody estimation, thyroid scan, serum cholesterol levels, and thyroid biopsy.

Measurement of thyroid hormones:

- T3 and T4 levels are estimated by ELISA technique.
- More importantly free T3 and free T4 levels are estimated.
- In primary hyperthyroidism T3 and T4 levels are increased and TSH levels are decreased.
- In primary hypothyroidism the opposite is seen.

Measurement of plasma TSH levels:

- It is an important test done to identify thyroid status.
- In primary hypothyroidism, TSH levels are high and T3 and T4 levels are low, but in

secondary hypothyroidism TSH, T3 and T4 are all low.
- TSH level is low in primary hyperthyroidism.

TRH response test:
- Normally on administration of TRH, it increases TSH production and thereby T3 and T4 levels are increased.
- But in primary hyperthyroidism as T3 negatively inhibits TSH production, the levels do not increase.

Radioiodine uptake studies:
- Iodine is usually taken up by the thyroid gland for formation of T3 and T4.
- So, the uptake of radioactive iodine gives an idea about the function of the gland.
- The radioactive forms used are ^{123}I and ^{131}I.
- The RAI is given with water and an x-ray counter is placed on the neck and the thyroid uptake is determined.
- In hyperthyroidism, it is increased and in hypothyroidism it is decreased.

Measurement of metabolic rate: Normal value is ± 20%, in hyperthyroidism it is increased up to 100% and in hypothyroidism it is decreased up to –30 to –40%.

Thyroid antibody detection:
- This test is done to identify antibodies in Grave's disease and Hashimoto's thyroiditis.
- In Grave's disease antibodies against TSH receptors are detected and in Hashimoto's disease antibodies against thyroglobulin molecule are detected.

Thyroid scan:
- Ultrasound scanning of the gland gives a clear idea about the nature of lesions in the gland, either cystic or solid lesions.
- CT scan and MRI scan are useful in determining retrosternal and retro tracheal extension of the gland.

Fine needle aspiration biopsy: It is done in patients with nodular goiter to identify malignancies.

---
16. Composition of semen.

- Semen as a white colored secretion ejected from the male urethra during sexual intercourse.
- It contains sperm and other secretions from seminal vesicles, prostate, urethral glands and Cowper's glands.
- The average volume in each ejaculation is 2.5–3.5 mL.
- The volume decreases after repeated ejaculation.
- There are 100 million sperms per ml of semen.

Composition of Semen
- pH 7.35–7.5
- Specific gravity –1.028
- Sperm count –100 million/mL, <20% abnormal forms

Other Components

From seminal vesicles:
- Phosphorylcholine
- Ergothioneine
- Ascorbic acid
- Flavins
- Prostaglandins

From prostate:
- Spermine
- Citric acid
- Cholesterol, phospholipids
- Fibrinolysin, fibrinogenase
- Zinc
- Acid phosphatase
- Phosphate
- Bicarbonate
- Hyaluronidase
- 60% of the sperms should show normal motility within 3 hours after collection.
- Abnormal sperms should not be more than 30–35%.

Semen analysis is used for:
- Assessing male fertility
- It reflects the normal functions of testes and accessory sex organs
- Infertility cases
- To find out the effectiveness of vasectomy
- For medico-legal cases like—rape, adultery, etc.

---
17. Pregnancy test.

The pregnancy tests are grouped as:
- **Biological tests:** Injection of urine of pregnant female containing hCG into

animals and look for presence of ovulation in female animals and shedding of sperm in male animals.
- **Immunological tests:** Antibodies are produced for hCG and mixed with urine of pregnant female and then RBC or latex particle coated with hCG. Presence of agglutination indicates negative for pregnancy and absence of agglutination indicates pregnancy.
- **One step immunoassay test (strip test):** The hCg antibody is mixed with a dye and is impregnated on a strip of paper. When the strip comes in contact with the urine containing hCG, a pink-purple band appears, indicating pregnancy.
- **Radiological test:** Pregnancy tests 1, 2 and 3 are based on the presence of the hormone hCG present in the urine of pregnant female. It is detected in urine as early as 9 days by radioimmunoassay.
  - *Enzyme-linked immunosorbent assay (ELISA):* It is a quantitative test where even minute levels of hCG can be identified to confirm pregnancy.
  - *Radioimmunoassay* can also be done.

18. Disseminated intravascular coagulation.

- It is a serious complication of septicemia, extensive tissue injury and other diseases.
- Fibrin is deposited in the vascular system and many small and medium-sized vessels are thrombosed.
- The increased consumption of platelets and coagulation factors causes bleeding to occur at the same time.
- The cause of such events is due to excessive generation of thrombin due to increased tissue phospholipid activity without adequate tissue factor inhibitory pathway activity.

19. Laws of blood grouping.

These are the Landsteiner's laws.
- **First law:** If an agglutinogen is present on the membrane of RBCs, the corresponding agglutinin will be absent in the plasma.
- For example, in A blood group, if A antigen is present on RBC membrane, its corresponding agglutinin, anti-A antibody will be absent in plasma.
- **Second law:** If an agglutinogen is absent on RBC membrane, the corresponding agglutinin will be present in the plasma. For example, in O blood group, since agglutinogens A and B are absent on RBC membrane but the agglutinins anti-A and anti-B are present in plasma.
Both the laws are applicable for the ABO system.
But for Rh system only the first law is applicable. This is because in Rh negative individual there are no preformed antibodies in plasma. They are formed later, if the person is exposed once to Rh antigen.

20. Law of gut.

- Peristaltic waves are stimulated by distension of intestines.
- The wave created by distension spreads on either direction but the wave towards the oral side dies out.
- Therefore, the peristaltic waves proceed only form oral to aboral direction and moves chyme only in the aboral direction.

21. Lung compliance.

- Stretchability or the recoiling tendency due to the elastic property of the lung is said to be the compliance.
- Compliance of the respiratory system is defined as the change in the lung volume per unit change in the airway pressure.
- It is given as $C = \Delta V / \Delta P$
  C = Compliance
  ΔV = Change in volume ΔP = Change in pressure
  It is expressed in L/cm H_2O
- Both the lungs and thoracic cavity are elastic and viscous in nature and therefore each of them has their own recoiling tendencies.
- Compliance of the lung is dependent on the elastic tissues in the lung and the presence of surfactant.
- Normal value of thoracic cavity and lungs together is 0.13 L/cm H_2O.
- It means, when there is an increase in airway pressure by 1 cm H_2O the volume of the lungs increases by 0.13 liters.

- Normal value of compliance of lung is 0.22 L/cm H_2O.
- Compliance is decreased in conditions like fibrosis, pleural effusion, pneumothorax, etc.
- It is increased in pneumothorax.

22. Exchange vessels

- Capillaries are the "exchange vessels" in the vascular system.
- The walls of the capillaries are lined by a single layer of endothelial cells.
- There are fenestrations or pores in between the capillaries are in varying dimensions.
- The presence of pores helps in exchange of nutrients and metabolic wastes between the blood and the interstitial tissue.
- Exchange of material takes place by filtration and diffusion, across the capillaries.

23. Functions of parietal lobe.

- Major functions of parietal lobe are somatosensory in nature. It is posterior to the frontal lobe and is posteriorly separated from occipital lobe by the calcarine fissure and laterally from temporal lobe by the sylvian fissure.
- The areas in this lobe are areas 3, 1, 2, 5, 7, SSII, 39, and 43.

Functions

- Perception of somatic sensations like touch, pressure, vibration, pain, etc.
- Spatial recognition, two-point discrimination, and tactile localization.
- Since taste area is in this lobe, perception of taste is a function.
- Area 39 helps in language and speech.
- Area 5 and 7 help in stereognosis and hand-eye coordination.
- Also involved in learning and memory.
- Helpful in recognition of different intensities of stimuli.

24. Waves of EEG.

Electroencephalogram

- This is a recording of spontaneous electrical activities generated in the cerebral cortex.
- These waves are recorded by placing electrodes on the scalp at various areas and also on the forehead.
- Neurons are known to generate impulses like AP and graded potentials—collectively called as brain waves (*refer* **Fig. 23**).

Waves of EEG

- Alpha waves
- Beta waves
- Theta waves
- Delta waves

Alpha waves:

- Occurs at a frequency of 8–13 per second. Amplitude 50–100 μV.
- Present in all normal individuals when they are awake and resting with closed eyes.

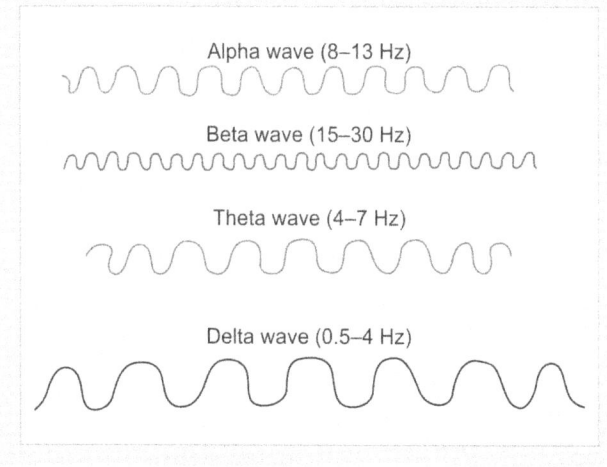

Fig. 23: EEG waves.

- Disappears entirely during sleep.
- It is found in the parieto-occipital region.
- Alpha block—alpha rhythm disappears on opening the eyes.
- Also called as desynchronization.
- Alpha rhythm affected by blood glucose levels, body temperature, and glucocorticoids.

Beta waves:
- Frequency between 14–30 Hz.
- Amplitude 5–10 µV.
- These waves appear when the nervous system is active.
- These waves appear in frontal regions.

Theta waves:
- At a frequency of 4–7 Hz. Amplitude is larger.
- Occurs normally in children and in adults at time of emotional stress.
- Found over parietal and temporal areas.
- Also occurs in many disorders of brain.

Delta waves:
- Frequency of these waves is 1–5 Hz.
- Amplitude is 20–200 µV.
- Delta waves occur in sleep in adults but present in infants during wakefulness.
- When present in an awake adult it indicates brain damage.

Uses of EEG
- Used to study normal functions of brain.
- To study the changes in brain activity during sleep.
- To diagnose various brain disorders like epilepsy, tumors, sites of trauma, degenerative diseases.

---

25. Referred pain.

Irritation of a vicus or viscera usually produces pain, which is not usually felt in the location of the viscus but in a somatic structure that is in a distance from the viscus. This is **referred pain**.

For example:
- Cardiac pain is usually referred to the inner aspect of the left arm or to the neck.
- When there is an irritation of central region of diaphragm there is pain in the tip of the shoulder.
- Pain in the testicle due to distension of ureter as in ureteric calculus.

Theories of Referred Pain
- The pain in viscera is usually referred to a somatic structure that has developed from the same embryonic segment or dermatome as the structure in which the pain originates—**dermatomal rule**.
- Theories of referred pain are—convergence theory and facilitation theory.

Convergence Theory
- Peripheral nerve fibers from the somatic and visceral structures converge on the same second order neuron present in lamina V of dorsal grey horn.
- The second order neuron is common for impulses from somatic and visceral structures.
- So, the tract carrying pain sensation from somatic structures also carry pain fibers from visceral structures.
- Cortex sometimes cannot differentiate from somatic and visceral inputs and so pain from visceral structure is referred to the somatic structure (*refer* **Fig. 24**).

Facilitation Theory
- The visceral afferent fibers on entering spinal cord give collaterals to afferents coming from the somatic structures.

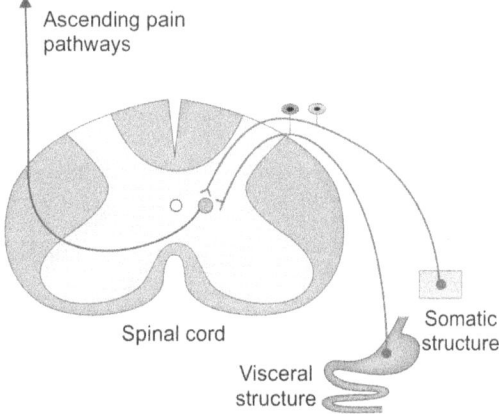

Fig. 24: Convergence theory of referred pain. Note the afferents from somatic and visceral structures converge on the same second order neuron.

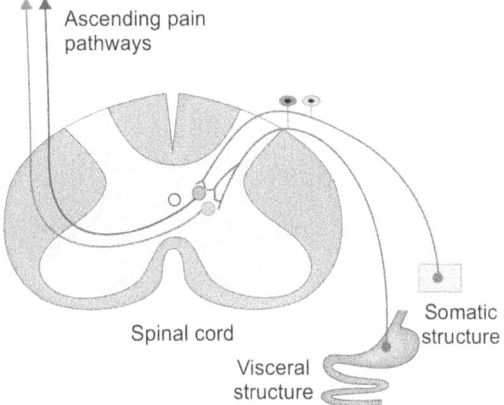

Fig. 25: Facilitation theory of referred pain. Note the visceral afferents give a collateral to second order neurons of somatic structure.

- So impulses coming from the visceral afferents facilitate and strengthen the impulses coming from the somatic structure.
- So a minor activity in the somatic afferents is facilitated by the visceral afferents and therefore pain is referred to the somatic structure (*refer* **Fig. 25**).

26. Circadian rhythm.

- It is a 24 hours fluctuation in the body functions.
- The rhythmic changes are seen in following conditions—sleep-wake cycle, secretion of ACTH and cortisol, body temperature, secretion of melatonin, etc.
- It is regulated by hypothalamus.
- The suprachiasmatic nucleus (SCN) in hypothalamus controls the circadian rhythm.
- SCN receives information about the day and night from retina through the retinohypothalamic tract.
- Efferents from SCN initiate neural and humoral signals that will regulate the various rhythmic activities in the body.
- Signals from SCN through sympathetic nerve to pineal gland regulates melatonin secretion in relation to day-night pattern.
- The diurnal changes in melatonin levels act as a timing signal for coordination of internal activities in relation to light-dark cycle in the environment.

27. Aphasia.

- Aphasias are abnormalities of language function that are not due to defects in vision or hearing or to motor paralysis. It is due to lesion in the categorical hemisphere.
- Common cause is due to emboli or thrombosis in the cerebral blood vessel supplying the speech areas.

There are four types:
1. Fluent or sensory aphasia
2. Nonfluent or motor aphasia
3. Global aphasia
4. Anomic aphasia

Fluent Aphasia or Wernicke's Aphasia

- It is also called as Wernicke's aphasia
- Lesion in the sensory speech area—Wernicke's area (area 22). It can happen due to blockage of vessels supplying the area or injury.
- Also called as fluent aphasia.
- Here the person is able to hear spoken words or identifying written words
- But cannot comprehend spoken or written words.
- Motor speech is intact. So, speech is not disturbed. Person speaks excessively.
- Impairment of written words as they are not able to comprehend written words also.

Nonfluent Aphasia or Broca's Aphasia

- In lesion of Broca's area there is normal comprehension of speech but there is poverty of speech.
- This type of aphasia is called as nonfluent aphasia or Broca's aphasia.
- Broca's area is the motor speech area (area 44) and is located in the foot of the primary motor cortex (area 4).
- In spoken speech, impulses from the ear are transmitted to the primary auditory area (area 42) in the temporal lobe.
- From area 42, the impulse reaches the auditory association areas and then to the sensory speech area—Wernicke's are (area 22). Here comprehension of speech happens.
- From the Wernicke's area impulses are transmitted to the Broca's area.

- It regulates the functions of the muscles of the lips, tongue, pharynx and larynx and it helps in vocalization of the reply.

Global Aphasia

- Lesion in both the Wernicke's area and Broca's area results in global aphasia.
- All aspects of speech are impaired.
- The patient is not able to comprehend or repeat words.

Anomic Aphasia

- It is a type of difficulty in speech due to lesion in the angular gyrus (area 39).
- The person has no difficulty in speech or understanding of auditory information.
- But there is trouble in understanding written language and pictures because the visual information is not processed and transmitted to Wernicke's area.
- It is also called as word blindness.

28. Kluver-Bucy syndrome.

- Lesions of the temporal lobe, especially the amygdala leads to temporal lobe syndrome or **Kluver-Bucy syndrome**.
- **Features of Kluver-Bucy syndrome are:**
  - Inability to identify objects visually, in spite of normal vision—**visual agnosia**.
  - Loss of hearing since the auditory area is in the temporal lobe
  - Tends to examine any object orally (oral tendencies)
  - Hyperphagia
  - Hypersexuality
  - Tends to show attention to all peripheral stimuli—hypermetamorphosis
  - Change in eating habits, monkeys start eating meat
  - Absence of fear, monkeys tend to handle the snakes
  - Loss of recent memory

29. Homunculus.

- Representation of the whole body in the somatosensory area 1 and primary motor cortex are called as sensory homunculus and motor homunculus respectively (*refer* **Fig. 26**).

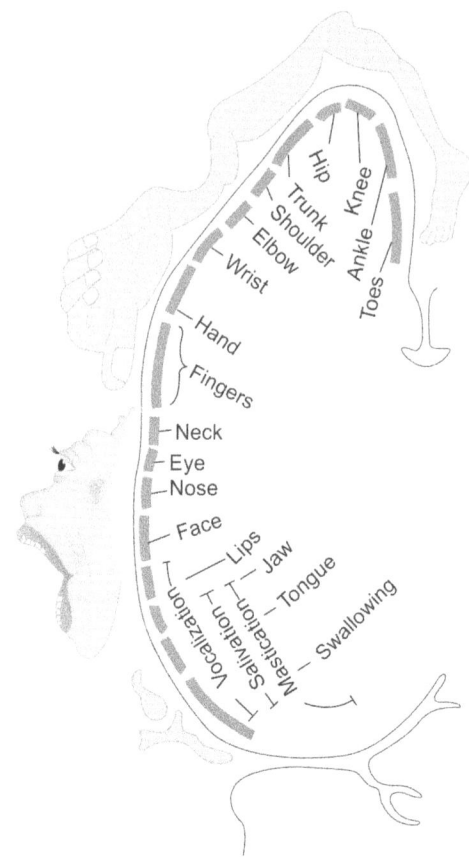

Fig. 26: Homunculus.

- The whole body is represented upside down in the homunculus.
- In sensory homunculus the body parts with a greater number of receptors have a larger representation. For example, the lips, fingers which have more numbers of receptors have a larger area of representation than the trunk and lower limbs.
- In motor homunculus the parts with fine, skilled movements have larger areas of representation, for example, hand, thumb, etc.

30. Sensation carried by posterior column.

- Posterior or the dorsal column is also called as the fasciculus gracilis and fasciculus cuneatus.
- The tract carries the following sensations:

- Fine touch
- Pressure
- Vibration sense
- Stereognosis
- Two-point discrimination
- Tactile localization
- Unconscious proprioception.

31. Receptor potential.

- Receptor potential is a graded potential.
- The experimental study to identify the receptor potential was done with the pacinian corpuscle.
- It is a receptor for touch and vibration.
- It is quite larger and therefore can be isolated and studied.
- Each capsule has concentric lamellae of connective tissue surrounding the unmyelinated ending of the sensory nerve fiber.
- Myelin sheath for the terminal starts within the corpuscle.
- The first node of Ranvier is also located inside the corpuscle and the second node is located at the point where the nerve leaves the corpuscle.
- On placing recording electrodes, over the nerve leaving the corpuscle and when graded pressure is applied, a non propagated depolarizing potential is recorded.
- It is said to be the generator potential or the receptor potential.
- As the pressure is increased the amplitude of the potential increases and as the potential reaches 10 mV an action potential is fired.
- It has been experimentally identified that the generator potential is generated in the unmyelinated nerve terminal of the sensory nerves.
- The receptor has converted the mechanical energy to electrical energy.
- The generator potential depolarizes the sensory nerve at the first node of Ranvier and generates the action potential there.

32. Reynolds number.

- Blood flow in a straight vessel is laminar or streamline. The velocity of blood flow in the center of the stream is greatest and lowest immediately below the vessel wall.
- Laminar flow occurs at velocities up to a level called as the **critical velocity**.
- At or above this velocity, the flow becomes turbulent.
- Laminar flow is silent but turbulent flow creates sounds.
- The probability of turbulence is also related to diameter of vessel and viscosity of blood.
- **This is given as the Reynolds number (Re)**
  $Re = \rho DV/\eta$
  - ρ = Density of fluid
  - D = Diameter of tube
  - V = Velocity of flow
  - η = Viscosity of fluid
- Higher the value of **Re** greater is the turbulence.
- When D is in cm, V is in cm/s^{-1}, η is in poises, flow is not turbulent if Re is <2000. When Re >3000 there is always a turbulent flow.

33. Artificial respiration.

When there is respiratory deficiency or respiratory arrest artificial respiration is given.

Conditions: Drowning, gas poisoning, electric shock, anesthesia, accidents, etc.

Methods: Instrumental and manual methods.

Instrumental Methods

- Used when there is a need for prolonged support.
- **Three types:**
  1. Positive pressure method
  2. Negative pressure method
  3. Boyle's apparatus

Positive Pressure Method

- Used in operation theaters
- Here air or O_2 mixture is used to inflate the lungs at positive pressures either continuously or intermittently.
- It impairs venous return.

Negative Pressure Method

- Achieved by alternate compression and relaxing the chest wall, externally.

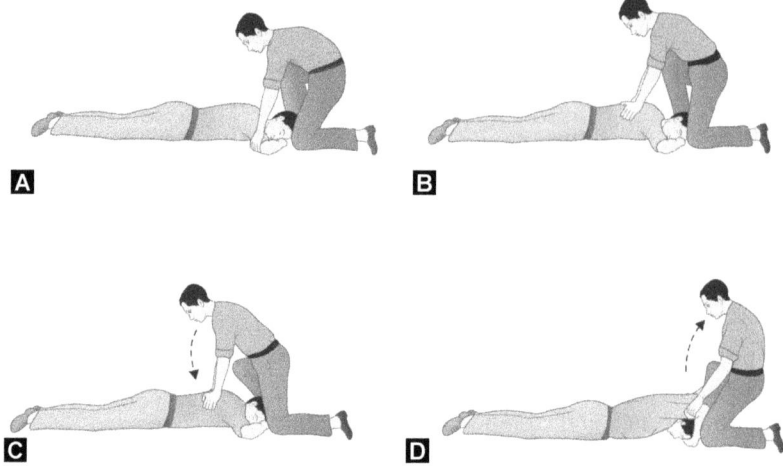
Fig. 27: Hoger-Neilson method of artificial respiration.

- **They are:**
  - Drinker's method (iron lung chamber).
  - Braggpaul method—use of hollow elastic rubber bag.
  - Others.

Drinker's Method (Iron Lung Method)

- The instrument contains an airtight iron chamber with a bellow on one side of the instrument.
- When the bellow moves in and out it creates a rise and fall of pressure inside the chamber.
- The person is placed inside the chamber with the head and neck outside the chamber.
- When the pressure rises inside the chamber expiration happens for the patient and when the pressure falls in the chamber there is inspiration.

Bragg Paul Method

- Here an elastic rubber bag is tied around the chest of the patient.
- The bag is connected to a pump which can inflate and deflate the bag.
- When the bag is inflated it compresses the chest and air is expired.
- When the pressure is released, the chest enlarges passively and air is drawn in.

Boyle's Apparatus

This apparatus is used in the hospitals for artificial ventilation. It is an automatic instrument in which rate and depth of ventilation and composition of inspired can be altered.

Manual Methods

Holger-Neilson Method

- The subject is made to lie prone and the head is turned to one side.
- The shoulder is abducted and flexed at the elbow and the hands are placed under the cheek.
- The operator is in kneeling position at the head of the patient and he places his hands spread on the back of the subject and bends forward to press on his back.
- The pressure on the back of the subject and compresses on the chest and expels the air out. Then he holds the arm above the elbow of the subject and pulls the arm forward.
- This enlarges the chest and results in inspiration. It is repeated 12/min. This is an exhaustive method for the examiner (*refer* **Fig. 27**).

Eve's Rocking Method

- Here the subject is made to lie prone on board which is rocketed on a pivot so that it can move up and down like a see-saw.
- When the board is tilted head down the abdominal organs push on the diaphragm resulting decrease in thoracic volume and expiration happens.
- When the board is tilted in the opposite direction the inspiration happens.

Mouth-to-mouth Respiration

- It can be direct or indirect method. In direct method the operator places his mouth directly on the subject's mouth and in indirect method it is done with a small tube.
- The subject is made to lie supine; the airway is kept clean from vomitus, foreign body, etc.
- The subject's head is extended, the operator sits on the side of the subject holds the lower jaw with his left hand and opens the mouth and with his right hand clips the nostrils.
- The operator then inhales deeply and places his mouth on the subject's mouth or the tube placed in the subject's mouth and blows into the subject's mouth smoothly, volume twice that of the tidal volume.
- This inflates the lungs of the subject and then the examiner removes his mouth from the subject's mouth and the lungs recoil resulting in expiration.
- It is repeated 12 times a minute.
- **Advantages:** Applied immediately, large tidal volume, CO_2 stimulates respiration, simple technique.
- **Disadvantages:** Infection may spread, volunteer may get exhausted.

34. Vital capacity.

It is the maximal volume of air which can be expired maximally following a maximal inspiration. The normal volume is 4800 mL in males and 3200 mL in females.

VC = TLC − RV
Or
VC = IRV + TV + ERV

- **VC** = Vital capacity
- **TLC** = Total lung capacity
- **RV** = Residual volume
- **IRV** = Inspiratory reserve volume
- **ERV** = Expiratory reserve volume
- **TV** = Tidal volume

It is measured by using a spirometer.

35. Errors of refraction.

Myopia—short-sightedness

Eyeball may be elongated and therefore parallel rays of light from a distant object are brought to focus in front of the retina. It may be genetic or acquired. It can be corrected by using biconcave lenses. The lens diverges the light rays before they strike the cornea and then they are converged by the lens in the eye, so that the object is focussed on the retina. It is the most common error of refraction (*refer* **Fig. 28**).

Hypermetropia—Far sightedness

Here the parallel rays of light from a distant object are brought to focus behind the retina. It occurs due to decrease in anteroposterior diameter of the eye. It can be corrected by using biconvex lenses so that they converge the light rays before they fall on the cornea and therefore the light rays fall on the retina.

Astigmatism

The problem here is the corneal surface is not spherical. One meridian of the cornea is different from the other. So, the parallel rays of light are not able to converge to a point of focus as there is unequal refraction from the different meridians. So, a blurred image is seen. It can be corrected using cylindrical lenses.

Presbyopia

- It is commonly seen in aged people above the age of 40 years.

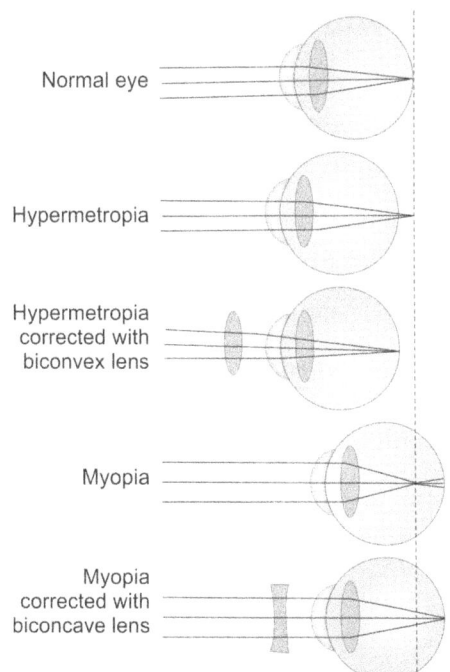

Fig. 28: Refractory errors of with corrections.

- The near point has receded beyond the normal reading distance due to loss of plasticity of lens. The loss of plasticity results in loss of accommodation property of the lens. It is corrected using convex lens for near work and plain glasses for far work and it is given as the bifocal lenses.

36. Functions of thalamus.

- Thalamus functions as a major relay station for most sensory impulses reaching the cortex.
- Thalamus acts as a crude center for sense perception like crude touch, pain, crude form of temperature sensation.
- It also contributes to motor function by relaying impulses from cerebellum and basal ganglia to motor cortex.
- Relays impulse between different areas of cortex.
- Contributes to regulation of autonomic activities and maintenance of consciousness.
- Due to the intimate connections of thalamus with frontal cortex and hypothalamus it is involved in various emotions.
- It is an integrating center for sleep, Intralaminar nuclei for non-rapid eye movement (NREM) sleep and lateral geniculate body for rapid eye movement (REM) sleep.
- Concerned with recent memory and emotions due to its involvement in Papez circuit.
- Concerned with language.
- Important role in genesis of synchronization of EEG waves and alertness of the individual. Induces alertness due to its connections with RAS.

37. Papez circuit.

- Hypothalamus along with limbic system participates in the expression of emotions.
- This relation is given as the Papez circuit which is responsible for emotions.

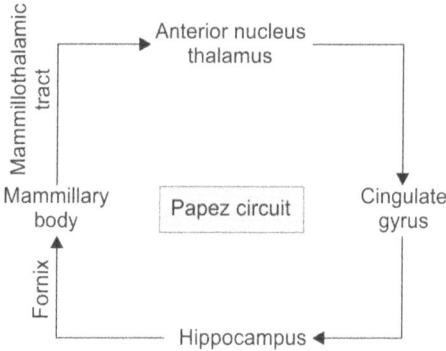

Fig. 29: Papez circuit.

- Papez circuit is also responsible for memory and learning.

Papez Circuit

- Hippocampus is connected to mamillary bodies through the fornix.
- Mamillary body is connected to the anterior thalamic nucleus through mammillothalamic tract.
- Anterior thalamic nucleus is connected to cingulate gyrus and it is in turn connected to hippocampus (*refer* **Fig. 29**).

38. Functions of cerebrospinal fluid.

- CSF offers mechanical protection by acting as a shock absorber.
- CSF offers the optimum chemical environment for accurate neuronal signaling.
- CSF acts as a circulating medium for exchange of nutrients and waste products between the blood and nervous tissue.
- Continuous formation and drainage removes metabolic wastes from brain.
- Acts as lymph.
- Provides nutrition.
- Reduces the weight of brain.

39. Bell-Magendie Law.

Bell-Magendie Law states that in the spinal cord the dorsal nerve roots are sensory and ventral nerve roots are motor.

Answers to 2021 Question Paper

ANSWER ALL QUESTIONS

I. Essay Questions   (15 Marks each)

1. Describe the physiological roles of the different types of leukocytes circulating in blood. Add a note on functions of lymphocytes in viral infection.
2. Describe the digestion and absorption of proteins in the digestive tract. Write a note on malabsorption.
3. Describe the mechanism of secretion of hydrochloric acid in the stomach. What are the factors regulating acid secretion? Add a note on peptic ulcer.
4. What is erythropoiesis? Describe the stages and factors regulating erythropoiesis. Add a note on anemias.
5. Name the functional divisions of the cerebellum. Describe the structure, connections and functions of cerebellum. Mention two signs of cerebellar lesions.
6. Describe the arterial blood pressure. Describe nervous regulation of arterial blood pressure.
7. Discuss about transport of oxygen in blood. Draw and explain oxygen—hemoglobin dissociation curve. Add a note on significance of P50.
8. Enumerate the ascending tracts of spinal cord. Explain in detail the pathway for pain. Add a note on analgesic system.

II. Short Notes   (5 Marks each)

1. Classify the fluid compartments of body giving their normal values, mention two methods to determine ECF volume.
2. Transport across cell membrane.
3. Structure and functions of neuromuscular junction.
4. Tissue macrophage system.
5. Non-excretory functions of kidney.
6. Cystometrogram and its significance.
7. Secretion of HCl in stomach and its regulation.
8. Regulations of blood calcium levels.
9. Spermatogenesis and seminal analysis.
10. Female contraceptive methods for birth control.
11. Classify diuretics and write a note on their sites of action.
12. Draw a neat labeled diagram of neuromuscular junction and explain the events in neuromuscular transmission.
13. Movements of small intestine.
14. Actions of parathormone.
15. Juxta glomerular apparatus.
16. Fibrinolytic system.
17. Functions of glucocorticoid.
18. Endometrial changes in menstrual cycle.
19. Active transport across cell membrane.
20. Digestion and absorption of fat.
21. Chloride shift.
22. Changes that occur in acclimatization.
23. Draw a normal spirogram and write about the volumes and capacities of lung.
24. Polysomnography.
25. Functions of hypothalamus.
26. Peculiarities of pulmonary circulation peculiarities of pulmonary circulation.
27. Hypovolemic shock.
28. Cardiopulmonary resuscitation.
29. Control of appetite.

30. Color vision.
31. Dark adaptation.
32. Baroreceptors.
33. Speech areas and aphasia.
34. Physiological changes in human body during exercise.
35. Acclimatization at high altitude.
36. Functions of hypothalamus.
37. Taste pathway.
38. Properties of cardiac muscle.
39. Hypoxia and its types.
40. Otolith organ.

I. ESSAY QUESTIONS

1. **Describe the physiological roles of the different types of leukocytes circulating in blood. Add a note on functions of lymphocytes in viral infection.**

The leukocytes are classified as granulocytes and agranulocytes:
- Granulocytes are—neutrophils, eosinophils and basophils (*refer* **Fig. 1**)
- Agranulocytes are—monocytes and lymphocytes.

Neutrophils

Physiological Roles of Neutrophils
- Neutrophils are the first line of defense
- It does the defense mechanism by phagocytosis.

Phagocytosis:
- Neutrophils are the first ones to reach the site of infection followed by macrophages (*refer* **Fig. 2**).
- They come out of the blood vessels by a process called **emigration**.
- Adhesion molecules like *selectins* and *integrins* help in emigration.
- Phagocytes are attracted to sites of infection or inflammation by chemotaxis.
- Substances inducing chemotaxis are called chemotaxins.
- On reaching the pathogens or tissue debris, phagocytes adhere to them—**adherence**.
- Then they put out processes—pseudopods and ingest the particles—**ingestion**.

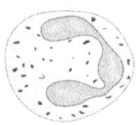 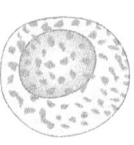 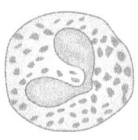

Neutrophil   Basophil   Eosinophil

Fig. 1: Granulocytes.

- The ingested particle is enclosed in a vesicle—**phagosome**.
- Phagosome attaches to lysosomes in the neutrophil to form—**phagolysosome**.
- The lysosomes put out hydrolytic enzymes like *lysozymes*.
- The phagocytes have oxidative enzymes in them which form lethal oxidative metabolites like— O_2^-, H_2O_2 and hypochlorite.
- Antimicrobials—**Defensins** in phagocytes kill the microorganisms.
- By all these killing mechanisms the microbes are killed and degraded or form **residual bodies**.

Other functions:
- Neutrophils release many chemical mediators like leukotrienes, thromboxane A2 which mediate inflammatory reaction.
- It mediates febrile response by releasing endogenous pyrogens.

Eosinophils

Structure of Eosinophils
- Size is same as that of neutrophils (10–14 µm)
- Bilobed nucleus and lobes are connected by thick chromatin strand—gives a spectacle shaped appearance.
- Cytoplasm has coarse, orange pink granules.
- Granules contain—eosinophil peroxidase, eosinophilic cationic protein, major basic protein, histaminase, catalase, etc.
- Mostly present in tissues.

Physiological Roles
- Leave the capillaries and enter tissue spaces where allergic reactions occur.
- Releases an enzyme, histaminase that combats the effects of histamine released by basophils.
- They inhibit mast cell degranulation

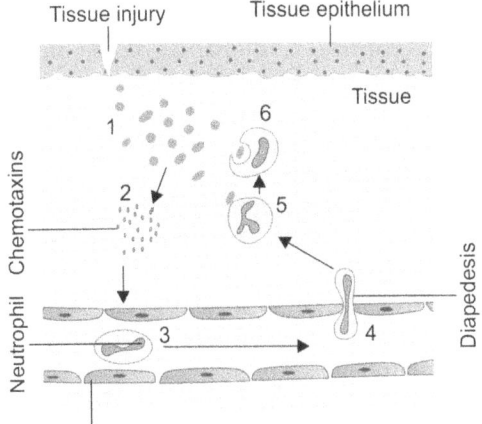

Fig. 2: Phagocytosis; neutrophils marginate towards the wall of capillary followed by diapedesis, chemotaxis and engulfing the microbes: (1) Entry of microorganisms; (2) Chemotaxis; (3) Margination; (4) Diapedesis; (5) Fusion of microbe with lysosome; (6) Formation of phagolysosome.

- They are weakly phagocytic and phagocytose Ag-Ab complexes
- Eosinophils also release substances (major basic protein) which kill the parasitic worms.
- So eosinophil counts increase in allergy and worm infestation.

Basophils
- They are similar to mast cells.
- They are mildly phagocytic
- They enter tissues at sites of infection or tissue damage and release histamine, heparin and serotonin.
- These chemicals are responsible for the inflammatory reactions.
- They also release eosinophilic chemotactic factor which attracts eosinophils to combat the inflammatory reactions by removing Ag-Ab complexes.
- Mast cells and basophils release the inflammatory mediators and are responsible for allergic reactions.
- Basophils release heparin which is an anticoagulant and thereby removes minute clots and prevents clotting of blood.

Monocytes
- Monocytes are formed in the bone marrow. They circulate in blood for 10–20 hours.
- They are the largest blood cells, 12–20 μm in size (2–2.5 times the size of RBCs).
- Nucleus occupies almost 50% of the cell volume and the rest is the cytoplasm. The granules in cytoplasm do not take the regular staining and therefore not visible. So is an agranulocyte.
- Monocytes after circulation, enter various tissues through the capillary membrane and swell up to become the macrophage.
- They live for months to years as a tissue macrophage.
- They exist as either fixed macrophages or mobile macrophage.
- The monocytes, macrophages and specialized endothelial cells in bone marrow, spleen and lymph nodes are grouped as reticulo-endothelial system.
- They are destroyed once their phagocytic action is over.
- Tissue macrophages are named according to the sites where they are present.

The macrophages have the following functions:
- **Phagocytosis:** As a phagocyte it is very powerful and it emigrates into the tissues following the bacterial invasion. But this happens 24 hours after the neutrophil action and therefore it is said to be the **second line of defense**. It engulfs the bacteria and digests it; the process of digestion of bacteria is similar to that of the neutrophils.
- **Secretory function:** Monocytes and macrophages secrete many chemicals like: Interleukins, IL-1, TNF-α, binding proteins like transferrin, lysozyme, proteases, acid hydrolase, etc.
- **Role in lymphocyte-mediated immunity:** Macrophages act as antigen presenting cells (APC) in immune reactions. It engulfs the microorganism and digests it and attaches the antigenic component to the MHC II molecule in the macrophage.

The antigen-MHCII complex now moves towards the membrane of the macrophage and is inserted there. This macrophage moves towards the lymph nodes and the antigen is presented to the Lymphocytes. The Lymphocytes with the receptor for the

antigen bind to the APC and is activated for further differentiation and division.
- **Monocyte-Macrophage** secretory products also play a *key role in healing and repair*.

Lymphocytes

- Lymphocytes are classified as two types of based on their formation, maturation and functions—T and B lymphocytes. They are involved in acquired immune mechanisms.
- **T lymphocytes** take part in cell-mediated immunity. They protect against intracellular pathogens like viral infections, destroy the cancer cells and are responsible for graft rejection. They also help in humoral immunity provided by the B lymphocytes.
- **B lymphocytes** take part in humoral immunity and they destroy the extracellular pathogens like bacteria.
- There are **natural killer cells (NK cells)** which also are a type of lymphocytes. They are involved in innate immune mechanisms.

Role of Lymphocytes in Viral Infections

- There are three types of T lymphocytes—helper T-lymphocytes, cytotoxic T-lymphocytes and memory T cells.
- **Helper T cells:** These cells have CD4 protein on their membrane and they help in cell-mediated as well as humoral immunity. There are two types—T_H1 and T_H2 cells. T_H1 cells help in cellular and T_H2 helps humoral immunity.
- **Cytotoxic T cells:** They have the CD 8 antigen on their cell membrane and they are the killer cells.
- **Memory T cells:** They are the memory cells and they live for many years in the tissues and when the same pathogens enter the host, they develop a swift and rapid response and eliminate the invader.

Mechanism of Cell-mediated Immunity

- Antigen presentation by the APCs
- Activation and proliferation of T cells
- Elimination of the invader

Antigen Presentation by APCs

- Macrophages, dendritic cells and B lymphocytes act as APCs.
- Macrophages phagocytose the antigens entering the body and breaks it down to peptide fragments.
- The antigenic fragment forms a complex with the MHC II protein present in macrophages.
- The antigen and MHC II complex are expressed on the membrane of macrophage.
- This macrophage moves to the lymph nodes and present the antigen to T Cells.

Activation and Proliferation of T Cells

- The T cells with the receptor for the antigen binds to it.
- After co-stimulation by the IL-2 secreted by Helper cells, T cells start to proliferate and differentiate and start forming a clone of similar cells.

The cytotoxic T cells eliminate the viruses by the following mechanisms:

- The activated CD8 cells synthesize and secrete proteins called "**perforins**" which are inserted into the membrane of the pathogen. The perforins are water channels which allow influx of water and thereby swelling of the microbe and cause its lysis (*refer* **Fig. 3**).
- Release of **lymphotoxins** by activated T cells. These cytokines destroy the microbes.
- Cytotoxic T cells secrete **interferons** which will favour the phagocytic activity of the neutrophils and macrophages by promoting opsonization.

---

2. Describe the digestion and absorption of proteins in the digestive tract. Write a note on malabsorption.

Digestion of Proteins

- Digestion of protein starts in the stomach where pepsins cleave the peptide bonds.
- Pepsin is secreted in the inactive form—pepsinogen.
- Pepsinogen is activated to pepsin by the hydrochloric acid present in stomach.

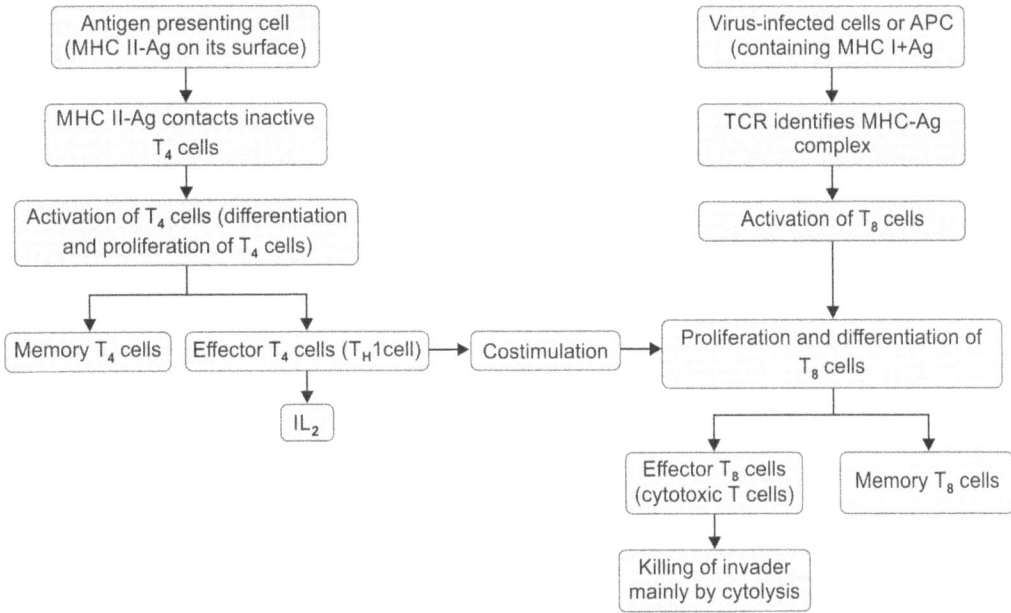

Fig. 3: Mechanism of cell-mediated immunity.

- The digestion of proteins by pepsin is terminated when the pH becomes higher as it enters the intestines.
- Pepsin digests proteins into polypeptides and they are further digested by the proteolytic enzymes in the pancreatic juice, trypsin, chymotrypsin and elastases. They act the interior peptide bonds—so called as endopeptidases.
- Carboxypeptidase, an exopeptidase hydrolyses the bonds in the terminals.
- Following the breakdown of peptides some of the free amino acids and are liberated in the intestinal lumen.
- Others are liberated close to the brush border by the action of aminopeptidases, carboxypeptidases, endopeptidases and dipeptidases which are brush border enzymes.
- So tri- and dipeptidases are hydrolyzed by intracellular peptidases in the enterocytes.
- Final digestion of proteins to amino acids take place in the intestinal lumen, brush border and inside the cells.

Absorption of Proteins

- There are seven different types of transporters to transport amino acids in the intestine.
- Five of them require Na^+ to co-transport amino acids. Two of these also require Cl.
- Two amino acid transporters are Na^+ independent.
- Di- and tri-peptides are transported into enterocytes along with H^+.
- The amino acids after the final intracellular digestion are transported across the basolateral sides through 5 transport systems.
- Two of these are Na^+ dependant and three are not.
- From there they enter the portal blood.
- Absorption of amino acids are rapid in duodenum and jejunum but slow in ileum.
- 50% of digested proteins come from ingested food, 25% from proteins in digestive juices and 25% from the desquamated epithelial cells.
- 2-5% of digested proteins enter colon and they are acted upon by the bacteria.

Defects in Protein Absorption

- **Hartnup disease:** Defect in absorption of neutral amino acids in the intestine and renal tubules.
- **Cystinuria:** It is due to congenital defect in transport of cysteine in intestinal renal tubules.

Malabsorption Syndrome

- Malabsorption syndrome occurs when more than 50% of the small intestine is resected or bypassed.
- The symptoms are due to defective absorption of nutrients and vitamins.

Defective absorption of bile salts:

- It occurs in conditions of resection of ileum.
- The bile slats are essential for absorption of lipids and lipid-soluble vitamins.
- This leads to steatorrhea.
- The presence of unabsorbed bile salts in the colon holds increases adenylyl cyclase activity and that leads to increased intestinal secretion.

The other complications are:

- Hypocalcemia and arthritis
- Hyperuricemia
- Fatty infiltration of liver and cirrhosis

Defective absorption of amino acids: Body wasting, hypoproteinemia and edema carbohydrate and fat absorption is also defective.

The common causes for malabsorption are:

- Tropical sprue
- Celiac disease
- Crohn's disease
- Larger resection of ileum leads to malabsorption syndrome.

---

3. Describe the mechanism of secretion of hydrochloric acid in the stomach. What are the factors regulating acid secretion? Add a note on peptic ulcer.

Composition of Gastric Juice

- 2–2.5 L/day
- pH 1-2
- Water—99.45%
- Solids—0.55%
- Electrolytes—Na^+, K^+, Mg^{2+}, Cl^-, HCO_3^-, HpO_4^-, SO_4^-
- Enzymes—pepsin, lipase, gelatinase
- Mucus—insoluble and soluble
- Intrinsic factor

Mechanism of HCl Secretion

- In stomach, hydrochloric acid is secreted by the parietal cells which are present in the main gastric glands in body of the stomach.
- Pure secretion from the parietal cell has a pH of 0.82 and is isotonic (150 mEq of H^+ and 150 mEq of Cl^+).
- Parietal cell is polarized with an apical side facing the lumen and a basolateral side facing the interstitium.
- There are many tubulovesicular structures in the parietal cell which are studded with H^+-K^+ ATPase which pump H^+ into the lumen in exchange for K^+.
- These cells are highly metabolizing and they put out lot of CO_2. The cell is also rich in the enzyme carbonic anhydrase (*refer* Fig. 4).

HCl secretion from the parietal cells happens in two steps:

1. Secretion of H^+ into the lumen
2. Secretion of Cl^- into the lumen.

The steps involved in HCl secretion are:

1. CO_2 in the cell is hydrated in the presence of Carbonic anhydrase, $CO_2 + H_2O \rightarrow H_2CO_3$
2. $H_2CO_3 \rightarrow H_2^+ + HCO_3^-$
3. The H^+ is pumped into the lumen by the H^+-K^+ ATPase pump on the apical side. For one H^+ pumped out of cell one K^+ is taken into the cell which later diffuses back into the lumen.

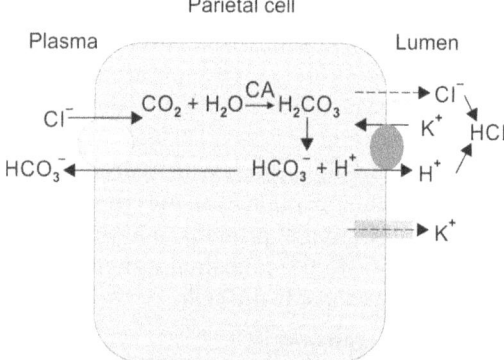

Fig. 4: Mechanism of HCl secretion.
(CA: carbonic anhydrase)

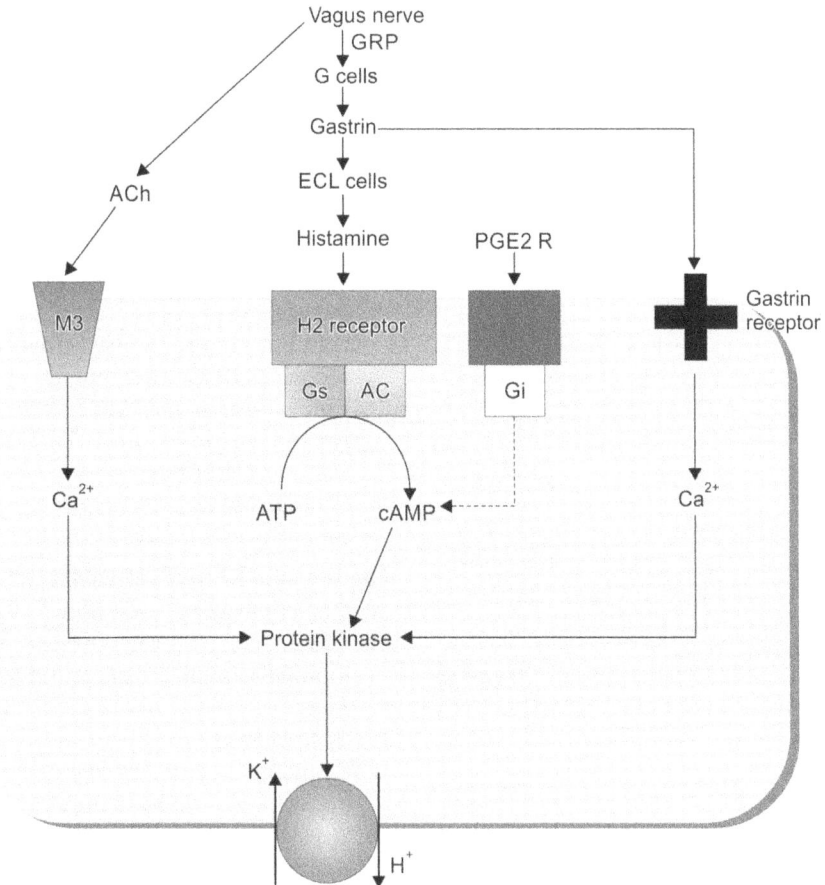

Fig. 5: Parietal cell with the regulating factors for HCl secretion.
(ACh: acetylcholine, ECL cells: enterochromaffin-like cells; GRP: gastrin releasing peptide; M3: muscarinic receptor; PGE2R: prostaglandin E2 receptor; Gs: G protein; AC: adenylyl cyclase; Gi: G protein)

4. HCO_3^- is extruded in the basolateral side through an anion exchanger in exchange for one Cl^-.
5. The Cl^- which enters the cell will diffuse across the apical membrane into the lumen.
6. So for every H^+ secreted, one Cl^- is also secreted into the lumen and one HCO_3^- is absorbed into the blood.

So when gastric secretion is increased after a meal, the HCO_3^- getting added to the blood is increased, thereby raising the pH of blood—**postprandial alkaline tide**.

Regulation of Gastric Secretion

Neural, humoral and reflex regulation of secretion (*refer* **Fig. 5**).

Factors that Stimulate
1. Vagus nerve
2. Gastrin
3. Histamine

Factors that Inhibit
1. Low pH in the stomach
2. Somatostatin
3. Prostaglandin E2

Regulation is Discussed in Terms of:
1. Cephalic phase
2. Gastric phase
3. Intestinal phase

Cephalic Phase
- Nearly 500 mL/hr (45% of total secretion)
- Initiated by thought, sight, smell, taste of food through vagus nerve

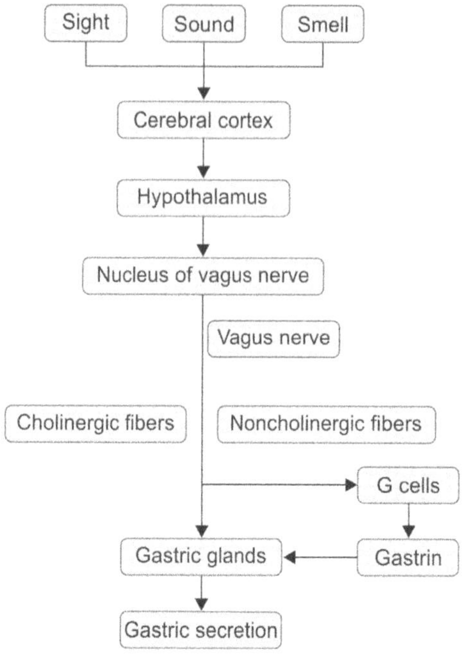

Fig. 6: Cephalic phase of regulation of HCl secretion. This phase of gastric secretion is regulated through vagus nerve.

- Emotions also affect secretion (*refer* **Fig. 6**).

Gastric Phase

50% of total secretion. Food in stomach induces secretion by:
- Distension of body of stomach (through reflexes—vagal reflex)
- Distension of antrum (through gastrin secretion)
- By products of partial digestion of protein (through gastrin secretion)

Intestinal Phase
- It begins when chyme enters the intestine.
- Intestinal influence is inhibited by:
  - *Enterogastric reflex:* By distension, presence of acid and products of digestion—inhibits secretion.
  - *Hormonal mechanism:* CCK, secretin, GIP, neurotensin, etc.—enterogastrone.

Peptic Ulcer

There are two types of ulcers:
1. **Duodenal ulcer**
2. **Gastric ulcer**

- Ulcer is due to disruption of the mucosal barrier or excess secretion of gastric juice.
- Acid or pepsin in gastric juice digests the mucosa leading to ulcer.

Mucosal barrier is formed by:
- **Mucus** secreted by the neck cells and surface mucosal cells in the mucosal lining. It also contains mucin, phospholipid, HCO_3^- and water.
- **Prostaglandins** secreted by epithelial cells have antisecretory activity (HCl) and increases HCO_3^- and mucus.
- **Epithelium of mucosa:** Low permeability, rapid turnover and HCO_3^-, mucus secretions from there.
- **Bicarbonate secretion** from gastric mucosal cells increases the pH.

Factors which Impair Mucosal Defense
- Defective mucus secretion
- Drugs like NSAIDs, cortisol, etc. They inhibit secretion of mucus and bicarbonate
- Alcohol
- Type of food
- Smoking – ↓ mucus and pancreatic secretions. Causes reflux of duodenal contents.
- Stress
- Reflux of gastric contents
- Delayed gastric emptying
- H. pylori infection—causes local inflammation in antral mucosa and disrupts the barrier.

Factors which Increase Secretion
- **Genetic factors:** Increased parietal cell mass, increased postprandial gastrin response
- **Psychosomatic factors:** Anxiety increases secretion
- **Food:** Alcohol, tea, coffee, spicy food
- Rapid gastric emptying
- **Zollinger-Ellison syndrome:** It is a gastrin secreting tumor of pancreas.

Symptoms of Peptic Ulcer
- The most common symptom is upper abdominal pain especially in empty stomach and is relieved after food intake.
- If the ulcer becomes erosive there will be features of hematemesis or malena (dark colored stools)

- If there is perforation of ulcer it can lead to peritonitis.

Physiological Basis of Treatment of Peptic Ulcer
- Antacids can be used and they coat the mucosal layer.
- H_2 receptor blockers like ranitidine, cimetidine and famotidine are used to block the actions of histamine. Histamine is a potent stimulator of parietal cells for HCl secretion.
- Proton-pump blockers like omeprazole, pantoprazole and rabeprazole are the various generations. They block the H^+-K^+ pump and thereby decrease HCl secretion.
- Sucralfate, forms a coating over the ulcer and prevents further erosion.
- Atropine antagonists are used to inhibit its action on the muscarinic receptors.
- Proglumide a gastrin inhibitor blocks the actions of gastrin.
- In *H.pylori* infections antibiotics can be used.
- NSAID-induced ulcers can be treated by stopping the usage of NSAIDs and administering prostaglandin antagonists like misoprostol.
- Gastrinomas can be removed surgically.
- Vagotomy—truncal, selective or highly selective vagotomy can be done to decrease secretion from the parietal cells.

---

4. What is erythropoiesis? Describe the stages and factors regulating erythropoiesis. Add a note on anemias.

- Erythropoiesis is production of RBCs. Life span of RBCs are 120 days.
- Hence continuous destruction and production of RBCs take place at a constant rate.

Site of Erythropoiesis
- **Mesoblastic stage:** In the embryonal stage-yolk sac.
- **Hepatic stage:** Later in the fetal stage upto 5 months—liver, spleen, thymus and lymph nodes.
- **Myeloid stage:** Three months before birth—red bone marrow of all bones.
- **Adult life:** Red bone marrow of flat bones and epiphysis of long bones.

Changes During Maturation
- Reduction in size of the cell.
- Cytoplasm increases in amount and nucleus decreases in size.
- Cytoplasm changes from basophilic nature to polychromatophilic and then to acidophilic nature due to hemoglobinization of cytoplasm.
- Disappearance of RNA.
- Loss of nucleoli and then nucleus.

Pronormoblast
- Large cell, diameter—20–25 µm.
- Cytoplasm is less.
- High concentration of polyribosomes.
- Large nucleus with multiple nucleoli.
- Hemoglobin not formed.

Early Normoblast
- Diameter of cell, 15–18 µm.
- Cell exhibits mitosis.
- Cytoplasm is still less, basophilic.
- Nucleus large, occupies 3/4th of cell.
- Heterochromatin clumps present.

Intermediate Normoblast
- The cell is smaller in size, 12–15 µm.
- Cytoplasm changes from blue to pink as hemoglobin starts to appear.
- Nucleus small, occupies half the cell. No nucleoli.
- Hemoglobin formation makes the cell acidophilic also—polychromatophilic cytoplasm.
- Mitosis is sluggish.

Late Normoblast
- Cell is smaller in size.
- Cytoplasm is deeply eosinophilic—orthochromatic erythroblast.
- Nucleus is small and pyknotic.
- Cart-wheel arrangement of chromatin.
- Hb synthesis increases.

Reticulocyte
- Cell size is 7.8 µm
- Nucleus is extruded
- Hemoglobin present
- Chromatin reticulum seen (*refer* **Fig. 7**).

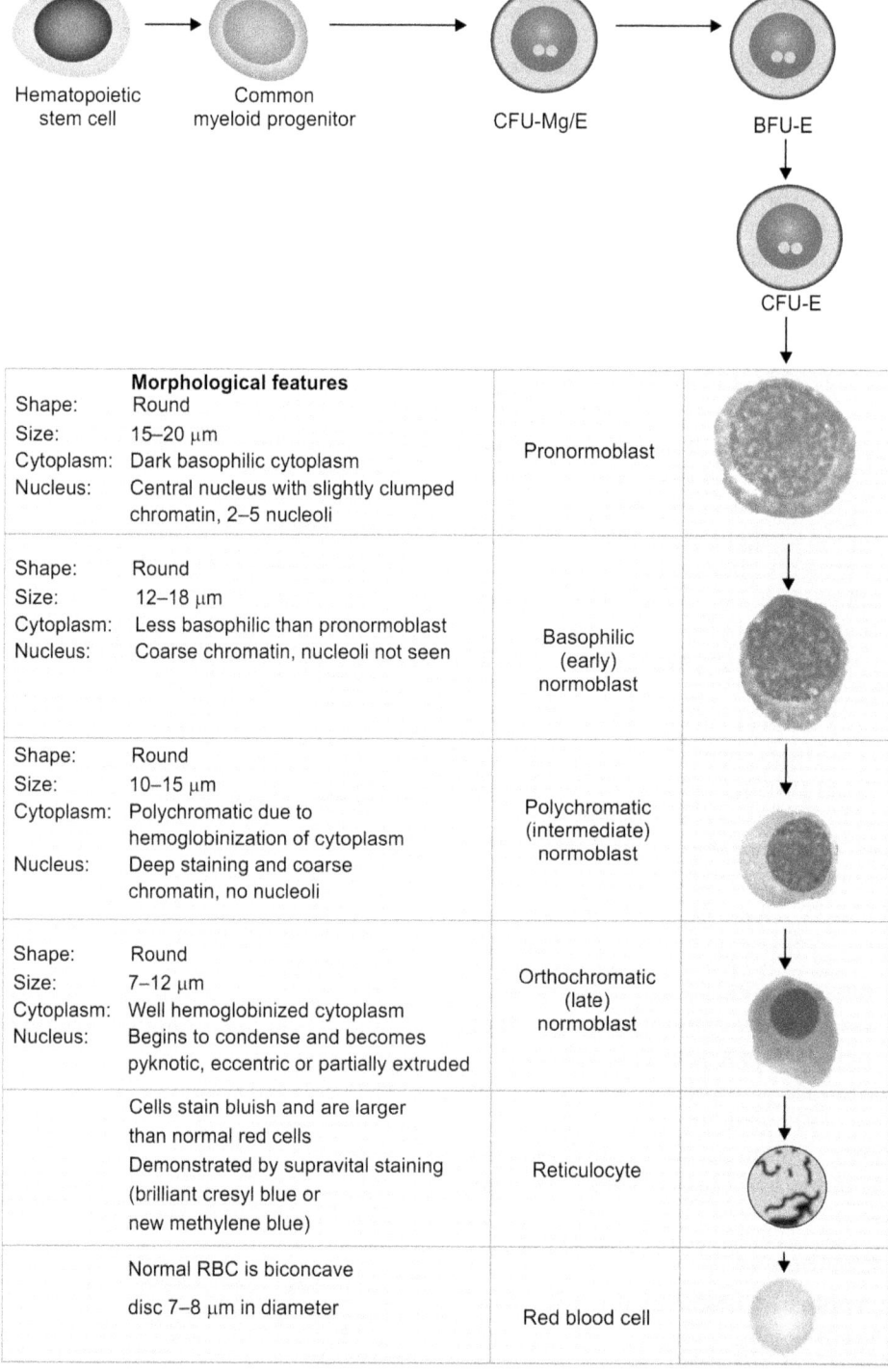

Fig. 7: Stages of erythropoiesis.
(CFU-Meg/E: colony forming unit—megakaryocyte/erythroid; BFU-E: blast forming unit-erythroid; CFU-E: colony forming unit-erythroid)

Mature RBC

- Cell size is 7.5 μm
- RBC is biconcave in shape
- Chromatin reticulum disappears.

The whole process of maturation from pronormoblast to reticulocyte takes 7 days. It takes 2 days for reticulocyte to mature as an RBC.

Regulation of Erythropoiesis

There are general and special factors regulating erythropoiesis.

General Factor—Hypoxia

- Major function of RBC is to carry oxygen to the tissues.
- So, when there is decrease in tissue oxygen levels, it induces production of RBCs.
- Hypoxia stimulates the interstitial cells of the kidneys to synthesize the hormone erythropoietin.
- It acts on bone marrow to stimulate the erythropoietin sensitive stem cells to become proerythroblasts and thereby stimulates formation of RBCs.
- It also increases the release of reticulocytes from the bone marrow.

Factors Increasing Erythropoietin Production

- Hypoxia
- Catecholamines
- Thyroxine
- Testosterone

Special Maturation Factors

Dietary factors:

- Proteins help in globin formation
- Iron helps in heme formation
- Copper, cobalt and nickel also helps in heme formation
- Calcium helps in absorption of iron from GIT
- Vitamin C also helps in iron absorption
- Vitamin B12 and folic acid helps in synthesis of nucleic acids and final maturation of RBC
- Intrinsic factor synthesized in the stomach by the parietal cells help in absorption of Vitamin B_{12}.

Anemia

- Anemia is defined as the decrease in red cell count or hemoglobin content in blood.
- Anemia is classified based on the **cause of anemia** and based on the **structure of red cells**.

Morphological Classification or Wintrobe's Classification

Based on the size and the presence of hemoglobin content inside the cell it is classified as:

1. **Normocytic normochromic anemia:** The RBC size (MCV) and the hemoglobin content (MCH and MCHC) is normal. It is seen in hemorrhagic anemia, hemolysis and aplastic anemia.
2. **Microcytic hypochromic anemia:** The cell volume and the hemoglobin content are decreased. MCV, MCH and MCHC are below normal. It is seen in iron deficiency anemia.
3. **Macrocytic anemia:** MCV is above normal range. There is macrocytosis and the hemoglobin concentration is normal. This type is normally seen in vitamin B_{12} and folic acid deficiency.

Etiological Classification or Wintrobe's Classification

Anemia is usually due to either decreased production from the bone marrow or increased destruction.

Classification of anemia:

1. **Decreased red cell production:**
   - Decreased production due to stem cell failure—aplastic anemia
   - *Dietary deficiencies:*
     - Iron deficiency anemia
     - **Megaloblastic anemia:** Due to deficiency of folic acid and vitamin B_{12} deficiency.
     - **Pernicious anemia:** Anemia due to vitamin B_{12} deficiency due to deficiency of Intrinsic factor.
     - Protein deficiency.
2. **Increased destruction of red cells:** Hemolytic anemias—congenital and acquired:

Congenital:
a. *Membrane defects:* Hereditary spherocytosis and hereditary elliptocytosis.
b. *Hemoglobin defects:*
   - Hemoglobinopathies (defects in hemoglobin): Sickle cell anemia (HbS, in the beta chain in the 6th position glutamic acid is replaced by valine), abnormal hemoglobin like HbC, HB E, Hb D.
   - Thalassemia (deficiency of hemoglobin: Deficiency of α or β chain)—major and minor.
c. *Enzyme defects:* Deficiency of glucose-6-phosphate dehydrogenase and pyruvate kinase.

Acquired:
- Due to antigen-antibody reactions—erythroblastosis fetalis, incompatible blood transfusions, etc.
- Infections—malaria
- Drug induced: Quinine, aspirin, etc.
- Snake venom
- Hypersplenism: Excessive destruction of RBCs
- Burns.

3. **Blood loss anemia:**
   - *Acute hemorrhage:* Trauma, surgery, etc.
   - *Chronic blood loss:* Menorrhagia, worm infestation.
4. **Anemia due to chronic renal failure:** Due to decreased production of erythropoietin.
5. Anemia associated with chronic diseases.

5. Name the functional divisions of the cerebellum. Describe the structure, connections and functions of cerebellum. Mention two signs of cerebellar lesions.

Anatomically each hemisphere of cerebellum is divided into three lobes by two transverse furrows into lobes—anterior lobe, posterior lobe and flocculonodular lobes (*refer* **Fig. 8**).

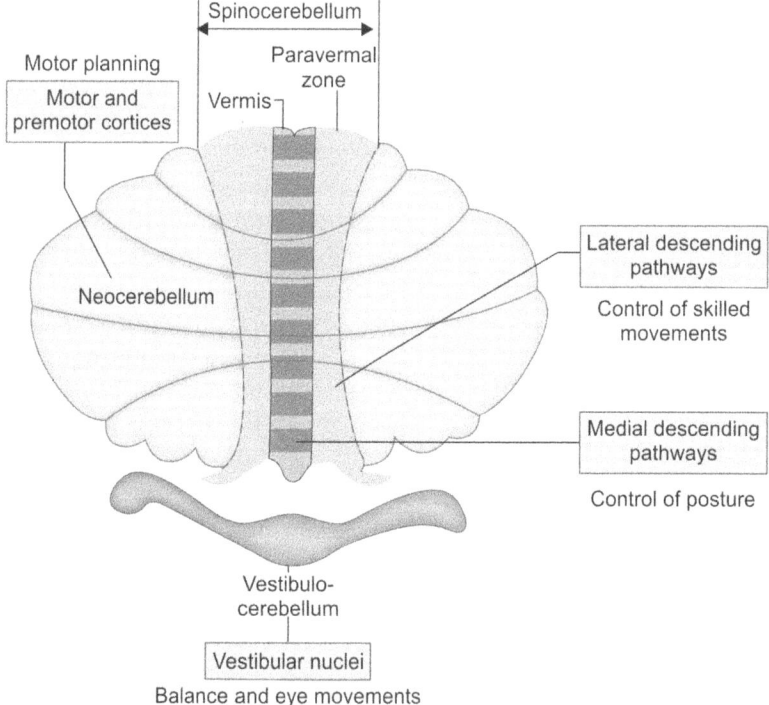

Fig. 8: Functional divisions of cerebellum with their connections and functions.

Functional Divisions

- The main functions of cerebellum are to maintain posture and balance and coordinate voluntary movements.
- Based on the functions it is divided into three parts:
  a. *Vestibulocerebellum:* Made up of the flocculonodular lobe.
  b. *Spinocerebellum:* Consists of vermis and the intermediate part of the cerebellar hemispheres (paravermal portion).
  c. *Neocerebellum:* Consists of the lateral parts of the hemispheres.

Connections and Functions of Cerebellum

- Connections include the afferents and efferents to cerebellum which enter cerebellum and leave, through the cerebellar peduncles.
- There are three cerebellar peduncles: Superior, inferior and middle cerebellar peduncles.

Afferent Connections

The afferents to cerebellum come through the climbing fibers and mossy fibers.

Climbing Fibers

- They contain the olivocerebellar tract which arises from the Inferior olivary nucleus in medulla.
- The olivary nucleus in turn receives proprioceptive inputs from all over the body.
- The climbing fibers end on the dendrites of Purkinje cells and they make one-to-one connection with the Purkinje cells and excite them.
- Collaterals from climbing fibers also excite the golgi cells and the deep nuclei of cerebellum.
- Climbing fibers enter the cerebellum through the inferior cerebellar peduncle. This peduncle brings in most of the other afferent fibers to cerebellum.

Mossy Fibers

- Mossy fibers include all the other afferents entering the cerebellum other than olivocerebellar tract.
- It includes—dorsal and ventral spinocerebellar tracts, vestibulocerebellar tract, reticulocerebellar tract, cuneocerebellar tract, tectocerebellar tract, rubrocerebellar tract and pontocerebellar tract.
  a. *Dorsal spinocerebellar tract:* It carries unconscious proprioceptive inputs and exteroceptive inputs from same side limbs and trunk of same side and they enter cerebellum through ipsilateral Inferior cerebellar peduncle. It ends on the spinocerebellum.
  b. *Ventral spinocerebellar tract:* It carries cutaneous and proprioceptive inputs from opposite side of the lower limbs and enters cerebellum through ipsilateral superior cerebellar peduncle and they are distributed to the hind limb area of spinocerebellum.
  c. *Vestibulocerebellar tract:* It carries impulses from the same side vestibular nucleus about information regarding the position of head in relation to body posture. It enters the cerebellum through ipsilateral inferior cerebellar peduncle. It ends in the flocculo nodular lobe (vestibulocerebellum).
  d. *Reticulocerebellar tract:* It arises from the lateral reticular nucleus and enters through inferior cerebellar peduncle and is distributed to all areas of cerebellar cortex.
  e. *Cuneocerebellar tract:* It arises from external arcuate nucleus and carries proprioceptive information from head, neck, upper limb and upper part of the body. It enters through ipsilateral inferior cerebellar peduncle and distributed to spinocerebellum.
  f. *Tectocerebellar tract:* It carries visual and auditory information from superior and inferior colliculi. It enters through superior cerebellar peduncle.

g. *Rubrocerebellar tract:* It arises from the red nucleus. It contains information from cerebral cortex. It has both crossed and uncrossed fibers. It enters through superior cerebellar peduncle and ends on dentate nucleus (one of the deep nuclei of cerebellum).
h. *Pontocerebellar tract:* These are fibers arising from motor area of cerebral cortex and end on pontine nuclei. From here they arise to form the pontocerebellar fibers. They cross to opposite side and enter through the opposite middle cerebellar peduncle and are distributed to all areas of cerebellar cortex.

Efferent Connections

- All the efferents from cerebellar cortex are through the Purkinje fiber output which ends on the deep cerebellar nuclei. Purkinje cell output is inhibitory in nature.
- The deep nuclei are: Dentate, emboliform, fastigial and globose. Emboliform and globose are together called as nucleus interpositus.
- The deep nuclei also receive collaterals from climbing and mossy fibers and both are excitatory in nature.
- The net effect of output from deep nuclei is excitatory to brain stem and thalamus.
- All parts of cerebellum, except the vestibulocerebellum exit the cerebellum through deep nuclei (*refer* **Fig. 9**)
  a. *Cerebellovestibular pathway-vestibulospinal tract:* It leaves the vestibulocerebellum and projects to the vestibular nuclei directly. It controls the activity of vestibulospinal tract.
  b. *Cerebelloreticular pathway-reticulospinal tract:* The vermal portion of spinocerebellum projects to pontine reticular formation through fastigial nucleus. From here the reticulospinal tract arises and through this tract cerebellum controls the anterior horn cells.
  c. *Paravermal portion* of spinocerebellum project to nucleus interpositus and this in turn projects to the red nucleus.

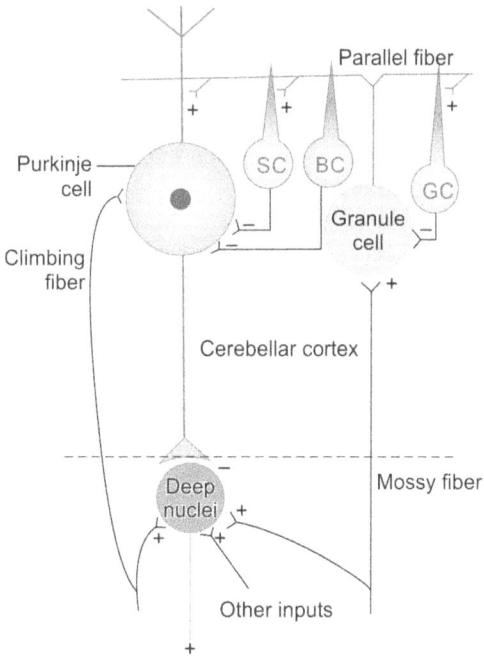

Fig. 9: Afferents to cerebellum through climbing and mossy fibers.
(SC: stellate cells; BC: basket cells; GC: Golgi cells; (−) inhibition; (+) stimulation)

Thereby cerebellum controls the rubrospinal tract.
  d. *Dentato-thalamo-cortical pathway:* Impulses from cerebrocerebellum end on dentate nucleus and from here it goes through thalamus and reaches motor cortex. From motor cortex corticospinal tract arises and ends on alpha motor neurons. Through this pathway cerebellum fine tunes the activity of corticospinal tract (*refer* **Fig. 10**).

Functions of Cerebellum

Control of Posture and Equilibrium

- Vestibulocerebellum or the flocculonodular lobe controls posture and equilibrium.
- It receives inputs from vestibular apparatus directly and also through vestibular nuclei about position of head and body.
- It sends efferents to vestibular nuclei from which the vestibulospinal tract arises to regulate posture.
- Vestibulocerebellum is also concerned with regulating vestibulo-ocular reflex.

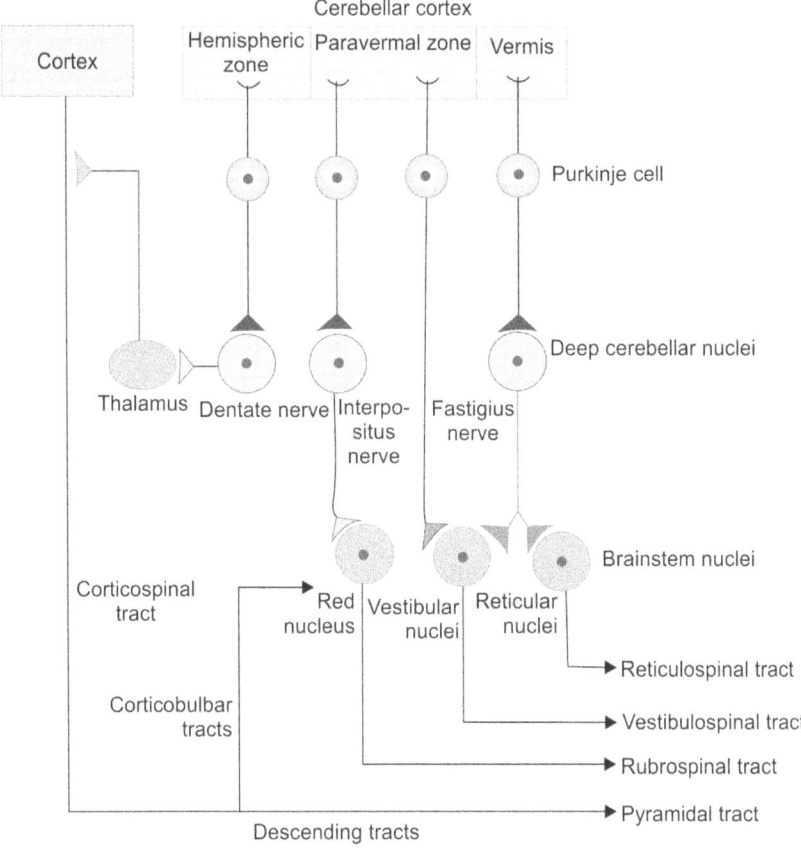

Fig. 10: Efferent connections from cerebellum through deep nuclei to brainstem.

Control of Muscle Tone and Stretch Reflex
- Spinocerebellum influences the muscle tone through its output via fastigial nucleus which in turn controls the vestibulospinal and reticulospinal tract (arising from pontine reticular formation).
- The major influence of cerebellum on tone is facilitatory.
- Vestibulospinal tract is facilitatory to α motor neurons and reticulospinal tract is facilitatory to γ motor neurons.
- Since control of cerebellum is on both α and γ motor neurons it has an important role in α-γ linkage.

Control of Voluntary Movements
- Paravermal portion of spinocerebellum controls skilled voluntary movements.
- It does not initiate movements but it coordinates voluntary movements.
- Coordination of movements is by regulating the time, rate, range, force and direction of movements.
- All three functional divisions of the cerebellum work together as "comparator of servomechanism".

Comparator servomechanism:
- Impulses for voluntary movements are planned and programmed in the premotor cortex and it is sequenced in primary motor area and the command to skeletal muscles is sent through the corticospinal tract.
- A copy of the plan or intended movement is also sent to the spinocerebellum.
- Cerebellum also gets feedback from the proprioceptors about the actual movement performed by the muscles and joints.
- It also receives other sensory inputs from eye, ear and vestibular apparatus.

- Now the cerebellum compares the intended movement and the executed movement along with other sensory inputs mentioned above.
- It thereby modifies appropriately the ongoing movement.
- If any corrections have to be done in programming of movements the error signals are sent to the motor cortex.

Control of Body Movements of One Side
- Motor cortex of one side is connected to opposite cerebellum through a closed feedback loop; cerebral-cerebellar-cerebral circuit, the cortico-ponto-dentato-thalamo-cortical pathway.
- So, each cerebellar hemisphere controls the opposite cerebral cortex.
- But the corticospinal tract descending down from the motor cortex decussates in medulla and controls the opposite side of the body.
- Since there is double decussation, it is that cerebellum controls same side of the body.

Planning and Programming of Movements
Cerebrocerebellum has extensive connections with motor cortex and therefore is involved in planning and programming of movements.

Learning of Skills
- Cerebellum always tends to make changes in ongoing movements and therefore it improves by learning.
- Another evidence is that there are increased activities in the climbing fibers when a new skill is learnt.
- So, cerebellum has a great role in learning skills.

Eyeball Movement
Pyramid of cerebellum is concerned with eyeball movement.

Signs of Cerebellar Lesions
- No paralysis
- No sensory deficits
- Deep reflexes not affected much except for pendular knee jerk
- Hypotonia
- All movements are characterized by ataxia.
- Ataxia: Defect in coordination due to errors in the rate, range, force and direction of movement.

It manifests as:
- Drunken gait
- Scanning speech
- Dysmetria
- Intention tremor
- Rebound phenomenon—pendular knee jerk
- Dysdiadochokinesia
- Decomposition of movements
- Nystagmus.

---

6. Describe the arterial blood pressure. Describe nervous regulation of arterial blood pressure.

BP is defined as the lateral pressure exerted by the moving column of blood on the vessel wall. Normal value = 120/80 mm Hg.

Components of BP:
- Systolic BP
- Diastolic BP
- Pulse pressure
- Mean arterial pressure

Neural Regulation of BP
- Regulation by autonomic nerves
- Regulation by medullary control centers
- Regulation by reflexes:
  - Baroreceptor reflex
  - Chemoreceptor reflex
  - CNS ischemic response

Regulation by Autonomic Nerves
- Blood vessels are supplied by sympathetic nerves.
- They are of two types—sympathetic vasoconstrictor and vasodilator fibers.
- Sympathetic VC fibers—in all blood vessels
- Sympathetic VD or cholinergic fibers—blood vessels of skeletal muscles, sweat glands and they originate from frontal

cortex to hypothalamus, midbrain medulla and end in the IML of SC.
- **Sympathetic stimulation results in:** Vaso- and venoconstriction, ↑ in HR and contractility and therefore the BP is increased.

Regulation by Medullary Control Centers
- There are two areas in the medulla which control the CVS.
- They are—vasomotor center (VMC) and cardiac vagal center (CVC).
- CVC—nucleus tractus solitarius, nucleus ambiguus
- Vagal center—dorsal motor nucleus of vagus.
- Stimulation of VMC—↑HR, contractility, vaso- and venoconstriction—↑BP and on inhibition vice versa.
- The final pathway from VMC is through sympathetic nerves to heart.
- Stimulation of CVC—↓HR, decreased vasoconstriction—↓BP.
- Final pathway is through vagus nerve to heart.
- There are inputs to VMC, from limbic centers through hypothalamus which are responsible for BP modulation in emotional states like anxiety (increase in BP and heart rate).

Reflex Regulation of BP
Baroreceptor reflex:

Baroreceptors:
- There are two types of baroreceptors (BRs). High pressure and low pressure baroreceptors.
- High pressure BRs are present in the carotid and aortic sinuses (*refer* **Fig. 11**).
- Low pressure BRs are present in the great veins, right and left atria.
- High pressure BRs are there to monitor and correct the day-to-day change in BP as in change of posture from supine to standing position.

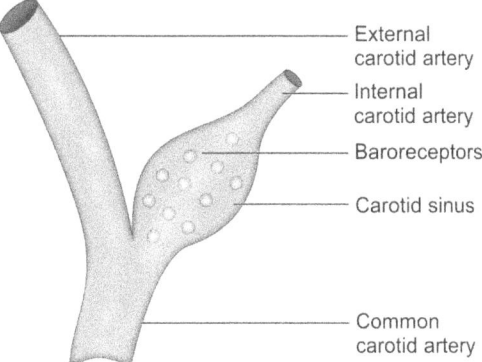

Fig. 11: Baroreceptor—carotid sinus.

- They regulate BP maximally when the MAP is between 70–110 mm Hg and stops firing when MAP falls <40 or rises above 150 mm Hg.

The reflex:
- Most important reflex to regulate BP
- Also called as sino-aortic reflex
- Receptor—carotid and aortic sinuses
- Stimulus—stretch of baroreceptors (as in increased BP)
- Afferents—IXth (supplies carotid sinus) and Xth cranial nerves (aortic sinus)
- Efferents—sympathetic nerves and vagus nerve
- Effector—heart and blood vessels
- Response—decrease in BP (*refer* **Figs. 12 and 13**).

Chemoreceptor reflex:
- Chemoreceptors are located in the carotid and aortic bodies.
- They sense the change in pO_2, pH and pCO_2 in arterial blood and stimulate respiration.
- They are supplied by IX and X cranial nerves.
- They usually project to respiratory centers and also to cardiovascular centers in medulla.
- They also send inputs to VMC and CVC and regulate BP.
- They are active within a range of 40–100 mm Hg MAP.

Decrease in BP MAP (40-100 mm Hg)
↓
Decreased blood flow to chemoreceptors
↓
Stimulation of chempreceptors
↓
Impulses carried through IXth and Xth cranial nerves to medulla

↓	↓	↓
Respiratory center	VMC	Cardiac vagal center (CVC)
↓	↓	↓
Hyperventilation, TC	Vasoconstriction, TC, Release of catecholamines	Bradycardia (BC)

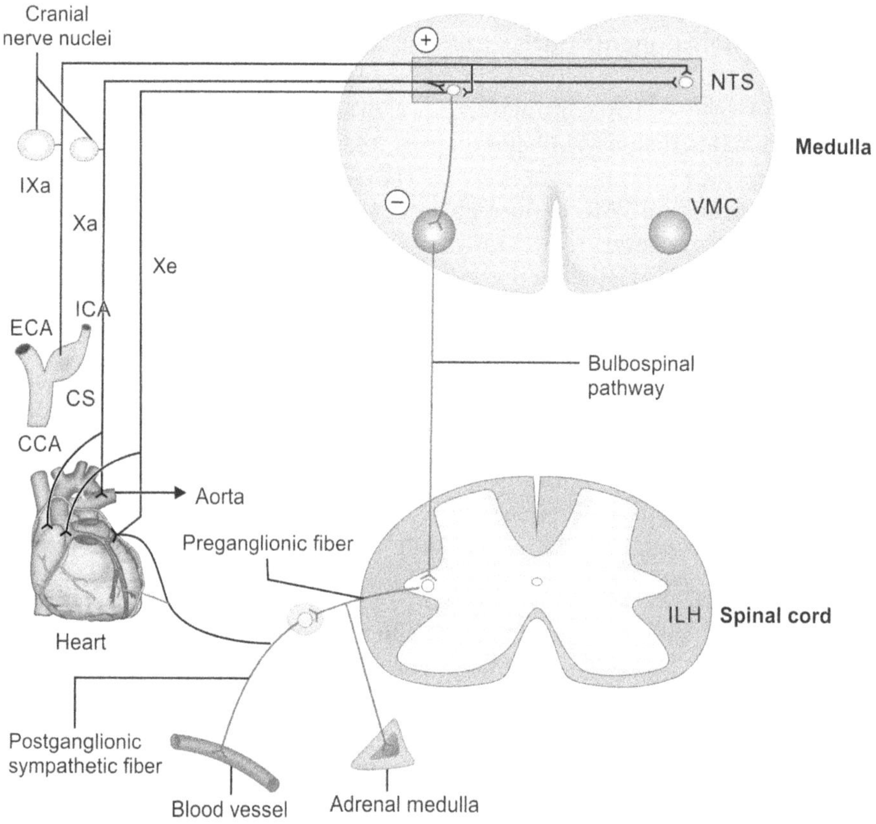

Fig. 12: Medullary cardiovascular centers and baroreceptor reflex pathway.
(CS: carotid sinus; CCA: common carotid artery; ECA: external carotid artery; Xa: afferents of vagus nerve; Xe: efferents of vagus nerve; IXa: afferents of glossopharyngeal nerve; VMC: vasomotor center; NTS: nucleus tractus solitarius; ILH: intermediolateral horn of spinal cord)

❏ The net effect is mild tachycardia and vasoconstriction → Increase in BP.

CNS ischemic response:
❏ It is activated when MAP falls below 40 mm Hg. It is said to be the "last ditch stand", the last effort put up by the body to try to correct the fall in BP.

Severe hypotension
↓
Decreased cerebral blood flow
↓

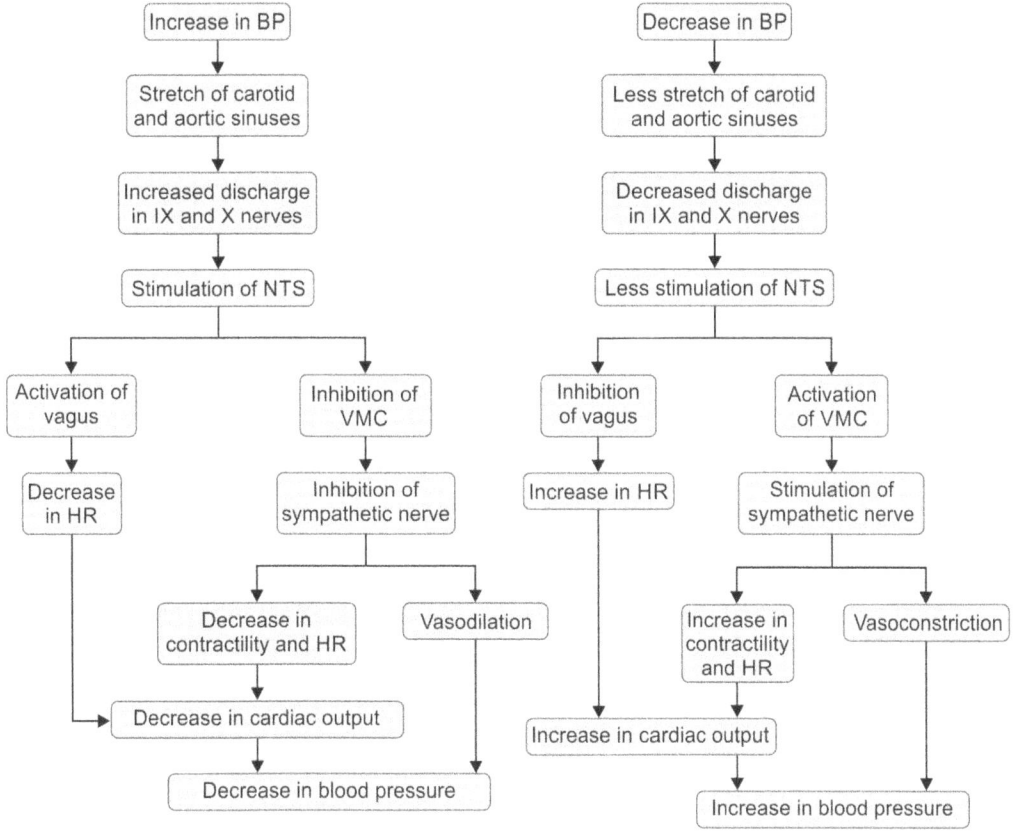

Fig. 13: Regulation of BP by baroreceptors.

Hypoxia and hypercapnia at VMC
↓
Strong stimulation of VMC
↓
Intense vasoconstriction
↓
↑BP

---

7. Discuss about transport of oxygen in blood. Draw and explain oxygen-hemoglobin dissociation curve. Add a note on significance of P50.

Transport of O_2

- O_2 is transported in blood in two forms.
- They are—dissolved form (2%) and as Oxy-Hb (98%)
- As O_2 enters the blood it gets saturated in plasma as dissolved O_2 and then there is a gradient between plasma and RBC → leads to entry of O_2 into RBC → as PO_2 increases inside the RBC, O_2 saturates Hb.

Dissolved O_2

- Dissolved O_2 is measured by the following equation.
- Dissolved O_2 = solubility of O_2 (0.003 mL/mm Hg) × arterial PO_2 (100 mm Hg) = 0.3 mL/dL
- Partial pressure of O_2 (PO_2) in blood is decided by the dissolved O_2 content of blood.

Oxy-hemoglobin

- Hemoglobin is an O_2 carrying protein in RBC.
- It increases the O_2 carrying capacity of blood by 70 times.
- Iron in the Hb is in ferrous form (Fe^{2+}) and combines with O_2 in appropriate affinity.
- O_2 + Hb ↔ HbO_2—oxygenation reaction **(it is not oxidation reaction)**
- If Fe^{2+} gets oxidized to Fe^{3+} methemoglobin is formed which does not release O_2.

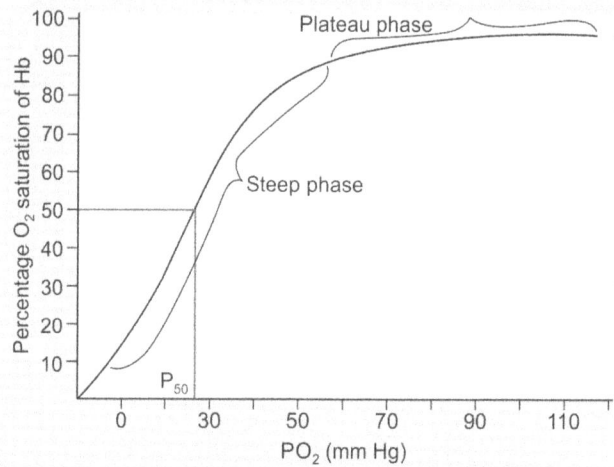

Fig. 14: Oxygen-hemoglobin dissociation curve.

- When the binding of O_2 with hemoglobin happens, affinity of Hb for O_2 increases gradually.
- Initially, Hb is in a tense configuration (T), as one molecule of O_2 combines, the Hb changes to relaxed configuration (R) and the affinity to O_2 increases to maximum when the 3rd O_2 molecule has combined.

O_2 Carrying Capacity of Blood

- Each gram of Hb carries 1.34 mL of O_2.
- Maximum amount of O_2 carried by Hb is the **O_2 carrying capacity of blood**.
- In a healthy individual, it is 20 mL/100 mL of blood (15 × 1.34 mL = 20.1 mL/dL).
- **O_2 content** is the amount actually bound to Hb.
- **% saturation of O_2 (SO_2)** = HbO_2 content/ HbO_2 capacity × 100.
- Normally in arterial blood % SO_2 is 98%.

O_2-Hb Dissociation Curve

- This curve compares the partial pressure of O_2 and % saturation of Hb with O_2.
- It is sigmoid in shape.
- The shape is sigmoid because of the change in configuration of hemoglobin from T to R state and therefore there is gradual increase in affinity for O_2 and then it gets saturated.
- It has a steep and plateau phase.
- 90% saturation of Hb takes place at a PO_2 of 60 mm Hg.
- P_{50} is the partial pressure at which 50% of the hemoglobin is saturated with oxygen.
- P_{50} is inversely related to the affinity of hemoglobin for oxygen.
- The steep phase denotes the unloading zone where even a minimum drop in PO_2 results in unloading of large amounts of oxygen to the tissues.
- The plateau phase denotes the loading zone, where O_2 is taken up by hemoglobin in the lungs and once all the four sites in Hb are loaded with O_2 there is no further uptake and thereby a plateau phase is reached (*refer* **Fig. 14**).
- The curve gets shifted to right are left in conditions of decreased or increase in affinity of hemoglobin for O_2 respectively.

Conditions where O_2-Hb dissociation curve is shifted to right:
- Hypoxia
- ↑PCO_2
- ↑temperature
- ↑2,3-DPG levels in RBC
- ↑H^+ concentration (acidosis)

Conditions where O_2-Hb dissociation curve is shifted to left:
- High PO_2
- Low PCO_2
- Low body temperature
- Presence of fetal hemoglobin
- Alkalosis

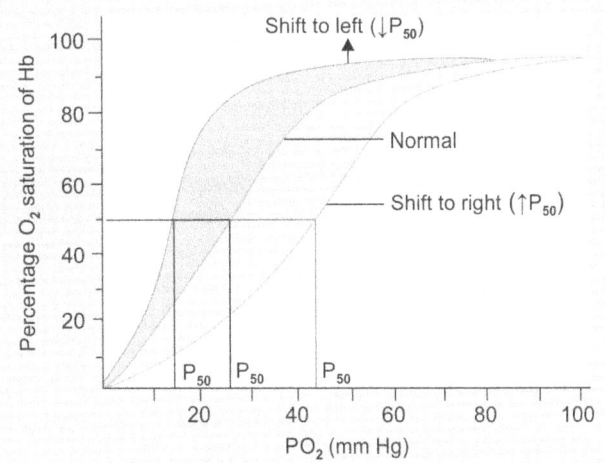

Fig. 15: Right and left shift of O_2-Hb dissociation curve. P_{50}, PO_2 at which hemoglobin is 50% saturated is 27 mm Hg.

- Low 2,3-DPG levels in RBC
- Carbon monoxide poisoning (*refer* **Fig. 15**).

8. Enumerate the ascending tracts of spinal cord. Explain in detail the pathway for pain. Add a note on analgesic system.

The ascending tracts in the spinal cord are:
- Dorsal column—fasciculus gracilis and fasciculus cuneatus
- Spinothalamic tracts—lateral and anterior spinothalamic tracts
- Spinocerebellar tracts—dorsal and ventral spinocerebellar tracts
- Spino-tectal tract
- Spino-olivary tract
- Spino-vestibular tract
- Spino-reticular tract.

Pain Pathway
- Pain sensation is carried by the lateral spinothalamic tract (LSTT).
- There are two types of pain—fast pain and slow pain.
- So, the LSTT has fibers for fast pain and for slow pain. There are separate pathways for fast and slow pain.

Fast Pain
- Fast pain is sensed by the free nerve endings of Aδ fibers.
- The pain sensation from periphery is carried through the Aδ fibers.
- Their cell bodies are present in the dorsal root ganglion.
- The fibers on entering spinal cord terminate on cells in laminae I and V of the dorsal grey horn.
- These are the second order neurons. Neurotransmitter released here is **glutamate**.
- Second order neurons cross to the opposite side and ascend up as **neospinothalamic tract** in the anterolateral column of spinal cord.
- Neospinothalamic tract reaches thalamus and ends on the ventral posterolateral nucleus of the thalamus (VPLN).
- The tract on its way to thalamus gives a few branches to periaqueductal grey (PAG) in midbrain.
- The third order neurons start from thalamus and reach somatosensory area I.
- This pathway is concerned with localization and interpretation of pain.

Slow Pain
- Slow pain is sensed by the free nerve endings of unmyelinated C fibers.
- Slow pain is carried by the same fibers to spinal cord and they terminate in the laminae II and III of dorsal grey horn.
- This is the first order neuron. The neurotransmitter released here is **substance-P**.

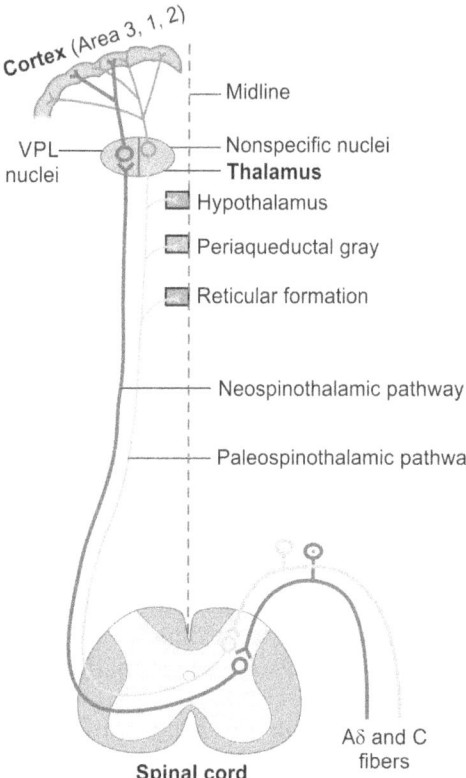

Fig. 16: Neospinothalamic and paleospinothalamic tracts.

- The second order neuron arises from laminae I and V and the fibers cross to the opposite side and ascends up as **paleospinothalamic tract** (*refer* **Fig. 16**).
- It ascends up along with neospinothalamic tract in the anterolateral column of spinal cord.
- This tract gives many fibers to PAG, Reticular formation and tectum.
- It then ends in the non-specific nucleus of thalamus.
- Third order neuron arises from here and is projected to entire cerebral cortex.
- This pathway is concerned with alertness, arousal and perception of pain rather than localisation of pain.

Analgesic System in the Brain

Pain modulation takes place in two places:
1. At the peripheral nerve endings
2. At the spinal cord level

Peripheral nerve endings:
Endorphins and enkephalins combine with nociceptors and decrease the response to stimuli.

At the spinal cord:
- **Peripheral mechanism: By gate control theory**—large Aβ fibers (when stimulated by touching or rubbing the painful area) ↓ nociception in C fibers.
- **Central pain suppressing mechanism:** Opioids secreted from areas in brain stem inhibit pain transmission in the spinal cord.

Gate control mechanism:
- Pain sensation is carried by Aδ and unmyelinated C fibers and they ascend up as spinothalamic tract.
- Touch and pressure sensations are carried by large myelinated Aβ fibers and they ascend up as dorsal column tract in spinal cord.
- Dorsal column fibers in the spinal cord give a branch to inhibitory interneurons which secrete enkephalins and which in turn end on the second order neurons in pain pathway.
- So, when there is pain in an area, touching or pressing that region stimulates the large Aβ fibers which in turn inhibit pain pathway and thereby there is decreased pain perception.
- So the large Aβ fibers gate the pain pathway.

Central pain suppressing mechanism:
- Pain pathway, as it ascends up gives branches to periaqueductal grey (PAG) in the midbrain.
- There is a pain suppressing descending pathway from PAG to medulla and to spinal cord.
- Axons of the neurons in PAG terminate on serotonergic neurons in raphe magnus nuclei in medulla.
- They secrete enkephalin here.
- Axons of serotonergic neurons in raphe magnus nuclei descend and terminate on the inhibitory interneurons in spinal cord (*refer* **Fig. 17**).
- They secrete serotonin and stimulate internuncial neurons which in turn inhibit

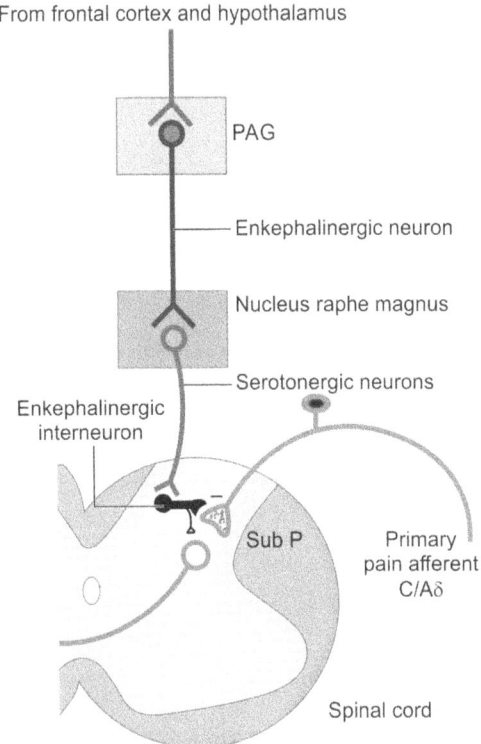

Fig. 17: Endogenous pain inhibition by spinal cord and brainstem structures.

second order neurons in the pain pathway by secreting enkephalin.

II. SHORT NOTES

1. Classify the fluid compartments of body giving their normal values, mention two methods to determine ECF volume.

Total body water is classified in two compartments:
- *Extracellular space:* Extracellular fluid—14 L (20% of body weight).
- *Intracellular space:* Intracellular fluid—28 L (40% of body weight).

Extracellular fluid is distributed as:
- Interstitial fluid—fluid present in between cells
- Intravascular—plasma
- Transcellular fluid—CSF, ocular fluid, peritoneal and pleural fluids, synovial fluid, ocular fluid, GIT secretion.
- Lymph—flows in the lymphatic channels.

Determination of ECF volume:
- ECF volume is measured by the indicator dilution technique.
- Substances used to measure ECF volume should remain only in the ECF. The substances used are inulin, mannitol, sucrose, sulfate, thiosulfate and thiocyanate.

Indicator dilution technique:
- A known volume of the substance (inulin) is injected into the blood. After sometime when the substance has uniformly distributed in the space, a sample of blood is taken and the concentration of substance in the blood is estimated using this formula:

$$\text{ECF volume} = \frac{\text{Amount of substance injected} - \text{amount excreted}}{\text{Average concentration of the substance}}$$

$$= \frac{150 \text{ mg} - 10 \text{ mg}}{1.01 \text{ mg/mL}}$$

$$= 14000 \text{ mL}$$

Similarly radioactive inulin can be used to measure ECF volume. It is done easily by counting the sample with radiation detectors.

2. Transport across cell membrane.

- The cell membrane, being a semi-permeable one, does not allow all substances to pass through it.
- It is easier for lipids and lipid soluble substances to pass through the bilipid layer.
- Water and water-soluble substances need channels/carriers to be transported across the membrane.
- Substances on either side of the membrane differ in their concentrations also, therefore they either move along the gradients or against the gradients.

So transport across the cell membrane is classified as:
- Active transport (*refer* **Fig. 18**)
- Passive transport
- Vesicle-mediated transport

```
                    Transport across membranes
                              │
            ┌─────────────────┴─────────────────┐
       Active transport                   Passive transport
            │                                   │
      ┌─────┴─────┐              ┌──────────────┼──────────────┐
   Secondary   Primary      Simple diffusion              Facilitated diffusion
            │                         │                        │
   Vesicle mediated    Solublizes in lipid—O₂, CO₂     Through channels
      │                                                        │
   ┌──┴───┐                                            ┌───────┴───────┐
Exocytosis Endocytosis                               Gated          Non-gated
                                                       │
                                    ┌──────────────────┼──────────────────┐
                              Voltage-gated       Ligand-gated     Mechanically-gated
                                                       │
                                                Carrier mediated
                                                       │
                                    ┌──────────────────┴──────────────────┐
                          Moves a single molecule            Transport 2 molecules in
                          in one direction (GLUT)            opposite directions (band)
                                (Uniport)                          (Anteport)
```

Fig. 18: Classification of transport across cell membrane.
(GLUT: glucose transporter)

Passive Transport

Here the movement of substances is along the concentration or electrical gradient and there is no energy expenditure.

Types:
1. Simple diffusion
2. Facilitated diffusion
3. Osmosis
4. Filtration
5. Bulk flow
6. Solvent drag

Simple Diffusion

- **Lipid soluble** substances diffuse by dissolving in the membrane and diffuse to either side of membrane—O_2, N_2, steroids, etc. (*refer* **Fig. 19**).
- **Water soluble** substances move through water filled channel proteins.
- No energy expenditure.
- Moves substances along concentration gradient.

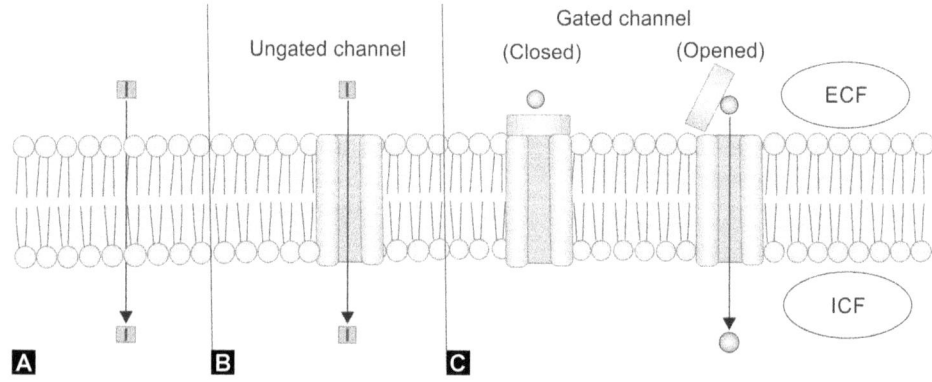

Figs. 19A to C: (A) Simple diffusion through lipid membrane; (B) simple diffusion through non-gated channels; (C) diffusion through gated channels.

Diffusion Through Channels

- Channels are water-filled pores.
- This allows water soluble substances to move across the membrane.
- The channels have selective permeability.
- They may be gated or non-gated
- Gates could be either change in—voltage, binding ligands or stretch (mechanical).

Factors Affecting Net Diffusion

- **Cell membrane permeability**
  - Thickness of membrane—inversely proportional
  - Lipid solubility—directly proportional
  - Distribution of protein channels in membrane
  - Temperature—directly proportional
  - Size of molecule—inversely proportional
  - Area of membrane—directly proportional.
- Concentration gradient—directly proportional
- Electrical gradient
- Pressure gradient—directly proportional.

Facilitated Diffusion

- Large water-soluble substances (e.g., glucose) are carried by a protein which changes configuration on binding (*refer* **Fig. 20**).
- This change in configuration shifts the molecule in or out.

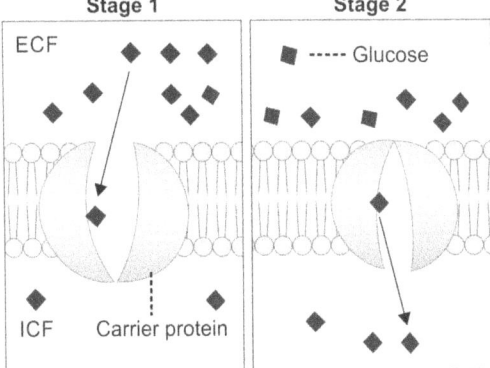

Fig. 20: Facilitated diffusion. A uniport transporting glucose molecules.

- Highly selective and specific.
- **Types:**
  - Uniport
  - Symport
  - Antiport
- **Characteristics:**
  - Specificity
  - Saturation
  - Competition

Osmosis

Diffusion of water or other solvent molecules through a semi-permeable membrane (i.e., membrane impermeable to solute and not to solvent) from a solution containing lower concentration of solutes to the solution containing higher concentration of solutes—**osmosis**.

Filtration and Bulk Flow

Filtration or movement of water and solutes through the capillary wall are examples of filtration.

If filtration involves movement of greater volume of water it is called bulk flow.

Solvent Drag

During bulk flow if solvents are carried along—solvent drag.

Active Transport

- It is also carrier mediated
- Moves substances uphill against concentration gradient.
- So associated with energy expenditure. Energy is derived from ATP, either directly or indirectly
- **Types:**
  - Primary active transport
  - Secondary active transport

Primary Active Transport

Here substances are moved uphill across the cell membrane with the help of pumps. It involves energy expenditure which is directly derived from break down of ATP.

Ex.
- $Na^+ K^+$ Pump
- $H^+ K^+$ Pump
- Ca^{++} ATPase

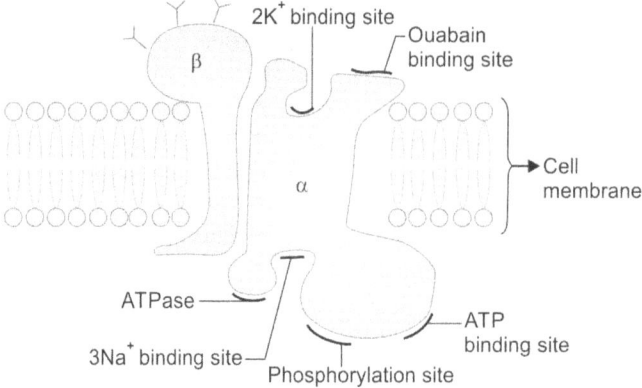

Fig. 21: Sodium-potassium pump; primary active transporter.

Na+- K+ Pump:

Sodium potassium ATPase is a ubiquitous pump. It pumps out three Na+ molecules from the cell in exchange for two K+ molecules into the cell. Na+ concentration is more in the ECF and K+ concentration is more in the ICF. So, both the ions are pumped against their concentration gradients out and in of the cell respectively. The pump is present in all the cells to maintain the cell volume and to maintain the membrane potential (*refer* **Fig. 21**).

Secondary Active Transport

In the secondary active transport, the substances are moved against the concentration gradient with the help of energy derived indirectly from the ATP. Na+-K+ pump, when it pumps out Na+ from the cell, creates a concentration gradient for Na+ into the cell. This gradient for Na+ is utilized for movement of other ions across the cell membrane. So the transporters of secondary active transport moves Na+ in exchange (sodium counter- transporter) or along (sodium cotransporter) with another molecule (both organic and inorganic substances) (*refer* **Fig. 22**).

Example:
- Na+-glucose symport
- Na+-amino acid symport
- Na+-H+ exchanger
- Na+-Ca+ exchanger

Vesicle-mediated Transport
- Large polar molecules—like protein hormones in endocrine glands are transported across the cell as membrane wrapped vesicles.
- **Types:**
  - Endocytosis
  - Exocytosis

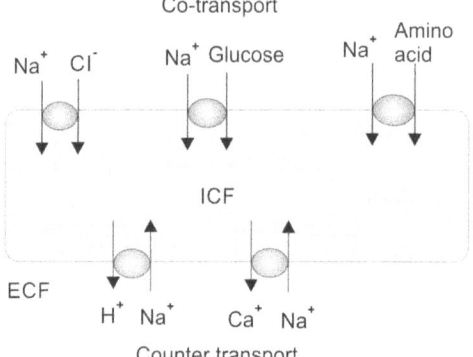

Fig. 22: Secondary active transporters; Na+-glucose symporter, Na+- amino acid symport, Na+-H+ exchanger, Na+- Ca2+ exchanger.

Endocytosis

It is the process by which substances are internalized within the cell. There are three types:
1. Phagocytosis
2. Pinocytosis
3. Receptor mediated endocytosis
1. **Phagocytosis:** Engulfing of solid substances (Cell eating) as that of microorganisms by the neutrophils (*refer* **Fig. 23**).
2. **Pinocytosis:** Engulfing the liquid components (cell drinking).

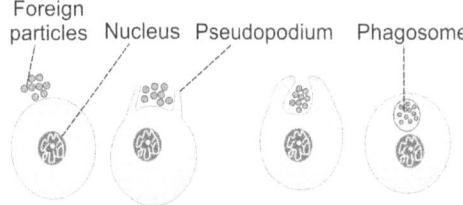

Fig. 23: Process of endocytosis.

3. **Receptor-mediated endocytosis:** Here the substances to be internalized get attached to a receptor protein present on the cell membrane and the whole complex is engulfed.

Exocytosis

It is the process by which substance are extruded from the cell. It is the reversal of endocytosis. The substances to be extruded are in the vesicle which moves towards the cell membrane and gets attached to the membrane and is later pinched out of the cell.

---

3. Structure and functions of neuromuscular junction.

It is the junction between the motor neuron and the muscle fiber it supplies.

Structure of NMJ

☐ The NMJ is formed by the axon terminal of the motor neuron.
☐ On approaching the muscle fiber, the axon it loses its myelin sheath and divides into many branches and the nerve terminals bulge to form the terminal buttons which approaches the muscle fiber at its center.
☐ NMJ has a presynaptic membrane, Synaptic cleft and postsynaptic membrane (*refer* **Fig. 24**).

Presynaptic Terminal

☐ It is the membrane of the terminal button of the axon.
☐ It has many ACh vesicles and mitochondria within the membrane.
☐ The membrane is studded with many Voltage-gated Ca^{2+} channels.

Synaptic Cleft

☐ It is a space of 50-100 nm width between the presynaptic and postsynaptic membranes.

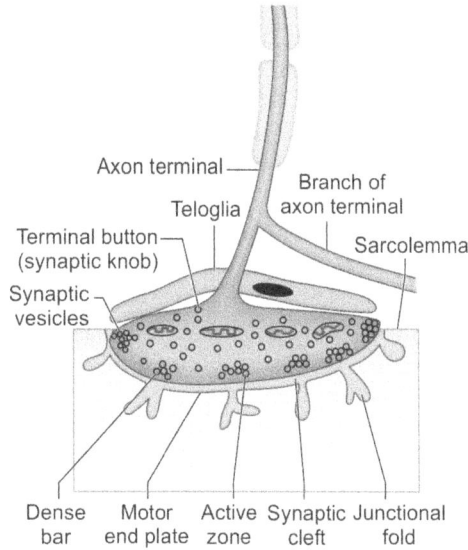

Fig. 24: Neuromuscular junction.

☐ It has ECF in it and acetylcholinesterase enzyme is present in it.

Postsynaptic Membrane

☐ It is the muscle membrane in contact with the nerve terminal and it is thrown into many folds—junctional folds and is thickened and deepened—synaptic trough.
☐ The muscle membrane here is called as the motor end plate.
☐ It contains the nicotinic acetylcholine receptors.

Impulse Transmission in NMJ

Stimulation of nerve fiber
↓
AP generated in nerve fiber
↓
Conduction of AP in nerve fiber
↓
Impulse reaches nerve terminal
↓
Voltage-gated Ca^{2+} channels in nerve terminal open
↓
Ca^{2+} influx into presynaptic membrane
↓
Exocytosis of ACh vesicles and ACh is released into synaptic cleft
↓

ACh moves across the cleft and binds to nicotinic ACh receptors in muscle membrane
↓
The receptor is a non-specific cation channel which opens on binding with ACh
↓
Influx of Na⁺ ions into postsynaptic membrane
↓
Local depolarization of muscle membrane— end plate potential
↓
Generation of action potential in the neighboring muscle membrane by the EPP

4. Tissue macrophage system.

- Monocytes are formed in the bone marrow. They circulate in blood for 10-20 hours.
- They are the largest blood cells, 12-20 μm in size (2-2.5 times the size of RBCs).
- Nucleus occupies almost 50% of the cell volume and the rest is the cytoplasm. The granules in cytoplasm do not take the regular staining and therefore not visible. So is an agranulocyte.
- Monocytes after circulation, enter various tissues through the capillary membrane and swell up to become the **macrophage**.
- They live for months to years as a tissue macrophage.
- They exist as either fixed macrophages or mobile macrophage.
- The monocytes, macrophages and specialized endothelial cells in bone marrow, spleen and lymph nodes are grouped as **reticuloendothelial system**.
- They are destroyed once their phagocytic action is over.
- Tissue macrophages are named according to the sites where they are present.

Following are the Tissue Macrophages

- **Pulmonary alveolar macrophage (PAM):** The PAMs are present in the walls of the alveolus. It is one of the routes of entry of microbes from the environment. Macrophages phagocytose the micro-organisms and if possible, digests them and release them into the lymph.
- **Kupffer cells in the liver sinusoids:** The other route of entry for microorganisms is through GIT. Bacteria absorbed from ingested food enters the portal circulation and reaches the liver and are phagocytosed and destroyed by kupffer cells lining the sinusoids.
- **Macrophages in the spleen and bone marrow:** Trabeculae of red pulp and sinuses of the spleen are lined by macrophages and they are very narrow passages and when blood squeezes through this path, unwanted debris and older cells like senile RBCs are phagocytosed and removed by the macrophages.

  In the bone marrow also there are macrophages to take care of micro organisms that enter through other routes of entry into the body.
- **Tissue macrophages in skin and subcutaneous tissues (histiocytes):** Normally skin forms a protective barrier to prevent entry of microorganisms, but in case of breakage of the protective skin barrier infections may enter and they are taken care by the skin macrophages.
- **Macrophages in lymph nodes:** There are macrophages in lymph nodes also.
- **Osteoclasts:** Osteoclasts also belong to the family of monocytes and when they come in contact with stromal cells of bone marrow, they get converted to osteoclasts and they erode the bone and help in its remodeling.
- **Microglia:** Microglia is a type of neuroglial cell and it belongs to the monocyte family and they have the property of scavenging foreign particles in the nervous system.

Functions of Monocyte-macrophage System

- Active phagocytosis, they are the second line of defence.
- They enter tissues to become macrophages. They are given different names in various tissues—kupffer cells in liver, PAM in lungs, etc.
- They also take part in immune response (as APCs).

- They synthesize many substances like IL1, TNF-α, lysozyme, proteases, etc.
- They also help in healing and repair of tissue.

5. Non-excretory functions of kidney.

- **Regulation of ECF volume:** Kidney is the major organ involved in the regulation of ECF volume. It is through the action of the hormones ADH, aldosterone, angiotensin II and ANP.
- **Regulation of plasma osmolality:** Changes in the plasma osmolality are sensed by the osmoreceptors present in hypothalamus and they stimulate or inhibit the secretion of ADH and thereby regulate the plasma osmolality at 290 mosm/L.
- **Regulation of blood pressure:** Kidneys play a major role in regulation of blood pressure through regulation of ECF volume by direct mechanism through regulation of GFR and tubular actions. It also regulates BP by indirect mechanism through actions of renin, angiotensin II and aldosterone.
- **Regulation of acid-base balance:** Kidneys play a major role in regulation of acid-base balance. This done by three mechanisms— reabsorption of HCO_3^-, secretion of H^+ and generation of new HCO_3^-.
- **Regulation of electrolytes in plasma:** Tubular reabsorption and secretion of electrolytes play a major role in regulating the serum electrolyte levels.
- **Endocrine functions of kidneys:** Kidneys secrete the following hormones:
  - *Erythropoietin:* It is secreted by the interstitial cells in the peritubular capillary bed in response to hypoxia. Thereby kidneys have a major role in regulation of erythropoiesis. In chronic renal failure the patients suffer from anemia.
  - *Renin:* It is a hormone secreted by the juxtaglomerular cells in response to decrease in ECF Volume or blood pressure. Renin activates the angiotensin system and thereby corrects the ECF volume and BP.
  - *Calcitriol:* Along with the skin and liver, kidneys synthesize 1,25 dihydroxy cholecalciferol.
- **Gluconeogenesis:** It happens in conditions of prolonged fasting.

6. Cystometrogram and its significance.

- Smooth muscles which make up the urinary bladder show the property of plasticity, a property when a muscle is stretched, the tension initially developed is not maintained. So, there is no length-tension relationship in the bladder wall muscle.
- A study is done to assess the relation between the intravesicular pressure and intravesicular volume. The bladder is catheterized and fully emptied. Then volumes of fluid in increments of 50 mL are filled into the bladder through the catheter. This test is said to be the *cystometry* (*refer* **Fig. 25**).
- A graph is plotted relating the intravesicular volume and intravesicular pressure, this is the cystometrogram.
- There are three components in this graph—Ia, Ib and II.
  - **Ia:** There is an initial rise in the pressure of 10 cm of H_2O when the bladder is filled with the first 100 mL of fluid.
  - **Ib:** Further increments of fluid up to 300–400 mL produces not much rise in the pressure and a flat segment is seen in the cystometrogram. This segment is said to follow the Law of Laplace which states that the distending pressure (P) in a spherical viscus is equal to twice wall tension (T) divided by the radius (r). P = 2T/r. As the bladder gets filled, the wall tension increases, so does the radius of the bladder and therefore the pressure increase is less till the organ is full.
  - **II:** As the volume in the bladder reaches 400 mL there is a sharp rise in the pressure resulting in initiation of the micturition reflex.
- Beyond 600 mL, the urge to empty the bladder is unbearable.

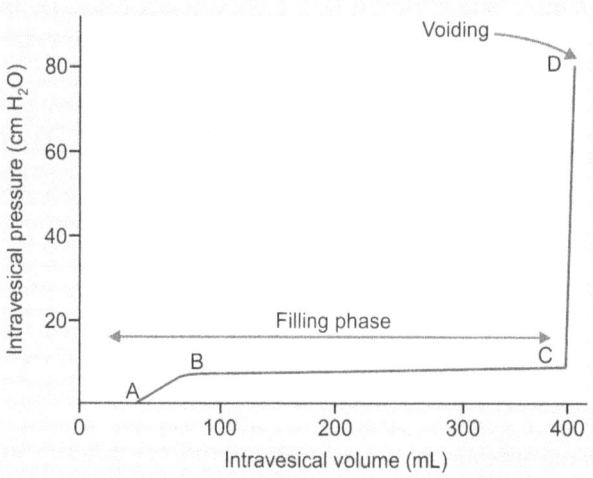

Fig. 25: Cystometrogram, Phases 1a (mild increase in pressure when 100 mL of water is infused into bladder), Phase 1b (not much rise in pressure from 100–400 mL intra-vesicular volume) and Phase II (steep rise in pressure when intra-vesicular volume reaches 400 mL and stimulates micturition reflex).

---

7. Secretion of HCl in stomach and its regulation.

Composition of Gastric Juice

- 2–2.5 L/day
- pH 1–2
- **Water:** 99.45%
- **Solids:** 0.55%
- **Electrolytes:** Na^+, K^+, Mg^{2+}, Cl^-, HCO_3^-, HpO_4^-, SO_4^-
- **Enzymes:** Pepsin, lipase, gelatinase
- **Mucus:** Insoluble and soluble
- **Intrinsic factor.**

Mechanism of HCl Secretion

- In stomach, hydrochloric acid is secreted by the Parietal cells which are present in the main gastric glands in body of the stomach.
- Pure secretion from the parietal cell has a pH of 0.82 and is isotonic (150 mEq of H^+ and 150 mEq of Cl^+).
- Parietal cell is polarized with an apical side facing the lumen and a basolateral side facing the interstitium.
- There are many tubulovesicular structures in the parietal cell which are studded with H^+-K^+ ATPase which pump H^+ into the lumen in exchange for K^+.
- These cells are highly metabolizing and they put out lot of CO_2. The cell is also rich in the enzyme carbonic anhydrase (*refer* Fig. 26).

HCl secretion from the parietal cells happens in two steps:

1. Secretion of H^+ into the lumen
2. Secretion of Cl into the lumen.

The steps involved in HCl secretion are:

1. CO_2 in the cell is hydrated in the presence of Carbonic anhydrase, $CO_2 + H_2O \rightarrow H_2CO_3$
2. $H_2CO_3 \rightarrow H^+ + HCO_3^-$
3. The H^+ is pumped into the lumen by the H^+K^+ ATPase pump on the apical side.

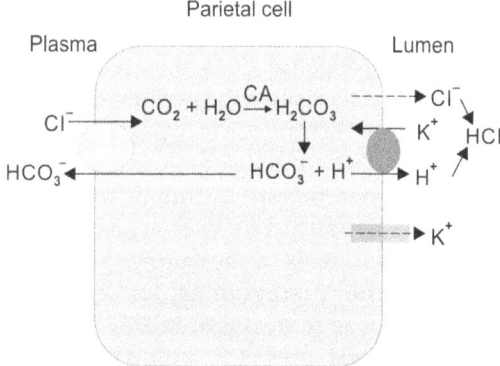

Fig. 26: Mechanism of HCl secretion.
(CA: carbonic anhydrase)

For one H⁺ pumped out of cell one K⁺ is taken into the cell which later diffuses back into the lumen
4. HCO_3^- is extruded in the basolateral side through an anion exchanger in exchange for one Cl⁻.
5. The Cl⁻ which enters the cell will diffuse across the apical membrane into the lumen.
6. So, for every H⁺ secreted, one Cl⁻ is also secreted into the lumen and one HCO_3^- is absorbed into the blood.

So, when gastric secretion is increased after a meal, the HCO_3^- getting added to the blood is increased, thereby raising the pH of blood—*postprandial alkaline tide*.

Regulation of Gastric Secretion

Neural, humoral and reflex regulation of secretion (*refer* **Fig. 27**).

Factors that Stimulate
1. Vagus nerve
2. Gastrin
3. Histamine

Factors that Inhibit
1. Low pH in the stomach
2. Somatostatin
3. Prostaglandin E2

Regulation is Discussed in Terms of:
❒ Cephalic phase
❒ Gastric phase
❒ Intestinal phase

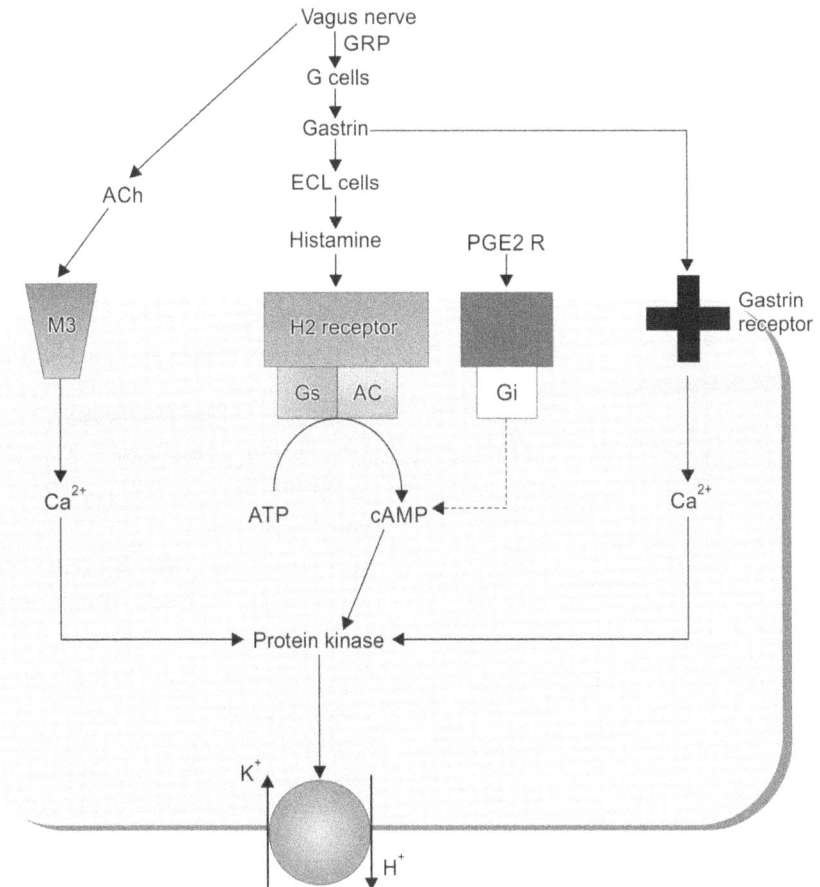

Fig. 27: Parietal cell with the regulating factors for HCl secretion.
(ACh: acetylcholine, ECL cells: enterochromaffin-like cells; GRP: gastrin releasing peptide; M3: muscarinic receptor; PGE2R: prostaglandin E2 receptor; Gs: G protein; AC: adenylyl cyclase; Gi: G protein)

Cephalic Phase
- Nearly 500 mL/hr (45% of total secretion)
- Initiated by thought, sight, smell, taste of food through vagus nerve.
- Emotions also affect secretion (refer **Fig. 28**).

Gastric Phase
50% of total secretion. Food in stomach induces secretion by:
- Distension of body of stomach (through reflexes—vagal reflex)
- Distension of antrum (through gastrin secretion)
- By-products of partial digestion of protein (through gastrin secretion).

Intestinal Phase
- It begins when chyme enters the intestine.
- Intestinal influence is inhibitory by:
  - Enterogastric reflex—by distension, presence of acid and products of digestion—inhibits secretion.
  - Hormonal mechanism—CCK, secretin, GIP, neurotensin, etc.—enterogastrone.

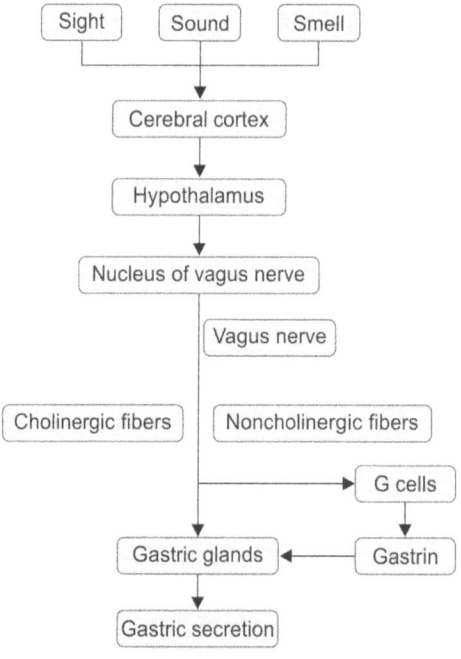

Fig. 28: Cephalic phase of regulation of HCl secretion. This phase of gastric secretion is regulated through vagus nerve.

8. Regulations of blood calcium levels.
- Normal plasma concentration of calcium is 10 mg/dL (5 mEq/L or 2.5 mmol/L). Plasm calcium is in bound form (non-diffusible) and in ionic and complexed form (diffusible)
- 99% of the body calcium is present in the bones. In the bone calcium pool is of two types—readily exchangeable reservoir and a stable pool.
- Calcium has various actions in the; acts as a second messenger, needed for muscle contraction, for coagulation.
- All these actions are done by ionic calcium. It is very important to regulate the ECF calcium levels as hypocalcemia increases neuromuscular excitability and may lead to tetany.
- In tetany the skeletal muscles go in for spasm and laryngospasm may lead to fatal asphyxia. So, the calcium levels are needed to be regulated.
- There are three hormones regulating blood calcium levels.

The hormones involved in calcium homeostasis are:
- Parathormone
- 1,25-Dihydroxycholecalciferol or calcitriol
- Calcitonin
- Parathormone and calcitriol increase serum calcium levels and calcitonin decreases calcium levels.
- Calcium homeostasis is done by these hormones.

Parathormone
The main actions of PTH are to increase blood calcium levels and decrease phosphate levels.

Effect on Bones
- It increases activity of both osteoclasts and osteoblasts.
- But the osteoclastic activity is the major effect resulting in resorption of bone and release of calcium and phosphates into the ECF.
- PTH stimulates the differentiation of precursors into osteoclasts, increases their numbers and size. The products of resorption are present in blood and are excreted in urine.

- **Action on osteoclasts:** This effect comes into action after a few days of exposure to PTH. The number and activity of osteoclasts are increased. Osteoclasts increase bone resorption and thereby increases calcium and phosphate levels in the blood. Also, levels of hydroxyproline and hydroxylysine are increased.
- **Action on osteoblasts:** At low doses PTH increases osteoblastic activity but in high doses it inhibits action of osteoblasts.

Action on Kidneys

There are three major actions on the kidneys:
1. Increased reabsorption of calcium in the Thick ascending limb of loop of Henle and DCT.
2. Decreases reabsorption of phosphate in the kidneys by its action on the PCT and induces phosphaturia. Serum phosphate levels are lowered by the action of PTH.
3. Stimulates the formation of 1,25-dihydroxycholecalciferol (calcitriol) by the kidneys. Calcitriol in turn increases reabsorption of calcium from GIT and kidneys.

Calcitriol

Calcitriol is the active form of vitamin D_3 and is also called as 1, 25 dihydroxycholecalciferol.

Actions of Calcitriol

- **Action on GIT:** It increases absorption of calcium from the GIT by increasing its permeability of brush border of the enterocytes. It also increases synthesis of Calbindin, a calcium binding protein in enterocytes.
- **Actions on bones:** It induces bone resorption and mineralization. In presence of PTH, calcitriol induces bone resorption.
- **Action on kidneys:** It increases reabsorption of calcium and phosphates from the renal tubules.

Calcitonin

- It is synthesized by the C cells or parafollicular cells in thyroid gland.
- It is also neural in origin.
- It is polypeptide in nature.
- It is secreted in response to increase in serum calcium levels.

Actions of Calcitonin

- It lowers circulating calcium and phosphate levels. Calcium is lowered by inhibition of bone resorption. It also inhibits activity of osteoclasts in vitro.
- It also increases calcium excretion via urine.
- It helps in bone development in young individuals.
- It protects against postprandial hypercalcemia.
- It protects the bones of mother from excess calcium loss during pregnancy.
- The process of formation of mature sperm is called spermatogenesis.

9. Spermatogenesis and seminal analysis.

Spermatogenesis

- It takes place in the seminiferous tubule. It happens in the wall of the tubule from basal lamina towards the lumen.
- The immature cells are present in the basal aspect of the tubule and the maturing cells move toward the adluminal compartment.
- Spermatogenesis involves both mitotic and meiotic divisions and spermiogenesis (*refer* **Fig. 12**).

Mitotic Division

- The primitive germ cell, spermatogonia, in the basal lamina of the seminiferous tubule undergoes mitotic divisions to form primary spermatocytes.
- Each spermatogonium divides 5 times to produce 32 spermatogonia.
- 32 spermatogonia (44 + X + Y) reach the adluminal side of the tubule and undergo mitosis to become 64 Primary spermatocytes (44 + X + Y).
- Primary spermatocytes are large cells with diploid number of chromosomes (2n) (*refer* **Fig. 29**).

Meiotic Divisions

- The primary spermatocytes with diploid number of chromosomes undergo the first meiotic division to form the secondary spermatocyte which is haploid in nature.

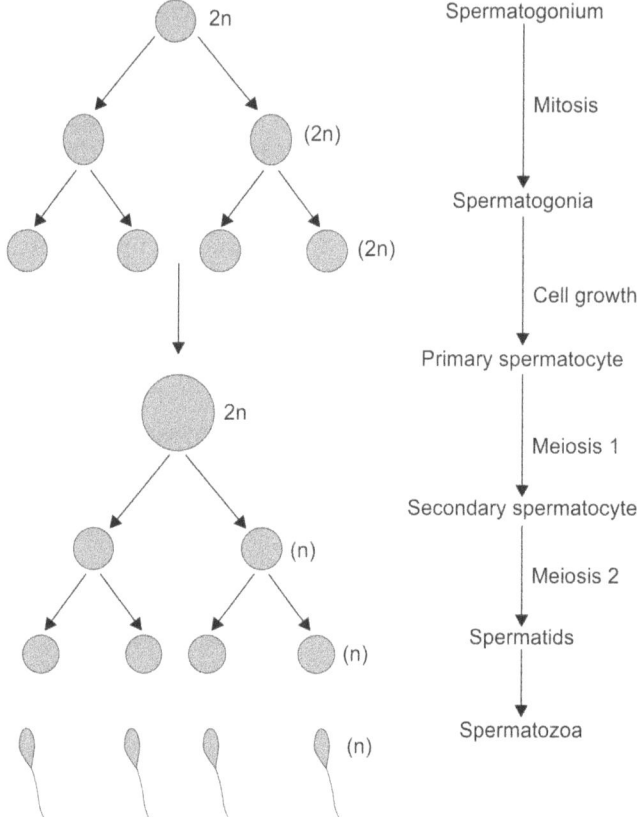

Fig. 29: Steps in spermatogenesis.
(2n: diploid number of chromosomes; n: haploid number of chromosomes)

- The second meiotic division results in formation of spermatids (22 + X or Y) (*refer* **Fig. 29**).
- A total of 512 spermatids are derived from single spermatogonia.

Spermiogenesis

- The spermatids do not undergo further divisions but structural changes take place as the spermatids mature into sperm—spermiogenesis.
- This process happens in the deep folds of Sertoli cells.

The changes taking place are:

- The amount of cytoplasm is reduced in spermatids
- The nucleus elongates to become the head of sperm
- The acrosomal cap is formed
- The tail and middle piece are formed.

Spermiation

- After the maturation the sperms stay attached to the sertoli cells.
- The release of sperms into the tubule is called spermiation.

Factors Regulating Spermatogenesis

Hormones regulating spermatogenesis are—androgens, gonadotrophins and estrogen.

Androgens: A high concentration of testosterone in the tubular fluid is essential for spermatogenesis. LH stimulates Leydig cells to secrete Testosterone. Sertoli cells secrete Androgen binding protein (ABP) to which testosterone binds and its levels are kept elevated.

Spermiogenesis is androgen dependent.

- **LH:** It stimulates Leydig cells to secrete testosterone and thereby is needed for spermatogenesis.

- **FSH:** Stimulates sertoli cells and sertoli cells help in conversion of spermatids to sperms, secretion of ABP and secretion of inhibin. It also increases LH receptors in leydig cells. It maintains gametogenic function of testis.
- **Estrogen** content is high in the fluid in rete testis and estrogen acts to increase fluid reabsorption and spermatozoa is concentrated. This is essential for fertility of an individual.
- **Body temperature:** Spermatogenesis takes place in a temperature less than the inner body temperature. The testes are kept at a temperature of 32°C. If the testes are exposed to higher temperatures the tubular walls degenerate and sterility results.

Semen Analysis

- Semen as a white colored secretion ejected from the male urethra during sexual intercourse.
- It contains sperm and other secretions from seminal vesicles, prostate, urethral glands and Cowper's glands.
- The average volume in each ejaculation is 2.5–3.5 mL.
- The volume decreases after repeated ejaculation.
- There are 100 million sperms per mL of semen.

Composition of Semen

- pH 7.35–7.5
- Specific gravity—1.028
- Sperm count—100 million/mL, <20% abnormal forms

Other Components
From seminal vesicles:
- Phosphorylcholine
- Ergothioneine
- Ascorbic acid
- Flavins
- Prostaglandins

From prostate:
- Spermine
- Citric acid
- Cholesterol, phospholipids
- Fibrinolysin, fibrinogenase
- Zinc
- Acid phosphatase
- Phosphate
- Bicarbonate
- Hyaluronidase
- 60% of the sperms should show normal motility within 3 hours after collection.
- Abnormal sperms should not be more than 30–35%.

Semen Analysis is Used for:
- Assessing male fertility
- It reflects the normal functions of testes and accessory sex organs
- Infertility cases
- To find out the effectiveness of vasectomy
- For medicolegal cases like—rape, adultery, etc.

10. Female contraceptive methods for birth control.

Contraception is prevention of pregnancy.

The needs for prevention of pregnancy are:
- To control population explosion
- To prevent pregnancy in mothers with heart diseases
- Certain methods prevent transmission of sexually transmitted diseases like AIDS

The methods can be:
- Temporary or spacing methods
- Terminal or permanent methods
  The methods are described as contraceptive methods in males and females.

Contraceptive Methods in Females
Spacing Methods
1. Rhythm method
2. Barrier method
3. Pills
4. Intrauterine contraceptive device
1. **Rhythm method:**
   - This method can be followed in females with regular menstrual cycles of 28–30 days.
   - During a normal menstrual cycle, ovulation happens on 14th day of the cycle.
   - The ovum stays viable for 48–72 hours after ovulation.

- After ejaculation, sperm stays viable in female reproductive tract for 24–48 hours.
- So pregnancy can happen if intercourse happens within this period.
- This is said to be the "dangerous period".
- So the days are calculated from first day of menstrual cycle and intercourse should be avoided in the dangerous period.
- 5-6 days after the bleeding phase and 5-6 days before the next menstruation is considered to be the "safe period".
- It can be utilized by females with regular cycles and who can keep a record of their time of ovulation by checking basal body temperature.

2. **Barrier method:**
   - Barriers can be mechanical or chemical barriers. They basically prevent the meeting of sperm and ovum.
   - Mechanical barrier—diaphragm and cervical caps
   - Chemical barriers—spermicidal agents like nonoxynol, ricinoleic acid in the form of jelly or foam is placed in the female reproductive tract before coitus.

3. **Pills:**
   - By pills we mean the oral contraceptive pills used for female contraception.
   - They are usually synthetic preparation of estrogen, progesterone or combination of both.
   - *The pills can be of different types:*
     a. Combined pill or classical pill
     b. Sequential pill
     c. Minipill
     d. Post-coital pill

     a. *Combined pill:*
     - It is a combination of estrogen and progesterone pill.
     - It contains a strip of 21 tablets and is consumed for 21 days from 5th day of menstrual cycle.
     - After 21 days, on stopping the tablets, withdrawal bleeding happens.
     - Again from 5th day, next cycle is started.

     It acts by:
     - Prevents ovulation, as the high estrogen levels disorganize the LH and FSH secretions.
     - Prevents implantation of fertilized ovum.
     - Progesterone makes the cervical mucus thick and prevents sperm penetration.

     b. *Sequential pill:*
     - It has high dose of estrogen and minimal amounts of progesterone.
     - It is not used nowadays as the high estrogen may induce endometrial cancer or breast cancer.

     c. *Minipill:*
     - It is progesterone only pill.
     - It does not affect ovulation but makes the cervical mucus thick and prevents sperm penetration.

     d. *Post-coital pill:*
     - It is used within 72 hours of unprotected intercourse.
     - It has high doses of estrogen and is given for 4–6 days.
     - High estrogen prevents implantation of the fertilized ovum.

     Depot preparation:
   - These are implants of progesterone and they are subdermally implanted and prevent pregnancy for 5 years.
   - The only problem is it can cause amenorrhea and irregular cycles.

4. **Intrauterine contraceptive devices:**
   These are small devices made of plastic or copper and placed in the uterus to prevent implantation of fertilized ovum.
   Lippe's loop:
   - It is a simple 'S'shaped plastic device with nylon threads.
   - Under aseptic precautions, the loop is inserted into the uterus and the thread is present in the vagina.
   - The loop is also impregnated with a small amount of barium sulphate for checking its presence by radiographs.

   Copper 'T':
   - It is a 'T' shaped device made of copper with nylon threads.

- They are inserted during the first 10 days of menstrual cycle.
- Copper prevents implantation of fertilized ovum by stimulating an aseptic inflammation of the endometrium.

Permanent Method
Tubectomy:
▫ It can be done by an open surgery or by laparoscopic surgery.
▫ Here the fallopian tubes are cut and ligated and buried.

11. Classify diuretics and write a note on their sites of action.

Diuretics are chemicals which increase excretion of Na^+ and water and thereby increase urine output.

Site of Action of Diuretics

Drugs Acting in Proximal Convoluted Tubule (PCT)

▫ **Carbonic anhydrase** inhibitors like acetazolamide, they inhibit carbonic anhydrase and thereby increases Na^+ excretion, decreases H^+ secretion and bicarbonate reabsorption. Since H^+ and K^+ compete with each other (for secretion) along with reabsorption of Na^+, there is increased K^+ secretion and excretion and therefore K^+ depletion occurs.
▫ **Osmotic diuretics** like mannitol and isosorbide. They are not reabsorbed in PCT and therefore are retained in the tubule along with water. This in turn alters the gradient for Na^+ reabsorption and therefore it inhibits Na^+ reabsorption.

Diuretics Acting on Loop of Henle

Loop diuretics like frusemide, bumetanide and ethacrynic acid: They act by inhibiting Na^+K^+-$2Cl^-$ transporter. They increase NaCl and K^+ excretion. K^+ depletion occurs while treating with these drugs.

Diuretics Acting on Distal Convoluted Tubule (DCT)

Thiazides: They act by inhibiting NaCl symport in DCT. They increase excretion of NaCl and K^+.

Diuretics Acting on Late DCT and Collecting Duct

K^+ sparing diuretics like spironolactone, Triamterene and amiloride act in late DCT and CD by inhibiting actions of aldosterone or epithelial sodium channel (ENaC). They increase excretion of Na^+ and retain K^+ and H^+.

12. Draw a neat labelled diagram of neuromuscular junction and explain the events in neuromuscular transmission.

Refer short note 3.

13. Movements of small intestine.

▫ **Five types of movements in the normal state:**
  1. Peristalsis—propulsive movement
  2. Mixing movements—segmentation contraction and tonic contraction
  3. Migrating motor complexes (MMC)
  4. Movements of villi
  5. Contractions of muscularis mucosa
▫ **Abnormal movements:** Peristaltic rushes.

MMC
▫ Migrating motility complexes are motility present in the interdigestive period.
▫ These are bursts of electrical and mechanical activities in GIT.
▫ It starts in the esophagus and spreads through the stomach and ileum to the ileocecal valve.
▫ Occurs once in 90 minutes and lasts for 10-20 min.
▫ It clears the GIT for the next meal.
▫ Occurs in 3 phases Phases I, II and III:
  - Phase I—no spike potential, no contractions
  - Phase II—irregular spike potentials and contractions
  - Phase III—regular spike potentials and contractions.

Mixing Movements

Segmentation Contractions

▫ These are ring like contractions present in short segments of the intestine of 1-2 cm.
▫ They are present in regular intervals.

- Their frequency matches the slow wave frequency.
- Slow waves are waves generated in the pace maker cells located in the wall of duodenum and it spreads through the muscular wall of the intestines.
- Strength of the contraction depends on the spike waves superimposed on the slow waves.
- These ring-like contractions appear in one segment and the nearby segment relaxes, this is followed by another set of contractions in the segments between the previous contractions.
- These contractions appear sausage shaped and they cut into the bolus and move it to and fro and increase their exposure to the absorptive surface of the mucosa.
- Therefore, these contractions help in mixing the bolus with digestive juices and in digestion and absorption of food.

Tonic Contractions
- These are prolonged contractions of one segment of intestine and the segment appears to be isolated from the rest of the ileum.
- Segmentation and tonic contractions delay the passage of chyme and thereby allow contact of chyme with enterocytes and favour absorption.

Peristalsis
- This is a type of propulsive movement which helps to move the chyme forward. It is a reflex initiated by the stretch of the intestinal wall following the entry of food.
- Stretch of the intestinal wall initiates a ring of constriction behind the bolus and a relaxation in front of the bolus.
- The ring of contraction behind pushes the bolus to the relaxed segment in front of the bolus.
- Next ring of contraction now appears in the previous relaxed segment and the bolus is pushed further.
- These waves always propel the contents from the oral to caudal direction and never in the opposite direction—*law of the gut*.
- These waves appear even in the absence of nerve supply but they can be modified by the autonomic nerves, parasympathetic nerves increase the activity and sympathetic nerves decrease the activity.
- The propelling speed varies from 2-25 cm/s.
- Sometimes the peristaltic waves can be very fast and they empty the contents faster—peristaltic rushes, seen in acute diarrhea.
- Antiperistalsis happens in vomiting.

Contractions of Muscularis Mucosa
- Irregular in nature.
- Occurs at a frequency of 3/sec.
- It helps in mixing the contents and in absorption.

Contraction of Villi
- The type of contraction seen as elongation and shortening of the villi.
- It helps in emptying of central lacteals of the villi and increases the absorptive surface area.
- It is stimulated by the hormone Villikinin.

Functions of Movements of Small Intestine
- Mixing the chyme with the digestive juices and helps in digestion
- Propelling the chyme forward
- Presenting the chyme to absorptive surface and helps for absorption.

14. Actions of parathormone.
- Parathormone is a polypeptide hormone with 84 AA secreted by the chief cells of the parathyroid gland.
- The main actions of PTH are to increase blood calcium levels and decrease phosphate levels.

Effect on Bones
- It increases activity of both osteoclasts and osteoblasts.
- But the osteoclastic activity is the major effect resulting in resorption of bone and release of calcium and phosphates into the ECF.
- PTH stimulates the differentiation of precursors into osteoclasts, increases their numbers and size. The products of

resorption are present in blood and are excreted in urine.
- **Action on osteoclasts:** This effect comes into action after a few days of exposure to PTH. The number and activity of osteoclasts are increased. Osteoclasts increase bone resorption and thereby increases calcium and phosphate levels in the blood. Also, levels of hydroxyproline and hydroxylysine are increased.
- **Action on osteoblasts:** At low doses PTH increases osteoblastic activity but in high doses it inhibits action of osteoblasts.

Action on Kidneys

There are three major actions on the kidneys:
a. Increased reabsorption of calcium in the Thick ascending limb of loop of Henle and DCT. 25-30% of the filtered Ca^{2+} is reabsorbed in the DCT and Loop of Henle by the action of PTH. 65% of filtered Ca^{2+} is reabsorbed in the PCT.
b. Decreases reabsorption of phosphate in the kidneys by its action on the PCT and induces Phosphaturia. Serum phosphate levels are lowered by the action of PTH.
c. Stimulates the formation of 1, 25 Dihydroxycholecalciferol (Calcitriol) by the kidneys. PTH stimulates the 1a Hydroxylation of 25 hydroxy cholecalciferol to form the active form of vitamin D3. Calcitriol in turn increases reabsorption of calcium from GIT and kidneys.

15. Juxtaglomerular apparatus.

- Juxtaglomerular apparatus is a combination of tubular cells and vascular cells.
- It is located near the glomerulus where the afferent arteriole enters and efferent arteriole leaves the glomerulus (*refer* **Fig. 30**).

It is made up of the following components:
- Juxtaglomerular cells
- Macula densa cells
- Lacis cells

Juxtaglomerular Cells

- These are myoepithelial cells lining the afferent arteriole just before it enters the glomerulus.

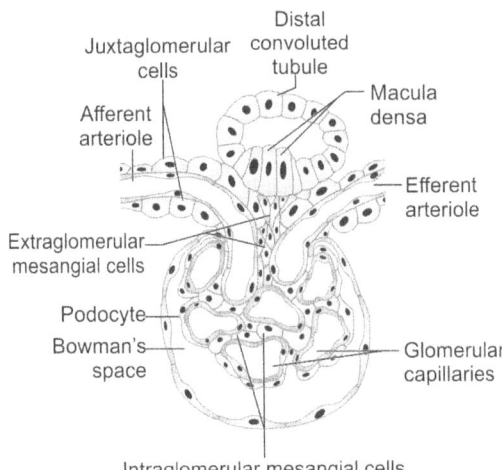

Fig. 30: JG apparatus.

- These cells are rich in endoplasmic reticulum and they secrete the hormone renin.
- They act as baroreceptors and they sense the change in the renal arterial pressure and respond to the pressure gradient between the afferent arteriole and the interstitium.
- When the renal arterial pressure drops JG cells release renin.
- These cells also sense the ECF volume and respond to hypovolemia by secreting renin.
- They are also supplied by sympathetic nerves and when the stimulation is there it releases renin.
- Renin converts angiotensinogen in plasma to angiotensin I
- Angiotensin I is converted to Angiotensin II by the action of angiotensin-converting enzyme (ACE) present abundantly in the liver.
- Angiotensin II is the most active substance and it has varied actions in the body (*refer* **Fig. 8**)

Macula Densa Cells

- They are present in the renal tubules at the junction of thick ascending limb of loop of Henle and the distal convoluted tubule.
- These cells are modified; they are more columnar and densely packed.

- They are in close contact with the mesangial cells and the JG cells.
- They act as chemoreceptors and they sense the NaCl content in the tubular fluid.
- They act through tubuloglomerular feedback and regulate the renal blood flow and GFR.

Mesangial Cells or Lacis Cells

- These are present in between the afferent and efferent arterioles and are in close contact with the JG cells and macula densa cells.
- They are contractile in nature and therefore they regulate GFR.
- They also secrete some amount of renin.

16. Fibrinolytic system.

- Tendency to form clot in an injured vessel is at the same time balanced by anticlotting or fibrinolytic pathways in the vessel to keep the lumen of blood vessel patent.
- Fibrinolytic system involves an important protease enzyme **plasmin** which is present in an inactive form as plasminogen in plasma.
- On activation, plasmin lyses the fibrin and fibrinogen to produce fibrin degradation products (FDP) which in turn inhibits thrombin (*refer* **Fig. 31**).
- Plasminogen is activated by thrombin, and there are plasminogen activators—the tissue type plasminogen activator (t-PA) and urokinase-type plasminogen activator (u-PA).
- Plasminogen receptors are also located on the endothelial cells and binding to the receptor, plasminogen is activated and prevents clot formation in intact vessels.
- There are also tissue plasminogen inhibitors in plasma which are regulated by protein C and its cofactor protein S.

17. Functions of glucocorticoid.

Metabolic actions of glucocorticoids are:
- **Effects on carbohydrate metabolism:**
  - Increases gluconeogenesis in liver → increased glycogen stores.
  - Antagonizes the action of insulin on muscle and adipose tissue—prevents glucose uptake.
  - This spares glucose for the brain.
  - Increases glucose output from liver.
  - Results in hyperglycemia
- **Effects on protein metabolism:**
  - It is proteolytic in action.
  - Breaks down proteins into AA and inhibits protein synthesis.
  - Amino acids are used for gluconeogenesis.

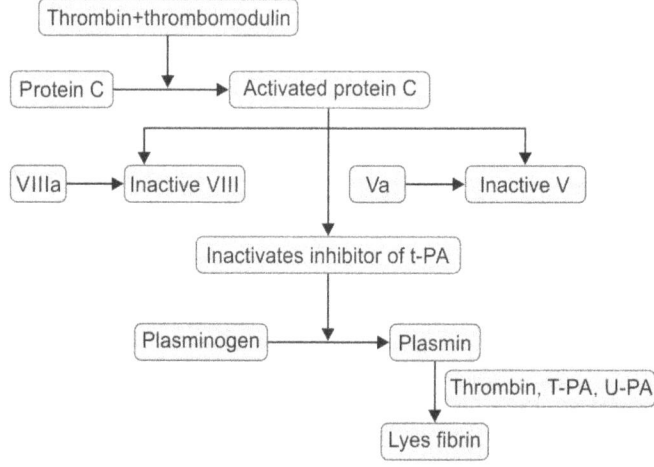

Fig. 31: Fibrinolytic system and its regulation.
(T-PA: tissue plasminogen activator, U-PA: urokinase activated plasminogen)

- Therefore, increased cortisol levels drain the protein stores in the body.
- **Effects on lipid metabolism:**
  - Cortisol is permissive for the lipolytic action of catecholamines.
  - But high cortisol levels increase total body fat by two mechanisms:
    1. Cortisol stimulates appetite → obesity due to increased caloric consumption.
    2. High cortisol →↑ blood glucose →↑ insulin secretion → lipogenesis.
- Pattern of fat distribution—**centripetal**—concentrated in trunk, but wasting is seen in arms and legs.

Permissive Action

- Cortisol amplifies effects of certain processes of other hormones where it does not act directly.
  Example:
  A. It does not induce glycogenolysis itself but augments glycogenolysis by glucagon.
  B. It also augments vasoresponsiveness of blood vessels to catecholamines.

Actions on Bones

Increases bone resorption by:

Cortisol decreases renal and GIT absorption of calcium
↓
Lowers serum calcium levels
↓
Parathyroid hormone secretion stimulated
↓
Mobilizes calcium from bone by resorption and demineralization

Also Inhibits action of osteoblasts and suppresses collagen formation. Hence high cortisol levels result in **osteoporosis**.

Actions on CVS

- Cortisol is permissive for the vasopressor effects of catecholamine and Ang ll.
- Hence it is necessary for maintenance of normal BP.
- Stimulates erythropoietin synthesis and so increases RBC production.

Actions on Connective Tissue

Cortisol inhibits fibroblast proliferation and collagen formation:

So excess cortisol levels
↓
Thinning of skin and walls of capillaries
↓
Easy damage to skin and easy bruising of capillaries
↓
Intracutaneous hemorrhage

Action on Kidneys

- Cortisol inhibits ADH secretion and action, so in absence of cortisol a water load leads to water intoxication.
- Cortisol also has a weak mineralocorticoid action →↑ Na^+ and H_2O reabsorption.
- **Increases GFR:**
  - By increasing cardiac output
  - By direct action on kidneys

Action on Muscles

- Cortisol has complex action on muscles.
- Excess cortisol results in muscle weakness due to:
  - Proteolysis
  - Hypokalemia

Actions on GIT

- Cortisol has a trophic action on GIT.
- It also increases appetite → weight gain in hypercortisolism.
- Increased acid secretion → acidity, gastritis.

Action on CNS

- Glucocorticoids alters mood and behavior.
- REM sleep ↓, but slow wave sleep ↑
- In excess—insomnia, elevated or depressed mood, ↓ memory.
- Frank psychosis occurs with excess or reduced cortisol levels.
- Dampens the acuity to olfactory, gustatory, auditory and visual stimuli.

Action in Fetus

- Facilitates maturity of CNS, retina, skin, GIT, and lungs.

- During the last week of pregnancy, the synthesis of surfactant is stimulated by cortisol.
- So if premature delivery suspected weekly doses of cortisol given to mother till delivery.

Action on Inflammation and Immune System

- Cortisol is frequently used clinically for its anti-inflammatory property.
- It inhibits synthesis of mediators of inflammation.
- Inhibits migration of leukocytes to site of injury.
- Decreases the number of circulating eosinophils.
- Inhibits fibroblast proliferation at inflammatory site which is a defense mechanism in the body to prevent spreading of infection.
- Excess cortisol inhibits normal defense mechanisms of body against infection.

Effect on Immune Response

- Cortisol inhibits immune response in the body.
- At high doses it decreases the number of T lymphocytes (helper tcells) and their migration to antigenic site.
- B lymphocytes and antibody production are not affected directly.
- Because of these effects, glucocorticoids are used for immunosuppression after organ transplantation.

Effect on Stress

- Protects the body against stress.
- During stress there is increased secretion of CRH from hypothalamus.
- This increases the secretion of ACTH from anterior pituitary.
- Therefore, glucocorticoid secretion increases.
- Cortisol facilitates lipolysis by catecholamine and increases release of free fatty acids which supplies the energy needed to cope up with stress.
- It is also permissive for the vasoconstriction induced by catecholamines which is needed for maintaining BP during stress.

18. Endometrial changes in menstrual cycle.

- Menstrual cycle is the female sexual cycle and it happens once in 28–30 days. It is associated with uterine bleeding—menstruation.
- It is a preparatory cycle for fertilization and implantation of the fertilized ovum
- Therefore, cyclic changes happen in the uterus, ovaries, cervix and vagina.
- All these changes are under the control of various hormones.
- The hormones regulating menstrual cycle are hypothalamic hormones (GnRH), anterior pituitary hormones (FSH and LH) and ovarian hormones (estrogen and progesterone).
- GnRH from hypothalamus is the key controller of gonadotrophin released from anterior pituitary.
- GnRH is secreted in pulsatile fashion and the pulsatility of GnRH is very important in regulating secretions of LH and FSH.
- GnRH pulsatility is in turn kept in check by levels of estrogen and progesterone. Just before LH surge, pulsatility of GnRH is increased by high levels of estrogen.
- We will be now discussing the hormonal regulation for ovarian changes and endometrial changes separately.

The uterine changes are given in 3 phases:
1. Proliferative phase
2. Secretory phase
3. Menstrual phase

Proliferative Phase

- This phase correlates with the follicular phase of ovarian cycle.
- Estrogen secreted from the follicle stimulates growth of uterine endometrium and therefore it thickens.
- Glands in the endometrium and the blood vessels in endometrium also grows.
- This phase is from day 5 till the day of ovulation (*refer* **Fig. 32**).

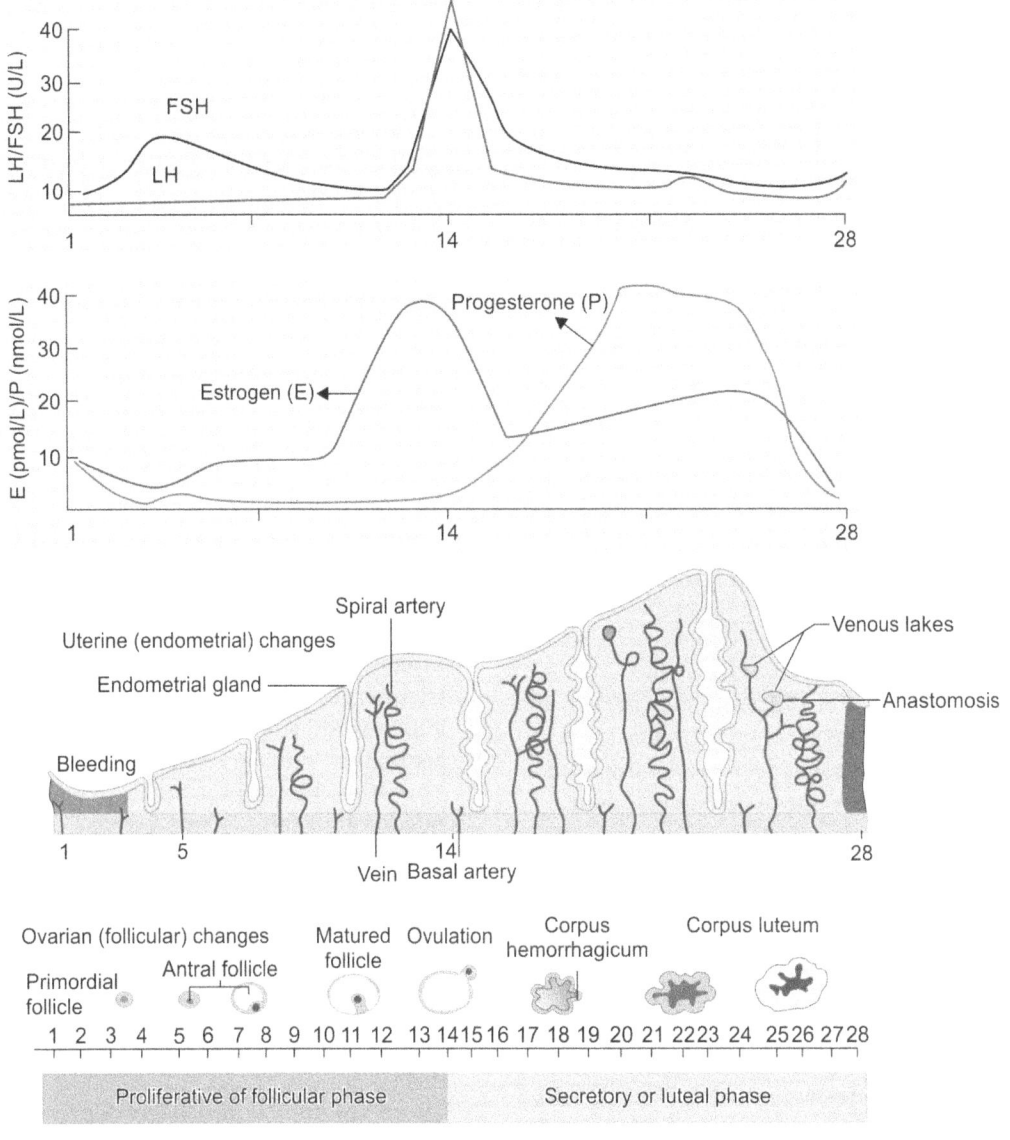

Fig. 32: Menstrual cycle. Hormonal changes, changes in endometrium and changes in ovary.

Secretory Phase

- This phase is from the day of ovulation to 25th day of the cycle.
- It correlates with the luteal phase in the ovarian cycle.
- Progesterone levels are high and they make the endometrium secretory by acting on the glands. Maximum action is 5–7 days after ovulation.
- The secretion from the endometrial glands is rich in glycogen and can nourish the fertilized ovum.
- The secretory endometrium is favorable for implantation of fertilized ovum.
- If fertilization does not happen, corpus luteum starts to regress and the progesterone and estrogen levels decrease.
- Withdrawal of hormonal support of the endometrium and release of prostaglandins

result in vasoconstriction of the spiral arteries → uterine ischemia happens and endometrial necrosis and shedding of endometrium happens resulting in bleeding.

Menstrual Phase

It starts with the menstrual bleeding with the shedding of outer 2/3rd of endometrium, unfertilized ovum and continues for 5 days.

19. Active transport across cell membrane.

Refer Short note 2.

20. Digestion and absorption of fat.

Dietary fat consists of neutral fats—triglycerides and also phospholipids, cholesterol, free fatty acids and lecithin. It also has fat-soluble vitamins.

Digestion of Fats

- There are fat-digesting enzymes in the mouth, stomach and pancreatic juice.
- Lingual lipase is secreted by the Ebner's gland on the dorsal surface of tongue.
- Lingual lipase starts its action while in the stomach and digests 30% of triglycerides. Gastric lipase is of little importance in digestion of fats except in conditions of pancreatic insufficiency.
- Most of the digestion of fats begin in the duodenum by the action of pancreatic lipase.
- It acts on the fats emulsified by bile salts.
- Action of lipase is potentiated by the action of colipase, an enzyme which is also present in the pancreatic juice.

Emulsification of Fats by Bile Salts

- Emulsification means breaking down of large fat molecules into smaller molecules by the detergent action (lowering of surface tension) of bile salts.
- The bile salts are amphipathic and their hydrophobic tails face the centre (where fat droplets are placed) and the heads are hydrophilic and they face the water in the lumen.
- This property along with the intestinal movements break the fat droplets to smaller molecules.
- The breaking down of fats into smaller molecules is essential as it increases the surface area on which the pancreatic lipase can act.
- Pancreatic lipase is water-soluble and it can act only on lipid-water interface of the fats.

Digestion of Fats by Lipolytic Enzymes

- Fat digestion begins mostly in duodenum by the action of pancreatic lipase.
- Pancreatic lipase is rich in enzymes and HCO_3^- and thereby it changes the pH of chyme from 6 to 7. This is the optimal pH for the action of lipases.
- Colipase is an enzyme secreted by pancreas which opens up a lid like structure in the amphipathic helix so that Lipase can act on triglycerides.
- Lipase acts on 1- and 3- bonds of triglycerides and on 2-bond at a low rate and the products of digestion are free fatty acids and 2-monoglycerides.
- The other lipase present in pancreatic juice is bile salt-activated lipase and it hydrolyses the cholesterol esters, esters of fat-soluble vitamins, phospholipids and triglycerides.
- Cholesteryl ester hydrolase in pancreatic juice hydrolyses cholesterol esters.
- Phospholipase A2 hydrolyses phospholipids and separates fatty acids from them.
- There are similar brush border lipases which act on the lipids in a similar way.

Absorption of Fats

- It starts in the duodenum and is completely absorbed by the time the fats reach jejunum.
- Absorption of fats is favoured by formation of micelles by the bile salts and lecithin.
- The lumen of intestine contains water and therefore movement of digested fats is favored only by micelle formation.
- On reaching enterocytes, fats move out of micelles and enter enterocytes by passive diffusion.

- The rate-limiting step in absorption of fats is formation and movement of micelles from the chyme in the lumen to the brush border.
- The bile salts forming the micelles, are absorbed in the terminal ileum.
- Fate of fats, entering the enterocytes is dependent on their size.
- Fats containing 10–12 carbon atoms, easily pass through the basal side of the enterocytes and enter the portal blood vessels as free fatty acids and are transported.
- Fatty acids with more than 12 carbon atoms are esterified to triglycerides and the absorbed cholesterol is also esterified and they are coated with protein (β lipoprotein), cholesterol and phospholipids to form **chylomicrons**.
- The chylomicrons now exocytosis through the basal side of the enterocytes to enter the lymphatics in the villus, the lacteal.
- They are transported in the lymphatics and are drained into the thoracic duct and finally they enter the blood circulation.
- Absorption of large chain fatty acids are more in the upper parts of the intestine and some amount of absorption happens in terminal parts also.
- In moderate fat intake, nearly 95% of ingested fats are absorbed.

Steatorrhea

- Steatorrhea is malabsorption of fats resulting in excretion of fat in stools.
- The indigested fats appear in stools and the stools are fatty, bulky and clay-colored. This is said to be steatorrhea.
- The faecal fat content is more than 40–50 g/day.
- It happens due to either destruction of exocrine pancreas, lipase deficiency or absence of bicarbonate in pancreatic juice which results in acidic environment in the intestine precipitating the bile salts.
- Acids also inhibit pancreatic lipase and therefore patients with gastrin-secreting tumor have steatorrhea.
- It is also seen in conditions with defective absorption of bile salts in terminal ileum.

21. Chloride shift.

- This happens when CO_2 is transported in blood from the tissues to the lung.
- The major part of CO_2 (70%) is transported as HCO_3^- in plasma. CO_2 diffuses from the tissues and enters the interstitial tissue and from there it enters the RBC due to the pressure gradient in these areas.
- Inside the RBC the enzyme carbonic anhydrase (CA) is present.
- CO_2 enters RBC and combines with H_2O in presence of CA to form H_2CO_3.
- H_2CO_3 dissociates immediately and splits into H^+ and HCO_3^-.
- HCO_3^- levels increase within the RBC and the excess of HCO_3 leaves the cell in exchange for an anion, Cl^- through the anion exchanger, Band 3 protein (*refer* **Fig. 33**).
- This exchange is called **chloride shift or Hamburger shift**.
- For each molecule of CO_2 added to a red cell there is an increase of one osmotically active particle in the cell either Cl^- or HCO_3^-.
- Therefore, the RBC takes up water and swells up and increases in size.
- This increases the hematocrit of venous blood by 3% than the arterial blood.

22. Changes that occur in acclimatization.

Physiological Changes at High Altitude

- Effects of high altitude is due to low barometric pressure →↓ P_{IO2}
- Hypoxic symptoms appear at 10,000 ft and are severe at 15,000 to 18,000 ft.
- There are various compensatory mechanisms by which the O_2 supply to tissue is increased. They are:

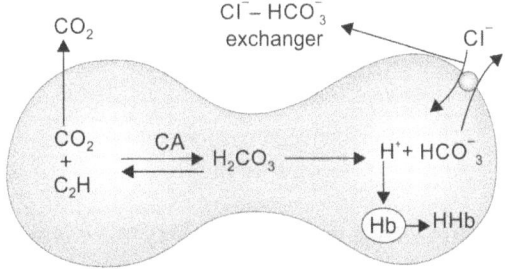

Fig. 33: Chloride shift.

- First and foremost—hyperventilation
- In high altitude, there is no drive for ventilation till PO_2 is <60 mm Hg (at 14,000 ft) and on reaching <60 mm Hg, there is hyperventilation, because:
  - **1st stage:** Hypoxia acts on peripheral chemoreceptors (PCR) → stimulation of ventilation → CO_2 blow out →↓ PCO_2 →↑ arterial pH →↓ ventilation.
  - **2nd stage:**
    - Ventilation slowly decreases and then increases and becomes stable after 8–10 hrs, due to: pH of CSF is more alkaline in the acute phase. But later ventilation increases by ↓pH, by movement of HCO_3^- out of CSF
    - There is renal compensation for the alkaline nature because the kidneys excrete more HCO_3^- into the urine →↓pH.

Acclimatization to High Altitude

☐ When a person ascends to high altitudes and stays there for some time, he gets adapted.
☐ It starts by 12 hours and takes several days.
☐ The maximum height up to which acclimatization possible is 18,000 ft.

Changes During Acclimatization to High Altitude

☐ **Respiratory changes:**
  - *Initial changes:*

Hyperventilation by hypoxia stimulating PCR
↓
CO_2 washout
↓
Renal compensation and HCO_3^- excretion out of CSF
↓
Stimulates central chemoreceptors and ↑ventilation
↓
After 4 days ventilation slowly increases and is dependent on altitude

☐ **Hematological changes:**
  - Hypoxia stimulates erythropoietin production by kidneys →↑RBC production (starts after 3 days) →↑O_2 delivery to tissues.
  - There is also increase in 2,3-DPG levels in RBC →↑O_2 delivery to tissues.

☐ **CVS changes:**
  - There is ↑in HR, cardiac output (CO) and BP due to activation of sympatho adrenal activity →↑CO and ↑HR →↑blood flow.
  - Vasodilatation due to hypoxia →↑ blood flow.

☐ **Changes in tissues:**
  - ↑in number of capillaries
  - ↑in number of mitochondria in cells
  - ↑in activity of oxidative enzymes like cytochrome oxidase
  - ↑in myoglobin content
  - Angiogenesis.

23. Draw a normal spirogram and write about the volumes and capacities of lung.

☐ Spirogram is a graphic recording of the various lung volumes and capacities other than residual volume, functional residual capacity and total lung capacity.
☐ The instrument is the spirometer.
☐ Spirometry is the recording of volume changes during the breathing events (*refer* Fig. 34).
☐ There are two types of spirometers—simple spirometer or a computerized spirometer.
☐ The spirogram shows the various lung volumes and capacities.
☐ Capacities are two or more lung volumes.

Tidal Volume (TV)

☐ It is the volume of air inspired or expired with each breath during normal breathing.
☐ Normal value –500 mL.

Inspiratory Reserve Volume (IRV)

☐ It is the maximal volume of air inspired with effort in excess of tidal volume.
☐ Normal value—2000 to 3200 mL
☐ IRV: From TV to TLC.

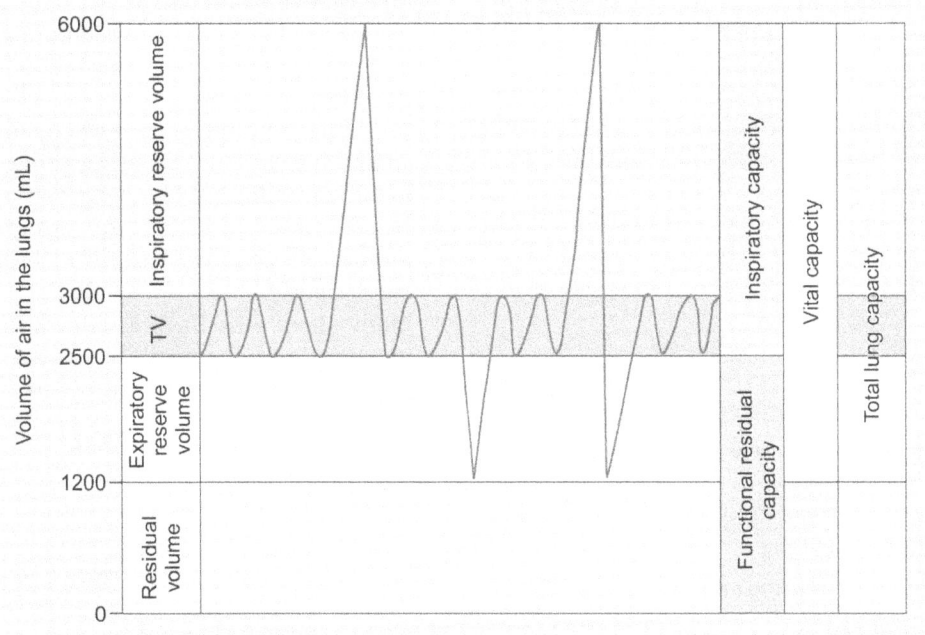

Fig. 34: Spirogram.
(TV: tidal volume)

Expiratory Reserve Volume (ERV)

- It is the maximal volume of air exhaled from the resting end-expiratory level. (volume expired by active expiration after passive expiration).
- Normal value—750 to 1000 mL.
- **ERV:** From TV to RV.

Residual Volume (RV)

- It is the volume of air remaining in the lungs at the end of maximal expiration. Normally it accounts for about 25% of TLC.
- Normal value—1200 mL
- This volume cannot be measured with spirometer.
- It is calculated from subtracting ERV from FRC.
- FRC is measured by helium dilution technique.

Inspiratory Capacity (IC)

- It is the maximal volume of air inspired from resting expiratory level.
- Normal value—3000 to 3500 mL.

IC = IRV + TV.

Functional Residual Capacity (FRC)

- It is the volume of air remaining in the lungs at the end of resting (normal) expiration. NV—2500 mL.
  FRC = RV + ERV.
- Is measured by Nitrogen washout technique or helium dilution technique.

Significance of FRC

- This volume of gas in the lung helps in continuous exchange of gases between breaths.
- Helps to Buffer the levels of concentration of O_2 and CO_2 in blood.

Total Lung Capacity (TLC)

- It is the total volume of air within the lung after maximum inspiration. (The maximum volume of air that the lung can contain).
  NV—**6000 mL**
  TLC = FVC + RV
  or
  TLC = RV + ERV + TV + IRV

TLC increased in airway narrowing with air trapping (bronchial asthma).

Vital Capacity

Maximum volume of gas completely expired from the lungs following a maximal inspiration.

NV – 4800 mL (in males) and 3200 mL (in females)

VC = TLC – RV

or

VC = IRV+TV+ERV

Factors that Influence VC

- Respiratory muscle power
- Airway patency
- Compliance of the lung
- Elasticity of lung

Conditions Increasing and Decreasing VC

- **Increased in:**
  - Swimmers and divers
  - Trained athletes
  - People living in high altitude
- **Decreased in:**
  - Old age
  - Lying posture
  - Pregnancy
  - Obesity
  - Diseases like poliomyelitis, pleural effusion, asthma, emphysema, etc.

24. Polysomnography.

- Polysomnography (PSG) is a laboratory based sleep study to study sleep disorders like obstructive sleep apnea, narcolepsy, insomnia, REM sleep disorders, periodic limb movement disorders, sleep-related hypoventilation/hypoxia, nocturnal seizures, etc.
- It is a non-invasive study and involves simultaneous recording of multiple physiological parameters in sleep and wakefulness.
- The PSG records—EEG, electrooculogram (EOG), electromyogram (EMG), ECG, pulse oximetry, respiratory efforts and air flow.
- The PSG is recorded with a minimal of 12 channels.
- There are three leads for ECG, two for EOG, one or two for chin muscle tone, one or two for leg movements, one or two to measure air flow, one for oxygen saturation, one belt each for chest movements and abdominal movements.
- The wires from the leads converge into a central box and that is in turn connected to the computer.
- During the recording the computer monitor displays the various recordings continuously.
- Many sleep labs have a video camera installed and the technician can also directly monitor the patient.

25. Functions of hypothalamus.

Functions

- Regulation of food intake
- Regulation of body temperature
- Regulation of thirst
- Regulation of anterior pituitary hormones
- Regulation of posterior pituitary hormones
- Regulation of sleep wake cycle
- Control of autonomic nervous system
- Control of reproduction
- Control of emotions
- Control of circadian rhythm
- Role in stress
- Role in visceral and somatic function
- Role in reward and punishment.

Regulation of Food Intake

- There are two groups of neurons involved in food intake:
  1. Ventromedial nucleus (satiety center)
  2. Lateral nucleus (feeding center)
- Feeding center stimulates appetite and increases food intake and satiety center inhibits feeding center and brings satiety.

Regulation of food intake:

These are the hypothesis regulating food intake:

- *Glucostatic hypothesis:* Activity of satiety center is regulated by glucose utilization of the neurons. When the glucose utilization is low their activity is less and vice versa. When satiety center activity is less the feeding center's activity is unchecked and the person feels hungry. When utilization

is high, the glucostats activity is unchecked and there is inhibition of feeding center and the person feels sated. Hypoglycemia is an appetite stimulant and the decrease in plasma glucose decreases the utilization of glucose by the cells.
- *Lipostatic hypothesis:* This hypothesis is based on the fact that the adipose tissues send humoral signals like leptin, a hormone secreted by adipose tissue. When fat depots are more, the leptin levels increase and it decreases food intake and increases energy output.
- *Gut-peptide theory:* After food intake, there are hormones released from the GIT which act on the hypothalamus and thereby inhibits food intake
- *Thermostatic theory:* Food intake is increased in cold weather and decreased in warm weather.

Hormones and neurotensin (NT) regulating food intake:
- **Hormones increasing food intake:**
  - Neuropeptide Y
  - Orexins
  - Ghrelin
  - Melanin-concentrating hormone (MCH)
  - Agouti-related protein (AgRP)
  - Galanin
  - Growth hormone releasing hormone (GHRH)
- **Hormones decreasing food intake:**
  - Estrogen
  - Dopamine
  - Alpha-melanocyte-stimulating-hormone (α-MSH)
  - Cocaine and amphetamine-regulated transcript (CART)
  - Corticotrophin releasing hormone (CRH)
  - Gut hormones
  - Cholecystokinin
  - Leptin

Temperature Regulation
- Humans need to maintain body temperature at 37°C.
- Preoptic region of anterior hypothalamus has a role in regulation of body temperature in warmth. When body temperature goes above set point it stimulates heat dissipating mechanisms like vasodilation and sweating.
- Posterior hypothalamus acts in cool temperature and involved in heat conserving mechanisms like vasoconstriction, piloerection and sympathetic stimulation.

Regulation of Thirst
- Thirst center is located in the hypothalamus.
- It is located in the lateral hypothalamus.
- It is stimulated by osmoreceptors in increase in tonicity of body fluids.
- A decrease in ECF volume also stimulates thirst center.

Regulation of ECF Volume
Achieved by regulation of ADH, aldosterone and thirst mechanism.

Regulation of Endocrine Functions
- Hypothalamus controls anterior pituitary and through anterior pituitary it regulates secretion of other endocrine glands.
- It secretes posterior pituitary hormones.
- Hypothalamus is considered to be the master of endocrine orchestra.
- It is a part of the brain and therefore is the link between neural and endocrine systems.

Control of Reproduction
- Hypothalamus releases GnRH which regulates the release of FSH and LH from anterior pituitary gland.
- They in turn control reproductive function in males and females.
- They regulate spermatogenesis, development of accessory sex organs in males and menstrual cycle and secondary sexual characteristics in females.
- Also the sexual behavior are influenced by hypothalamus (preoptic and anterior hypothalamus).

Regulation of Sleep Wake Cycle

- Hypothalamus regulates sleep wake cycle.
- There are two sleep centers:
  1. Diencephalic sleep zone
  2. Basal forebrain sleep zone
- Stimulation of these areas at the frequency of 8 Hz induces slow wave sleep.

Control of Autonomic Nervous System (ANS)

- Hypothalamus controls and integrates the activities of ANS.
- Through ANS it is a major regulator of visceral activities.
- Stimulation of posterior hypothalamus results in increase in HR, BP, pupillary dilatation, piloerection (sympathetic system stimulated).
- Stimulation of anterior hypothalamus results in decreased HR, increased HCl secretion, urination, etc. (parasympathetic system stimulated).

Regulation of Emotional and Behavioral Patterns

- With the limbic system it participates in the expressions of emotions.
- The circuit given below is responsible for emotions (*refer* **Fig. 35**).

Regulation of Circadian Rhythm

- The suprachiasmatic nucleus establishes patterns of awakening and sleep that occur on a circadian (daily) schedule.
- This is mediated through retino-hypothalamic tract.
- **Example:**
  - Cortisol secretion
  - Body temperature
  - ACTH secretion
  - Melatonin secretion
  - Sleep-wakefulness

Regulation of Reward and Punishment Areas

- Hypothalamus along with LS and cortex integrate and bring about smooth responses for reward and punishment.
- VM nucleus is associated with reward and posterior and lateral nucleus of hypothalamus with punishment.

26. Peculiarities of pulmonary circulation.

- It is a low pressure and low resistance system (MAP – 15 mm Hg)
- Pulmonary arteries have less amount of smooth muscles in their walls and they are more compliant → can accommodate more blood without much raise in pressure.
- Pulmonary arterioles are also thin-walled and have lesser amounts of smooth muscles.
- Pulmonary capillaries are arranged in a network around the alveolus so that blood flows in a thin sheet through them. The capillary walls are thin and can be collapsed when the alveolar pressure rises.
- In response to hypoxia, the pulmonary arterioles undergo vasoconstriction whereas in systemic vessels, hypoxia induces vasodilatation and thereby increases blood flow to hypoxic areas.
- Hypoxia occurs when the alveoli are ill ventilated and therefore vasoconstriction in the supplying vessels diverts the blood to the vessels supplying the neighboring well-ventilated alveoli.
- Blood flow in pulmonary capillaries is decided by the pulmonary—arterial and venous and alveolar pressures.
- Pulmonary vascular resistance falls as the pulmonary arterial pressure increases as in conditions like increase in cardiac output.
- **This is because of two reasons:**
  1. Recruitment of capillaries (opening of capillaries which are kept collapsed)

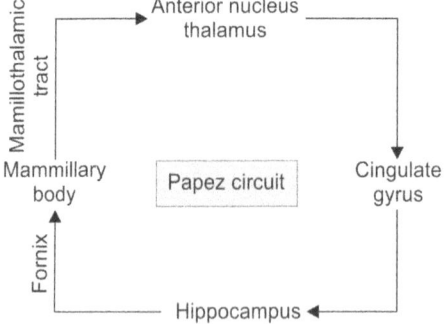

Fig. 35: Papez circuit.

2. Capillary distension (distension of already patent capillaries).

27. Hypovolemic shock.

❒ Shock is a syndrome in which there is inadequate tissue perfusion related with absolute or relative decrease in Cardiac output. It is also called as 'cold shock'
❒ **Types of shock:**
  1. Hypovolemic shock
  2. Distributive shock
  3. Cardiogenic shock
  4. Obstructive shock

Hypovolemic Shock

Causes for Hypovolemic Shock
❒ Trauma
❒ Hemorrhage
❒ Surgery
❒ Burns
❒ Fluid loss due to vomiting or diarrhea

Symptoms are
❒ Hypotension
❒ Rapid thready pulse
❒ Skin is cold and clammy with greyish tinge
❒ Intense thirst
❒ Rapid breathing
❒ Restlessness
❒ Increased lactic acid production

Stages of Shock
Reversible and irreversible shock
1. **Reversible or non-progressive shock:**
   - It is a stage in shock where the amount of blood lost is less than 1 L and various body mechanisms try to compensate the decrease in circulatory volume and to correct and cause full recovery without any treatment.
   - It is also called as compensated stage.
   The following are the compensatory mechanisms:
   - Immediate tachycardia and increase in pulse rate—due to decrease in blood volume baroreceptors are inhibited which results in sympathetic nerves stimulation.
   - Sympathetic stimulation causes vasoconstriction in all the vessels except cerebral and coronary vasculature.
   - Sympathetic nerves also cause venoconstriction which results in increased venous return and thereby increased cardiac output and blood pressure.
   - Due to loss of RBC and stagnant blood flow and acidosis, chemoreceptors are stimulated → Tachypnoea → Thoracic pumping → Increase VR and thereby CO and BP.
   - Restlessness due to release of adrenaline from adrenal medulla → Acts on reticular formation → skeletal muscle activity → increase in VR.
   - Movement of interstitial fluid into capillaries → increases blood volume.
   - Increased secretion of renin, angiotensin II and aldosterone → reabsorption of electrolytes and water from tubules → increase in blood volume.
   - Increased secretion of ADH.
   - Long term compensations are increase in erythropoiesis and plasma protein synthesis.
2. **Refractory shock:**
   - Depending upon the amount of blood lost many patients die soon after the blood loss.
   - Some recover with the compensatory mechanisms and with appropriate treatment.
   - But some patients the shock persists for hours and it progresses to there is no improvement with treatment, cardiac output stays decreased.
   - This condition is said to be refractory shock or Irreversible shock
   - This happens because of operation of various positive feedback mechanisms.
   - Severe blood loss → Depression of vasomotor center → Vasodilatation and decrease in heart rate → further drop in BP → further drop in cerebral blood flow → further depression of VMC and cardiac areas.
   - Severe shock → coronary blood flow is decreased due to hypotension and tachycardia → decrease myocardial

contractility → further decrease in cardiac output → further decrease in coronary blood flow.
- Acidosis makes the situation worse.

If no treatment advocated it leads to refractory shock resulting in:
- Depletion of ATP
- Tissue damage and necrosis
- Acute tubular necrosis in kidneys
- Respiratory distress—shock lung syndrome.

Treatment

Treatment should aim at correcting the cause and restoring the circulatory volume.
- **General treatment:**
  - Patient should be kept at room temperature.
  - Raise the foot end of patient's bed to increase venous return.
- **Treating the cause:**
  - In hemorrhagic, traumatic and surgical shock the cause is blood loss, so immediately compatible whole blood should be transfused.
  - IV fluids can be given temporarily.
  - In burn shock, plasma is lost and there is hemoconcentration. So, plasma should be infused. Plasma expanders which hold the fluid in the capillary can also be given.

---

28. Cardiopulmonary resuscitation.

- Cardiopulmonary resuscitation is a procedure to support ventilation and cardiac activity in persons with cardiac and ventilatory arrest.
- It is indicated in the following conditions—drowning, electrocution, cardiac arrest, cardiac arrhythmias like ventricular fibrillation, arrhythmias following acute MI, anaphylactic shock, etc.

Steps in Performing CPR
- First assess the state of the patient for the following—level of consciousness, respiratory movements, arterial pulse and color of skin.
- If there is no respiratory movement, immediately start ventilatory support by—mouth to mouth respiration, mouth to nose respiration, Holger-Nielsen method or other manual methods.
- If there are no palpable pulsations then the ventilatory support is alternated with external cardiac massage.

Ventilatory Support

Mouth to Mouth Respiration
- Patient is placed on a flat, firm surface
- Check the oral cavity for foreign body, vomitus, blood, debris, etc., if present the oral cavity is cleared.
- The neck is extended by placing the palm of the examiner on the forehead and pressing the head down. This extends the neck and the airway patency is established.
- The chin is lifted with the other hand by placing the hand below the chin. This chin lift prevents the tongue from obstructing the airway.
- The nostril of the patient is clipped with the thumb and index finger of the examiner.
- The examiner takes a deep inspiration and places his mouth over the mouth of the patient and blows into the mouth maximally.
- Check for the chest expansion and abdominal distension.
- Wait for expiration to occur passively.
- Then repeat the procedure 10–15 times per minute.
- In children instead of mouth to mouth, mouth to nose respiration is performed. The steps are similar as mentioned above.

External Cardiac Massage
- Check for cardiac activity by palpating the carotid pulsations.
- If absent the ventilatory support is alternated with cardiac massage.
- The patient is made to lie on a flat firm surface.
- The person conducting the cardiac massage places the heel of one hand on the xiphoid process and the heel of the other hand on top of the first hand.
- Pressure is applied on the heel of the hand to depress the sternum by 4 or 5 cm towards the spine.

- This procedure is repeated 80–100 times per minute.
- The compression and ventilation are done at the rate of 1:5 ratio.
- If pulses return, ventilation is continued.

Once help arrives, the patient is immediately shifted to the hospital and advanced life support in the form of defibrillation, airway management and oxygen therapy is given.

29. Control of appetite.

- Appetite, food intake is controlled by hypothalamus.
- In hypothalamus, there are two centers to regulate food intake, they are—feeding and satiety centers.
  - These are two groups of neurons involved in food intake:
    1. Ventromedial nucleus (satiety center)
    2. Lateral nucleus (feeding center)
  - Feeding center stimulates appetite and increases food intake and satiety center inhibits feeding center and brings satiety.
  - Feeding center is chronically active and its activity is transiently inhibited by activity in the satiety center after ingestion of food.
- Lesion of feeding center causes severe anorexia.
- Lesion of satiety center leads to hyperphagia and over eating results in hypothalamic obesity.
- There are various hormones and neurotransmitters regulating the appetite.
- The following are:
  - *Hormones increasing food intake:*
    - Neuropeptide Y
    - Orexins
    - Ghrelin
    - Melanin-concentrating hormone (MCH)
    - Agouti-related protein (AgRP)
    - Galanin
    - Growth hormone releasing hormone (GHRH)
  - *Hormones decreasing food intake:*
    - Leptin
    - Estrogen
    - Dopamine
    - α-Melanocyte stimulating hormone
    - Cocaine- and amphetamine regulated transcript (CART)
    - Corticotrophin releasing hormone (CRH)
    - Gut hormones
    - Cholecystokinin (CCK)
- There are four hypotheses by which appetite is regulated by action of the above hormones and neurotransmitters on the feeding and satiety centers.

They are:
1. *Glucostatic hypothesis:* Blood glucose levels affects the appetite. The neurons in the satiety center are activated by the blood glucose levels. When the blood glucose levels are low the neuronal uptake of glucose decreases and the feeding center is stimulated resulting in hunger and food intake. When glucose utilisation increases the satiety center is activated and feeding center is inhibited.
2. *Lipostatic hypothesis:* The amount of adipose tissue affects the food intake by a proportional amount of humoral signal, Leptin. As the leptin level increases it decreases the appetite and food intake and increases energy output and vice versa.
3. *Gut-peptide theory:* Food in the gastrointestinal tract causes release of one or more polypeptides like CCK-PZ which acts on the hypothalamus to inhibit food intake.
4. *Thermostatic theory:* A fall in body temperature below the set point stimulates appetite and a rise above the set point inhibits appetite.

30. Color vision.

- Color has three attributes—hue, intensity and saturation.
- Each color has a complementary color and when it is mixed with it, produces white color.
- Cones are the receptors for color vision.
- There are three primary colors—red (723–647 nm), green (575–493 nm), blue (492–450 nm).

- Young-Helmholtz have postulated that there are 3 types of cones each responding to a particular wavelength of light (*refer* **Fig. 36**).
- They are maximally sensitive to each of the primary colors due to presence of three types of photopigments and therefore three types of cones—S (Blue), L (Red) and M (Green) cones.
- The L, M and S cones show maximal response to wavelengths of 560 nm, 530 nm and 420 nm respectively (*refer* **Fig. 10**).
- Different color sensations are perceived by determining the relative frequencies of impulses from each cone system.
- The color perceived is also dependent on the level of illumination and also the background color.
- Different shades of colors perceived also depend on the intensity of the color.
- Based on Young-Helmholtz theory, for perceiving a color at least two cone types are needed.
- The visual cortex compares the relative frequency of action potentials in the activated cone pathways and finds the wavelength and thereby identifies the color.
- Change in intensity is appreciated by change in wavelength.
- Color vision is a function of fovea as it has densely packed cones and this are can get details of the object rather than discrimination of colors.
- Gene for rhodopsin is on chromosome 3 and gene for S-cone pigment is on chromosome 7 and for green and red pigment it is on X chromosome.

Neural Mechanisms

- Color impulses are mediated by P type of ganglion cells by subtracting input from one cone type to other.
- From lateral geniculate body (LGB) impulses travel to cortex in 3 pathways:
  1. A red-green pathway—signals differences between L and M cones.
  2. A blue-yellow pathway—signals differences between S and sum of L and M cones.
  3. Luminance pathway—signals sum of L and M cones.
- They project to 4C layer and blobs in layer 2 and 3 of Area 17 (V1) → then projects to V8.
- **Color blindness** may be only for some colors—due to absence of one or more types of cones.
- The suffix 'anopia' is used for color blindness.
- The suffix 'anomaly' is used to denote color weakness.
- The prefixes 'prot, deuter, trit' are used to for 'red, green and blue' colors.

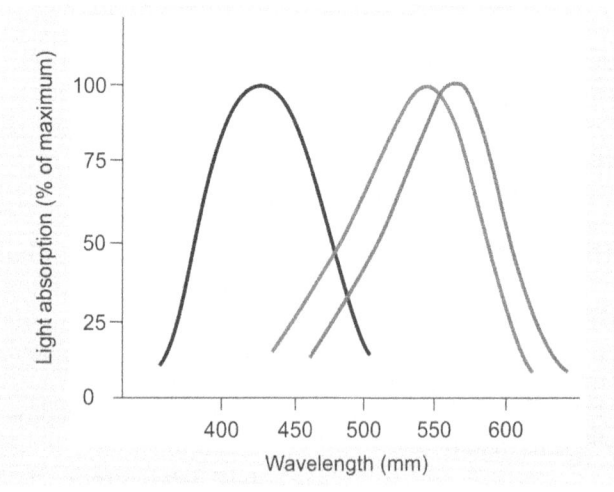

Fig. 36: Three cones and their sensitive wavelength.

- If only 2 cones are present and one cone is absent (**dichromats**)—**protanopia** (red blindness), **deuteranopia** (green color blindness) or **tritanopia** (blue color blindness).
- **Trichromats:** Have all 3 cones, but one is weak.
- **Monochromats** are individuals with only one cone system. They do not appreciate any colors. They see only black, white and shades of grey.

31. Dark adaptation.

- When a person moves from a brightly illuminated place to a dark environment, he is not able to see anything. But gradually the eyes get accommodated to the darkness and his vision improves. This is said to be dark adaptation. Complete adaptation happens in 20 minutes.
- The changes happening in the eye in darkness are—dilatation of pupil, shifting of cone vision to rod vision and regeneration of rhodopsin in darkness.
- The changes happening are discussed under neural adaptation and chemical adaptation.

Neural Adaptation

- The dark adaptation happens in two phases.
- The first phase is due to cone adaptation and it happens in the first 5–10 minutes.
- This increases the retinal sensitivity to light 100 times.
- In the second phase of adaptation the rod sensitivity to light increases and the retinal sensitivity increases by 1000–10,000 times.
- Once rod adaptation has happened even a single photon of light is visible to the eye.

Chemical Adaptation

- When a person stays in bright light, the rod pigment rhodopsin is bleached and is converted to all-trans-retinal and opsin.
- Therefore rods are insensitive to light and do not respond to light.
- The rod sensitivity can increase only when the rhodopsin is resynthesized and this takes several minutes to happen.

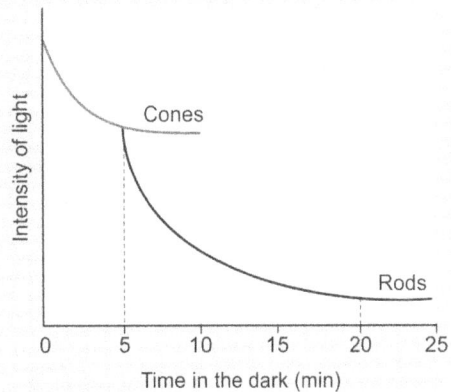

Fig. 37: Dark adaptation curve. There are two curves, red curve shows cone adaptation and violet curve shows rod adaptation.

- That is why the dark adaptation by rods takes 20 minutes.
- The rods are present in the retina 15–20 degrees away from the fovea. That is the reason there is dilatation of the pupil to expose the retina rich in rods to light.
- The time taken for dark adaptation depends on the degree of brightness of light to which the eye is exposed and for how long it is being exposed.
- Brighter the light and longer the duration later it takes for dark adaptation (*refer* **Fig. 37**).

32. Baroreceptors.

- There are two types of baroreceptors (BRs). High pressure and low pressure baroreceptors.
- High pressure BRs are present in the Carotid and aortic sinuses (*refer* **Fig. 38**).

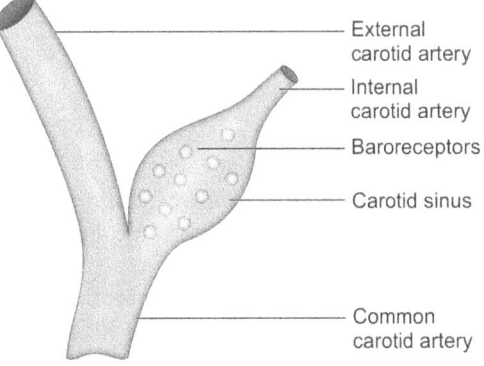

Fig. 38: Baroreceptor—carotid sinus.

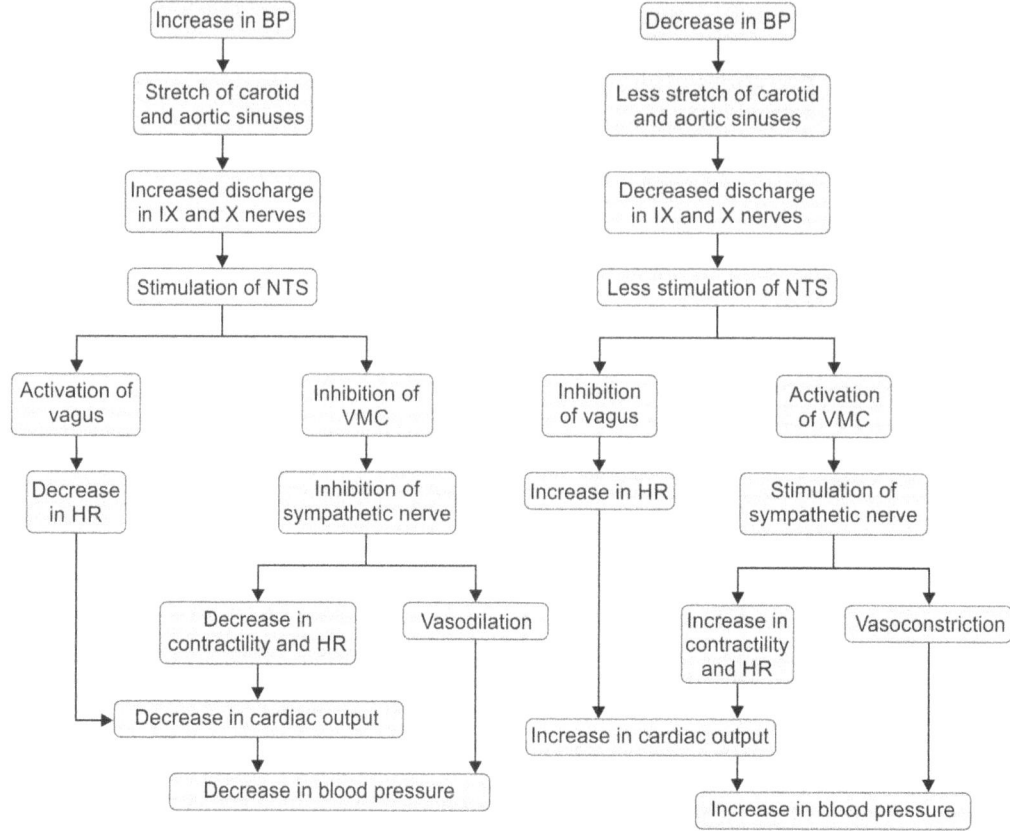

Fig. 39: Regulation of BP by baroreceptors.

- Low pressure BRs are present in the great veins, right and left atria.
- High pressure BRs are there to monitor and correct the daytoday change in BP as in change of posture from supine to standing position.
- They regulate BP maximally when the MAP is between 70–110 mm Hg and stops firing when MAP falls <40 or rises above 150 mm Hg.

Baroreceptor Reflex

It is a most important reflex to regulate BP.
- Also called as sino-aortic reflex
- Receptor—carotid and aortic sinuses
- Stimulus—stretch of baroreceptors (as in increased BP)
- Afferents—IXth (supplies carotid sinus) and Xth cranial nerves (aortic sinus)
- Efferents—sympathetic nerves and vagus nerve
- Effector—heart and blood vessels
- Response—decrease in BP

The reflex is explained in the **Figure 39**.

33. Speech areas and aphasia.

- Understanding spoken and written words and to express ideas in speech and writing is language.
- It is a role of the dominant or categorical hemisphere.
- It is one of the higher functions of cerebral cortex.
- Speech is thought to be a mode of communication between human beings.
- There are two forms of speech—written words and spoken words.

- Speech involves coordinated activities of central and peripheral speech apparatus.

Areas Involved in Language

- All areas for language are around the sylvian fissure. They are:
  - **Wernicke's area (area 22):** Comprehension of auditory and visual information.
  - **Broca's area (area 44):** Processes the information comprehended by Wernicke's area into a coordinated pattern for vocalization.
  - **Arcuate fasciculus:** Transmits information from area 22 to 44.
  - **Angular gyrus (area 39):** Processes information from that are read and converted to auditory form of words in area 22 (*refer* **Fig. 40**).
  - **Motor area.**

Aphasia

It is inability to communicate in the form of spoken or written language due to defects in the speech areas of categorical hemisphere.

Fluent Aphasia or Wernicke's Aphasia

- Lesion in the sensory speech area—Wernicke's area (area 22). It can happen due to blockage of vessels supplying the area or injury.
- Also called as fluent aphasia.
- Here the person is able to hear spoken words or identifying written words.
- But cannot comprehend spoken or written words.
- Motor speech is intact. So, speech is not disturbed. Person speaks excessively.
- Impairment of written words as they are not able to comprehend written words also.

Non-fluent Aphasia or Broca's Aphasia

- In lesion of Broca's area there is normal comprehension of speech but there is poverty of speech.
- This type of aphasia is called as nonfluent aphasia.
- Broca's area is the motor speech area (area 44) and is located in the foot of the primary motor cortex (area 4).
- In spoken speech, impulses from the ear are transmitted to the primary auditory area (area 42) in the temporal lobe.
- From area 42, the impulse reaches the auditory association areas and then to the sensory speech area—Wernicke's are (area 22). Here comprehension of speech happens.
- From the Wernicke's area impulses are transmitted to the Broca's area.
- It regulates the functions of the muscles of the lips, tongue, pharynx and larynx and it helps in vocalization of the reply.

Global Aphasia

- Lesion in both the Wernicke's area and Broca's area results in Global aphasia.
- All aspects of speech are impaired.
- The patient is not able to comprehend or repeat words.

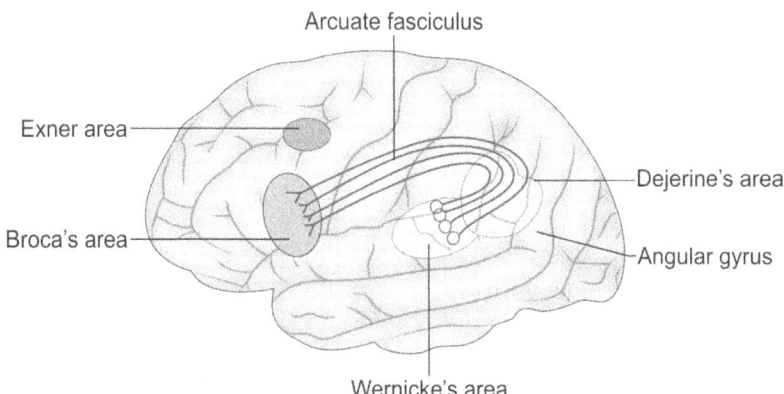

Fig. 40: Speech areas in cerebral cortex.

Anomic Aphasia

- It is a type of difficulty in speech due to lesion in the angular gyrus (area 39).
- The person has no difficulty in speech or understanding of auditory information.
- But there is trouble in understanding written language and pictures because the visual information is not processed and transmitted to Wernicke's area.
- It is also called as word blindness.

---

34. Physiological changes in human body during exercise.

Exercises are of two types, based on the types of muscle contraction. They are classified as isotonic and isometric exercises.

Isometric Exercise

- In this type of exercise, the muscle length remains the same and the force generated is increased.
- Since no shortening of muscle happens there is no work being done.
- Examples are—pushing against the wall and holding the weight as in weight lifting.

Isotonic Exercise

- In this type of exercise there is shortening of muscle fiber and therefore external work is done.
- Here tension in the muscle remains the same.
- Examples are—walking, running, jogging, etc.

Physiological Changes During Exercise

- Exercise is a type of stress to the body and therefore there are many physiological changes happening in the body to face this stress.
- The changes are happening to provide additional amount of energy needed for the exercising muscle and to remove waste metabolites put out by the working muscles.
- So bodily changes happen at the level of O_2 uptake, cardiovascular changes, respiratory changes and changes in the muscles and other tissues.

O_2 Uptake

- Normal O_2 uptake at rest is 250 mL/min. It can increase to 3L/min during exercise.
- So it is given as the maximum amount of O_2 consumed by an individual during exercise or VO_2 max.
- VO_2 max is the product of maximal cardiac output and maximal O_2 extraction by the tissues.
- VO_2 max improves with training. In a sedentary individual it is around 3L/min and in athletes it is upto 5L/min.
- There is a linear increase in O_2 uptake in the initial phases of exercise and it reaches the VO_2 max. But as the severity of exercise increases and as the VO_2 max is reached, there is no further increse in O_2 uptake.
- So the excess energy requirement is dealt by utilization of anaerobic glycolytic pathway of metabolism and also break down of creatinine phosphate for energy.
- This results in production of lactic acid and the blood pH decreases resulting in hyperventilation. This further limits the production of lactic acid.
- Increase in O_2 uptake continues to be increased even after termination of exercise and the extra O_2 consumed, is used to repay the O_2 debt.
- This O_2 debt is used to remove the lactic acid, replenish ATP and phosphoryl creatine and the O_2 store in myoglobin.

Changes in the Respiratory System

- Changes happening in RS during exercise is to supply the extra amount of O_2 needed by the muscles and to remove the extra CO_2 put out by the working muscles.
- Hyperventilation during exercise helps to achieve this demand and also to maintain pO_2 and pCO_2 at normal levels in arterial blood.

Increased Ventilation During Exercise

- Increase in ventilation matches the energy requirement of working muscles.
- Increase in ventilation is by increasing the depth and rate of respiration.

- Normal rate of respiration is 12–18 cycles/min and the depth of respiration is assessed by the tidal volume and it is 500 mL at rest. So the minute ventilation is around 6L/min.
- During exercise, tidal volume and rate increases, initially both are increased and once TV reaches its saturation, further increase is by increasing the rate of respiration. It can be increased to 80–100 L/min.
- The **pattern of increase in ventilation** is by an abrupt increase in the beginning followed by a small pause then a gradual increase and after stopping the exercise there is an abrupt decrease in ventilation followed by a gradual decline to baseline level.
- The initial abrupt increase is due to psychic stimuli from the cortex followed by neural stimuli arising from the proprioceptors in muscles, joints and tendons.
- The gradual increase in ventilation is due to the chemical changes happening in the PO_2, PCO_2 levels and pH in arterial blood.
- Arterial PO_2 and PCO_2 levels remain the same, even in severe exercise, but the stimulation of chemoreceptors happen because of increase in sensitivity of the chemoreceptors for the normal fluctuations in the levels of PO_2 and PCO_2.
- The other important mechanism by which ventilation increases is due to increase in body temperature.
- Increase in plasma K^+ levels in blood following its release from the exercising muscles, also stimulates respiration.

Increase in O_2 Uptake

O_2 uptake increases following exercise from 250 mL/min to 4000 mL/min.

This is happening because of:
- **Increased blood flow to lungs** as the cardiac output increases, due to increase in heart rate and stroke volume.
- **Increase in pO_2 gradient** between the alveolus and pulmonary arterial blood. Exercising muscles extract more O_2 from arterial blood and therefore the venous blood reaching the pulmonary artery has low PO_2. This increases the gradient for O_2 movement.
- **Increase in diffusion capacity** of the respiratory membrane. Most of the pulmonary capillaries remain closed in resting states. During exercise these capillaries also open up and therefore the surface area across which exchange happens increases.

Changes in the Cardiovascular System

Changes in the CVS happen to supply the extra O_2 needed by the exercising muscles.

This happens by:
- Increase in heart rate, increase in cardiac output, increase in blood flow to skeletal muscles, decreased blood flow to other organs.
- The cardiovascular change during exercise depends on the type of exercise being performed.

Isometric Exercise

There is a prompt increase in heart rate (HR) on the start of exercise.

Causes for Increase in HR:
- HR rises even before starting the exercise due to psychic stimuli.
- The increase is mainly due to decreased vagal tone and increase in sympathetic discharge to the heart.
- Impulses from joints and muscles increase HR and rise in body temperature also increases HR.
- Release of catecholamines from adrenal medulla also increases HR.
- The maximum increase in HR is a good indicator of fitness and it is based on the basal heart rate.
- The target heart rate achieved during exercise in the adults is 195/min and in children it is 200/min and above. With advancing age it declines.

Changes in BP
- There is an increase in systolic and diastolic blood pressure following isometric exercise.
- Systolic pressure increases due to increase in HR.

- Diastolic pressure increases due to compression of the blood vessels by the contracting muscles.
- There is not much change in stroke volume.
- Blood flow to the steadily contracting muscle is decreased.

Isotonic Exercise

There is increase in HR and the causes are the same as the above.

Changes in BP

- Systolic BP rises moderately.
- Diastolic BP remains same or decreases as the peripheral resistance decreases.
- Peripheral resistance decreases due to vasodilatation.
- Vasodilatation is due the vasodilator metabolites ($\uparrow PCO_2$, $\downarrow PO_2$, lactate, adenosine, etc.) produced by the working muscle.
- Stroke volume is increased.

Changes in Cardiac Output

- Cardiac output (CO) increases to supply the extra demand faced by the body.
- It decides the O_2 delivery to the tissues and rise in cardiac output is the rate limiting step for O_2 extraction.
- CO increases from 5L/min at rest to 25L/min during exercise.
- CO increase is due to both, increase in HR and stroke volume.
- Increase in stroke volume is due to – increase in myocardial contractility following sympathetic stimulation and increase in EDV due to activation of skeletal muscle pump, thaoracic pump and abdominal pump.

Skeletal Muscle Blood Flow

The blood flow to the exercising muscles increases 30 times from the baseline value. At rest the muscle blood flow is 2–4 mL/100 g/min.

The causes for increase in muscle blood flow:

- The increase happens even before start of exercise due to a neural mechanism. It involves the sympathetic cholinergic system.
- This is followed by the local mechanisms. As the exercise progresses the working muscle put out vasodilator metabolites— $\downarrow PO_2$, $\uparrow PCO_2$, $\uparrow K^+$, lactate, etc. These chemicals dilate the blood vessels.
- The heat generated by the contracting muscles increses the blood flow by dilating the vessels.

O_2 **extraction by the muscles** is also increased as the metabolites and increased body temperature and 2,3,DPG levels shift the O_2-Hb dissociation curve to the right and thereby liberates O_2 to the muscles.

Redistribution of Blood Flow

- As the blood flow to exercising muscles increase, there is a compromise in blood flow to certain organs and increased blood flow to other organs.
- So the redistribution also contributes to the increase in skeletal muscle flow along with the increased cardiac output.

Redistribution

- Blood flow to the visceral organs is decreased.
- Blood flow to skin is also decreased initially but as the exercise progresses, the rise in body temperature causes vasodilataion and increased blood flow to skin helps in losing the body heat.
- Cerebral blood flow is maintained.
- Coronary blood flow increases by neural and local mechanisms.
- Blood flow to adipose tissues increase to mobilize fatty acids.

35. Acclimatization at high altitude.

Refer Short note 22.

36. Functions of hypothalamus.

Refer Short note 25.

37. Taste pathway.

The taste receptors are present in the taste buds which are located on the tongue in the papillae.

- There are 10,000 taste buds.
- Taste buds are located in—fungiform, foliate and vallate papillae.

- Cells in taste buds—type 1 and 2—supporting cells.
- Type 3 cells—receptor epithelial cells has microvilli projecting into taste pore.
- They are receptors are replaced constantly in 10 days.
- Each bud is innervated by 50 nerves at bases of receptor cells.
- Each nerve innervates 5 taste buds.
- The sensory fibers from the taste buds travel through 3 nerves—chorda tympani branch of facial nerve (from anterior 2/3rd of the tongue), glossopharyngeal nerve (from posterior 1/3rd of the tongue) and vagus nerve from epiglottis, pharynx and palate.
- They all reach the medulla and terminate on the same side nucleus tractus solitarius.
- From here the second order neurons travel along with medial lemniscus to reach ventral posteromedial nucleus of ipsilateral thalamus (*refer* **Fig. 41**).
- Some fibers from medulla go to the vomiting center, hypothalamus, limbic system and salivary nucleus.
- The 3rd order neurons arise from the thalamus and they reach the foot of post central gyrus on the same side (area 43).
- From there impulses are also transmitted to the insula and lateral orbitofrontal cortex.

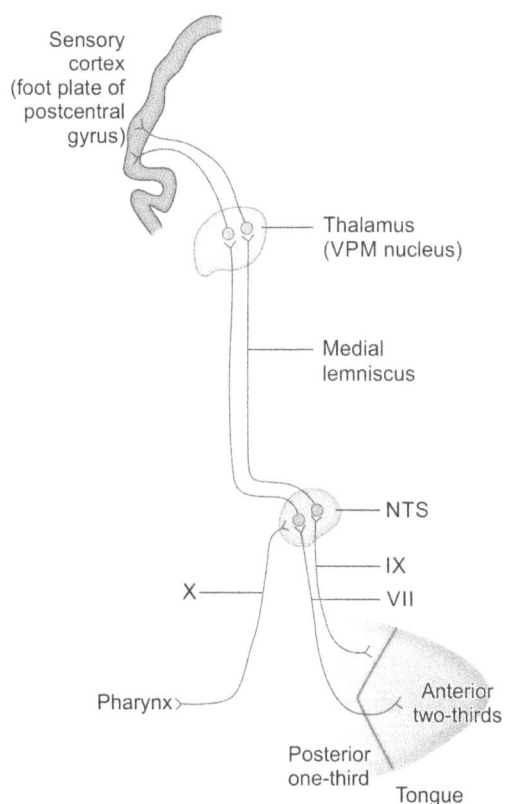

Fig. 41: Taste pathway.

38. Properties of cardiac muscle.

Properties of cardiac muscle are classified as electrical and mechanical properties.
- Electrical properties are—automaticity, rhythmicity, excitability, conductivity, refractory period.
- Mechanical properties are—contractility, staircase phenomenon, all or none law and length-tension relationship.

Electrical Properties

Automaticity
- It is the property of initiation of impulses automatically even in the absence of any stimulus.
- The heart has the ability to beat continuously even after it is denervated and removed from the body and kept in a solution resembling the ECF.
- It is due to the presence of the pacemaker tissue, the SA node which can generate impulses automatically, the pacemaker potential.
- Other structures in the heart, the AV node, His bundle, Purkinje fibers and the ventricular tissue also have the ability to generate their own impulses.

Rhythmicity
- The automatic generation of impulses from the SA Node is rhythmic in nature.
- Rhythmicity means, the impulses produced from the pacemaker, the SA Node is in regular intervals and is constant. Since it is generated from the SA node, it is said to be the sinus rhythm.
- The normal rate of impulse generation from SA node is 60–100 per minute. It is the highest rate generated by the tissues of the heart.

- In conditions of disease in SA node, the impulse generation starts in the other tissues like the atrium, AV node His-Purkinje fibers and ventricular tissue.
- The order or hierarchy of taking over the role of pacemaking is determined by the rate of generation of impulses.
- The rate of AV node is 45-60 per minute and in disease of AV node the impulses from the infranodal tissue is 45 per minute and if the ventricle is the pacemaker the rate is 35 per minute.

Excitability
- It is the property of the cardiac muscle to respond to stimuli in the form of impulse generation or contraction.
- In response to impulse generation from the SA node the other tissues of the conducting system—atria, AV node, His bundle, Purkinje fibers and ventricular muscles respond by developing action potentials and conduction of AP—impulse generation.
- Atrial and ventricular musculature respond to the AP and contract.
- Excitability of cardiac muscle is affected by concentration of ions in the ECF and the influence of sympathetic and parasympathetic nerves.

Conductivity
- It is the property of cardiac muscle to conduct the impulses generated in SA node to the ventricular musculature.
- The conduction of impulses occurs in the following pathway:

SA node
↓
Right atrial musculature and Internodal tracts
↓Interatrial bundle   ↓
Left atrium   AV node
↓
His bundle
↓
Purkinje fibers
↓
Ventricular musculature

Refractory Period
- Refractory period is the time period in the muscle action potential during which the muscle does not respond to the second stimulus, no matter how strong is the stimulus.
- It is of two types—absolute refractory period (ARP) and relative refractory period (RRP).
- The duration of refractory period is longer in cardiac muscles.
- The ARP is 200 ms and RRP is 50 ms.
- The contractile period of the cardiac muscle falls within the refractory period and therefore another impulse cannot stimulate the cardiac muscle and it can never be tetanized.

Mechanical Properties

Contractility
It is the ability of cardiac muscles— atrial and ventricular tissues to contract following excitation:
- It is called as inotropism.
- The contraction of the heart results in systole following which blood is pumped into the circulatory system.
- The increase in contractility results in increase in stroke volume and thereby increase in cardiac output and vice versa.
- Factors which enhance the contractility are called as positive inotropic agents—sympathetic stimulation, digitalis, etc.
- Factors which decrease the contractility are called as negative inotropic agents—hypoxia, hypercapnia, acidosis, etc.

Stair-case Phenomenon
- It is also called as the Bowditch phenomenon. In a quiescent heart if stimuli are given continuously within 10 seconds, there is gradual increase in force of contraction for the first 3-4 stimuli and after that it becomes a constant.
- It is due to the beneficial effect of the first stimulus for the next stimulus.

It is explained by the following reasons:
- The increased availability of calcium ions for the second contraction as there is no time to pump back calcium into the SR following the first contraction.

- The rise in temperature following first contraction enhances the enzyme actions.
- The initial contraction alters the viscoelastic property of cardiac muscle, may be due to increase in temperature.

All-or-none Law

- If a quiescent heart is stimulated with stimuli of varying intensity, the heart does not respond to subthreshold stimuli and the response to threshold stimulus is the optimum and if suprathreshold stimulus is given the magnitude of response remains the same as that for threshold stimulus and there is no further increase in magnitude of response.
- This is called as all-or-none law.
- In cardiac muscle if threshold stimulus is given the whole ventricular musculature contracts as a single unit because of the syncytial nature of cardiac muscles, which in turn is due to the presence of gap junctions between the muscle fibers.

Length-tension Relationship

- Length-tension relationship of cardiac muscle is similar to that of the skeletal muscles.
- It is given by the Frank-Starling's law, which states that, the force of contraction is directly proportional to the initial length of the muscle fiber within physiological limits.
- The initial length is the muscle length before it starts to contract and it is equal to the preload.
- If the preload increases, the force of contraction increases and the stroke volume increases within physiological limits.
- It is due to the optimal interaction between the actin and cross-bridges which produces maximal tension following contraction.

39. Hypoxia and its types.

- Hypoxia is defined as deficiency of O_2 at tissue level.
- **Types:**
  - Hypoxic hypoxia
  - Anemic hypoxia
  - Stagnant hypoxia
  - Histotoxic hypoxia

Hypoxic Hypoxia

- Arterial pO_2 is low, therefore tissue pO_2 is less
- **Mechanism of hypoxia:** pO_2 of arterial blood is low due to either ↓O_2 in inspired air or disease of respiratory apparatus.
- **Conditions:**
  - Low pO_2 in inspired air (as in high altitude)
  - Hypoventilation
  - Diffusion defects
  - Ventilation/perfusion mismatch
  - A-V shunt

Anemic Hypoxia

- It is due to decreased O_2 carrying capacity of blood and so ↓O_2 content in blood. pO_2 is normal.
- **Conditions:** Anemia, CO poisoning, presence of altered Hb (methemoglobin), etc.
- In mild conditions the 2,3-DPG levels increase in the RBC → easy dissociation of O_2

Stagnant Hypoxia

- Hypoxia due to decreased blood flow to tissues. Also called as ischemic hypoxia.
- **Mechanism:** O_2 content and pO_2 are normal in arterial blood. Hypoxia is due to stagnation of blood → circulatory hypoxia.
- **Seen in:**
  - Heart failure
  - Shock
  - Vascular obstruction

Histotoxic Hypoxia

- Tissues cannot utilize O_2 in spite of normal O_2 supply as in cyanide poisoning.
- Venous pO_2 is high (> 46 mm Hg)
- Cyanide poisoning is treated with methylene blue or nitrites → forms methemoglobin → reacts with cyanide → cyanmethemoglobin. It is less poisonous.
- Hyperbaric O_2 is also used for treatment.

40. Otolith organ.

- The vestibular apparatus in the inner ear consists of—3 semicircular canals and 2 sac like structures—utricle and saccule.

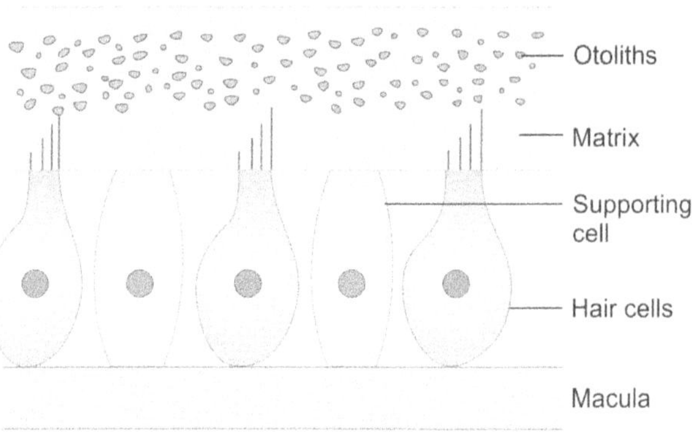

Fig. 42: Otolithic organ.

- The receptors for vestibular sensation are the hair cells and they are located in the cristae in the ampulla of semicircular canals and the macula or otolithic organ of the utricle and saccule.
- The receptors in the canals and the utricle and saccule are the hair cells located in unique structures.
- The hairs of the hair cells are embedded in thick gelatinous substance called the cupula.

Receptors in Utricle and Saccule

- The receptor organ in utricle and saccule is called the macula.
- Macula in utricle is in horizontal plane and in saccule in vertical plane.
- The macula is an elevation in the sacs.
- It is made of epithelial cells with hair cells interspersed.
- The hair is embedded in the cupula.
- Cupula in utricle and saccule are embedded with calcium carbonate crystals–otoliths (*refer* **Fig. 42**)
- So, these organs are called as otolithic organs.

Mechanism of Action of Otolithic Organs

- Hair cells in the otolithic organ is oriented in different directions.
- They are stimulated as the head is tilted in any direction.
- The maculae are receptors of static equilibrium and some amount of dynamic equilibrium.
- It provides information about the position of head in space and essential for maintaining appropriate balance.
- Also used for detecting linear acceleration and deceleration, either vertical or horizontal.
- As the head is tilted forward, the otolithic organ is tilted to the front due to gravity, pulling the hairs and depolarizing the nerves.
- Linear acceleration: As travelling in a car, as it starts with a jerk, there is a thrust to forward direction.
- The otolithic organ lags behind due to inertia and pulls on the hair and bends them.
- This initiates impulses in the nerves.
- The person bends forward to correct the position.

Functions of Otolithic Organ

Utricle and saccule (otolithic organ) detect linear acceleration and position of head in relation to gravity.

Physiology Topic-wise University Questions (from 2011–2021 Papers)

CHAPTER 1: GENERAL PHYSIOLOGY

Homeostasis
- Milieu interior (2011)
- Negative feedback mechanism with example (2011, 2020)
- Positive feedback mechanism (2015, 2017)

Cell Physiology
- Endoplasmic reticulum (2016)
- Functions of mitochondria (2012)
- Apoptosis (2013, 2019)

Transport Across Cell membrane
- A transport across cell membrane (2014, 2021)
- Secondary active transport (2011, 2014)
- Na^+-K^+ pump (2011, 2012, 2013, 2017, 2018)
- Facilitated diffusion (2013, 2016, 2019)
- Primary active transport (2013, 2017)
- Endocytosis (2018, 2020)
- Passive transport (2018)
- Active transport across cell membrane (2021)

Membrane Potentials

Resting membrane potential (2011, 2015, 2019)

Body Fluids
- Classify body fluid compartments, give their normal values, methods to determine ECF volume (2018, 2021)
- ECF volume and blood volume in a 70 kg adult male (2013)
- Concentration of Na^+ and K^+ in intracellular and extracellular fluids (2014)

CHAPTER 2: BLOOD

Plasma Proteins
- Types and functions of plasma proteins (2011, 2012, 2014, 2020)
- Albumin: Globulin ratio (2014)
- Colloid oncotic pressure and its importance (2014)

Red Blood Cells
- Erythropoiesis – Stages and regulation (2011, 2012, 2015, 2016)
- Significance of ESR (2012, 2015, 2021)
- Red cell indices (2015)
- Shape of erythrocytes (2019)

Anemia and Polycythemia
- Anemia (2014, 2021)
- Sickle cell anemia (2012)
- Types of Polycythemias and its complications (2014, 2016, 2017)
- Reticulocyte response (2017)
- Megaloblastic anemia (2019)

WBCs
- Phagocytosis (2016)
- Cytokines (2011)
- Opsonization (2012)
- Functions of different granulocytes in circulating blood (2014)
- Functions of different types of leucocytes in blood (2021)
- Functions of macrophages (2014)
- Opsonins (2014)
- Tissue macrophage system (2014, 2019, 2021)
- Functions of lymphocytes (2015)
- Functions of lymphocytes in viral infections (2021)
- Functions of neutrophil (2020)

Lymph and Edema
- Mechanism of edema in congestive heart failure (2013)
- Extracellular edema (2015)
- Functions of lymph (2019)

Immunity

- Cell mediated immunity (2017)
- Essay on immunity (2013, 2017, 2020)
- T Lymphocytes (2018)
- Formation and functions of immunoglobulins (2012)
- Autoimmune disease (2011, 2013, 2020)
- Helper cells (2011, 2017)
- Immunological memory (2012)
- Cells which express MHC II (2014)
- Complement system for antibody action (2018)
- Mast cells (2019)

Platelets

- Structure and functions of platelets (2012, 2014, 2020)

Hemostasis

- Mechanism of coagulation (2011, 2013, 2015, 2018, 2020)
- Anticoagulants (2012, 2016, 2019)
- Hemophilia (2011, 2012, 2016)
- Fibrinolysis (2011, 2018, 2021)
- Role of vitamin K in the body (2013)
- Vitamin K dependent coagulation factors (2013, 2014)
- Finding of tests of hemostasis in hemophilia (2014)
- Clot retraction (2017)
- Disseminated intravascular coagulation (2020)

Blood Groups

- Erythroblastosis fetalis (2013, 2019)
- Blood groups (2013, 2015)
- Landsteiner's laws (2020)
- Kernicterus (2011)
- Rh blood group (2012, 2016)
- Rh status of mother, father and child for occurrence of Rh incompatibility (2013)
- Indications and complications of blood transfusion (2015)
- Bombay blood group (2017)
- Cross-matching (2018)

CHAPTER 3: NERVE MUSCLE PHYSIOLOGY

Nerve

- Nerve action potential (2017, 2020)
- Compound action potential (2016)
- Saltatory conduction in nerve fibers (2012, 2017)
- Chronaxie (2012, 2013, 2015)
- Rheobase (2015)
- Refractory period (2014, 2020)
- Define all or none law, its application in skeletal and cardiac muscle (2015)
- Classification of nerve fibers (2012)
- Role of myelin sheath in conduction of nerve impulse (2013, 2014)

Neuromuscular Junction

- Neuromuscular junction (2011, 2015, 2016, 2021)
- Myasthenia gravis (2011, 2012, 2014)
- Type of acetylcholine receptor on skeletal muscle and its function (2013)
- Neuromuscular blockers (2018)
- Mechanism of action of botulinum toxin (2018)

Muscle Physiology

- Excitation-contraction coupling (2017)
- Electron microscopic structure of skeletal muscle and molecular mechanism of muscle contraction (2011, 2012, 2019)
- Multi-unit smooth muscle (2011)
- Sarcomere (2011)
- Rigor mortis (2011, 2017, 2019)
- Sliding filament hypothesis and cross-bridge cycling (2012)
- Isotonic and isometric contraction (2013, 2016)
- Motor unit (2013, 2014, 2020)
- Calcium transporters in membrane of Sarcoplasmic reticulum (2013)
- Role of tropomyosin in muscle contraction (2013)
- Membrane transporters involved in clearance of cytoplasmic calcium (2014)
- Role of ATP in muscle relaxation (2014)
- Draw a schematic diagram of sarcomere and label the parts (2014)
- Name the muscle proteins. What is the role of troponin C in muscle contraction (2015, 2017)
- Properties of smooth muscle (2018)
- Physiological basis of length-tension relationship (2019)

- Energy sources in muscle (2019)
- Heat production in skeletal muscle (2020)

CHAPTER 4: GASTROINTESTINAL SYSTEM

Introduction

Enteric nervous system (2018, 2020)

Salivary Secretion

Composition, regulation and functions of saliva (2011, 2013, 2014, 2016)

Deglutition

Deglutition (2014, 2015, 2016)

Esophagus and Applied Aspects

Achalasia cardia (2017, 2019)

Stomach—Secretion and Motility

- Composition, mechanism and regulation of gastric secretion (2011, 2012, 2014, 2015, 2016, 2018, 2019, 2021)
- Experimental evidences for gastric secretion (2015)
- Gastric emptying (2013, 2018)
- Pathophysiology of peptic ulcer (2014, 2015, 2020, 2021)
- Role of *H. pylori* in peptic ulcer (2017)
- Functions of stomach (2020)

Pancreatic Secretions

- Composition, function and regulation of pancreatic secretion (2011, 2013, 2018)
- Enzymes of exocrine pancreas (2014)
- Intestinal phase of pancreatic secretion (2015)

Liver, Gallbladder and Bile Secretion

- Functions of liver and jaundice (2018)
- Enterohepatic circulation of bile (2013, 2014, 2016, 2019)
- Cholelithiasis (2012, 2020)
- Functions of bile salts (2012)
- Composition of bile and physiological role of its components (2014)

Small intestine—Secretion and Motility

- Succus entericus (2015)
- Movements of small intestine (2011, 2012, 2015, 2021)
- Migrating myoelectric complex (2017)
- APUD cells (2011)
- Law of intestine (2011, 2016, 2020)
- Counter-current blood flow in the villi (2012)
- Enterogastric reflex (2012)
- Peristaltic rush (2012)
- Peristalsis (2013)

Large intestine—Secretions and Motility

- Functions of large intestine (2011, 2017)
- Dietary fiber (2011, 2015)
- Gastrocolic reflex (2017)
- Physiological basis of treatment of diarrhea (2017)

GI Hormones

- Gastrointestinal hormones (2020)
- Gastrin (2016)
- Secretin (2018)

Principles of Digestion and Absorption of Carbohydrates, Fats and Proteins and Applied Aspects

- Steatorrhea (2011, 2013, 2018)
- Digestion and absorption of fat (2013, 2016, 2021)
- Enzymes involved in fat digestion (2014)
- Absorption of carbohydrates in the food (2019)
- Digestion and absorption of proteins (2021)
- Malabsorption syndrome (2021)

CHAPTER 5: RENAL SYSTEM

Introduction to Renal System and Functional Anatomy of Kidneys

- Functions of Juxtaglomerular apparatus (2013, 2017, 2021)
- Renin-Angiotensin system (2015)
- Macula densa (2012)
- Non-excretory functions of kidneys (2014, 2019, 2021)
- Peculiarities of renal blood flow (2018)

Glomerular Filtration

- Definition, factors affecting and measurement (2011, 2013, 2014, 2016, 2020)
- Autoregulation of GFR (2013, 2014)

- Clinical tests to assess GFR (2014)
- Filtration fraction (2019)

Tubular Functions

- Tubuloglomerular feedback (2012, 2017)
- Types of water absorption (2011)
- Aquaporins (2012)
- Transport maximum (2013)
- Renal glycosuria (2013)
- Proximal tubular events (2015)
- Renal threshold and tubular maximum for glucose (2018)
- Glucose transporters (2019)
- Bartter's syndrome (2019)

Concentration of Urine

- Counter-current exchangers in kidney (2013, 2015)
- Counter-current mechanism (2018)

Acidification of Urine

- Renal contribution of pH regulation (2012)
- Anion gap (2012, 2017)
- Mechanism of generation of HCO3- in distal tubule (2013)

Kidney Function Tests

- Inulin clearance (2012, 2015)
- Free-water clearance (2020)

Diuresis and Diuretics

- Osmotic diuresis (2013)
- Diuretics and their sites of action (2016, 2018, 2020, 2021)

Dialysis

Artificial kidney (2013)

Nerve Supply of Urinary Bladder, Cystometrogram, Micturition Reflex and Bladder Disorders

- Cystometrogram (2014, 2021)
- Nerve supply of urinary bladder and micturition reflex (2011, 2012, 2015, 2016, 2020)
- Atonic bladder (2014, 2019)

Skin

- Functions of skin (2014)

CHAPTER 6: ENDOCRINOLOGY

Introduction to Endocrinology and Second Messengers

- Name the second messengers (2011, 2012)
- Second messengers (2018)
- G protein (2012)
- G-Protein coupled receptors (2013)
- cAMP signaling pathway with an example (2014)
- Radioimmunoassay (2017)

Hypothalamic Hormones

- Name the hormones of hypothalamus (2013)

Pituitary Hormones—Anterior and Posterior Pituitary Hormones

- Actions of growth hormone (2020)
- List the hormones of anterior pituitary, Mechanism of action of growth hormone, acromegaly (2017)
- Regulation of growth hormone secretion (2017)
- Milk ejection reflex (2019)
- Neuroendocrine reflex (2011, 2018)
- Acromegaly (2013, 2014, 2015)
- Differences between cretinism and dwarfism (2017)
- Dwarf (2011, 2015)
- Name the hormones involved in growth (2011)
- Houssay animal (2011)
- Laron dwarf (2012)
- Progeria (2012)
- Oxytocin (2012)
- Somatomedins (2013, 2015)
- Functions of any one hormone of posterior pituitary (2014)
- Hypersecretion of growth hormone (2014, 2018)
- Diabetes insipidus (2015, 2017)
- Gigantism (2019)

Thyroid Hormones

- Thyroid function tests (2012, 2020)
- Hypothyroidism (2015)
- Synthesis and functions of thyroid hormones (2013, 2015, 2016, 2018)
- Cretinism (2013, 2014)

- Regulation of thyroid hormones (2015)
- Action of thyroxine on CVS (2015)
- Hyperthyroidism (2017)
- Cretinism (2018, 2020)

Adrenocortical Hormones

- Actions, regulation and applied aspects of glucocorticoids (2012, 2014, 2015, 2021)
- Cushing's syndrome (2015, 2017)
- Actions and regulation of secretion of Aldosterone (2013, 2019)
- Conn's syndrome (2012, 2013, 2020)
- Aldosterone escape (2011, 2019)
- Permissive action (2012, 2014)
- Hormones of adrenal cortex (2013)
- Addison's disease (2013)
- Addisonian crisis (2016)
- Compare the actions of adrenaline and Nor-adrenaline on heart and blood vessels (2018)

Endocrine Pancreas

- Glucose homeostasis, GTT and diabetes mellitus (2013)
- Name hyperglycemic hormones, Actions of hypoglycemic hormone, GTT, diabetes mellitus (2018)
- Glucagon (2011, 2019)
- Pathophysiology of diabetes mellitus (2011, 2012)
- Normal blood sugar levels, hormonal regulation of blood glucose levels (2012)
- Pancreatic C-peptide and its significance as a laboratory test (2013)
- Significance of glycosylated hemoglobin (2014, 2015)
- Control of insulin secretion (2016)

Calcium Regulating Hormones

- Actions and regulation of parathormone (2013, 2020, 2021)
- Regulation of serum calcium levels (2021)
- Hormones involved in calcium regulation (2011, 2014)
- Calcitriol (2012)
- Tetany (2012, 2013)
- Normal blood calcium level (2013)
- Role of Vitamin D in calcium homeostasis (2014)
- Vitamin D deficiency (2019)

Other Hormones

- Erythropoietin (2016)

CHAPTER 7: REPRODUCTIVE SYSTEM

Sex Determination and Differentiation

- What is Turner's syndrome, give three features (2011)
- Puberty (2012)
- Menarche (2013)
- Female pseudo hermaphroditism (2019)

Male Reproductive System

- Spermatogenesis (2011, 2013, 2014, 2019, 2021)
- Functions of Sertoli cells (2012, 2015)
- Composition of semen and its use as a diagnostic tool (2020, 2021)
- Cryptorchidism (2013)
- Influence of temperature on spermatogenesis (2015, 2018)
- Functions of prostate gland (2016)

Female Reproductive System

Menstrual Cycle

- Menstrual cycle, hormonal regulation (2011, 2013, 2014)
- Indicators of ovulation (2013, 2015)
- Corpus luteum (2013, 2014)
- LH surge (2013, 2020)
- Endometrial changes in menstrual cycle (2021)

Ovarian Hormones

- Functions of estrogen (2016)
- Actions of relaxin and inhibin (2016)
- Effect of estrogen on uterine endometrium (2015)

Pregnancy

- Pregnancy tests (2020)
- Parturition (2013)

Placental functions

- Functions of placenta (2011, 2012, 2020)
- Fetoplacental unit (2011, 2015, 2017)
- Placental hormones (2012, 2013, 2015)

Lactation

- Why are ovarian cycles suppressed during lactation? (2013)

Contraception

- Contraceptives (2013)
- Female contraceptive methods (2018, 2021)
- Pills (2012)
- Contraception in males (2014, 2017)
- Oral contraceptives (2015, 2018)

CHAPTER 8: CARDIOVASCULAR SYSTEM

Properties of Cardiac Muscle

- Pacemaker potential (2012, 2013, 2015, 2017, 2020)
- List the properties of cardiac muscle (2011)
- SA node as pacemaker (2013)
- List the calcium transporters on the sarcoplasmic reticulum membrane in ventricular muscle (2013)
- Auto rhythmicity of heart (2016)
- Ventricular action potential (2018)
- Properties of cardiac muscle (2021)

Conducting System of Heart

- Origin and spread of cardiac impulse (2015, 2017, 2020)
- Structure and function of conducting system of heart (2011)
- AV Nodal delay (2015)

Electrocardiogram

- Draw an ECG, cause for each wave (2018)
- Kirchhoff's law and Einthoven's law (2016, 2018)
- Normal ECG in lead II (2011, 2012, 2014, 2017, 2020)
- PR interval (2012, 2013, 2016)
- J Point (2012)
- Extrasystole (2012)
- 3 Bipolar limb leads of ECG, significance of PR segment and ST segment in ECG (2014)
- What is myocardial infarction? State one ECG change in this condition. (2014)
- Clinical uses of ECG (2018)
- Heart block (2019)
- AV Nodal delay (2019)

Cardiac Cycle and Heart Sounds

- Define cardiac cycle (2013, 2014, 2016)
- Pressure-volume changes in left ventricle, left atrium and aorta in cardiac cycle (2013, 2014)
- Heart sounds (2012, 2013, 2014, 2015, 2020)
- Events of cardiac cycle (2016)

Cardiac Output

- Cardiac index (2013)
- Define cardiac output, factors regulating cardiac output (2011, 2012, 2013, 2015, 2018, 2020)
- Fick's principle (2011)
- State Frank-Starling's law of heart (2011, 2012, 2013)
- Cardiac reserve (2012, 2015))
- Methods of determining cardiac output (2012, 2013
- Significance of ejection fraction in ventricular function (2012, 2015)
- End diastolic volume (2013)
- Discuss the terms cardiac output and Total peripheral resistance and discuss their determinants (2014)
- Define preload and state its effects on cardiac function (2014)
- Venous return (2018)
- Determinants of force of contraction of heart (2019)
- Two examples for high cardiac output and low cardiac output states (2019)

Arterial and Venous Pulse

- Jugular venous pulse (2017, 2019)
- Dicrotic notch (2012)

Vascular System

- Windkessel effect (2013)
- Exchange vessels (2020)

Hemodynamics of Circulation

Reynold's number (2012, 2017, 2018, 2020)

Blood Pressure and Hypertension

- Define blood pressure, normal values (2013, 2014, 2017)
- Describe arterial blood pressure (2021)
- Nervous regulation of blood pressure (2021)
- Baroreceptor mechanism of regulation of blood pressure (2014, 2015, 2019, 2021)

- Regulation of blood pressure (2013)
- Korotkov's sounds (2014)
- Short term and long-term regulation of blood pressure (2017)
- List short-term regulation of blood pressure (2011)
- Determinants of blood pressure (2013, 2014, 2015)
- Add a note on hypertension (2014, 2017)
- Bain-bridge reflex (2016, 2017)
- Mean arterial pressure (2016, 2018)

Special Circulation

- Fetal circulation (2018)
- Regulation of coronary circulation (2011)
- Special features of coronary circulation (2011, 2017, 2019),
- Triple response (2017, 2018)
- Blood-brain barrier (2018)
- Phasic changes in coronary circulation (2012, 2015)
- Splanchnic circulation (2015)
- Physiology of fetal circulation before and after birth (2019)
- Myocardial infarction (2019)

Pathophysiology of Shock

- Non-progressive shock (2012)
- Hypovolemic shock (2012, 2021)
- List the types of shock (2014)
- Features of shock (2015)
- Anaphylactic shock (2018)

Others

- Effects of Positive 'g' (2015)

CHAPTER 9: RESPIRATORY SYSTEM

Functional Anatomy of Respiratory System

Non-respiratory functions of lungs (2011, 2018, 2020)

Mechanics of Breathing

- Compliance of lungs (2011, 2017, 2020)
- Surfactant (2013, 2015, 2016, 2019)
- Physiological dead space (2018)
- Respiratory distress syndrome (2019)
- Intrapleural pressure (2011)
- Dead space and its normal value (2011, 2013, 2014, 2017, 2018)
- Muscles of inspiration (2013)
- Muscle actions responsible for (a) Normal expiration, (b) Forced expiration (2014)
- Transpulmonary pressure (2016)
- Measurement of dead space (2019)

Lung Volumes and Capacities

- Definition and measurement of Functional residual capacity (2011, 2013)
- Clinical importance of FRC (2011)
- Timed vital capacity (2012)
- FEV1 (2012)
- Peak expiratory flow rate (2015)
- Vital capacity (2017, 2020)
- Residual volume (2017)
- Lung volumes and capacities (2018)
- Normal spirogram, lung volumes and capacities (2021)

Diffusion of Gases

- Diagram of alveolo-capillary membrane and write the thickness of it (2011)
- Respiratory membrane (2013)

Pulmonary Circulation and V/Q Ratio

- Peculiarities of pulmonary circulation (2021)
- Ventilation/perfusion ratio (2012, 2019)

Transport of Gases

- Oxygen transport (2012, 2016)
- Fetal hemoglobin (2016)
- Oxygen-dissociation curve (2012, 2014, 2016, 2020, 2021)
- Double Bohr Effect (2011)
- Chloride shift (2013, 2021)
- Haldane's effect (2019)
- Bohr's effect and its significance (2012, 2017, 2019)
- CO_2 transport (2011, 2013)
- P50 (2013, 2018, 2021)
- What is the effect of 2,3 DPG on Oxy-Hb dissociation curve? Does it help in loading or unloading of oxygen? (2013)
- Oxygen carrying capacity of blood (2014)
- Respiratory exchange ratio (2018)

Regulation of Respiration

- Chemical regulation of respiration (2012, 2013, 2014, 2015)

- Neural regulation of regulation (2013, 2014, 2018, 2020)
- Who discovered J receptors? What is its physiological significance? (2011)
- Pneumotaxic center (2012)
- Hering–Breuer inflation reflex (2012, 2014, 2016)
- Respiratory failure (2014)
- Hypoxic vasoconstriction—Where does it occur and what are its complications? (2014)
- Periodic breathing (2019)

Hypoxia
- Hypoxic hypoxia (2017, 2019)
- Hypoxia (2013, 2014, 2018, 2021)
- Define histotoxic hypoxia with an example (2011, 2019)
- Oxygen toxicity (2015)
- Hyperbaric oxygen therapy (2017)

High Altitude Physiology
Acclimatization to high altitude (2015, 2021)

Deep Sea Physiology
- Decompression sickness/Dysbarism/Caisson's disease (2011, 2012, 2013, 2015, 2016, 2019)
- SCUBA diving (2011)
- Nitrogen narcosis (2015)

Abnormal Respirations
- Stages of asphyxia (2012)
- Periodic breathing (2015)

Pulmonary Function Tests
- Name two pulmonary function tests to detect obstructive pulmonary disease (2014)

Artificial Respiration
- Artificial respiration (2011, 2015, 2017, 2020)
- Mouth to mouth respiration (2019)
- Cardiopulmonary resuscitation (2021)

CHAPTER 10: NERVOUS SYSTEM

Synapse and Neurotransmitters
- What is summation? Mention its types (2011, 2012, 2013)
- What are cholinergic and adrenergic receptors? (2011)
- Dopamine (2012)
- Define synapse and describe its properties (2013, 2017, 2020)
- Name the facilitatory and inhibitory neurotransmitters and their sites of actions (2017)
- Denervation hypersensitivity (2019)
- Synaptic plasticity (2019)

Sensory System—Sensory Modalities, Sensory Cortex
- Bell-Magendie law (2011, 2012, 2020)
- What is stereognosis? Where is its center? (2011)
- Functions of somatosensory area (2017)

Receptors
- What is Monro-Kellie doctrine (2011)
- What are mechanoreceptors? Give an example. (2011)
- Receptor potential (2014, 2018, 2020)
- Law of projection (2018)

Ascending Pathways
- Enumerate the ascending pathways (2012, 2021)
- Discuss the posterior column with a diagram (2012, 2018)
- Name of tracts made up by second order neurons in the pathway for—fine touch and pain (2013)
- Trace the pathway for perception of fine touch (2014)
- Draw the diagram of crude touch pathway and label it (2014)
- Sensations carried by posterior column (2017, 2020)

Pain
- Referred pain and its theories (2011, 2013, 2015, 2020)
- Brown-Sequard syndrome (2011, 2012, 2014, 2019)
- Pathway for pain (2012, 2013, 2021)
- Classify pain (2012)
- Receptors for pain (2012)
- Analgesic system in the pain (2012, 2013, 2015, 2021)

- Gating of pain (2013)
- Endogenous opioid peptides (2014, 2019)

Thalamus
- Functions of thalamus (2013)
- Thalamic syndrome (2019)

Motor system—Motor cortex
- Motor homunculus (2014)

Reflexes—Classification, Stretch Reflex
- Stretch reflex (2017)
- Reflex arc (2013)
- Mass reflex (2015)
- Properties of reflex (2015)
- Golgi tendon reflex (2016)

Muscle spindle and Golgi tendon
- Physiological roles of muscle spindle (2013)
- Define muscle tone and discuss the phenomenon responsible for it, what conditions lead to alteration of tone (2014)

Descending Tracts—Pyramidal and Extrapyramidal Tracts
- Describe corticospinal tract and effect of lesions at various levels (2015, 2019)
- Differences between UMN and LMN lesions (2015, 2019)
- Babinski sign (2015)
- Differences between spasticity and rigidity (2011)
- Cog wheel rigidity (2012)
- Conditions where plantar reflex is 'extensor' (2014)

Regulation of Posture and Movement
- Righting reflexes (2013)
- Decerebrate rigidity (2011, 2013)

Thalamus
- Functions of thalamus (2011, 2018, 2020)
- Thalamic syndrome (2013)

Basal Ganglia
- Connections and functions of basal ganglia, clinical disorders and physiological basis of treatment (2013, 2020)
- Parkinson's disease (2012, 2014, 2017)
- Putamen circuit of basal ganglia (2016)

Cerebellum
- Connections and functions of cerebellum (2011, 2017, 2018, 2021)
- Clinical features of cerebellar lesion (2011, 2013, 2014, 2021)
- Functional divisions of cerebellum (2011, 2021)
- Role of Purkinje cells of cerebellum (2012)
- Vestibulocerebellum (2013)
- Functions and tests of cerebellum (2014, 2020)

Vestibular Apparatus
- Otolith organ—mechanism of action and functions (2011, 2021)
- Receptors for vestibular sensation (2013)
- Components of vestibular apparatus (2014)
- Functions of utricle and saccule (2016)

Hypothalamus
- Explain auditory pathway with neat hypothalamus (2013, 2015, 2017, 2021)
- Fever (2012)
- Heat loss mechanisms (2013)
- Control of food intake (2021)
- Name the nuclei responsible for hunger and satiety in human beings (2013)
- Circadian rhythm (2020)

Limbic System
- Functions of limbic system (2018)
- Papez circuit (2015, 2017, 2020)
- Reward and punishment centers (2016)

EEG and Sleep
- Berger's rhythm (2012, 2016, 2020)
- Alpha block (2011)
- Compare REM and NREM sleep (2015)
- Rapid eye movement sleep (2011, 2017)
- Delta waves in EEG (2011)
- Stages of sleep (2014, 2017, 2019)
- Sleep-wake theory (2016)
- Polysomnography (2021)

Reticular Formation
- Four functions of reticular activating system (2011)

- Functions of ascending reticular activating system (2012, 2014)

Learning and Memory

- Conditioned reflex (2015)
- Types of memory (2013)
- Operant conditioning (2014)
- Antegrade amnesia (2018)
- Implicit memory (2019)

Language and Sleep

- Anomic aphasia (2012)
- Physiology of speech (2013)
- Aphasia (2014, 2020, 2021)
- Fluent aphasia (2014)
- Wernicke's and global aphasia (2016)
- Speech areas (2021)

Cerebral Cortex

- Functions of parietal lobe (2020)
- Functions of prefrontal lobe (2011, 2013)
- Functions of frontal lobe (2011)
- Betz cells (2012)
- Homunculus (2012, 2020)
- Klüver-Bucy syndrome (2013, 2020)
- Connections and functions of temporal lobe (2016)
- Prefrontal lobotomy (2019)

Cerebrospinal Fluid

- Describe formation, circulation and functions of CSF (2012, 2013, 2014, 2015, 2020)

CHAPTER 11: SPECIAL SENSES

Vision

- Accommodation for near vision (2015, 2016, 2016, 2019)
- Visual pathway and lesions (2014, 2015, 2019)
- Refractory errors of eye (2011, 2012, 2013, 2014, 2020)
- Dark adaptation (2011, 2013, 2015, 2017, 2021)
- Color vision (2011, 2021)
- Defect in astigmatism and correction (2012, 2013)
- Draw the structure of rods and cones (2011)
- Ocular dominance columns (2012)
- Perimetry (2013)
- Photochemical mechanism of vision (2013)
- Visual field defect when the optic chiasma is cut in the middle (2013)
- What is 'Blind spot'? (2013)
- Presbyopia (2016)
- Trichromatic theory of color vision (2016)
- Astigmatism (2018)
- Red-green color blindness (2018)

Hearing

- Functions of middle ear (2012, 2013, 2014, 2015, 2017)
- Travelling wave theory (2012, 2019)
- Explain auditory pathway with neat diagram (2015, 2020)
- Theories of hearing (2011)
- What is endocochlear potential? (2011, 2016)
- Attenuation reflex/Stapedial reflex (2013, 2014, 2017, 2018)
- Region of the cochlea which vibrates most for the highest sound frequency in the audible range. (2013)
- Discuss the phenomenon by which sound waves in air induce action potentials in the cochlear nerve (2014)
- Finding in Weber's test in conduction deafness of the left ear (2014)
- Impedance matching (2015)
- Types of deafness (2018)

Taste

- Taste pathway (2011, 2012, 2014, 2019, 2021)
- Gustatory receptors (2016)
- Primary taste sensations (2018)

CHAPTER 12: EXERCISE PHYSIOLOGY

- VO_2 max (2015)
- O_2 debt (2015)
- Changes in cardiac output in exercise (2016)
- Physiological changes in human body during exercise (2021)

EU GSPR Authorised Reprsentative
Logos Europe, 9 rue Nicolas Poussin
1700, La Rochelle, France
Phone: +33 (0) 6 67 93 73 78
E-mail: contact@logoseurope.eu

www.ingramcontent.com/pod-product-compliance
Ingram Content Group UK Ltd.
Pitfield, Milton Keynes, MK11 3LW, UK
UKHW050455150426
5217IPUK00025B/1702